Venereal Disease

Bibliography

1966–1970

Venereal Disease Bibliography 1966–1970

compiled by
Stephen H. Goode

The Whitston Publishing Company
Incorporated
Troy, New York
1972

© Copyright 1972
Stephen H. Goode

Library of Congress Catalog Card Number: 71-189843

ISBN 0-87875-023-1

Printed in the United States of America

PREFACE

This is a five-year near-complete world bibliography of venereal disease literature covering the period, 1966-1970. Annual supplements will appear beginning with that of 1971 and will appear serially in the fall of each succeeding year. The bibliography is divided into two sections: a title section arranged alphabetically; and a subject section, arranged alphabetically by subject and alphabetically by title within subjects. Titles and subjects are provided so that researchers who do not trust subject assignments, which are always arbitrary and unique to the individual compiler, can conduct their own to-some-extent original literature search. Especial care has been taken to develop subject headings meaningful to the user: entries are broken down into almost 300 subject categories; even so, it is regrettable that, for example, "Syphilis: Serodiagnosis" is altogether too large. The distinction among immunology, serodiagnosis, serology, et al., however, is very fine and impossible very often to arrive at. In such instances entries are duplicated as often as feasible in other applicable categories-- and ample "See" and "See Also" references are cited at the beginning of the subject heads.

The bibliography is designed to serve the needs of different kinds of researchers from medical scientists to those with only superficial or beginning interests in this very major socio-medical problem; it should be of service to the undergraduate, graduate, and professional medical scientist, nurse, psychologist, theoretical and applied sociologist, political scientist, and so forth.

The following bibliographies and serials indexes have been searched in compiling this bibliography: BIBLIOGRAPHIC INDEX; BOOKS IN PRINT; CANADIAN PERIODICAL INDEX; CUMULATIVE BOOK INDEX; CUMULATIVE INDEX TO NURSING LITERATURE; CURRENT INDEX TO JOURNALS IN EDUCATION; CURRENT LITERATURE OF VENEREAL DISEASE; EDUCATION INDEX; INDEX TO LEGAL

PERIODICALS; INDEX MEDICUS; INDEX TO PERIODICAL ARTICLES RELATED TO LAW; INTERNATIONAL NURSING INDEX; PUBLIC AFFAIRS INFORMATION SERVICE; READERS GUIDE TO PERIODICAL LITERATURE; SOCIAL SCIENCES AND HUMANITIES INDEX. Thus, such a gathering from so wide and disparate a series of indexes and bibliographies obviates a large amount of searching, even if the user's library is large enough to offer such diverse holdings.

There are two interesting observations to emerge from the compiling of this particular bibliography. Although the especially helpful and pertinent bibliographies, INDEX MEDICUS and CURRENT LITERATURE OF VENEREAL DISEASE would be assumed to either duplicate each other or be mutually exclusive, neither is the case; large percentages of entries appear in only one and not the other. Second, it is apparent in dealing with such a literature search as this that the United States has for some time, until recently, neglected its interest in venereal disease in comparison with, for example, the USSR, Italy, Czechoslovakia, Poland, and so forth. Only immediately and minimally is the United States assuming any renewal of interest in the control of these insidious diseases.

This current volume and its annual supplements, then, already assumes largest importance as necessity forces our attention to what is now the third or fourth major socio-medical concern--behind only those caused by cancer and cardiovascular ailments.

In using the subject section, the following reminders are of importance:

1. "Neonatal" entries are not reproduced under "Congenital" subject heads.

2. Compounds, such as penicillin compounds or ampicillin compounds, are found under the root compound unless a number of entries are involved; but specific derivatives, such as Doxycycline derived from Tetracycline, have their own heads.

3. The Jarisch-Herxheimer reaction, although it might more logically be found under "Syphilis: Serodiagnosis," is found in this bibliography under the subject heading, "Reactions: Jarisch-Herxheimer," etc.

4. Entries involving the fetus will be found under "Pregnancy".

5. Not all possible "See Also" subject heads are listed; that is, for "Non-gonococcal Infections and Diseases," for example, "Giardiasis" is not listed, but "Minor Venereal Diseases and Infections are, together with "Mycoplasmas," "Urethritis, Non-Gonococcal," etc.

6. It did not seem proper to split "Education" as it pertained to such as "High School Education" away from "Education" as it applied to Medical Schools.

7. In some instances one will find entries under "See Also" headings duplicated in the referred-to subject areas, because of the certainty of the connection of the entries with that subject head; but if they are only tangentially related, the entry is not duplicated.

8. The most important thing to remember is that the subject head, for example, "Treatment," is listed in several separate respects: under "Treatment," meaning general or generic, applying to venereal disease as a whole or to both gonorrhea and syphilis; under "Syphilis: Treatment," under "Gonorrhea: Treatment;" under "Trichomoniasis: Treatment," etc., so that if the searcher is looking for all aspects of, for a further example, the history of all venereal diseases, he must look under "Syphilis: History;" under "Gonorrhoea: History;" under the subject heading cited simply as "History," and so forth.

Stephen H. Goode

LIST OF ABBREVIATIONS
AND PERIODICALS

Abbreviation	Title
Acta Allergol also: Acta Allerg	Acta Allergologica (Kobenhavn)
Acta Cytol	Acta Cytologica (Baltimore)
Acta Derm	Acta Dermatologica (Kyoto) in Japanese: Hifuka Kiyo
Acta Dermatovener	Acta Dermato-Venereologica (Stockholm)
Acta Med Okayama	Acta Medicinae Okayama
Acta Med Scand	Acta Medica Scandinavica
Acta Microbiol Acad Sci Hung	Acta Microbiologica Academiae Scientiarum Hungaricae (Budapest)
Acta Neurol	Acta Neurologica (Napoli)
Acta Neurol Belg	Acta Neurologica Belgica (Bruxelles) formerly Acta Neurologica et Psychiatrica Belgica
Acta Neurol Lat Amer	Acta Neurologica Latinoamericana (Montevideo)
Acta Obstet Gynec Scand	Acta Obstetricia et Gynecologica Scandinavica (Lund)
Acta Ophthal	Acta Ophthalmologica (Kobenhavn)
Acta Orthop Belg	Acta Orthopaedica Belgica (Bruxelles)
Acta Paediat Scand	Acta Paediatrica Scandinavica (Stockholm) formerly Acta Paeditrica
Acta Paediat Sinica	Acta Paediatrica Sinica (Taipei) title in Chinese: Hsiao erh K'O I Hsueh Hui Tsa Chih
Acta Path Microbiol Scand	Acta Pathologica et Microbiologica Scandinavica Section A: Pathology (Kobenhavn) formerly Acta Pathologica et Microbiologica Scandinavica Section B: Microbiology & Immunology (Copenhagen)
Acta Psychiat Scand	Acta Psychiatrica Scandinavica (Kobenhavn)
Acta Soc Ophthal Jap	Acta Societatis Ophthalmologicae Japonicae (Tokyon) title in Japa-

	nese: Nippon Ganka Gakkai Zasshi
Acta Trop	Acta Tropica (Basel)
Acta Urol Belg	Acta Urologica Belgica (Bruxelles)
Actas Dermosif	Actas Dermo-Sifilio Graficas (Madrid)
Advances Pharmacol	Advances in Pharmacology (New York) merged with advances in Chemotherapy To Form Advances in Pharmacology and Chemotherapy (New York)
Aero-Space Med	Aerospace Medicine (St. Paul)
Akush Ginek	Akusherstvo i Ginekologiia (Moscow)
Akush Ginek	Akusherstvo i Ginekologiia (Sofiia) formerly Akusherstvo i Ginekologiia supplement to Suvremenna Meditsina (Sofia)
Alergia	Alergia Revista Iberoamericana de Alergologia (Mexico)
Am Anthrop	American Anthropologist (Washington)
Am Druggist	American Druggist (New York)
Am J Sociol	American Journal of Sociology (Chicago)
Amer Heart J	American Heart Journal (St. Louis)
Amer J Cardiol	American Journal of Cardiology (New York)
Amer J Clin Path	American Journal of Clinical Pathology (Baltimore)
Amer J Dis Child	American Journal of Diseases of Children (Chicago)
Amer J Epidem	American Journal of Epidemiology (Baltimore)
Amer J Med	American Journal of Medicine
Amer J Med Sci	American Journal of Medical Sciences American Journal of the Medical Sciences (Philadelphia)
Amer J Med Techn	American Journal of Medical Technology (Houston)
Amer J Obstet Gynec	American Journal of Obstetrics and Gynecology (St. Louis)
Amer J Ophthal	American Journal of Ophthalmology (Chicago)
Amer J Psychiat	American Journal of Psychiatry (Hanover, N.H.)
Amer J Public Health	American Journal of Public Health and the Nation's Health (New York)
Amer Rev Resp Dis	American Review of Respiratory Disease (Baltimore)
An Brasil Derm	Anais Brasileiros De Dermatologia

An Esc Nac Saude Publica Med Trop	(Rio de Janeiro) formerly Anais Brasileiros De Dermatologic E Sifilografia Anais Da Escola Nacional De Saude Publica E De Medicina Tropical (Lisboa) supersedes Anais Do Instituto De Medicina Tropical
Anaesthesist	Anaesthesist (Berlin)
Anesth Analg	Anesthesia and Analgesia Current Researches (Cleveland)
Anesthesiology	Anesthesiology (Philadelphia)
Angiologia	Angeiologie (Paris)
Ann Allerg	Annals of Allergy (St. Paul)
Ann Biol Clin	Annales De Biologie Clinique (Paris)
Ann Chir Gynaec Fenn	Annales Chirurgiae Et Gynaecologiae Fenniae (Helsinki)
Ann Clin Res	Annals of Clinical Research (Helsinki) formed by merging of Annales Medicinae Internal Fenniae and Annales Paediatriae Fenniae
Ann Derm Syph	Annales De Dermatologie et Syphiligraphie (Paris)
Ann Inst Pasteur	Annales De L'Institut Pasteur (Paris)
Ann Intern Med	Annals of Internal Medicine (Philadelphia)
Ann Ital Chir	Annali Italiani Di Chirurgia (Bologna)
Ann Med Nav	Annali Di Medicina Navale (Roma)
Ann N Y Acad Sci	Annals of the New York Academy of Sciences (New York)
Ann Oculist	Annals of the New York Academy of Sciences (Paris)
Ann Ostet Ginec	Annali Di Ostetricia E Ginecologia (Milano)
Ann Ottal	Annali Di Ottalmologia E Clinica Oculistica (Parma)
Ann Paediat Fenn	Annales Paediatriae Fenniae (Helsinki)
Ann Rev Med	Annual Review of Medicine (Palo Alto)
Ann Rheum Dis	Annals of the Rheumatic Diseases (London)
Ann Sanit Pubblica	Annali Della Sanita Pubblica (Roma)
Ann Thorac Surg	Annals of Thoracic Surgery (Boston)
Antibiotica	Antibiotica (Rome)
Antibiotiki	Antibiotiki (Moscow

Antimicrob Agents Chemother	Antimicrobial Agents and Chemotherapy (Detroit)
Appl Microbiol	Applied Microbiology (Baltimore)
Appl Ther	Applied Therapeutics (Toronto)
Arch Argent Pediatr	Archivos Argentinos De Pediatria (Buenos Aires)
Arch Derm	Archives of Dermatology (Chicago)
Arch Environ Health	Archives of Environmental Health (Chicago)
Arch Franc Mal Appar Dig	Archives Francaises Des Maladies De L'Appareil Digestif (Paris)
Arch Franc Pediat	Archives Francaises De Pediatrie (Paris)
Arch Fund Roux Ocefa	Archivos De La Fundacion Roux-Ocefa (Buenos Aires)
Arch Hist Med	Archiwum Historii Medycyny (Warsaw)
Arch Hyg Bakt	Archiv Fur Hygiene Und Bakteriologie (Munich)
Arch Immun Ther Exp	Archivum Immunologiae Et Therapiae Experimentalis (Warsaw)
Arch Inst Cardiol Mex	Archivos Del Instituto De Cardiologia De Mexico
Arch Intern Med	Archives of Internal Medicine (Chicago)
Arch Ital Derm Vener	Archivio Italioano Di Dermatologia Venereologia E Sessuologia (Bologna)
Arch Klin Exp Derm	Archiv Fur Klinische Und Experimentelle Dermatologie (Berlin)
Arch Mal Coeur	Archives Des Maladies Du Coeur Et Des Vaisseaux (Paris)
Arch Maragliano Pat Clin	Archivio E Maragliano Di Patologia E Clinica (Geneva)
Arch Ophthal	Archives of Ophthalmology (Chicago)
Arch Orthop Unfallchir	Archiv Fur Ortho Paedische Und Unfall-Chirugie (Munchen)
Arch Otolarng	Archives of Otolaryngology (Chicago)
Arch Path	Archives of Pathology (Chicago)
Arch Phys Med	Archives of Physical Medicine and Rehabilitation (Chicago)
Arch Psychiat Nervenkr	Archiv Fur Psychiatrie Und Nervenkrankheiten Vereinigt Mit Zeitschrift Fur Die Gesamte Neurologie Und Psychiatrie (Berlin)
Arch Roum Path Exp Microbiol	Archives Roumaines De Pathologie Experimentale Et De Microbiologie (Bucuresti)

Arch Sci Med	Archivio Per Le Science Mediche (Torino)
Arch Surg	Archives of Surgery (Chicago)
Arizona Med	Arizona Medicine (Scottsdale)
Arkh Pat	Arkhiv Patologii (Moscow)
Arq Brasil Cardiol	Arquivos Brasileiros De Cardiologia (Sao Paulo)
Arthritis Rheum	Arthritis and Rheumatism (New York)
Arzneimittelforschung	Arzneimittel-Forschung (Aulendorf)
Atti Accad Med Lombard	Atti Della Accademia Medica Lombarda (Milano)
Attualita Ostet Ginec	Attualita De Ostetricia E Ginecologia (Padova)
Aust Ann Med	Australian Annals of Medicine (Sydney)
Aust J Derm	Australian Journal of Dermatology (Sidney)
Beitr Orthop Trauma	Beitraege zur Orthopaedie und Traumatologie (Berlin)
Berlin Munchen Tieraerztl Wschr	Berliner Und Munchener Tieraerztliche Wochenschrift (Berlin)
Bibl Gynaec	Bibliotheca Gynaecologica supplementa Ad Gynaecologia (Basel)
Bibl Haemat	Bibliotheca Haematologica supplementa Ad Acta Haematologica (Basel)
Biol Med	Biologie Medicale (Paris)
Bol Asoc Med P Rico	Boletin De La Asociacion Medica De Puerto Rico (Santurce)
Bol Chile Parasit	Boletin Chileno De Parasitologia (Santiago)
Bol Inst Puericult	Boletim Do Instituto De Puericultura E Pediatria (Rio de Janeiro)
Bol Ofic Sanit Panamer	Boletin De La Oficina Sanitaria Panamericana (Washington)
Boll Soc Ital Biol Sper	Bollettino Della Societa Italiana Di Biologia Sperimentale (Napoli)
Bordeaux Med	Bordeaux Medical
Bratisl Lek Listy	Bratislavske Lekarske Listy (Bratislava)
Bristol Medicochir J	Bristol Medico-Chirurgical Journal
Brit J Clin Pract	British Journal of Clinical Practice (London)
Brit J Derm	British Journal of Dermatology (London)
Brit J Ophthal	British Journal of Ophthalmology (London)

Brit J Oral Surg	British Journal of Oral Surgery (Edinburgh)
Brit J Prev Soc Med	British Journal of Preventive and Social Medicine (London)
Brit J Psychiat	British Journal of Psychiatry (London)
Brit J Radiol	British Journal of Radiology (London)
Brit J Soc Clin Psychol	British Journal of Social and Clinical Psychology (Cambridge)
Brit J Urol	British Journal of Urology (London)
Brit J Vener Dis	British Journal of Venereal Diseases (London)
Brit Med J	British Medical Journal (London)
Bruxelles Med	Bruxelles-Medical (Bruxelles)
Bull Acad Nat Med	Bulletin De l'Academie Nationale de Medicine (Paris)
Bull Fed Gynec Obstet Franc	Bulletin De La Federation Des Societes De Gynecologie Et D'Obstetrique De Langue Francaise (Paris)
Bull Hopkins Hosp	Johns Hopkins Hospital Bulletin (Baltimore)
Bull Hyg	Bulletin of Hygiene (London)
Bull Inst Nat Sante	Bulletin De l'Institute National De La Sante Et De La Recherche Medicale (Paris)
Bull Inst Natl Sante Rech Med	Bulletin De l'Institute National De La Sante Et De La Recherche Medicale (Paris)
Bull Ophthal Soc Egypt	Bulletin of the Ophthalmological Society of Egypt (Cairo)
Bull Pharm Res Inst	Bulletin of Pharmaceutical Research Institute (Takatsuki)
Bull Soc Franc Derm Syph	Bulletin De La Societe Francaise De Dermatologie Et De Syphiligraphie (Paris)
Bull Soc Med Afr Noire Lang Franc	Bulletin De La Societe Medicale d'Afrique Noire De Langue Francaise (Dakar)
Bull Soc Ophtal Franc	Bulletin Des Societes d'Ophtalmologie De France (Paris)
Bull Soc Path Exot	Bulletin De La Societe De Pathologie Exotique Et De Ses Filiales (Paris)
Bull Soc Roy Belg Gynec Obstet	Bulletin De La Societe Royale Belge De Gynecologie Et d'Obstetrique (Bruxelles)
Bull Who	Bulletin of the World Health Organization (Geneva)

C R Acad Sci	Comptes Rendus Herdomadaires des Seances De l'Academic Des Sciences D: Sciences Naturelles (Paris)
Calif Med	California Medicine (San Francisco)
Canad J Med Techn	Canadian Journal of Medical Technology (Hamilton)
Canad J Public Health	Canadian Journal of Public Health (Toronto)
Canad Med Ass J	Canadian Medical Association Journal (Toronto)
Cancer Res	Cancer Research (Chicago)
Cardiol Prat	Cardiologia Pratica (Firenze)
Cas Lek Cesk	Casopis Lekaru Ceskych (Praha)
Cent Afr J Med	Central African Journal of Medicine (Salisbury)
Cesk Derm	Ceskoslovenska Dermatologie (Praha)
Cesk Epidem	Ceskoslovenska Epidemiologie Mikrobiologie Imunologie (Prague)
Cesk Gynek	Ceskoslovenska Gynekologie (Prague)
Cesk Oftal	Ceskoslovenska Oftalmologie (Prague)
Cesk Pediat	Ceskoslovenska Pediatrie (Prague)
Cesk Zdrav	Ceskoslovenska Zdravotnictvi (Prague)
Chem Phys Lipids	Chemistry and Physics of Lipids (Amsterdam)
Chemotherapy	Chemotherapy (Basel)
Chir Narzad Ruchu Ortop Pol	Chirugia Narzadow Ruchu i Ortopedia Polska (Warsaw)
Chirurg	Chirurg (Berlin)
Clin Endocr	Clinical Endocrinology (Tokyo) In Japanese: Horumon To Rinsho
Clin Exp Immun	Clinical and Experimental Immunology (Oxford)
Clin Orthop	Clinical Orthopaedics and related Research (Philadelphia)
Clin Pediat	Clinica Pediatrica (Bologne)
Clin Pediat	Clinical Pediatrics (Philadelphia)
Clin Pharmacol Ther	Clinical Pharmacology and Therapeutics (St. Louis)
Clin Proc Child Hosp DC	Clinical Proceedings of Childrens Hospital of the District of Columbia (Washington)
Clin Radiol	Clinical Radiology (London)
Clin Ter	Clinica Terapeutica (Rome)
Conn Med	Connecticut Medicine (New Haven)
Curr Ther Res	Current Therapeutic Research (New York)

Czas Stomat	Czasopismo Stomatologiczne (Warsaw)
Danish Med Bull Suppl	Danish Medical Bulletin (Kobenhavn)
Dapim Refuiim	Dapim Refuiim (Tel-Aviv)
Delaware Med J	Delaware Medical Journal
Dent Assist	Dental Assistant (New York)
Dent Dig	Dental Digest (Pittsburgh)
Derm Int	Dermatologia Internationalis (Philadelphia)
Derm Mschr	Dermatologische Monatsschrift (Basel)
Derm Wschr	Dermatologische Wochenschrift (Leipzig)
Dermatologica	Dermatologica (Basel)
Deutsch Gesundh	Deutsche Gesundheitswesen (Berlin)
Deutsch Med Wschr	Deutsch Medizinische Wochenschrift (Stuttgart)
Deutsch Z Nervenheilk	Deutsche Zeitschrift Fur Nervenheilkunde (Berlin)
Deutsch Zahnaerztl Z	Deutsche Zahnaerztliche Zeitschrift (Munchen)
Dis Colon Rectum	Diseases of the Colon and Rectum (Philadelphia)
Dis Nerv Syst	Diseases of the Nervous System (Galveston)
District Nurs	District Nursing (London)
Duodecim	Duodecim (Helsinki)
E Afr Med J	East African Medical Journal (Nairobi)
Ed Res	Educational Researcher (Washington)
Ergebn Chir Orthop	Ergebnisse Der Chirurgie Und Orthopaedie (Berlin)
Experientia	Experientia (Basel)
Feldsh Akush	Fel'dsher I Akusherka (Moscow)
Fertil Steril	Fertility and Sterility (New York)
The Filter	The Filter (Oakland)
Folia Allerg	Folia Allergologica (Rome)
Folia Cardiol	Folia Cardiologica (Milano)
Folia Med Cracov	Folia Medica Cracoviensia
Forecast Home Econ	Forecast for Home Economics (New York)
Fortschr Arzneimittelforsch	Fortschritte Der Arzneimittelforschung (Basel)
Fortschr Roentgenstr	Fortschritte Auf Dem Gebiete Der Roentgenstrahlen Und Der Nuklearmedizin (Stuttgart)
Fracastoro	Fracastoro (Fracastoro)

Friuli Med	Friuli Medico (Voine)
GP	GP (Kansas City)
G Batt Virol Immun	Giornale Di Batteriologia Virologia Ed Immunologia (Turin)
G Clin Med	Giornale Di Clinica Medica (Bologna)
G Ital Derm	Giornale Italiano Di Dermatologia-Minerva Dermatologica (Torino) formed by merging Giornale Italiano Di Dermatolgia (Milan) and Minerva Dermatologica (Torino)
G Mal Infett	Giornale Di Malattie Infettive E Parassitarie (Torino)
G Psichiat Neuropat	Geornale Di Psichiatria E Di Neuropatologia (Ferrara)
Gac Med Mex	Gaceta Medica De Mexico
Geburtsh Frauenheilk	Geburtshilfe Und Frauenheilkunde (Stuttgart)
Geriatrics	Geriatrics (Minneapolis)
German Med Monthly	German Medical Monthly (Stuttgart)
Ginec Obstet Mex	Ginecologia Y Obstetricia De Mexico (Mexico City)
Ginek Pol	Ginekologia Polska (Lodz)
God Sborn Med Fak Skopje	Godisen Zbornik Na Medicinskiot Fakultet Vo Skopje
Good H	Good Housekeeping
Gynaecologia	Gynaecologia (Basel)
Gynec Prat	Gynecologie Pratique (Paris)
Hautarzt	Hautarzt (Berlin)
Hawaii Med J	Hawaii Medical Journal
Health Bull	Health Bull (Edinburgh)
Health Lab Sci	Health Laboratory Science (New York)
Helv Med Acta	Helvetica Medica Acta (Basel)
Helv Paediat Acta	Helvetica Paediatrica Acta (Basel)
Hindustan Antibiot Bull	Hindustan Antibiotics Bulletin (Primpri)
Hippokrates	Hippokrates (Stuttgart)
HNO	HNO Wegweiser Fur Die Fachaerztliche Praxis (Berlin)
Hospital	Hospital (Rio de Janeiro)
Immunology	Immunology (Oxford)
Indian Heart J	Indian Heart J (Calcutta)
Indian J Derm	Indian Journal of Dermatology (Calcutta)
Indian J Med Res	Indian Journal of Medical Research (New Delhi)
Int Arch Allerg	International Archives of Allergy

	and Applied Immunology (Basel)
Int J Derm	International Journal of Dermatology (Philadelphia)
Int J Leprosy	International Journal of Leprosy (Washington)
Int Psychiat Clin	International Psychiatry Clinics (Boston)
Int Surg	International Surgery (Chicago)
Int Z Klin Pharmakol Ther Toxik	Internationale Zeitschrift Fur Kinische Pharmakologie Therapie Und Toxikologie (Munchen)
Invest Urol	Investigative Urology (Baltimore)
Iryo	Iryo (Tokyo)
JAMA	Journal of the American Medical Association (Chicago)
J Abnorm Psychol	Journal of Abnormal Psychology (Washington)
J All India Ophthal Soc	Journal of the All-India Ophthalmological Society (Bombay)
J Allerg	Journal of Allergy (St. Louis)
J Amer Coll Health Ass	Journal of the American College Health Association (Ithaca)
J Amer Dent Ass	Journal of the American Dental Association (Chicago)
J Amer Geriat Soc	Journal of the American Geriatrics Society (Baltimore)
J Amer Med Wom Ass	Journal of the American Medical Womens Association (Nashville)
J Amer Osteopath Ass	Journal of the American Osteopathic Association (Chicago)
J Amer Vet Med Ass	Journal of the American Veterinary Medical Association (Chicago)
J Antibiot	Journal of Antibiotics (Tokyo)
J Bact	Journal of Bacteriology (Baltimore)
J Belg Rhum Med Phys	Journal Belge De Rhumatologie Et De Medecine Physique (Bruxelles)
J Bone Joint Surg	Journal of Bone and Joint Surgery American Volume (Boston) Journal of Bone and Joint Surgery British Volume (London)
J Clin Invest	Journal of Clinical Investigation (Boston)
J Clin Path	Journal of Clinical Pathology (London)
J Dent Res	Journal of Dental Research (Chicago)
J Florida Med Ass	Journal of the Florida Medical Association (Jacksonville)
J Formosan Med Ass	Journal of the Formosan Medical

	Association (Taipei)
J Gen Virol	Journal of General Virology (London)
J Hyg Epidem	Journal of Hygiene Epidemiology Microbiology and Immunology (Praha)
J Immun	Journal of Immunology (Baltimore)
J Indian Med Ass	Journal of the Indian Medical Association (Calcutta)
J Infect Dis	Journal of Infectious Diseases (Chicago)
J Invest Derm	Journal of Investigative Dermatology (Baltimore)
J Iowa Med Soc	Journal of the Iowa Medical Society (Des Moines)
J Jap Ass Infect Dis	Journal of the Japanese Association For Infectious Disease (Tokyo) Title In Japanese: Kansenshogaku Zasshi
J Jap Med Ass	Journal of the Japan Medical Association (Tokyo) In Japanese: Nippon Ishikai Zasshi
J Jap Obstet Gynec Soc	Journal of the Japanese Obstetrical and Gynecological Society (Tokyo) In Japanese: Nippon Sanka-Fujinka Gakkai Zasshi (Tokyo)
J Kansas Med Soc	Journal of the Kansas Medical Society (Topeka)
J Kentucky Med Ass	Journal of the Kentucky Medical Association (Louisville)
J Lab Clin Med	Journal of Laboratory and Clinical Medicine (St. Louis)
J Laryng	Journal of Laryngology And Otology (London)
J Maine Med Ass	Journal of the Maine Medical Association (Brunswick)
J Med Ass Alabama	Journal of the Medical Association Of The State Of Alabama (Montgomery)
J Med Ass Georgia	Journal of the Medical Association Of Georgia (Atlanta)
J Med Bordeaux	Journal De Medecine De Bordeaux Et Du Sud-Ouest
J Med Educ	Journal Of Medical Education (Chicago)
J Med Genet	Journal Of Medical Genetics (London)
J Med Lab Techn	Journal Of Medical Laboratory Technology (London)
J Med Lyon	Journal De Medecine De Lyon

J Med Microbiol	Journal Of Medical Microbiology (Edinburgh)
J Mount Sinai Hosp	Journal Of The Mount Sinai Hospital (New York)
J NY Sch Nurse-Teach Ass	Journal Of The School Nurse-Teacher Association (East Greenbush)
J Nat Med Ass	Journal Of The National Medical Association (New York)
J Neurol Neurosurg Psychiat	Journal Of Neurology Neurosurgery And Psychiatry (London)
J Neurol Sci	Journal Of The Neurological Sciences (Amsterdam)
J Neurosurg	Journal Of Neurosurgery (Chicago)
J Obstet Gynaec Brit Comm	Journal Of Obstetrics And Gynaecology Of The British Commonwealth (London)
J Okla Med Ass	Journal Of The Oklahoma State Medical Association (Oklahoma City)
J Oral Surg	Journal Of Oral Surgery (Chicago)
J Oslo City Hosp	Journal Of The Oslo City Hospitals
J Pediat	Journal Of Pediatrics (St. Louis)
J Periodont	Journal Of Periodontology (Indianapolis)
J Pharmacol Exp Ther	Journal Of Pharmacology And Experimental Therapeutics (Baltimore)
J Psychiat Nurs	Journal Of Psychiatry Nursing (New Jersey)
J Radiol Electr	Journal De Radiologie d'Electrologie Et De Medecine Nucleaire
J Roy Coll Gen Pract	Journal Of The Royal College Of General Practitioners (Dartmouth, England)
J Roy Nav Med Serv	Journal Of The Royal Naval Medical Service (Alverstoke)
J S Carolina Med Ass	Journal Of The South Carolina Medical Association (Florence)
J Sch Health	Journal Of School Health (Columbus)
J Sci Med Lille	Journal Des Sciences Medicales De Lille
J Sec Ed	Journal Of Secondary Education (Burlingame, California)
J Tenn Med Ass	Journal Of The Tennessee Medical Association (Nashville)
J Trop Med Hyg	Journal Of Tropical Medicine And Hygiene (London)
J Urol	Journal Of Urology (Baltimore)
J Urol Nephrol	Journal d'Urologie Et De Nephro-

Jap J Bact	logie (Paris) Japanese Journal Of Bacteriology (Tokyo) Nippon Saikingaku Zasshi
Jap J Clin Med	Japanese Journal Of Clinical Medicine (Osaka) Nippon Rinsho
Jap J Clin Path	Japanese Journal Of Clinical Pathology (Tokyo) Rinsho Byori
Jap J Exp Med	Japanese Journal Of Experimental Medicine (Tokyo)
Jap J Med Sci Biol	Japanese Journal Of Medical Science And Biology (Tokyo)
Jap J Nurs Art	Japanese Journal Of Nursing Art (Tokyo)
Jap J Urol	Japanese Journal Of Urology (Tokyo) Nippon Hinyokika Gakkai Zasshi (Tokyo)
Johns Hopkins Med J	Johns Hopkins Medical Journal (Baltimore)
Kango	Kango
Kardiol Pol	Kardiologia Polska (Warsaw)
Klin Khir	Klinicheskaia Khirurgiia (Kiev)
Klin Mbl Augenheilk	Klinische Monatsblaetter Fur Augenheilkunde (Stuttgart)
Klin Med	Linicheskaia Meditsina (Moscow)
Klin Oczna	Klinika Oczna: Acta Ophthalmologica Polonica (Warsaw)
Klin Wschr	Klinische Wochenschrift (Berlin)
Lab Delo	Labortornoe Delo (Moscow)
Lahey Clin Found Bull	Lahey Clinic Foundation Bulletin (Boston)
Lakartidningen	Lakartidningen (Stockholm)
Lancet	Lancet (London)
Landarzt	Landarzt: Zeitschrift Fur Allgemeinmedizin (Stuttgart)
Lebensversicherungsmedizin	Lebensversicherungsmedizin (Karlsruhe)
Leprosy Rev	Leprosy Review (London)
Lijecn Vjesn	Lijecnicki Vjesnik (Zagreb)
Lille Med	Lille Medical
Lyon Med	Lyon Medical
Maroc Med	Maroc Medical (Casablanca)
Marseille Med	Marseille Medical
Maryland Med J	Maryland State Medical Journal
Massachusetts Gen Pract News	Massachusetts General Practice News (American Academy Of General Practice Massachusetts Chapter)
Matern Child Hlth	Maternal & Child Health (Chicago)
Mayo Clin Proc	Mayo Clinic Proceedings (Rochester, Minnesota)

Med Ann DC	Medical Annals Of The District Of Columbia
Med Clin N Amer	Medical Clinics Of North America (Philadelphia)
Med Glas	Medicinski Glasnik (Beograd)
Med Intern	Medicina Interna (Bucuresti)
Med J Aust	Medical Journal Of Australia (Sydney)
Med Klin	Medizinische Klinik (Munchen)
Med Leg Domm Corpor	Medecine Legale Et Dommage Corporel (Paris)
Med Lett Drugs Ther	Medical Letter On Drugs And Therapeutics (New York)
Med Mschr	Medizinische Monatsschrift (Stuttgart)
Med Parazit	Meditsinskaia Parazitologiia i Parazitarnye Bolezni (Moscow)
Med Serv J Canada	Medical Services Journal Of Canada
Med Times	Medical Times (Manhasset)
Med Trop	Medicina Tropical (Madrid)
Med Trop	Medecine Tropicale: Revue Du Service De Sante Des Troupes De Marine (Marseille)
Med Welt	Medizinische Welt (Stuttgart)
Mediscope	Mediscope: Journal Of Medicine And Surgery (Madras)
Mich Med	Michigan Medicine (East Lansing)
Microbiologia	Microbiologia Parazitologia Epidemiologia (Bucharest)
Milit Med	Military Medicine (Washington)
Minerva Cardioangiol	Minderva Cardioangiologica (Torino)
Minerva Derm	Minerva Dermatologica (Torino)
Minerva Ginec	Minderva Ginecologica (Torino)
Minerva Med	Minerva Medica (Torino)
Minerva Nipiol	Minerva Nipiologica (Torino)
Minerva Ortop	Minerva Ortopedica (Torino)
Minerva Pediat	Minderva Pediatrica (Torino)
Minn Med	Minnesota Medicine (St. Paul)
Missouri Med	Missouri Medicine (St. Paul)
Mod Treatm	Modern Treatment (New York)
Mschr Kinderheilk	Monatsschrift Fur Kinderheilkunde (Berlin)
Mschr Ohrenheilk	Monatsschrift Fur Ohrenheilkunde Und Laryngorhinologie (Wien)
Mt Sinai J Med	Mount Sinai Journal Of Medicine (New York)
Munca Sanit	Munca Sanitara Nursing Care (Bucharest)
Munchen Med Wschr	Muenchener Medizinische Wochen-

N M	
N Carolina Med J	North Carolina Medical Journal (Winston-Salem)
Naika	Naika (Tokyo)
Nations Sch	Nation's Schools (Chicago)
Nature	Nature (London)
Nauch Tr Vissh Med Inst Sofiia	Nauchni Trudove Na Visshia Meditsinki Institut Sofiia
Nebraska Med J	Nebraska State Medical Journal (Lincoln)
Nederl T Geneesk	Nederlands Tijdschrift Voor Geneeskunde (Amsterdam)
Nederl T Verlosk	Nederlandsch Tijdschrift Voor Verloskunde En Gynaecologie (Haarlem)
Neurocirugia	Neurocirugia (Santiago)
Neurol India	Neurology India (Bombay)
Neurol Neurochir Pol	Neurologia I Neurochirurgia Polska (Warsaw)
Neurol Neurochir Psychiat Pol	Neurologia Neurochirurgia I Psychiatria Polska (Warsaw)
Neurologia	Neurologia Psihiatria Neurochirurgia (Bucuresti)
Neurology	Neurology (Minneapolis)
New Eng J Med	New England Journal Of Medicine (Boston)
New York J Med	New York State Journal Of Medicine (New York)
New Zeal Med J	New Zealand Medical Journal (Wellington)
New Zealand Nurs J	New Zealand Nursing Journal (Wellington)
Newsweek	Newsweek
Nippon Ika Daig Z	Nippon Ika Daigaku Zasshi (Tokyo)
Nord Med	Nordisk Medicin (Stockholm)
Northwest Med	Northwest Medicine (Seattle)
Nunt Radiol	Nuntius Radiologicus (Roma)
Nuovi Ann Ig Microbiol	Nuovi Annali D'Igiene E Microbiologia (Roma)
Nurs Mirror	Nursing Mirror & Midwive's Journal (London)
Nurs Times	Nursing Times (London)
Obstet Gynec	Obstetrics And Gynecology (New York)
Oeff Gesundheitwesen	Oeffentliche Gesundheitswesen (Stuttgart)
Oest Z Stomat	Oesterreichische Zeitschrift Fur Stomatologie (Wien)
Ohio Sch	Ohio Schools (Columbus)

Nursing Mirror — appears above "North Carolina Medical Journal" as translation of "N M"

Oral Surg	Oral Surgery Oral Medicine And Oral Pathology (St. Louis)
Orv Hetil	Orvosi Hetilap (Budapest)
Osped Ital Chir	Ospedali d'Italia: Chirurgia (Firenze)
Otolaryngology	In Japanese: Jibinkoka (Tokyo)
Pa Sch J	Pennsylvania School Journal (Harrisburg)
Parents Mag	Parents Magazine And Better Family Living (New York)
Path Biol	Pathologie Et Biologie (Paris)
Pediat Akush Ginek	Pediatriia Akusherstvo I Ginekologiia (Kiev)
Pediat Clin N Amer	Pediatric Clinics Of North America (Philadelphia)
Pediat Pol	Pediatria Polska (Warsaw)
Pediatria	Pediatria (Bucharest)
Pediatrics	Pediatrics (Springfield, Illinois)
Penn Med	Pennsylvania Medicine (Harrisburg)
Pieleg Poloz	Pielegniarka I Polozna (Warsaw)
Pol Med J	Polish Medical Journal (Warsaw)
Pol Przegl Chir	Polski Przeglad Chirugrgiczny (Warsaw)
Pol Tyg Lek	Polski Tygodnik Lekarski (Warsaw)
Policlinico	Policlinico Sezione Pratica (Rome)
Postgrad Med	Postgraduate Medicine (Minneapolis)
Postgrad Med J	Postgraduate Medical Journal (London)
Poznan Two Przyjac Nauk Wydz Lek	Poznanskie Towarzystwo Przyjaciol Nauk Wydzial Lekarski Prace Komisji Medycyny Doswiadczalnj D Lekarskiej (Poznan)
Practitioner	Practitioner (London)
Praxis	Praxis (Bern)
Prensa Med Argent	Prensa Medica Argentina (Buenos Aires)
Presse Med	Presse Médicale (Paris)
Probl Tuberk	Problemy Tuberkuleza (Moscow)
Proc Roy Soc Med	Proceedings Of The Royal Society Of Medicine (London)
Proc Soc Exp Biol Med	Proceedings Of The Society For Experimental Biology And Medicine (New York)
Prophyl Sanit Morale	Prophylaxie Sanitaire Et Morale (Paris)
Przegl Derm	Przeglad Dermatologieczny (Warsaw)
Przegl Lek	Przeglad Lekarski (Krakow)

Psychiat Clin	Psychiatria Clinica (Basel)
Psychiat Neurol Med Psychol	Psychiatrie Neurologie Und Medizinische Psychologie (Leipzig)
Psychiat Neurol Neurochir	Psychiatria Neurologia Neurochirurgia
Psychoanal Rev	Psychoanalytic Review (New York)
Public Health Rep	Public Health Reports (Washington)
Quad Clin Ostet Ginec	Quaderni Di Clinica Ostetrica E Ginecologica (Parma)
RN	RN; National Magazine For Nurses (Oradell, New Jersey)
Rad Med Fak Zagreb	Radovi Medicinskog Fakulteta U Zagrebu
Radiology	Radiology (Syracuse)
Rass Int Clin Ter	Rassegna Internazionale Di Clinica E Terapia (Napoli)
Reumatologia	Reumatologia (Warsaw)
Rev Ass Med Brasil	Revista Da Associacao Medica Brasileira (Sao Paulo)
Rev Bras Med	Revista Brasileira De Medicina (Rio de Janeiro)
Rev Chile Obstet Ginec	Revista Chilena De Obstetricia Y Ginecologia
Rev Chile Pediat	Revista Chilena De Pediatria (Santiago)
Rev Clin Esp	Revista Clinica Espanola (Madrid)
Rev Columbia Obstet Ginec	Revista Colombiana De Obstetricia Y Ginecologia (Bogota)
Rev Corps Sante Armees	Revue Des Corps De Sante Des Armees Terre Mer Air (Paris)
Rev Dent Liban	Revue Dentaire Libanaise (Beirut)
Rev Ecuat Hig	Revista Ecuatoriana De Higiene Y Medicina Tropical (Guayaquil)
Rev Esp Enferm Apar Dig	Revista Espanola De Las Enfermedades Del Aparato Digestivo (Madrid)
Rev Franc Odontostomat	Revue Francaise d'Odontostomatologie (Paris)
Rev Franc Transfus	Revue Francaise De Transfusion (Paris)
Rev Inst Med Trop S Paulo	Revista Do Instituto De Medicina Tropical De Sao Paulo
Rev Invest Salud Publica	Revista De Investigacion En Salud Publica (Mexico)
Rev Laryng	Revue De Laryngologie (Bordeaux)
Rev Lat Amer Microbiol	Revista Latinoamericana De Microbiologia (Mexico)
Rev Med Suisse Rom	Revue Medicale De La Suisse Romande (Lausanne)
Rev Medicochir Iasi	Revista Medico-Chirurgicala A

Rev Neurol	Societatii Di Medici Si Naturalisti Din Iasi Revue Neurologique (Paris)
Rev Obstet Ginec Venez	Revista Obstetricia Y Ginecologia De Venezuela (Caracas)
Rev Otoneuroophtal	Revue d'Oto-Neuro-Ophtalmologie (Paris)
Rev Paul Med	Revista Paulista De Medicina (Sao Paulo)
Rev Rhum	Revue Du Rhumatisme Et Des Maladies Osteo-Articulaires (Paris)
Rev Sanid Milit Argent	Revista De La Sanidad Militar Argentina (Buenos Aires)
Rev Saude Publica	Revista De Saude Publica (Sao Paulo)
Rev Stomat	Revue De Stomatologie Et De Chirur Gie Maxillo-Faciale (Paris)
Rev Venez Urol	Revista Venezolana De Urologia (Caracas)
Rheumatol Phys Med	Rheumatology And Physical Medicine (London)
Riv Ist Sieroter Ital	Revista Dell'Istituto Sieroterapico Italiano (Naples)
Roczn Pom Akad Med Swierczewski	Rocznik Pomorskiej Akademii Medycznej Imienia Generala Karola Swierczewskiego W Szczedinie
Roy Soc Health J	Royal Society Of Health Journal (London)
Rum Med Rev	Rumanian Medical Review (Bucharest)
S Afr Med J	South African Medical Journal (Capetown)
S Carolina Dent J	South Carolina Dental Journal (Greenwich)
S Carolina Nurs	South Carolina Nursing (Columbia)
S Dakota J Med	South Dakota Journal Of Medicine (Sioux Falls)
Saishin Igaku	Saishin Igaku (Osaka)
Salud Publica Mex	Salud Publica De Mexico (Mexico City)
Sanfujin Jissai	Sanfujinka No Jissai (Tokyo)
Sat R	Saturday Review (New York)
Sborn Ved Prac Lek Fak	Sbornik Vedeckych Praci Lekarske Fakulty Karlovy University (Hradec Kralove)
Scand J Haemat	Scandinavian Journal Of Haematology (Kobenhavn)
Sch And Com	School And Community (Columbia, Missouri)
Schweiz Med Wschr	Schweizerische Medizinische Wochenschrift (Basel)

Sci N	Science News (Washington)
Sci Rep Res Inst Tohoku Univ	Science Reports Of The Research Institutes Tohoku University Series C: Medicine (Sendai)
Science	Science (Washington)
Scot Med J	Scottish Medical Journal (Glasgow)
Sem Hop Paris	Semaine Des Hopitaux De Paris
Sem Ther	Semaine Therapeutique (Paris)
Sightsav Rev	Sight-Saving Review (New York)
Sotilaslaak Aikak	Sotilaslaaketieteellinen Aikakauslehti (Helsinki)
Southern Med J	Southern Medical Journal (Birmingham)
Sovet Med	Sovetskaia Meditsina (Moscow)
Sovet Zdravookhr	Sovetskoe Zdravookhranenie (Moscow)
Srpski Ark Celok Lek	Srpski Arkiv Za Celokupno Lekarstvo (Beograd)
Statist Bull Metrop Life Insur Co	Statistical Bulletin Metropolitan Life Insurance Company (New York)
Sudhoff Arch	Sudhoffs Archiv Zeitschrift Fur Wissenshafts-Geschichte (Wiesbaden)
Surg Clin N Amer	Surgical Clinics Of North America (Philadelphia)
Surg Gynec Obstet	Surgery Gynecology And Obstetrics (Chicago)
Survey Ophthal	Survey Of Ophthalmology (Baltimore
T Norsk Laegeforen	Tidsskrift For Den Norske Laegeforening (Oslo)
T Sygepl	Tidsskrift For Sygepleje (Copenhagen)
Techn Bull Regist Med Techn	Technical Bulletin Of The Registry Of Medical Technologists (Baltimore)
Ter Arkh	Terapevticheskii Arkhiv (Moscow)
Texas Med	Texas Medicine (Autin)
Ther Gegenw	Therapie Der Gegenwart (Berlin)
Ther Umsch	Therapeutische Umschau (Bern)
Thorac Surg	Thoracic Medicine And Surgery (Mexico)
Thoraxchirurgie	Thoraxchirurgie Und Vaskulaere Chirurgie (Stuttgart)
Time	Time (Chicago)
Tip Fak Mec	Tip Fakultesi Mecmuasi (Istanbul)
Tohoku J Exp Med	Tohoku Journal Of Experimental Medicine (Sendai)
Trans Amer Acad Ophthal Otolaryng	Transactions Of The American Academy Of Ophthalmology and

	Otolaryngology (Rochester, Minnesota)
Trans Amer Ophthal Soc	Transactions Of The American Ophthalmological Society (New York)
Trans Ophthal Soc Uk	Transactions Of The Ophthalmological Societies Of The United Kingdom (London)
Trans Pacif Coast Otoophthal Soc	Transactions Of The Pacific Coast Oto-Ophthalmological Society
Trans Roy Soc Trop Med Hyg	Transactions Of The Royal Society Of Tropical Medicine And Hygiene (London)
Trans St John Hosp Derm Soc	Transactions Of The St. John's Hospital Dermatological Society (London)
Transfusion	Transfusion (Philadelphia)
Triangle	Triangle: Sandoz Journal Of Medical Science (Basel)
Trop Geogr Med	Tropical And Geographical Medicine (Haarlem)
Turk Hij Tecr Biyol Derg	Turk Hijiyen Ve Tecrubi Biyoloji Dergisi (Ankara)
Turk Tip Cem Mec	Turk Tip Cemiyeti Mecmuasi (Istanbul)
UN Med Canada	Union Medicale Du Canada (Montreal)
U S Naval Med Field Res Lab	U S Naval Medical Field Research Laboratory (Camp Lejeune, North Carolina)
Ugeskr Laeg	Ugeskrift For Laeger (Kobenhavn)
Ukranian Pediat Akush Ginek	Ukranian Pediat Akush Ginek (Kiev)
Ulster Med J	Ulster Medical Journal (Belfast)
Univ Mich Med Cent J	University Of Michigan Medical Center Journal (Ann Arbor)
Urol Nefrol	Urologiia I Nefrologiia (Moscow)
Vestn Derm Vener	Vestnik Dermatologii I Venerologii (Moscow)
Vestn Akad Med Nauk Ssr	Vestnik Akademii Nauk Sssr (Moscow)
Virchow Arch	Virchows Archiv: Abteilung A: Pathologische Anatomie (Berlin)
Virginia Med Monthly	Virginia Medical Monthly (Richmond)
Vnitrni Lek	Vnitrni Lekarstvi (Praha)
Voennomed Zh	Voenno-Meditsinskii Zhurnal (Moscow)
Vojnosanit Pregl	Vojnosanitetski Pregled (Beograd)
Vop Okhr Materin Dets	Voprosy Okhrany Materinstva I

	Detstva (Moscow)
Vop Revm	Voprosy Revmatizma (Moscow)
Vrach Delo	Vrachebnoe Delo (Kiev
WHO Chron	WHO Chronicle (Geneva)
W Indian Med J	West Indian Medical Journal (Kingston)
W Virginia Med J	West Virginia Medical Journal (Charleston)
West Afr Med J	West African Medical Journal (Ibadan)
Wiad Lek	Wiadomsci Lekarskie (Warsaw)
Wiad Parazyt	Wiadomosci Parazytologiczne (Wroclaw)
Wien Klin Wschr	Wiener Klinische Wochenschrift (Vienna)
Wien Z Nervenheilk	Wiener Zeitschrift Fur Nervenheilkunde Und Deren Grenzgebiete
Wisconsin Med J	Wisconsin Medical Journal (Madison)
World Health	World Health (Geneva)
Yng Laeg	Yngre Laeger (Kobenhavn)
Yonsei Med J	Yonsei Medical Journal (Seoul)
Z Aerztl Fortbild	Zeitschrift Fur Aerztliche Fortbildung (Jena)
Z Allgemeinmed	Zeitschrift Fur Allgemeinmedizin: Der Landarzt
Z Geburtsh Gynaek	Zeitschrift Fur Geburtshilfe Und Gynaekologie (Stuttgart)
Z Ges Inn Med	Zeitschrift Fur Die Gesamte Innere Medizin Und Ihre Grenzgebiete (Leipzig)
Z Haut Geschlechtskr	Zeitschrift Fur Haut-Und Geschlechts-Krankheiten (Berlin)
Z Immunitaetsforsch	Zeitschrift Fur Immunitaetsforschung Allergie Und Klinische Immunologie (Stuttgart)
Z Kinderheilk	Zeitschrift Fur Kinderheilkunde (Berlin)
Z Med Mikrobiol Immun	Zeitschrift Fur Medizinische Mikrobiologie Und Immunologie (Berlin)
Z Orthop	Zeitschrift Fur Orthopaedie Und Ihre Grenzgebiete (Stuttgart)
Z Tropenmed Parasit	Zeitschrift Fur Tropenmedizin Und Parasitologie (Stuttgart)
Z Urol	Zeitschrift Fur Urologie Und Nephrologie (Leipzig)
ZBL Bakt	Zentralblatt Fur Bakteriologie Parasitenkunde Infektionskrankheiten Und Hygiene: Erste Abteilung: Originale (Stuttgart)

Zbl Chir	Zentralblatt Fur Chirurgie (Leipzig)
Zbl Gynaek	Zentralblatt Fur Gynaekologie (Leipzig)
Zbl Veterinaermed	Zentralblatt Fur Veterinaermedizin: Reihe B: Infektions Und Invasionskrankheiten, Bakteriologie Virologie Parasitologie Hygiene Lebensmittelhygiene Pathologie (Berlin)
Zdrow Publiczne	Zdrowie Publiczne (Warsaw)
Zh Mikrobiol	Zhurnal Mikrobiologii Epidemiologii I Immunobiologii (Moscow)
Zh Nevropat Psikhiat Korsakov	Zhurnal Nevropatologii I Psikhiatrii Imeni S. S. Korsakova (Moscow)
Zh Ushn Nos Gorl Bolez	Zhurnal Ushnykh Nosovyky I Gorlovykh Boleznei (Kiev)

SUBJECT HEADINGS USED IN THIS BIBLIOGRAPHY

ACD Preparations
ACTH
Acetazolamide
Adolescents & Venereal Disease
Adoption
Albothyl
Allergy
Alphachloromethyl-2-methyl-5-nitro-1-imidazole ethanol
Amphotericin B
Ampicillin
Ano-Rectal
Antimicrobial Treatment
Aortitis
Arthritis
Atricana
Balanoposthitis
Bedsoniae
Bejel
Bibliography
Bicillin
Bismuth

Blennorrhagia
Blood Donors and Transfusions
Cancer & Pre-Cancer
Candidiasis
Carbamazepine
Cefazolin
Cellini, B.
Cephalexin
Cephaloridine
Cephalosporins
Cephalothin
Chagas' Disease
Chancroid
Charcot's Joints
Children
Chloramphenicol
Chlorocide
Chloroquine
Chlorosulfonamides
Cirrhosis, Hepatic
Citral
Clinics, Institutes & Societies
Clomocycline

Colpitis
Conferences
Contraception
Copper Oxidase
Crede's Prophylaxis
Debecillin
Deflamon
Demethylchlortetracycline
Dentistry
de Santa Cruz y Espejo, Francisco Xavier Eugenio
Detromycin
Diabetes
Diagnosis
Dimethyl Sulfoxide
Diribiotine
Donovanosis
Doxicillin
Doxycycline
Drug Addiction
Ecmonovocillin
Education
Ehrlich, Paul
Enduracidin
Enzymology
Epilepsy
Erythromycin
Flagyl
Frambesia
Furacin
Furadonin
Furazolidone
Fusidic Acid
Geriatrics
Giardiasis
Glitisol
Gonorrhea
Gonorrhea: Ano Rectal
Gonorrhea: Arthritic
Gonorrhea: Bartholinitis
Gonorrhea: Cardiovascular
Gonorrhea: Children
Gonorrhea: Complications
Gonorrhea: Contraception
Gonorrhea: Diagnosis
Gonorrhea: Education
Gonorrhea: Endocarditis
Gonorrhea: Experimental
Gonorrhea: Hepatic
Gonorrhea: History
Gonorrhea: Immunology
Gonorrhea: Microbiology
Gonorrhea: Morphology
Gonorrhea: Neonatal
Gonorrhea: Occurrence
Gonorrhea: Ophthalmology
Gonorrhea: Penile
Gonorrhea: Peritonitis
Gonorrhea: Pharyngeal
Gonorrhea: Pregnancy
Gonorrhea: Prevention & Control
Gonorrhea: Prostitutes
Gonorrhea: Pseudogonorrhea
Gonorrhea: Serodiagnosis
Gonorrhea: Serology
Gonorrhea: Servicemen
Gonorrhea: Sociology
Gonorrhea: Tongue
Gonorrhea: Treatment
Gonorrhea: Youth
Granuloma Inguinale
Granuloma Venerum Tropical
Hamycin
Herpes
Hetacillin
History
Homosexuality
Hutchinson, Jonathan
Imidazole
Immunology
Infants
Infertility
Institutes
Interstitial Keratitis
Iodinol
Iodopovidone
Jacksons Syndrome
Jarisch-Herxheimer Reaction
Jasomycin
Kanamycin
Klion
Law
Ledermycin
Leprosy
Leukoplakia
Leutic Glossitis
Levorin
Lincomycin
Lupus Erythematosus
Lymphogranuloma Venereum

Macmiror
Magmilor
Marcus Gunn Phenomenon
Medical Doctors & Venereal Disease
Megaclor
Methacycline
Metronidazole
Minocycline
Minor Venereal Infections & Diseases
Monomycin
Mononucleosis
Mycoplasmas
Mycoses
Naxogin
Neisser, Albert
Neonatal
Nifuratel
Niridazole
Nitrimidazine
Nitrofuran
Nitroimidazole
Non-Gonorrheal Infections & Diseases
Non-Gonorrheal Urethritis
Obstetrics
Occurrence
Oleandomycin
Oletetrin
Ophthalmia Neonatorum
Ophthalmology
Oral
Oxygen Therapy
Oxyguinoline
Oxyterracine
Oxytetracycline
Paresis
Paretics
Paromycin
Pasomysin
Pavlov, Sergei T.
Pediculosis
Penicillin
Phosphonomycin
Pimafucin
Pimaricin
Pinta
Polyradiculneuritis
Prednisone
Pregnancy

Prevention & Control
Probenecid
Prodigiosane
Prostitution
Psoriasis
Psychiatry
Pyrogenale
Q Fever
Reactions
Reactions: Ampicillin
Reactions: Antibiotics
Reactions: Antimicrobial
Reactions: Bicillins
Reactions: Cephaloridine
Reactions: Cephalothin
Reactions: Cephalosporins
Reactions: Jarisch-Herxheimer
Reactions: Novocain
Reactions: Penicillin
Reactions: Streptomycin
Reiter's Disease
Reverin
Ricord, Philippe
Rifampicin
Rifomycin
Rimactan
Rondomycin
Rovamycin
Salpingitis
Scabies
Scientific Society of Dermatologists-Venerologists
Serodiagnosis
Serology
Servicemen
Sex Research
Sigmamycin
Smallpox
Societies, Clinics, & Institutes
Sociology & Behavior
Spectinomycin
Spiramycin
Spondylitis
Statistics
Sterility
Streptomycin
Sulphamethoxazole
Sulfanilamide
Sulfisoxazole
Sulphonamides

Symposia
Syphilis
Syphilis: Ano-Rectal
Syphilis: Arthritic
Syphilis: Arthropathy
Syphilis: Aural
Syphilis: Bibliography
Syphilis: Cardiovascular
Syphilis: Cerebrospinal
    Fluid
Syphilis: Children
Syphilis: Complications
Syphilis: Congenital
Syphilis: Cutaneous
Syphilis: Dentistry
Syphilis: Diagnosis
Syphilis: Diagnosis: Cere-
    brospinal Fluid
Syphilis: Experimental
Syphilis: Gastrointestinal
Syphilis: Geriatrics
Syphilis: History
Syphilis: Homosexuality
Syphilis: Immunology
Syphilis: Infants
Syphilis: Jaundice
Syphilis: Kidney
Syphilis: Liver
Syphilis: Lung
Syphilis: Lymph
Syphilis: Meningitis
Syphilis: Metabolism
Syphilis: Microbiology
Syphilis: Nasopharyngeal
Syphilis: Neonatal
Syphilis: Nephrosis
Syphilis: Neurosyphilis
Syphilis: Occurrence
Syphilis: Ophthalmology
Syphilis: Oral
Syphilis: Osseous
Syphilis: Pathology
Syphilis: Penile
Syphilis: Pregnancy
Syphilis: Prevention-Control
Syphilis: Pseudo-Syphilis
Syphilis: Pulmonary
Syphilis: Renal
Syphilis: Serology and Sero-
    diagnosis
Syphilis: Servicemen
Syphilis: Treatment
Syphilis: Vocal Cords
Tabes
Tegretol
Terramycin
Tetracycline
Tetraverin
Tetroid Lactic
Thiamphenicol
Thiophenicol
Thrush Colpitis
Thyadione
Thyroid
Tinidazole
Treatment
Triacetyloleandomycin
Tricho-Kolpicortin
Trichomoniasis
Trichomoniasis: Children &
    Infants
Trichomoniasis: Complications
Trichomoniasis: Diagnosis
Trichomoniasis: Experimental
Trichomoniasis: Occurrence
Trichomoniasis: Pregnancy
Trichomoniasis: Treatment
Trichopol
Trimethoprim-Sulphonamide
2-Mercaptoethanol
Urethritis:Non-Gonococcal
Usnic Acid
Uveitis
Vaccination
V-cillin
Venereal Disease
Venereological Institutes
Veterinary
Vibramycin
Viruses
Vulcacycline
Yaws
Yaws: Occurrence
Yaws: Prevention & Control
Yaws: Treatment
Youth

TABLE OF CONTENTS

Preface..i
List of Abbreviations...................................v
Subject Headings Used in This Bibliography..........xxvi
Books...1
Periodical Literature:
    Title Index..5
    Subject Index....................................249
Author Index..584

BOOKS

Amelar, R. D. INFERTILITY IN MEN. Philadelphia: Davis, 1966.

American Association for Health, Physical Education and Recreation. VENEREAL DISEASE; RESOURCE UNIT [for] HIGH SCHOOL. Washington, D.C.: The Association, 1967.

The American Social Health Association. TODAY'S VENEREAL DISEASE CONTROL PROBLEM. A JOINT STATEMENT. New York: The Association, 1966.

Behrman, S. J. and R. W. Kistner, editors. PROGRESS IN INFERTILITY. Boston: Little, 1968.

Blanzaco, Andre, et al. VD: FACTS YOU SHOULD KNOW. New York: Lothrop, 1970.

Brown, William J. et al. SYPHILIS & OTHER VENEREAL DISEASES. (Vital & Health Statistics Monographs, American Public Health Association Ser). Cambridge: Harvard University Press, 1970.

Catterall, R. Duncan. THE VENEREAL DISEASES. New York: International Publications Service, 1967; New York: Evans, 1967.

Chesser, Eustace. UNMARRIED LOVE. New York: Pocket Books, 1966.

Davis, Maxine. SEX & THE ADOLESCENT. New York: Pocket Books, 1968.

Deschin, Celia S. THE TEENAGER AND VD; A SOCIAL SYMPTOM OF OUR TIMES. New York: Rosen, 1969.

Fink, Paul and Van Buren O. Hammett. SEXUAL FUNCTION & DYSFUNCTION. Philadelphia: Davis Co., 1969.

Fribourg, Arlette. EVERY GIRL'S BOOK OF SEX. New York: Arc Books, 1967.

Frieboes, W. and W. H. P. Schonfeld. ATLAS DER HAUT-UND GESCHLECHT-SHRANKHEITEN. Fortgefuhrt von Joseph Kimmig and Michael Janner. 3rd rev. ed. Stuttgart:

Thieme, 1966.

--COLOR ATLAS OF DERMATOLOGY. Philadelphia: Saunders, 1966.

Griffith, Edward F. MARRIAGE & THE UNCONSCIOUS. 2nd ed. Springfield: C. C. Thomas, 1967.

Hirsch, E. W. IMPOTENCE AND FRIGIDITY. New York: Citadel, 1966.

Israel, S. L. DIAGNOSIS AND TREATMENT OF MENSTRUAL DISORDERS AND STERILITY. 5th ed. New York: Harper, 1967.

Johnson, J. DISORDERS OF SEXUAL POTENCY IN THE MALE. Elmsford: Pergamon, 1968.

King, Ambrose and Claude Nicol. VENEREAL DISEASES. 2nd ed. New York: Davis, 1970.

Kleegman, S. J. and S. A. Kaufman. INFERTILITY IN WOMEN. New York: Davis, 1966.

Luger, Anton, editor. CURRENT PROBLEMS IN DERMATOLOGY Vol. 2: ANTIBIOTIC TREATMENT OF VENEREAL DISEASES. White Plains: Phiebig, 1968.

McCary, James L. HUMAN SEXUALITY. New York: VanN-Rein, 1967.

McLachlan, A. E. W. MCLACHLAN'S HANDBOOK OF DIAGNOSIS & TREATMENT OF VENEREAL DISEASE. 5th ed. Baltimore: Williams & Wilkins, 1970.

Mali, J. W., editor. CURRENT PROBLEMS IN DERMATOLOGY. Vol. 3. White Plains: Phiebig, 1970.

Miller, A., et al. A SYNOPSIS OF RENAL DISEASES AND UROLOGY. Baltimore: Williams & Wilkins, 1966.

Minnesota. Department of Health. Section of Public Health Education. VENEREAL DISEASE EDUCATION; A TEACHING GUIDE. St. Paul: The Section, 1966.

Morton, Robert S. VENEREAL DISEASES. [Pelican Book A 819]. Baltimore: Penguin, 1966.

Podair, S. VENEREAL DISEASE. Palo Alto: Fearon, 1966.

Robinson, J. O. MODERN UROLOGY FOR NURSES. New York:

Heinemann, 1968.

Roland, M. MANAGEMENT OF THE INFERTILE COUPLE. Springfield: C. C. Thomas, 1968.

Schwartz, Benjamin. CLINICAL VENEREOLOGY, FOR NURSES & STUDENTS. Elmsford: Pergamon, 1966.

Schwartz, Bernard. SYPHILIS AND THE EYE. Baltimore: Williams & Wilkins, 1970.

Smith, J. Lawton. SPIROCHETES IN LATE SERONEGATIVE SYPHILIS PENICILLIN NOT WITHSTANDING. Springfield: C. C. Thomas, 1969.

Taymor, M. L. THE MANAGEMENT OF INFERTILITY. Springfield: C. C. Thomas, 1969.

U.S. Public Health Service. Bureau of Disease Prevention and Environmental Control. CURRENT LITERATURE ON VENEREAL DISEASE, ABSTRACTS AND BIBLIOGRAPHY. [Atlanta, Georgia]. See Numbers.

Vermes, Jean C. POT IS ROT: AND OTHER HORRIBLE FACTS ABOUT BAD THINGS. New York: Association Press, 1969.

Warner, M. P. MODERN FERTILITY GUIDE. New York: Funk, 1969.

Wykes, A. THE DOCTOR AND HIS ENEMY. New York: Dutton, 1966.

YEAR BOOK OF UROLOGY. 1964-1965 to 1965-1966. 2v. Chicago: Year Book Medical, 1966.

--1966-1967. Chicago: Year Book Medical, 1967.

--1967-1968. Chicago: Year Book Medical, 1968.

PERIODICAL LITERATURE

"ABO and rhesus blood group distribution among patients attending venereal diseases clinics," by C. B. Schofield. J MED GENET (London). 3:101-103, June, 1966.

"ABO blood groups and acute biologic false positive serological tests for syphilis," by A. I. Morrison. BRIT J VENER DIS. 42:37-39, March, 1966.

"ACTH as a prophylactic against the Jarisch-Herxheimer reaction," by E. Sylvester. Z HAUT GESCHLECHTSKR. 44:125-126, February 15, 1969.

"AMA national symposium on venereal disease control. Introductory speech," by J. H. Sterner. ARCH ENVIRON HEALTH (Chicago). 13:352, September, 1966.

--"Opening address," by A. W. Christensen. ARCH ENVIRON HEALTH (Chicago). 13:354-356, September, 1966.

--"Welcoming address," by C. C. Edwards. ARCH ENVIRON HEALTH (Chicago). 13:353, September, 1966.

"APHA conference report, 1968. Laboratory." PUBLIC HEALTH REP. 84:272-279, March, 1969.

"Abdominoperineal resection of the rectum," by R. K. Gilchrist. SURG CLIN N AMER. 46:1191-1199, October 1966.

"Abnormal bleeding in women with trichomonas vaginalis infection," by G. Terzano, et al. WIAD PARAZYT. 15:331-332, 1969.

"Absence of syphilis in the population of Chipaya (Bolivia)," by P. Cirera, et al. BULL SOC PATH EXOT. 61:849-852, November-December, 1968.

"Absorbed fluorescent treponemal antibody (FTA-ABS) test. Comparison with the FTA-200 and TPI tests on 1,056 problem sera," by N. A. Johnston, et al. BRIT J VENER DIS. 44:287-290, December, 1968.

"Accidental human infection in the laboratory with Nichols rabbit-adapted virulent strain of treponema pallidum," by C. W. Chacko. BULL WHO. 35:809-810, 1966.

"Accidents during the treatment of neurosyphilis," by J. Roland. MAROC MED. 45:221-222, March, 1966.

"Achievements in the field of gonorrhea control," by I. M. Porudominskii, et al. VESTA DERM VENER. 41:27-36, October, 1967.

"Achievements in Soviet syphilidology," by M. A. Rozentul, et al. VESTN DERM VENER. 41:12-20, October, 1967.

"Achievements of famous Polish surgeons in venerology in the 19th century," by K. Lejman. PRZEGL DERM. 55:621-629, September-October, 1968.

"Action and secondary action of metronidazol in the therapy of trichomoniasis," by K. Wiesner, et al. FORTSCHR ARZNEIMITTELFORSCH. 9:361-391, 1966.

"Action of primaricin on postpartum mycoses," by M. E. Rochet, et al. LYON MED. 216:1179-1183, November 20, 1966.

"Active detection of patients with trichomoniasis," by L. M. Korik, et al. VESTN DERM VENER. 42:90-92, January, 1968.

"Activities of the board of all-Russian scientific society of dermatologists-venereologists," by B. M. Pashkov. VESTN DERM VENER. 43:75-79, June, 1969.

"Activities of the board of the all-union scientific medical society of dermatologists-venereologists for 1966-1968," by A. A. Studnitsin, et al. VESTN DERM VENER. 43:69-74, June, 1969.

"Activities of the Minsk dermatologists," by AIa. Prokopchuk. VESTN DERM VENER. 43:3-6, May, 1969.

"The activities of the Moscow scientific society of dermatologists and venereologists (1917-1967)," by V. A. Rakhmanov, et al. VESTN DERM VENER. 41:73-77, October, 1967.

"Activity of nifuratel against infective vulvovaginitis due to yeasts, trichomonas and bacteria," by J. E. Murphy. BRIT J CLIN PRACT. 22:431-432, October, 1968.

"Activity of the V. M. Tarnovskii Leningrad dermatological and venereal society during World War II," by G.

V. Shiman. VESTN DERM VENER. 45:52-54, December, 1969.

"Acute and subacute demyelination of the optic nerves," by W. H. Melanowski. KLIN OCZNA. 37:517-525, 1967.

"Acute bilateral perivasculitis retinae probably of a a gonococcal origin," by S. Kamel. BULL OPHTHAL SOC EGYPT. 59 Suppl 63:107+, 1966.

"Acute conjunctivitis among Cairo adult inhabitants. Increase in bacteriologically negative cases," by A. Mortada. BULL OPHTHAL SOC EGYPT. 58:37-45, 1965.

"Acute conjunctivitis among Cairo children. Decrease in K.W. and gonococcal infections and increase in bacteriologically negative cases," by A. Mortada, et al. BULL OPHTHAL SOC EGYPT. 58:25-35,1965.

"Acute embolic-toxic induced incident in treatment of stomach syphilis with penicillin," by W. Lindheimer. THER GEGENW. 106:755-759, June, 1967.

"Acute gonococcal urethritis: failure of response to phosphonomycin therapy," by P. M. Southern, Jr., et al. ANTIMICROB AGENTS CHEMOTHER. 9:343-345, 1969.

"Acute, non-allergic reactions following I.M. administration of clemizole-penicillin G and streptomycin," by K. Bornemann, et al. MUNCHEN MED WSCHR. 108:834-837, April 15, 1966.

"Acute psychotic reactions to aqueous procaine penicillin," by P. M. Utley, et al. SOUTHERN MED J. 59:1271-1274, November, 1966.

"Acute vaginitis and its treatment by a gynecologic terramycin foam. Clinical study and therapeutic results," by P. Magnier. GYNEC PRAT. 17:315-335, 1966.

"An additional case of pulmonary syphilis," by J. Horak. VNITRNI LEK. 13:848-852, September, 1967.

"Additional information on the TPIT in congenital syphilis," by L. Pospisil, et al. CESK DERM. 41:97-101, April, 1966.

"Adolescent coitus and cervical cancer: associations of related events with increased risk," by I. D. Rotkin. CANCER RES. 27:603-617, April, 1967.

"The adolescent's crisis today. Sex and the adolescent," by G. B. Blaine. NEW YORK J MED. 67:1967-1975, July 15, 1967.

"Advances in bacteriologic diagnosis of gonorrhea," by U. Berger. DEUTSCH MED WSCHR. 92:847-850, May 5, 1967.

"Advances in the treatment of venereal diseases," by C. B. Schofield. PRACTITIONER. 119:506-512, October, 1967.

"Advantage of a routine Reiter protein complement-fixation test in the serodiagnosis of syphilis in pregnancy," by C. A. Morris. J CLIN PATH. 21:731-734, November, 1968.

"Adverse reactions to penicillin," by J. Silverio. J AMER DENT ASS. 77:17, July, 1968.

"Ageing and false positive reactions for syphilis," by D. L. Tuffanelli. BRIT J VENER DIS. 42:40-41, March, 1966.

"Agglutination of particulate antigens in agar gel," by F. Milgrom, et al. J IMMUN. 98:102-109, January, 1967.

"Agglutination of Reiter's spirochete in serodiagnosis of syphilis," by G. Mariani. MINERVA MED. 58:3583-3585, October 20, 1967.

"Agglutination of spirochetes in the blood with the Roemer and Schlipkoeter method. Contribution to the serodiagnosis of syphilis," by G. Bratina. MINERVA MED. 58:3245-3247, September 22, 1967.

"Agranulocytosis with monohistiocytosis associated with ampicillin therapy," by M. Graf, et al. ANN INTERN MED. 69:91-95, July, 1968.

"Alabama Department of Public Health: state activates gonorrhea control project," by C. G. Lamar. J MED ASS ALABAMA. 38:631-632, January, 1969.

"An alarming problem in syphilography: the irreductible serologic reactions," by P. Rimbaud. PRESSE MED. 76:2471-2472, December 28, 1968.

"Albert Neisser (1855-1916) the discoverer of the diplococcus of gonorrhea," by E. Stocki. WIAD LEK. 20:397-398, February 15, 1967.

"Alcoholic lymphalgia in early syphilis," by D. J. Wright. POSTGRAD MED J. 45:191-192, March 1969.

"Alertness, awareness and responsibility." S CAROLINA DENT J. 26:12-12, January, 1968.

"Alfred Klopstock," by W. Pagel. INT ARCH ALLERG. 35:308, 1969.

"Allergenic factors in penicillins and cephalosporins," by G. T. Stewart. AMER HEART J. 75:429-431, March, 1968.

"Allergic cutaneous reactions to penicillin and their mechanisms," by M. J. Fellner, et al. DERMATOLOGICA. 135:362-368, 1967.

"Allergic reaction during repeated administration of penicillin," by D. I. Khozeniuk. VRACH DELO. 11:141-142, November, 1967.

"Allergic reactions in patients with syphilis treated with penicillin," by L. Ciecierski, et al. PRZEGI DERM. 53:189-192, March-April, 1966.

"Allergic reactions to antibiotics," by J. E. Kasik, et al. MED CLIN N AMER. 54:59-73, January, 1970.

"Allergic reactions to penicillins. Advances in understanding and management," by A. L. De Weck, et al. MINN MED. 52:137-150, January, 1969.

"Allergy to antibiotics. 1. Fact and conjecture on the sensitizing contaminants of penicillins and cephalosporins," by J. G. Feinberg. INT ARCH ALLERG. 33:439-443, 1968.

"Allergy to antibiotics. II. Comparative immunogenicity of some penicillins," by J. G. Feinberg. INT ARCH ALLERG. 33:444-453, 1968.

"Allergy to penicillin. Clinical study of 105 patients tested with penicilloyl-polylysine," by E. B. Negreiros. REV BRASIL MED. 25:597-600, September, 1968.

"Allergy to penicillin in children," by J. Charles, et al. ARCH FRANC PEDIAT. 25:955-956, October, 1968.

"Alphachloromethyl-2-methyl-5-nitro-1-imidazole ethanol (RO 7-0207), a substance exhibiting antiparasitic activity against amoebae, trichomonads, and pinworms," by E. Grunberg, et al. PROC SOC EXP BIOL MED. 133: 490-492, February, 1970.

"Ambulatory treatment of trichomonas infections in industrial and rural population," by T. Lopatecki. WIAD LEK. 22:11-13, January 1, 1969.

"The amoebicidal, trichomonicidal, and antibacterial effects of niridazole in laboratory animals," by F. Kradolfer, et al. ANN NY ACAD SCI. 160:740-748, October 6, 1969.

"Ampicillin in the treatment of gonorrhoea," by A. Finger. MED J AUST. 2:250-251, August 1, 1970.

"Ampicillin in the treatment of granuloma inguinale," by M. A. Thew, et al. JAMA. 210:866-867, November 3, 1969.

"Ampicillin in the treatment of 'penicillin-resistant' gonorrhea," by E. B. Smith. MILIT MED. 131:345-347, April, 1966.

"Anabolic hormones and gamma globulins in the course of experimental syphilis," by I. Orhel. RAD MED FAK ZAGREB. 15:203-211, 1967.

"Anaerobic pelvic infections and developments in hyperbaric oxygen therapy," by R. T. Parker, et al. AMER J OBSTET GYNEC. 96:645-659, November 1, 1966.

"Anal syphilis," by O. Delzant. ARCH FRANC MAL APPAR DIG. 59:Suppl 7-8:13+, July-August, 1970.

"Analysis of the antigenic structure of the Reiter strain of Treponema pallidum and significance of the strain in the syphilis serologic reaction," by Y. Saijo. JAP J BACT. 22:510-518, September, 1967.

"Analysis of the causes for the increase of gonorrhea in Slovakia," by E. Hegyi, et al. BRATISL LEK LISTY. 47:341-354, March 31, 1967.

"Analysis of morbidity to venereal diseases in Poland in 1966," by J. Bachurzewski. PRZEGL DERM. 54:641-50, November-December, 1967.

"An analysis of some characteristics of males with gonorrhoea," by L. H. Glass. BRIT J VENER DIS. 43:128-132, June, 1967.

"Anamnestic reactions in syphilis serology," by A. Lassus,

et al. INT ARCH ALLERG. 36:394-398, 1969.

"Anaphylactic reactions after intradermal diagnostic tests with penicilloyl-polylysin. Preliminary report," by J. Bowszyc. PRZEGL DERM. 55:307-309, May-June, 1968.

"Anaphylactic reactions after penicillin as a clinical and medicolegal problem," by Z. Starzycki. PRZEGL DERM. 55:559-563, July-September, 1968.

"Anaphylactic shock after intra-muscular administration of penicillin," by V. N. Groshev. TER ARKH. 39:122, February, 1967.

"Anaphylactic shock and its treatment in field practice," by Z. Balcar. SBORN VED PRAC LEK FAK KARLOV UNIV. 11:665-675, 1968.

"Anaphylactic shock caused by the use of bicillin forte," by M. V. Ignat'ev. KLIN MED. 46:138, May, 1968.

"Anaphylactic shock during skin test with antibiotics," by I. U. A. Tereshchenko. SOVET MED. 32:137-139, August, 1969.

"Anaphylactic shock following administration of penicillin," by P. M. Liashuk, et al. VRACH DELO. 1:139, January, 1968.

"Anaphylactic shock in the administration of penicillin," by M. P. Golovinskii. VRACH DELO. 3:146-147, March, 1966.

"Anaphylactic shock in antibiotic therapy," by V. V. Kuptsov. VRACH DELO. 7:127-128, July, 1968.

"Anaphylactic shock in penicillin and streptomycin therapy," by B. V. Smirnov, et al. SOVET MED. 30:135-136, February, 1967.

"Anatomoclinical case of secondary papulotuberculous syphilis," by P. Le Coulant, et al. BULL SOC FRANC DERM SYPH. 75:367-368, 1968.

"An anatomo-clinical case of tabes and syphilitic aneurysm of the aorta. Its course under treatment," by M. Giroud, et al. LYON MED. 215:1603-1609, June 5, 1966.

"Ancillary investigations in neurological diagnosis," by J. M. Sutherland, et al. MED J AUST. 2:452-546, September 16, 1967.

"Aneurysm of the ascending aorta. Recession and direct anastomosis. Report of a case," by J. F. Saadi, et al. ARQ BRASIL CARDIOL. 21:215-220, June, 1968.

"Aneurysms of the descending thoracic aorta," by M. L. Dillon, et al. THORAC SURG. 3:430-438, May, 1967.

"Aneurysms of the thoracic and abdominal aorta. I. Incidence of aortic aneurysm in 10,392 autopsies," by P. Tala, et al. ANN CHIR GYNAEC FENN. 56:270-277, 1967.

"Angiographic demonstration of aortic aneurysm," by E. Lohr, et al. FORTSCHR ROENTGENSTR. 110-71-78, January, 1969.

"Angiographic demonstration of coronary ostial stenosis. Report of a case probably due to syphilis," by C. A. Macleod, et al. AMER J CARDIOL. 22:122-125, July, 1968.

"Anogenital cutaneous lesions," by R. R. Kierland. JAMA. 203:213-218, January 15, 1968.

"Anogenital sinuses and polypi. Crohn's disease," by B. A. Thomas. BRIT J DERM. 80:414-415, June, 1968.

"Ano-rectal gonococcia," by J. Soullard, et al. ARCH FRANC MAL APPAR DIG. 59:Suppl 7-8:31+, July-August, 1970.

"Ano-rectal syphilis," by O. Delzant. ARCH FRANC MAL APPAR DIG. 59:Suppl 7-8, 13+, July-August, 1970.

"Anorectal syphilis," by B. Samenius, et al. NORD MED. 76:813, July 14, 1966.

"Anorectal venereal diseases," by J. Lentini. REV ESP ENFERM APAR DIG. 30:339-355, February 1, 1970.

"Another look at the Morbus Gallicus," by R. S. Morton. BRIT J VENER DIS. 42:174-177, June, 1968.

"Anti-anginal activity of a beta-adrenergic blocking agent, butydrine, alone and in association with pentaerythritol tetranitrate, in the aged," by A. Gatti, et al. CLIN TER. 41:363-374, May 31, 1967.

"Antibiotic sensitivity of gonococcal strains isolated in the south-east Asia and western Pacific regions in 1961-1968," by A. Reyn. BULL WHO, 40:257-262, 1969.

"Antibiotic sensitivity of gonococci and treatment of gonorrhoea in Uganda," by O. P. Arya, et al. BRIT J VENER DIS. 46:149-152, April, 1970.

"Antibiotic sensitivity of gonococci in Kampala," by I. Phillips, et al. E AFR MED J. 46:38-45, January, 1969.

"Antibiotic sensitivity of gonococci in women with various forms of gonorrhea," by Z. A. Pesina, et al. ANTIBIOTIKA. 10:852-855, September, 1965.

"Antibiotic sensitivity of Neisseria gonorrhoeae strains in the Essen area with special reference to penicillin sensitivity," by D. Hantschke. Z HAUT GESCHLECHTSKR. 45:49-62, January 1, 1970.

"Antibiotic susceptibilities of niesseria gonorrheae isolates," by A. Ronald, et al. NORTHWEST MED. 66:352-356, April, 1967.

"Antibiotics other than penicillin in the treatment of syphilis," by F. P. Merklen, et al. SEM THER 42:93-95, February, 1966.

"Antibodies in human sera against antigens in gonococci, demonstrated by a passive haemolysis test," by J. A. Maeland. ACTA PATH MICROBIOL SCAND. 67:102-110, 1966.

"Antibodies of the IgG, IgM, and IgA classes in newborn and adult sera reactive with gram-negative bacteria," by I. R. Cohen, et al. J CLIN INVEST. 47:1053-1062, May, 1968.

"The antibody pattern in representative groups of Ethiopian village children," by T. Mellbin, et al. ACTA PAEDIAT SCAND. 57:385-394, September, 1968.

"Anticomplement fluorescent antibody technic in experimental studies and serodiagnosis of syphilis," by N. M. Ovchinnikov, et al. VESTN DERM VENER. 42:33-38, December, 1968.

"Anticomplementary activity in serological tests for syphilis as a clue to connective tissue diseases of an auto-immune nature," by A. Lassus, et al. ANN CLIN RES. 1:74-76, May, 1969.

"Anticomplementary reactions and their relation to some auto-immune phenomena in syphilitic infection," by

A. Lassus, et al. ACTA DERMATOVENER. 49:519-523, 1969.

"Antigenic characteristics of nucleic acids of cultivable treponemes," by K. Király, et al. Z IMMUNITAETSFORSCH. 131:434-443, December, 1966.

"Antigenic community between the galactodiglyceride of Treponema Reiteri and cerebrosides," by P. Dupouey, et al. C R ACAD SCI. 270:1541-1544, March 16, 1970.

"Antigenic determinants of aqueous ether extracted endotoxin from Neisseria gonorrhoeae," by J. A. Maeland. ACTA PATH MICROBIOL SCAND. 76:475-483, 1969.

"Antigenic properties of various preparations of Neisseria gonorrhoeae endotoxin," by J. A. Maeland. ACTA PATH MICROBIOL SCAND. 73:413-422, 1968.

"Antigenic relationships of 14 treponemes demonstrated by immunofluorescence," by P. E. Meyer, et al. J BACT. 93:784-789, March, 1967.

"Antigenic structure of Treponema pallidum, Nichols strain. II. Extraction of a polysaccharide antigen with "strain-specific" serological activity," by J. N. Miller, et al. J BACT. 99:132-135, July, 1969.

"Antigens of Neisseria gonorrhoeae: Characterization by gel filtration, complement fixation, and agar-gel diffusion of antigens of gonococcal protoplasm," by D. G. Danielsson, et al. J BACT. 97:1012-1017, March, 1969.

"Antimicrobial polypeptide synthesized by mucor pusillus NRRL 2543," by G. A. Somkuti, et al. PROC SOC EXP BIOL MED. 133:780-785, March, 1970.

"Antimicrobial therapy in patients allergic to penicillin," by P. A. Bunn. NEW YORK J MED. 69:1859-1865, July 1, 1969.

"Antinuclear factors in sera from chronic false positive seroreactors for syphilis," by K. K. Mustakallio, et al. ACTA PATH MICROBIOL SCAND. 69:614-615, 1967.

"Antinuclear factors, rheumatoid factors and Bordet-Wassermann reaction in chronic and systemic lupus erythematosus," by J. Strejcek, et al. ACTA DERMATOVENER. 48:198-202, 1968.

"Antiprotozoan activity of nitroimidazoles," by I. De Carneri. ARZNEIMITTELFORSCHUNG. 19:382-386, March, 1969.

"Antitreponemic immunoglobulins and immunoantibodies. Chromatographic and immunoelectrophoretic preliminary research," by A. Buzzoni. G ITAL DERM. 108:401-410, September-October, 1967.

"Anti-vaccination and syphilis," by D. Green. MED J AUST. 1:500-501, March 7, 1970.

"Antivenereal fight in the Western Bohemian Region," by V. Resl. CESK DERM. 43:43-45, February, 1968.

"Aortic aneurysm and block of the right branch in a 22-year-old man. Syphilis?," by G. Heuillet, et al. MARSEILLE MED. 106:437-444, 1969.

"Aortic arch replacement in leutic aneurysm," by G. Heberer, et al. CHIRURG. 40:174-179, April, 1969.

"Aortic root aneurysm, Diagnosis and treatment," by H. Najafi. JAMA. 197:133-134, July 11, 1966.

"Aortic valve insufficiency in geriatrics. 3. Clinical observations on 206 cases over 60 years of age," by H. Ueda, et al. SAISHIN IGAKU. 22:2738-2744, December 10, 1967.

"Aortitis," by I. Ito. NAIKA. 19:1116-1118, June 1967.

"Applied immunofluorescence in dermato-venereology," by J. Thivolet, et al. G MAL INFETT. 20:109-118, January, 1968.

"Apropos of a case of balanitis," by A. Siboulet. BULL SOC FRANC DERM SYPH. 74:339-342, 1967.

"Apropos of a case of osseous syphilis," by M. Ruelle. J BEIG RHUM MED PHYS. 21:11-14, January-February, 1966.

"Apropos of a case of specific arteritis," by A. Luise. CARDIOL PRAT. 17:215-220, April, 1966.

"Apropos of a case of syphilitic reinfection," by P. Caubet. BULL SOC FRANC DERM SYPH. 73:110-111, January-February, 1966.

"Apropos of a case of tabetic arthropathy of both shoulders," by S. D. E. Seze, et al. REV RHUM. 35:551-554, October, 1968.

"Apropos of false specific serology in a woman presenting habitual abortions," by G. Zographos, et al. BULL FED GYNEC OBSTET FRANC. 18:299-301, June-August, 1966.

"Apropos of the pathogenesis of trichomonas vaginitis," by D. Cazzola, et al. ANN OSTET GINEC. 88:683-691, September, 1966.

"Apropos of serological reactivations caused by injection of 'luetin'. Further series of cases," by G. Tramier, et al. BULL SOC FRANC DERM SYPH. 74:596-598, 1967.

"Apropos of the treatment of late syphilis," by A. Meyer. PRESSE MED. 74:1306, May 21, 1966.

"Apropos of an unusual case of penicillin allergy," by M. Zivkovic. SRPSKI ARH CELOK. 95:297-300, May, 1967.

"Apropos of uveitis in childhood, by S. Braun-Vallon, et al. ANN OCULIST. 200:764-777, July, 1967.

"Are there any scientific and practical reasons for objections against the current instructions and schedules for the treatment of gonorrhea?," by I. M. Porudominskii. VEST DERM VENER. 39:48-53, October, 1965.

"Are venereal diseases increasing? A change of legislation on the control of venereal diseases," by W. Becker. MED KLIN. 64:609-611, March 28, 1969.

"Argyll Robertson pupil," by D. Leak. NM 123: iv+, February 17, 1967.

"The Argyll Robertson pupil, 1869-1969. A critical survey of the literature," by I. E. Loewenfeld. SURVEY OPHAL. 14:199-200, November, 1969.

"Arteriographic findings in an atrophic tabetic arthropathy," by H. J. Maurer, et al. Z ORTHOP. 107:139-144, November, 1969.

"Arthritis and gonococcal infection". NEW ENG J MED. 279:268, August 1, 1968.

"Arthritis associated with gonorrhoea," by J. O. Partain, et al. ANN RHEUM DIS. 27:156-162, March, 1968.

"Arthritis gonorrhoea. Report of a case in pregnancy with negative GR in serum and positive GR in the synovial fluid," by A. Nielsen. UGESKR LAEG. 130:1867-1868, October 31, 1968.

"Arthrodesis in tabetic arthropathy," by G. Friedebold. ARCH ORTHOP UNFALLCHIR. 59:272-285, 1966.

"Artificial immunization of rabbits against syphilis. I. Effect of increasing doses of treponemes given by the intramuscular route," by M. Metzger, et al. BRIT J VENER DIS. 45:308-312, December, 1969.

"Aspects of endemic syphilis among the Tuaregs of Niger," by A. Basset, et al. BULL SOC PATH EXOT. 62:80-92, January-February, 1969.

"Assessment of the 'Luotest' in late syphilis," by S. M. Laird, et al. BRIT J VENER DIS. 42:119-121, June, 1966.

"An assessment of the Reiter protein complement fixation (RPCF) test," by E. Fowler, et al. CANAD J PUBLIC HEALTH. 59:6-9, January, 1968.

"Assessment of various technics of the immunofluorescence test in the serological diagnosis of syphilis," by N. M. Ovchinnikov, et al. VESTN DERM VENER. 42:40-45, February, 1968.

"Association of carcinoma of the uterine cervix and trichomonas vaginalis infestations. Frequency of trichomonas vaginalis in preinvasive and invasive cervical carcinoma," by O. Berggren. AMER J OBSTET GYNEC. 105:166-168, September, 1969.

"The association of genital herpesvirus with cervical atypia and carcinoma in situ," by I. Royston, et al. AMER J EPIDEM. 91:531-538, June, 1970.

"The association of herpesvirus type 2 and carcinoma of the uterine cervix," by W. F. Rawls, et al. AMER J EPIDEM. 89:547-554, May, 1969.

"The association of syphilis with hepatic cirrhosis: a report of six cases and a review of the literature," by G. Karmi, et al. POSTGRAD MED J. 45:675-679, October, 1969.

"Asymptomatic gonorrhea," by R. W. Thatcher, et al. JAMA. 210:315-317, October, 1969.

"Asymptomatic gonorrhea, the gonococcal carrier state, and gonococcemia in men," by A. B. Ackerman, et al. JAMA. 196:101-103, April 4, 1966.

"Atrophic luetic glossitis. Report of a case," by A. M. Captine, et al. ORAL SURG. 30:192-195, August, 1970.

"Attempt at classification of skin and venereal diseases," by J. Danda. CESK DERM. 42:167-172, June, 1967.

"Attempt at the evaluation of the influence of environment on the incidence of syphilis in soldiers of obligatory service," by J. Lańcucki, et al. PRZEGL DERM. Suppl: 93-99, 1969.

"Attempt at simplification of the TPI test," by S. Stoyanoff, et al. MAROC MED. 45:216-220, March, 1966.

"Attempt to induce in vitro penicillin resistance in Neisseria gonorrhoeae," by F. Vymola, et al. J HYG EPIDEM. 12:426-430, 1968.

"An attempt to revise the opinion on the sensitivity of Nelson's test and the possibility of its spontaneous rejection," by J. Lesinski. CESK DERM. 41:289-295, October, 1966.

"Attempted simplification of Nelson's test," by S. Stoyanoff, et al. MAROC MED. 45:216-220, March, 1966.

"Attempts at the increase of sensitivity of the treponema pallidum immobilization test," by K. Kiraly. DERM WSCHR. 151:2035-2041, September 25, 1965.

"Attempts for speeding up the development of experimentally maintained specific orchitis in rabbits, contaminated with 'Nichols' strain," by D. Naumova. NAUCH TR VISSH MED INST SOFIIA. 48:45-53, 1969.

"Attempts to standardize the trichomonas laboratory diagnosis," by W. A. Muller. DEUTSCH GESUNDH. 23:2041-2043, October 24, 1968.

"Attitudes of college students in East Africa to sexual activity and venereal disease," by O. P. Arya, et al. BRIT J VENER DIS. 44:160-166, June, 1968.

"Attitudes of prospective school teachers on teaching venereal disease information," by W. B. Neser. PUBLIC HEALTH REP. 82:917-920, October, 1967.

"Attitudes toward venereal disease," by W. L. Porter. DELAWARE MED J. 40:373-375, December, 1968.

"Atypical FTA-ABS test fluorescence in lupus erythematosus patients," by S. J. Kraus, et al. JAMA 211:2140-2141, March 30, 1970.

"Atypical serology in neurosyphilis," by K. Dewhurst. J NEUROL NEUROSURG PSYCHIAT. 31:496-500, October, 1968.

"Atypical sub-periosteal abscess simulating a syphilitic gumma," by J. M. Meshaka, et al. REV DENT LIBAN. 17:26-30, April-September, 1967.

"August Von Wassermann (1866-1925). Wassermann reaction," JAMA. 204:1000-1001, June 10. 1968.

"Aural condylomata in secondary syphilis," by J. F. Jarvis, et al. J LARYNG. 82:157-159, February, 1968.

"The Austin Flint murmur in cardiac diagnosis," by D. N. Wysham, et al. INDIAN HEART J. 19:238-246, July, 1967.

"Autoimmune phenomena in patients with old treated syphilis nonreactive to the treponema pallidum immobilization test," by A. Lassus, et al. ACTA PATH MICROBIOL SCAND. 69:613-614, 1967.

"Autoimmune phenomena in syphilitic infection: rheumatoid factor and cryoglobulins in different stages of syphilis," by K. K. Mustakallio, et al. INT ARCH ALLERG, BASEL. 31:417-426, 1967.

"Autoimmune serologic reactions with lipid antigen," by R. L. Kahn. AMER J MED TECHN. 32:57-68, January-February, 1966.

"Auto-immune serum factors and IgA elevation in lymphogranuloma venereum," by A. Lassus, et al. ANN CLIN RES. 2:51-56, March, 1970.

"Automated fluorescent treponemal antibody test: instrument and evaluation," by J. S. Lewis, et al. APPL MICROBIOL. 19:898-901, June, 1970.

"Automated instrument for the fluorescent treponemal antibody-absorption test and other immunofluorescence tests," by G. F. Binnings, et al. APPL MICROBIOL. 18:861-868, November, 1969.

"Automated, quantitative microhemagglutination assay for treponema pallidum antibodies," by P. M. Cox, et al. APPL MICROBIOL. 18:485-489, September, 1970.

"The automated reagin test: results compared with VDRL and FTA-ABS tests," by R. W. Stevens, et al. AMER J CLIN PATH. 53:32-34, January, 1970.

"Automatic apparatus for Wassermann and Reiter complement-fixation tests utilizing the 'discrete-analysis' principle," by R. E. Trotman. AMER J CLIN PATH. 22:501-503, July, 1969.

"Automation of a flocculation test for syphilis," by B. E. McGrew, et al. AMER J CLIN PATH. 50:52-59, July, 1968.

"Autopsy case of congenital syphilis with jaundice," by Y. Ishiwata, et al. J CLIN MED. 24:784-790, April, 1966.

"Bacterial endocarditis due to Neisseria perflava in a patient hypersensitive to penicillin," by A. B. Breslin, et al. AUST ANN MED. 16:245-249, August, 1967.

"Bacteriologic studies on the etiology of colpitis," by M. Pinter. GEBURTSH FRAUENHEILK. 26:27-31, January, 1966.

"Bacteriological diagnosis and treatment of gonococcal urethritis in the male," by Oliva J. Bravo, et al. MED TROP. 43:143-151, March-April, 1967.

"Balanoposthitis of bifid urethra," by L. Linguiti. NUNT RADIOL. 34:1839-1845, December, 1968.

"Balneotherapy in trichomonas vaginitis," by R. Dionigi. QUAD CLIN OSTET GINEC. 21:1258-1268, December, 1966.

"The bases of a suitable marital and premarital education in Turin. Activities of the AIEMP," by I. Terzi, et al. G BATT VIROL IMMUN. 62:703-709, September-October, 1969.

"Basophil degranulation test in penicillin sensitivity," by Z. Rumbolt, et al. LIJECNV JESN. 88:619-625, June, 1966.

"Be alert to the dental patient with venereal disease," by D. R. Wallace. DENT ASSIST. 35:23, November, 1966.

"A Bedsonia isolated from a patient with clinical-lymphogranuloma venereum," by J. Schachter. AMER J OPHTHAL. 63:1049-1053, May, 1967.

"Bedsoniae inclusions in two newborn infants in Lebanon," by N. A. Haddad. AMER J OPHTHAL. 64:124-128, July, 1967.

"Beginning of dermatological and venerological instruction at the University of Halle," by W. Kaiser, et al. MED MSCHR. 23:352-358, August, 1969.

"Behavior of cardiolipin and protidic antigens toward carate serums," by J. Breuillaud, et al. BULL SOC PATH EXOT. 61:190-194, 1968.

"Behavior of serum mucoproteins in the course of some skin diseases and in early syphilis," by Z. Cygan, et al. PRZEGL DERM. 56:1-5, January-February, 1969.

"Behavior of treponema pallidum under the effect of various antibiotics in the secretion from lesions in early syphilis in man," by K. Lejman, et al. PRZEGL DERM. Suppl:13-27, 1969.

"Behavior of trichomonas vaginalis in women treated with radiation energy and cytostatic drugs," by J. Zawadzki, et al. WIAD PARAZYT. 13:729-732, 1967.

"Behavior of the VDS test and intradermoreaction with old tuberculin in subjects affected by non-tuberculous pulmonary diseases," by Z. Garnuszewski, et al. CLIN PEDIAT. 48:55-58, February, 1966.

"The behavioural diseases. 2. The venereal diseases," by R. D. Catterall. NURS TIMES. 64:1041-1043, August 2, 1968.

"Bejel in Sheffield," by P. M. Wray. BRIT J VENER DIS. 42:25-27, March, 1966.

"Benign gonococcaemia," by J. Verbov, et al. BRIT MED J. 3:407, August 15, 1970.

"Benign gonococcal sepsis. A report of 36 cases," by A. Bjornberg. ACTA DERMATOVENER. 50:313-316, 1970.

"Benign gonococcal sepsis with skin lesions," by A. Bjornberg, et al. BRIT J VENER DIS. 42:100-102, June, 1966.

"Bicillin in the treatment of acute gonorrhea," by V. F. Maksimov. VESTN DERM VENER. 41:86-87, April, 1967.

"Bicillin-6 in therapy of gonorrhea in women," by F. V. Potapnev, et al. VESTN DERM VENER. 43:52-55, January, 1969.

"Bicillin-6 in the treatment of gonorrhea in men," by M. U. Mirsagatov, et al. VESTN DERM VENER. 41:70-72, October, 1967.

"Bicillin-6 therapy in combination with pyrogenale and prodigiosane of patients with contagious forms of syphilis," by O. K. Loseva, et al. VESTN DERM VENER. 42:71-75, 1968.

"Bilateral recurrent laryngeal nerve paralysis in early childhood following congenital syphilis," by B. Fioresi. MSCHR OHRENHEILK. 101:375-377, 1967.

"The biological false positive reaction to serological tests for syphilis," by M. F. Garner. J CLIN PATH. 23:31-34, February, 1970.

"Biologic false-positive reactions and infectious mononucleosis," by H. A. Cabrera, et al. TECHN BULL REGIST MED TECHN. 38:261-263, October, 1968.

"Biologic false-positive reactions for syphilis," by W. L. Palmer. JAMA. 204:833, May 27, 1968.

"The biological false positive reaction to serological tests for syphilis," by M. F. Garner. J CLIN PATH. 23:31-34, February, 1970.

"Biological false positive Wassermann reactions in Uganda," by W. D. Foster, et al. BRIT J VENER DIS. 42:272-275, December, 1966.

"Biologically false-positive serologic tests for syphilis due to smallpox vaccination," by L. J. Grossman, et al. AMER J CLIN PATH. 51:375-378, March, 1969.

"A biomathematical model for prevalence of trichomonas vaginalis," by J. Ipsen, et al. AMER J EPIDEM. 91:175-184, February, 1970.

"Biologic false positive syphilis reactions," by L. Kornstad. T NORSK LAEGEFOREN. 86:1724-1728, December 15, 1966.

"Blitz on syphilis in Alabama," by W. H. Smith. J MED ASS. 36:505 passim, November, 1966; also in; PUBLIC HEALTH REP ALABAMA. 81:835-841, September, 1966.

"A blood bank microscope," by T. E. Allen. AMER J MED TECHN. 32:421, November-December, 1966.

"Blood properidin in recent syphilis," by D. Bubola, et al. G ITAL DERM. 107:223-30, May-June, 1966.

"Bone lesions observed in serological trepanematosis. Study of 267 patients," by R. P. Delahaye, et al. SEM HOP PARIS. 46:189-194, January 14, 1970.

"Bone marrow inhibition in latent syphilis," by J. Jedličková, et al. VNITRNI LEK. 16:798-801, August, 1970.

"Boswell's clap," by W. B. Ober. JAMA. 212:91-95, April 6, 1970.

"Boswell's gonorrhea," by W. B. Ober. BULL NY ACAD MED. 45:587-636, June, 1969.

"Brain tumor syndrome in syphilitic arteritis," by R. Suchenwirth. DEUTSCH Z NERVENHEILK. 190:338-348, 1967.

"Breakthrough in VD education in Los Angeles county," by E. Reinig, et al. PUBLIC HEALTH REP. 82:505-512, June, 1967.

"A brief review of syphilis serology," by W. J. Brown, et al. J AMER OSTEOPATH ASS. 66:1112-1118, June, 1967.

"The British venereal diseases service, 1916-1966." BRIT J VENER DIS. 42:223-224, December, 1966.

"Broad spectrum antibiotics. The editors view," by E. J. Best. DENT DIG. 74:268, June, 1968.

"Brucellosis, treponematosis, rickettsiosis, and psittacosis in Surinam. A serological survey," by P. Kody. TROP GEOGR MED. 22:172-178, June, 1970.

"C-reactive protein in skin and venereal diseases (a review of the literature)," by V. N. Mikhailov, et al. VESTN DERM VENER. 40:48-53, October, 1966.

"Campaign for eradication of yaws in Indonesia," by M. D. Tverskoi. MED PARAZIT. 36:103-106, January-February, 1967.

"Can syphilis be controlled through treatment and epidemiology," by J. F. Donohue. REV AGRUP ODONT ARGENT. 20:1201-1203, 1968.

"Can treatment and epidemiology control syphilis?," by J. F. Donohue. SALUD PUBLICA MEX. 10:607-610, September-October, 1968.

"Can we really stamp out VD?," by H. S. Gorlick. RN. 29:39-45, April, 1966.

"Cancriform pyoderma," by L. V. Vallejo, et al. PRENSA MED ARGENT. 55:624-627, May 31, 1968.

"Candida albicans and the contraceptive pill," by R. D. Catterall. LANCET. 2:830-831, October 15, 1966.

"Candidamycoses. Candidiasistinea (Candidamycetica) of the skin including genitalia," by H. Grimmer. Z HAUT GESCHLECHTSKR. 40:15-26, January 15, 1966.

"Candidiases of the skin and mucosae," by D. Grigoriou. REV MED SUISSE ROM. 86:619-631, September, 1966.

"Canine venereal lymphoma as a model of experimental cancer," by H. Márquez-Monter. GAC MED MEX. 100:168-183, February, 1970.

"Carbamazepine for tabetic pain," by D. Alarcon-Segovia, et al. JAMA. 203:57, January 1, 1968.

"Cardiac asystole following intravenous administration of aqueous potassium penicillin." ANESTH ANALG. 48:55-57, January-February, 1969.

"Cardio-aortic syphilis." PENN MED. 72-75, February, 1969.

"Cardiolipin antigen in syphilis serodiagnosis according to data of the central dermatologic-venereological institute (1954-1965)," by L. S. Reznikova, et al. VESTN DERM VENER. 41:62-66, November, 1967.

"Cardiovascular and neurological findings in Ethiopians with syphilitic heart disease," by D. Vukotich, et al. TROP GEOGR MED. 22:45-52, March, 1970.

"Cardiovascular syphilis in a 20-year old man," by C. Hiltenbrand, et al. ARCH MAL COEUR. 60:1041-1048, July, 1967.

"Case contribution to the problem of penicillin resistance in gonorrhea," by E. Friedrich, et al. Z HAUT GESCHLECHTSKR. 40:194-200, March 15, 1966.

"Case contribution to tabetic arthropathy of the spine and of both elbow joints," by K. Wallmann. BEITR ORTHOP TRAUMA. 14:441-448, August, 1967.

"Case-finding in venereal disease control with special reference to the District of Columbia Department of Public Health," by C. W. Freeman. MED ANN DC. 38:183-186 passim, April, 1969.

"Case-finding through ante-natal serological tests for syphilis," by J. A. Burgess. BRIT J VENER DIST. 42:116-118, June, 1966.

"A case of acquired syphilis revealed by unilateral keratitis," by P. Desbordes, et al. MED TROP, (Marseilles). 28:230-232, March-April, 1968.

"A case of anaphylactic shock after penicillin and novocain injection," by A. G. Ostrovskii. ANTIBIOTIKI. 12:338-339, April, 1967.

"A case of anaphylactic shock in a pregnant woman with nephropathia after the administration of penicillin," by T.A. Avksent'Eva. AKUSH GINEK. 42:43, December, 1966.

"A case of (and for) syphilis maligna and negative serology," by D. J. Cripps, et al. ARCH DERM. 100:122-124, July, 1969.

"A case of chronic gonococcal folliculitis," by M. Skencić, et al. SRPSKI ARH CELOK LEK. 94:403-407, April, 1966.

"A case of congenital paresis in 1966," by M. M. Carruthers, et al. ANN INTERN MED. 66:1204-1206, June, 1967.

"A case of delayed diagnosis of tabetic arthropathy," by P. F. Triapichnikov. VESTN DERM VENER. 42:86-88, 1968.

"A case of diffuse syphilitic osteoperiostitis," by R. Quilichini, et al. MARSEILLE MED. 107:499-503, June, 1970.

"A case of early malignant syphilis," by S. Boulle, et al. BULL SOC FRANC DERM SYPH. 74:32-34, 1967.

"A case of early malignant syphilis," by P. Laugier, et al. BULL SOC FRANC DERM SYPH. 77:15-16, July, 1970.

"Case of fatal anaphylactic shock caused by the administration of antibiotics," by E. M. Deliagina. KLIN MED. 48:129-131, March, 1970.

"A case of generalized thrombocytopenic diathesis after local application of crystalline penicillin solution," by T. Pytel-Dabrowska. PEDIAT POL. 43:73-74, January, 1968.

"Case of hepatic syphilis," by Y. Salembier. LILLE MED. 12:1215-1216, November, 1967.

"A case of intravital diagnosis of dissecting aneurysm of the abdominal aorta," by E. B. Shnaider. KLIN MED. 44:124-125, January, 1966.

"A case of malignant syphilis," by A. Zanca, et al. MINERVA DERM. 42:462-467, September, 1967.

"A case of Marcus Gunn phenomenon with oculomotor paralysis," by J. Kaouzny. KLIN OCZNA. 37:389-393, 1967.

"A case of polyarthropathy of cryptogenic tabetic type," by L. Canet, et al. REV RHUM. 36:613-615, November, 1969.

"A case of pyloric stenosis due to syphilis," by W. Straczkowski, et al. WIAD LEK. 20:893-894, May 1, 1967.

"A case of renal lesion in secondary recurrent syphilis," by B. Batko, et al. WIAD LEK. 23:1043-1045, June 15, 1970.

"A case of rupture of an aortic aneurysm into the trachea," by Z. S. Chichinadze. ZH USHN NOS GORL BOLEZ. 26:82-83, September-October, 1966.

"A case of syphilitic anterior uveitis with posterior chamber hemorrhage," by C. S. Kalidasan. J ALL INDIA OPHTHAL SOC. 17:123-124, June, 1969.

"A case of tabetic mandibular fracture," by J. F. Laroche, et al. REV STOMAT. 71:74-76, January-February, 1970.

"A case of thrombosis of the left median cerebral artery with active syphilis of the vessels," by Z. Konopka, et al. PRZEGL DERM. 54:343-346, May-June, 1967.

"A case of trichomonas vulvovaginitis in the newborn," by B. I. Bondarenko. PEDIAT AKUSH GINEK. 5:62-63, September-October, 1966.

"A case of triple fusiform aneurysym of the aortic arch successfully operated with resection and grafting," by D. Guilmet, et al. MINERVA CARDIOANGIOL. 15:175-181, February, 1967.

"A case of undetected syphilis of the stomach," by L. A. Shifrin. KLIN KHIR. 8:61-63, August, 1966.

"Case records of the Massachusetts General Hospital. Weekly clinicopathological exercises. Case 52-1969," NEW ENG J MED. 281:1414-1419, December 18, 1969.

"A case report of gangrenous balanitis in progressive reaction in leprosy," by D. S. Chaudhury, et al. LEPROSY REV. 37:225-226, October, 1966.

"Case reports from the Institute of Venereology (India). Uncommon features of donovanosis," by P. N. Rangiah, et al. MEDISCOPE. 8:658-662, February, 1966.

"Juvenile GPI: A case study," by G. C. Kanjilal. NURS TIMES. 65:1066-1067, August 21, 1969.

"Casuistic contribution on the practical significance of so-called pseudogonorrhea," by H. J. Conraths. ARCH KLIN EXP DERM. 227:645-650, 1966.

"Catamnestic remarks on the therapy of gonorrhea in 572 cases," by D. Kiesewalter. DEUTSCH GESUNDH. 23:1408-1412, July 25, 1968.

"Catamnestic studies of syphilis patients treated with arsenobenzene-penicillin-bismuth," by J. Rossberg. DERM WSCHR. 153:161-164, February 18, 1967.

"Causes of treatment failure in the penicillin therapy of gonorrhea," by J. Meyer-Rohn. ANTIMICROB AGENTS CHEMOTHER. 5:721-723, 1965.

"Cefazolin, a new semisynthetic cephalosporin antibiotic.

II. In vitro and in vivo antimicrobial activity," by M. Nishida, et al. J ANTIBIOT. 23:137-148, March, 1970.

"Cellini and his syphilis. Malevolent mercurial cure?," by G. W. Geelhoed. JAMA. 204:Suppl:245-246, May 13, 1968.

"Centers of rickettsiosis and treponematosis in the east of the Central African Republic (Bangassou, 1966)," by A. Retel-Laurentin. BULL SOC PATH EXOT. 61:321-339, 1968.

"Central nervous system toxicity secondary to massive doses of penicillin 'G' in the treatment of overwhelming infections," by D. F. Cohill, et al. AMER J MED SCI. 254:692-694, November, 1967.

"Cephalexin and cephaloglycin activity in vitro and absorption and urinary excretion of single oral doses in normal young adults," by P. Braun, et al. APPL MICROBIOL. 16:1684-1694, November, 1968.

"Cephalexin - a new oral antibiotic," by A. Bailey, et al. POSTGRAD MED J. 46:157-158, March, 1970.

"Cephalexin, a new oral antibiotic," by A. Bailey, et al. POUMON COEUR. 26:299-303, 1970.

"Cephaloridine in early syphilis," by L. Z. Oller. POSTGRAD MED J. 43:Suppl 43:128-129, August, 1967.

"Cephaloridine in gonorrhoea in females," by A. Jouhar, et al. BRIT J VENER DIS. 44:223-225, September, 1968.

"Cephaloridine in the treatment of non-gonococcal urethritis," by G. W. Csonka, et al. POSTGRAD MED J. 43:Suppl 43:123-124, August, 1967.

"Cephaloridine treatment of experimental rabbit syphilis," by S. Kuwahara, et al. POSTGRAD MED J.(Minneapolis). 43:Suppl:43:130-133, August, 1967.

"Cephaloridine treatment of gonorrhoea in the female," by D. G. McLone, et al. BRIT J VENER DIS. 44:220-222, September, 1968.

"Cephalothin in gonococcal urethritis," by E. B. Smith. CURR THER RES. 9:79-81, February, 1967.

"Cerobrospinal fluid electrolyte disturbances in neurological disorders: with special reference to inorganic phosphate," by U. Breyer, et al. NEUROLOGY. 20:247-253, March, 1970.

"Cerebrospinal fluid findings after treatment of early syphilis with penicillin. A further series of 80 cases," by W. L. Fernando. BRIT J VENER DIS. 42: 134-135, June, 1968.

"Cerobrospinal fluid findings in ophthalmology. In eye diseases (Japanese)," by S. Shimizu. ACTA SOC OPHTHAL JAP. 71:1825-1845, October, 1967.

"Certain peculiarities of the clinical aspects and course of the initial period of syphilis at the present time," by V. A. Rakhmanov, et al. VESTN DERM VENER. 41:36-40, March, 1967.

"Certain problems of deontology," by A. A. Studnitsin. VESTN DERM VENER. 43:7-12, November, 1969.

"Certain problems of dispensarization and treatment of trichomoniasis in males," by M. G. Manikhas, et al. VESTN DERM VENER. 43:60-62, November, 1969.

"Certain problems of preventive therapy of syphilis," by L. A. Shteinlukht, et al. VESTN DERM VENER. 41:62-65, September, 1967.

"Cervical and peritoneal bacterial flora associated with salpingitis," by J. Lip, et al. OBSTET GYNEC. 28: 561-563, October, 1966.

"Cervical cytology of patients attending a venereal disease clinic," by A. J. Lucas, et al. J OBSTET GYNAEC BRIT COMM. 74:104-110, February, 1967.

"Chacko-Nair egg-enriched selective medium in the diagnosis of pathogenic Neisseriae," by C. W. Chacko, et al. BRIT J VENER DIS. 44:67-71, March, 1968.

"The chain of venereal disease control," by C. W. Freeman. MED ANN DC. 35:355-356, 374, July, 1966.

"Chancriform gumma developing in 20 years at the site of former primary syphiloma," by B. S. Pankov. VESTN DERM VENER. 40:89-91, October, 1966.

"The change of the ground substance of the aorta in syphilitic aortitis," by L. Józsa, et al. VIRCHOW ARCH 345:324-330, 1968.

"The changes in age structure of patients with gonorrhea during the past years," by V. Sedláček. CESK DERM. 42:108-114, April, 1967.

"Changes in the ECG during penicillin shock," by A. M. Korepanov. TER ARKH. 39:118-121, June, 1967.

"Changes in the nuclear ultrastructure observed in trichomonas vaginalis after treatment with metronidazole," by D. Panaitescu, et al. MICROBIOLOGIA. 15:43-48, January-February, 1970.

"The changes in the pH levels of the vagina in infections with trichomonas vaginalis and candida," by H. Spitzbart. ZBL GYNAEK. 88:1680-1683, December 3, 1966.

"Changes in vaginal microbial flora during treatment with progestational hormones," by B. Ferrari, et al. QUAD CLIN OSTET GINEC. 21:1001-1008, December, 1966.

"Changes occurring in the composition of the vaginal bacterial flora accompanying trichomonas vaginalis in women treated with gamma and x-rays," by E. Slowakiewicz, et al. WIAD PARAZYT. 15:449-451, 1969.

"Changing clinical picture of neurosyphilis (letter to ed.)," by B. Levy. BRIT MED J. 2:491-492, May 25, 1968.

"Changing clinical picture of neurosyphilis: report of seven unusual cases," by R. Joffe, et al. BRIT MED J. 1:211-212, January 27, 1968.

"Changing pattern of morbidity at Groote Schuur Hospital, 1939-1965," by J. F. Brock. S AFR MED J. 41:739-747, August 12, 1967.

"Changing patterns of late syphilis," by J. Towpik, et al. BRIT J VENER DIS. 46:132-134, April, 1970.

"Characteristics of allergic reactions in Bicillin therapy for the prevention of rheumatic exacerbations," by O. A. Kuvaldina. VOP REVM. 8:83-85, April-June, 1968.

"Characteristics of the colpocytological changes in women infested with trichomonas vaginalis donne," by J. Teras, et al. WIAD PARAZYT. 15:327-329, 1969.

"Charcot joint of the lumbar spine," by D. P. McNeel, et al. J NEUROSURG. 30:55-61, January, 1969.

"Charcot joints," by G. O. Storey. RHEUMATOL PHYS MED. 10:312-320, August, 1970.

"Chemistry and biology of phospholipids from an unclassified mycobacteria," by M. Motomiya, et al. CHEM PHYS LIPIDS. 3:159-167, April, 1969.

"Chemotherapy of chlamydial infections," by E. Jawetz. ADVANCES PHARMACOL. 7:253-282, 1969.

"Chemotherapy of trichomoniasis," by R. M. Michaels. ADVANCES CHEMOTHER. 3:39-108, 1968.

"Chiasmal arachnoiditis as a manifestation of generalized arachnoiditis in systemic vascular disease. Clinicopathological report of two cases," by M. Oliver, et al. BRIT J OPHTHAL. 52:227-235, March, 1968.

"Chinaroot in the 'Epistola de radicis Chinae usu' of Andreas Vesalius (1546)," by R. Schmitz, et al. SUDHOFF ARCH. 51:217-228, September, 1967.

"Cholesterol embolism in the course of antiluetic therapy," by P. H. Berghuis, et al. NEDERL T GENEESK. 113:2046-2049, November 15, 1969.

"Cholesterol embolism in the course of antiluetic therapy," by D. J. Vermeer. NEDERL T GENEESK. 114:172, January 24, 1970.

"Christopher Columbus and the history of syphilis," by E. H. Hudson. ACTA TROP. 25:1-16, 1968.

"Chronic biologic false positive seroreactions for syphilis as a harbinger of systemic lupus erythematosus," by T. Putkonen, et al. ACTA DERMATOVENER. 47:83-88, 1967.

"Chronic syphilitic multiple subdural meningitis," by G. Lemercier, et al. BULL SOC MED AFR NOIRE LANG FRANC. 11:62-65, 1966.

"Circumscribed non-gummous mandibular osteitis as primary organic manifestation of tertiary syphilis," by M. Strassburg. DEUTSCH ZAHNAERZTL Z. 22:1052-1056, August, 1967.

"Classroom sex education," by A. E. Gravatt. J AMER COLL HEALTH ASS. 15:61-65, May, 1967.

"Clinic for dermatologic and venereal diseases." GOD

ZBORN MED FAK SKOPJE. 14:51-53, 1968.

"Clinical and epidemiologic impact of penicillins old and new," by G. T. Stewart. PEDIAT CLIN N AMER. 15:13-29, February, 1968.

"Clinical and experimental studies on the thrombosis formation influenced by penicillin," by B. Nagay. ROCZN POM AKAD MED SWIERCZEWSKI. 13:289-306, 1967.

"Clinical and laboratory diagnosis of venereal diseases," by M. B. Moore, Jr. BOL OFIC SANIT PANAMER. 60:316-327, April, 1966.

"Clinical and laboratory studies on vaginal trichomoniasis," by C. N. Nagesha, et al. AMER J OBSTET GYNEC. 106:933-935, March 15, 1970.

"A clinical and laboratory study of trichomoniasis of the female genital tract," by H. E. Hughes, et al. J OBSTET GYNAEC BRIT COMM. 73:821-827, October, 1966.

"Clinical and laboratory study of vaginitis. Evaluation of diagnostic methods and results of treatment, by S. G. Burgess, et al. NEW YORK J MED. 70:2086-2091, August 15, 1970.

"Clinical and serological profiles in leprosy," by L. J. Matthews, et al. LANCET. 2:915-917, November 6, 1965.

"Clinical and virologic study of patients seen in the Yale-New Haven hospital women's clinic (1963-1964)," by M. E. Wade, et al. AMER J OBSTET GYNEC. 99:595-597, October 15, 1967.

"Clinical application of methyldichlorophenylisoxazolyl penicillin (dicloxacillin, staphcillin A) for urinary tract infections, especially for non-gonorrheal urethritis," by J. Ishigami, et al. J ANTIBIOT. 19:354-357, October, 1966.

"Clinical aspects of ascending gonorrhea in women during the past 18 years (1947-1964)," by A. V. Chastikova. VESTN DERM VENER. 41:54-57, June, 1967.

"Clinical aspects of the dissecting aortic aneurysum," by M. I. Gorbunova. KLIN MED. 48:133-135, January, 1970.

"Clinical bacterial study of drug resistance of gonococci.

Preliminary note," by M. Fazio, et al. G ITAL DERM. 45:163-164, March, 1970.

"Clinical course and treatment of female gonorrhea," by J. Obrtel. CESK GYNEK. 33:463-467, July, 1968.

"Clinical course of gonorrhea combined with trichomoniasis in males," by Ia. I. Khasin, et al. VESTN DERM VENER. 41:69-70, December, 1967.

"Clinical criterion of cure in syphilis. Statistical method," by C. Rabito. MINERVA DERM. 42:238-243, July, 1967.

"The clinical diagnosis of penicillin allergy," by J. Pedersen-Bjergaard. ACTA ALLERGOL. 25:89-130, June, 1970.

"Clinical evaluation of metronidazole 'Polfa' in the treatment of trichomoniasis in women," by C. Zwierz, et al. WIAD PARAZYT. 15:387-388, 1969.

"Clinical evaluation of treatment of gonorrhea in the female," by L. H. Shapiro, et al. AMER J OBSTET GYNEC. 97:968-973, April 1, 1967.

"Clinical experience with ampicillin and probenecid in the management of treponeme-associated uveitis," by J. N. Goldman. TRANS AMER ACAD OPHTHAL OTOLARYNG. 74:509-514, May-June, 1970.

"Clinical experience with a new antibiotic in blenorrhagic infections," by N. M. Prandini. HOSPITAL. 74:1327-1331, October, 1968.

"Clinical experience with nifuratel," by J. Wainstock, et al. REV BRAS MED. 26:675-681, November, 1969.

"Clinical experience with sigmamycin in skin and venereal diseases," by E. Heinke. MED WELT. 5:265-269, February 4, 1967.

"Clinical experience with spiramycin in the 'minute therapy' of gonorrhea," by E. Heinke, et al. DEUTSCH MED WSCHR. 94:1182-1185, May 30, 1969.

"Clinical experimentation with a new urinary antibiotic: thiamphenicol," by L. Timmermans, et al. ACTA UROL BELG. 34:349-353, July, 1966.

"Clinical experimentation with rifomycin in dermatologic

and venereal diseases," by L. Rasponi. G CLIN MED. 50:896-903, October, 1969.

"Clinical experiments with diribiotine tablets," by J. Govers. THER UNSCH. 23:149-150, April, 1966.

"Clinical findings using demethylchlortetracycline in acute gonococcal urethritis," by J. Berger. REV BRASIL MED. 26:249-250, April, 1969.

"Clinical forms of gonococcal arthritis," by H. Keiser, et al. NEW ENG J MED. 279:234-240, August 1, 1968.

"Clinical investigation of inflammatory polyradiculoneuritis in France," by P. Castaigne, et al. REV NEUROL. 115:849-872, October, 1966.

"Clinical investigations on a new treatment of vaginal trichomoniasis," by F. Destro, et al. HOSPITAL. 75:1065-1072, March, 1969.

"Clinical manifestations and criteria for diagnosis of yaws. (Based on a study in Dudhi Tehsil of District Mirzapur, U.P., India in 1954-1956)," by B. L. Taneja. INDIAN J MED RES. 56:100-113, January, 1968.

"Clinical manifestations and diagnosis of penicillin allergy and other penicillin side effects," by N. Sonnichsen, et al. DERM MSCHR. 155:739-750, 1969.

"Clinical manifestations and treatment of frambesie," by S. N. Strakhov. KLIN MED. 44:120-127, November, 1966.

"Clinical manifestations of visceral lues," by P. Kop. SRPSKI ARH CELOK LEK. 94:143-149, February, 1966.

"Clinical neuropathological conference," by S. M. Aronson, et al. DIS NERV SYST. 28:688-694, October, 1967.

"Clinical observation of early congenital syphilis," by F. C. Yu, et al. ACTA PAEDIAT SINICA. 8:93-101, April-June, 1967.

"Clinical observations on the problem of penicillin allergy," by P. Sunder-Plassmann. MED KLIN. 61:892, June 3, 1966.

"Clinical observations on symptomatic neurosyphilis," by D. Loesch. NEUROL NEUROCHIR PSYCHIAT POL. 16:1047-

1056, September, 1966.

"Clinical peculiarities of skin and venereal diseases detected among persons arriving from tropical countries," by R. S. Babaiants. VESTN DERM VENER. 43:18-23, July, 1969.

"The clinical picture of adnexitis as a complication of female gonorrhea," by J. Divis, et al. CESK GYNEK. 35:1-4, February, 1970.

"The clinical picture of gonorrhea with special reference to infections of eye in newborn infants," by V. Resl. CESK OFTAL. 22:333-334, September, 1966.

"Clinical picture of sepsis in a two-month-old infant. What could be the cause of edema, ascites, icteris and anemia?." CLIN PEDIAT. 9:214-225, April, 1970.

"Clinical picture of syphilitic lesions in 22 men infected by the same female partner," by M. Borkowski. PREGL DERM. Suppl:111-4, 1969.

"Clinical picture of trichomonas hominis colitis and its differential diagnosis," by L. Cziraki, et al. ORV HETIL. 108:1850-1852, September 24, 1967.

"Clinical relapse in early syphilis: unusual skin lesion following inadequate treatment," by R. H. Kampmeier, et al. J TENN MED ASS. 59:146-150, February, 1966.

"Clinical, serological and epidemiological features of Framboesia tropica (yaws) and its control in rural communities," by T. Guthe. ACTA DERMATOVENER. 49: 343-368, 1969.

"Clinical significance of chronic biologic false positive Wassermann reaction and 'antinuclear factors'," by S. Berglund, et al. ACTA MED SCAND. 180:407-412, October, 1966.

"Clinical significance of lincomycin-resistant Neisseria gonorrhoeae," by E. Kutscher, et al. ANTIMICROB AGENTS CHEMOTHER. 8:331-334, 1968.

"Clinical significance of nonspecific syphilis serological reaction," by K. Király, et al. ORV HETIL. 107: 1441-1448, July 31, 1966.

"Clinical significance of the rheumatoid factor in old age," by Z. Hrncir, et al. CAS LEK CESK. 106:257-

263, March 10, 1967.

"Clinical statistics in the department of urology of Kanazawa University during the last 10 years (1955-1964)," by K. Kuroda, et al. JAP J UROL. 57:773-794, July, 1966.

"Clinical studies of alimentary system disorders in trichomonas infections in women," by C. Todea. PRZEGL LEK. 23:565-568, July, 1967.

"Clinical studies on chewable triacetyloleandomycin," by O. Kitamoto, et al. J ANTIBIOT. 20:410-414, December, 1967.

"Clinical studies on gonococcal arthritis and Reiter's syndrome and measurement of gonococcal and Bedsonia antibodies," by J. T. Sharp, et al. ARTHRITIS RHEUM. 11:569-578, August, 1968.

"Clinical studies on trichomonas infections in girls," by I. Sipowicz, et al. WIAD PARAZYT. 15:337-339, 1969.

"Clinical studies on trichomonas vaginalis," by A. Motobayashi. J JAP OBSTET GYNEC SOC. 20:199-203, March, 1968.

"Clinical studies on trichomonas vaginitis," by S. Nohara. J ANTIBIOT. 19:253-268, August, 1966.

"A clinical study of the efficacy of Levorin in urogenital trichomoniasis," by I. I. Il'in. VESTN DERM VENER. 41:87-88, September, 1967.

"Clinical syndromes with mycoplasma infections," by D. A. Tyrrell. POSTGRAD MED J. 43:104-106, March, 1967.

"Clinical test of a drug: nitroimidazine (1-N-Beta-Ethyl-morpholin-5-Nitroimidazole) in genital trichomoniasis," by J. E. Zuniga, et al. REV COLUMBIA OBSTET GINEC, 21:193-196, March-April, 1970.

"Clinical tests using iodopovidone in patients with vaginal trichomoniasis," by A. A. Rustrian, et al. GINEC OBSTET MEX. 27:467-470, April, 1970.

"Clinical treatment of patients with post-penicillin reactions after early syphilis therapy," by J. Bowszyc. PRZEGL DERM. 54:585-589, September-October, 1967.

"Clinical trial of clomocycline (Megaclor) in gonococcal and non-gonococcal urethritis," by G. S. Andrew, et al. BRIT J VENER DIS. 45:154-156, June, 1969.

"Clinical use of pimaricin in parasitic vaginitis," by D. Colavita, et al. MINERVA GINEC. 18:473-476, May 15, 1966.

"Clinical verification of the phenomenon of chemical saturation of antibodies during allergic shock caused by penicillin," by E. Seropian. MED INTERNA. 22:997-1000, August, 1970.

"Clinically useful antimicrobial agents. Untoward reactions," POSTGRAD MED (Minn.). 42:396-419, November, 1967.

"Clinico-laboratory studies of syphilis patients treated with bicillin-6," by A. A. Akovbian, et al. VESTN DERM VENER. 41:63-67, July, 1967.

"Clinicopathologic conference," by D. Jones, et al. TEXAS MED. 62:92-96, October, 1966.

"Clinicopathologic conference," by E. H. Eigenbrodt, et al. TEXAS MED. 65:84-90, July, 1969.

"Clinicopathologic conference. Case presentation (JHH 631077)," by V. A. McKusick, et al. BULL HOPKINS HOSP. 119:150-160, August, 1966.

"Clinico-pathological aspects of the neurosyphilitic psychoses," by K. Dewhurst. POSTGRAD MED J. 44:898-902, December, 1968.

"A clinico-serologic study of pinta in the Alto Beni Region, Bolivia," by W. F. Edmundson, et al. DERM INT. 6:64-76, April-June, 1967.

"Collapse after penicillin injection," by K. Naess. T NORSK LAEGEFOREN. 90:324-325, February 1, 1970.

"Colonial morphology of Neisseria gonorrhoeae isolated from males and females," by P. F. Sparling, et al. J BACT. 93:513, January, 1967.

"Colonization of newborn infants by mycoplasmas," by J. O. Klein, et al. NEW ENG J MED. 280:1025-1030, May 8, 1969.

"The colored treponemal intradermal test seen from the present immunologic standpoint," by G. Cocuzza, et al. DERM WSCHR. 152:699-702, July 2, 1966.

"Colposcopic and cytological picture in 2 cases of primary luetic infection of uterine cervix," by J. Zadjelović. LIJECN VJESN. 90:433-437, May, 1968.

"Colposcopic examination of patients with and after infection with trichomonas vaginalis," by K. J. Verschoof. NEDERL T VERLOSK. 68:269-272, August, 1968.

"Colposcopy and photo-colposcopy in the diagnosis of trichomonal colpitis," by F. A. Syrovatko, et al. AKUSH GINEK. 9:27-35, 1970.

"Colposcopy in the diagnosis of trichomonas vaginitis," by P. G. Kalov. AKUSH GINEK. 45:17-21, August, 1969.

"The combination of hetacillin and kanamycin in the treatment of gonococcal urethritis," by D. C. Rodriguez, et al. REV VENEZ UROL. 21:136-141, January-June, 1969.

"A combined epidemic of scabies and syphilis. What therapeutic course to follow?," by R. Rollier. LYON MED. 222:953-954, November 23, 1969.

"Combined use of fluorescent antibody technique and culture on selective medium for the identification of Neisseria gonorrhoeae," by I. Lind. ACTA PATH MICROBIOL SCAND. 76:279-287, 1969.

"Comments on the paper of Z. Truksa, P. Belák, P. Havlík: 'Contribution to the problem of supplementing the conventional diagnosis of gonorrhea by the fluorescent antibody technic'," by A. Kabátová. CESK EPIDEM. 17:63-64, January, 1968.

"Comparative assessment of the treatment of syphilis patients with bacillin-3, -4 and -6," by A. A. Akovbian, et al. VESTN DERM VENER. 43:44-48, November, 1969.

"Comparative assessment of the treatment of trichomonadurethritis in males with iodinol and ACD preparations," by L. M. Korik, et al. VESTN DERM VENER. 40:62-65, March, 1966.

"Comparative assessment of various methods of laboratory diagnosis of trichomonas infections," by G. A. Voskresenskaia. VESTN DERM VENER. 40:48-53, December, 1966.

"Comparative cutaneous sensitivity studies in man with benzylpenicillin and its purified counterpart," by

O. P. Robinson. ANTIMICRO AGENTS CHEMOTHER. 7:550-552, 1967.

"Comparative cyto-histological studies on the precancerous and early stages of cervix carcinoma with simultaneous trichomonas vaginitis," by E. Boquoi. Z GEBURTSH GYNAEK. 169:59-74, 1968.

"Comparative efficacy of the use of metronidazole of diverse manufacture in the treatment of patients with trichomoniasis," by M. M. Dadashzade. UROL NEFROL. 32:39-41, July-August, 1967.

"Comparative evaluation of serological reactions in syphilis," by F. Osada, et al. JAP J CLIN PATH. 15:435-438, June, 1967.

"Comparative experiments on syphilis serodiagnosis--results of the 1st and 2nd national quality control of syphilis serodiagnosis at the National University Laboratories," by Y. Fukuoka, et al. JAP J CLIN PATH. 16:365-372, April, 1968.

"Comparative serological diagnosis by classical and specific methods," by G. Elste, et al. DERM MSCHR. 155:535-544, 1969.

"Comparative studies in syphilis among the RPR (rapid plasma reagin) card test, classical serology, the FTA test and the TPI test)," by A. G. Bellone, et al. G ITAL DERM. 107:99-104, March-April, 1966.

"Comparative studies of cardiolipin and lipoid antigens in the diagnosis of syphilis," by D. Naumova. NAUCH TR VISSH MED INST SOFIIA. 48:55-62, 1969.

"Comparative studies of the value of methods used in the diagnosis of penicillin allergy," by E. Maciejowska. DERM MSCHR. 155:761-770, 1969.

"Comparative studies on the haemolytic and treponema pallidum immobilizing complement activity in the serum of different species," by F. Muller, et al. IMMUNOLOGY. 18:13-18, January, 1970.

"Comparative studies on the value of culture media Roiron, diamond and CPLM modified by Stepkowski in laboratory diagnosis of trichomoniasis," by B. Hoffmann, et al. WIAD PARAZYT. 15:271-274, 1969.

"Comparative study of cerebrospinal fluid and blood in

syphilis and cerebral cysticercosis," by E. Oberhauser, et al. NEUROCIRUGIA. 27:61-68, January-September, 1969.

"Comparative study of the composition of groups of patients with gonorrhea who came for treatment in 1954-1956 and 1964-1966," by C. H. Beek. NEDERL T GENEESK. 112:989-991, May 25, 1968.

"Comparative study of the sensitivity of gonococci to various antibiotics," by S. S. Lur'e, et al. VESTN DERM VENER. 43:46-49, February, 1969.

"Comparative study of the therapeutic effect of a single dose of hetacillin and ampicillin in gonococcal urethritis," by D. C. Rodriguez, et al. REV VENEZ UROL. 21:143-151, January-June, 1969.

"Comparative study of the therapeutic effects of a single dose of hetacilline and ampicillin in gonococcal urethritis," by D. C. Rodriguez, et al. HOSPITAL. 75:979-986, March, 1969.

"Comparative study of two therapies for gonorrhea," by M. Nelson. PUBLIC HEALTH REP. 84:980-984, November, 1969.

"A comparative study of unheated serum reagin (USR) VDRL and CF tests for syphilis," by R. S. Saxena, et al. INDIAN J MED RES. 57:2203-2204, December, 1969.

"Comparison between the results of the Brewer rapid plasma reagin card test and other tests for syphilis," by B. S. Tio. BRIT J VENER DIS. 46:287-289, August, 1970.

"Comparison of culture media for the growth of trichomonas vaginalis," by C. F. Rayner. BRIT J VENER DIS. 44:63-66, March, 1968.

"Comparison of fluorescent and conventional darkfield methods for the detection of treponema pallidum in syphilitic lesions," by R. Jue, et al. TECHN BULL REGIST MED TECHN. 37:123-125, May, 1967.

"Comparison of the fluorescent treponemal antibody absorption and treponema pallidum immobilization tests on serums from 1182 diagnostic problem cases," by R. M. Wood, et al. TECHN BULL REGIST MED TECHN. 37:55-58, March, 1967.

"Comparison of four culture media for the isolation of Neisseria gonorrhoeae: Correlation with the direct smear method," by S. A. Grady. CANAD J MED TECHN. 32:119-126, June, 1970.

"Comparison of inconclusive smears from gynecological and obstetrical clinics of Johns Hopkins Hospital," by M. B. Skrocka. J MAINE MED ASS. 58:79-83, April, 1967.

"Comparison of procedures for laboratory diagnosis of oculogenital infections with inclusion conjunctivitis agents," by J. Schachter, et al. AMER J EPIDEM. 85:453-458, May, 1967.

"A comparison of results of RPCF and TPHA with those of STS," by H. Usui, et al. BULL PHARM RES INST. 77:9-10, November, 1968.

"Comparison of the TPHA reaction with various syphilis serodiagnostic tests and its clinical significance," by A. Ozawa, et al. JAP J CLIN PATH. 16:911-916, December, 1968.

"Comparison of VDRL, RPCF, and FTA-ABS tests for syphilis," by R. H. Tanimoto, et al. HAWAII MED J. 28:33-36, September-October, 1968.

"Comparison of the VDRL slide, TPI, and FTA-ABS tests in experimental syphilis in rabbits," by S. M. Mothershed, et al. BRIT J VENER DIS. 43:267-271, December, 1967.

"Comparison of various immunofluorescent procedures in the serological diagnosis of syphilis," by K. Király, et al. DERMATOLOGICA. 135:443-450, 1967.

"Complement and lysozyme requirements for spirochetolysis in guinea pig serum," by T. A. Nevin, et al. J BACT. 1388-1393, November, 1967.

"Complement fixation reaction with antigens prepared from T. Pallidum," by K. Király. HAUTARZT. 19:36-42, January, 1968.

"Complement fixation test at cold temperature in the diagnosis of syphilis," by MIa. Gol'dberg. VESTN DERM VENER. 42:41-46, January, 1968.

"Complement-fixing and hemagglutinating antibodies to treponema microdentium," by C. R. Ghosh, et al. PROC

SOC EXP BIOL MED. 124:559-562, February, 1967.

"Complement fixing antibodies against miyagawanella ornithosis in a group of subjects in Accra (Ghana)," by V. Russo, et al. ANN MED NAV. 73:437-443, September-October, 1968.

"Complement-fixing antibodies to Bedsonia organisms in Reiter's syndrome and ankylosing spondylitis," by T. D. Kinsella, et al. ANN RHEUM DIS. 27:241-244, May, 1968.

"A complex diagnostic problem: the differentiation among gonococcal arthritis, Reiter's syndrome, and rheumatoid arthritis," by J. C. Brooks, Jr. J MED ASS. GEORGIA. 56:291-296, July, 1967.

"Complex shape and variability of the diastolic murmur of aortic regurgitation," by W. Dressler, et al. AMER J CARDIOL. 18:616-621, October, 1966.

"Complications after modern gonorrhea therapy," by J. Soltz-Szots. ARCH KLIN EXP DERM. 227:652-656, 1966.

"Complications of gonorrhea." BRIT MED J. 3:420-422, August 22, 1970.

"Complications of gonorrhea," by V. Starck. NORD MED. 76:811-812, July 14, 1966.

"The composition of the cerebrospinal fluid in the neurosyphilitic psychoses," by K. Dewhurst. ACTA NEUROL SCAND. 45:119-123, 1969.

"Concerning congenital syphilis in infants," by J. P. Soares. BOL INST PUERICULT. 22:123-134, August-December, 1965.

"Conclusions of the venerological conference held during the period of May 24-30, 1969 at Destný, Orlické Hory," by J. Obrtel. J CESK DERM. 45:145-153, August, 1970.

"Conditions of genital organs in women working in foundries," by R. Wawryk, et al. POL TYG LEK. 22:1208-1211, August 7, 1967.

"Condylomata acuminata," by B. A. Teokharov. AKUSH GINEK. 42:41-44, February, 1966.

"Condylomata acuminata--past and present," by B. Bafverstedt. ACTA DERMATOVENER. 47:376-381, 1967.

"Congenital luetic hearing impairment. Treatment with prednisone," by M. E. Patterson. ARCH OTOLARYNG. 87:378-382, April, 1968; also in TRANS PACIF COAST OTOOPHTHAL SOC. 51:235-246, 1967.

"Congenital luetic macrogiobulinemia and cryoglobulinemia. Literature review and personal contribution," by A. G. Marchi, et al. G MAL INFETT. 20:249-251, March, 1968.

"Congenital ocular syphilis," by W. G. Nicol, et al. AMER J OPHTHAL. 68:467-471, September, 1969.

"Congenital parenchymal dystrophy of the cornea (on 2 personal cases)," by A. Scialfa. ANN OTTAL. 92:383-393, June, 1966.

"Congenital syphilis," by M. Hart. ARCH DERM. 100:260. August, 1969.

"Congenital syphilis," by R. C. Robinson. ARCH DERM. 99:599-610, May, 1969.

"Congenital syphilis: a continuing problem," by A. J. Strauss, Jr. et al. VIRGINIA MED MONTHLY. 94:684-687, November, 1967.

"Congenital syphilis: a description of 18 cases and re-examination of an old but ever-present disease," by F. Saxoni, et al. CLIN PEDIAT. 6:687-691, December, 1967.

"Congenital syphilis has many faces," by R. McDonald. CLIN PEDIAT. 9:110-114, February, 1970.

"Congenital syphilis in an infant of a seronegative mother," by J. Hallock, et al. OBSTET GYNEC. 32:336-338, September, 1968.

"Congenital syphilis in the Istituto Provinciale Assistenza all' Infanzia of Rome. Comparison between the decade 1943-52 and that of 1957-66. Statistical clinical, therapeutic and prophylactic considerations," by V. Menichella, et al. MINERVA NIPIOL. 19:35-39, January-February, 1969.

"Congenital syphilis: observations on laboratory diagnosis of intrauterine infection," by B. D. Ackerman. J PEDIAT. 74:459-462, March, 1969.

"Congenital syphilitic labyrinthitis," by A. G. Kerr, et al. ARCH OTOLARYNG. 91:474-478, May, 1970.

"Conjugal blastomycocis," by M. W. Craig, et al. AMER REV RESP DIS. 102:86-90, July, 1970.

"Connective tissue disease and the chronic biologic false-positive test for syphilis (BFP reaction)," by A. M. Harvey, et al. MED CLIN N AMER. 50:1271-1279, September, 1966.

"Consent for care," by D. A. Dukelow. J SCH HEALTH. 40:223, May, 1970.

"Consequences of a diagnostic error--ulcus durum diagnosed as erosion of cervix uteri," by P. Botsov, et al. AKUSH GINEK. 9:58-60, 1970.

"Considerations in counselling teen-agers on sexual matters," by H. P. Coppolillo. MED TIMES. 95:580-585, May, 1967.

"Considerations on a case of primary syphiloma of the cervix uteri in pregnancy, with special reference to the differential diagnosis from cervical carcinoma," by E. Rocco. MINERVA GINEC. 19:30-34, January 15, 1967.

"Considerations on cerebellar atrophies," by A. F. Thompson. ARCH FUND ROUX OCEFA. 1:3-16, January-March, 1967.

"Considerations on a current problem. Syphilitic reinfections," by G. Tramier, et al. PRESSE MED. 74:2085-2090, October 1, 1966.

"Considerations on cutaneous reactivity in syphilis and its importance in the diagnosis of recovery," by A. Sapuppo. MINERVA DERM. 42:243-247, July, 1967.

"Considerations on the evolution of cardio-aortic and nervous syphilis in the city of Birlad in the past 15 years (1953-1967)," by I. Graur, et al. REV MEDICOCHIR IASI. 73:127-131, January-March, 1969.

"Considerations on the failure to eradicate gonorrhoea and syphilis," by N. Danbolt. TRIANGLE. 8:2-6, 1967.

"Considerations on some helpful measures in the propaganda against venereal diseases. (On experiences in the high schools of the Province of Venezia," by A.

Serena. ARCH ITAL DERM VENER. 34:395-398, 1966.

"Contact investigation of male West Indian patients with gonorrhoea," by R. R. Willcox, et al. BRIT J VENER DIS. 42:167-170, September, 1966.

"Contemporary principles and methods in treatment of syphilitic aortitis," by M. P. Frishman. VESTN DERM VENER. 44:47-51, May, 1970.

"Continuity in American sex research," by A. Kirch. PSYCHOANAL REV. 53:233-254, Summer, 1966.

"Contractures of the fingers associated with framboesial palmar hyperkeratosis," by S. G. Browne. DERM INT. 7:104-108, April-June, 1968.

"Contribution of cerebrospinal fluid electrophoresis to clinical diagnosis," by U. Consbruch, et al. DEUTSCH MED WSCHR. 93:2168-2172, November 8, 1968.

"Contribution of observations on the cases of male infertility," by L. Semmola. MINERVA DERM. 42:393-397, August, 1967.

"Contribution on lues visceralis," by N. Kraus, et al. Z GES INN MED. 21:443-445, July 15, 1966.

"Contribution to the bacterial diagnosis of gonorrhea," by M. Miljkovic, et al. VOJNOSANIT PREGL. 24:328-330, June, 1967.

"Contribution to the etiology of nonspecific urethritis," by J. Frantoz, et al. LIJECN VJESN. 90:1173-1181, 1968.

"Contribution to the evaluation of immobilism titre in the serologic diagnosis of syphilis," by I. Orhel. PRZEGL DERM. 53:705-714, November-December, 1966.

"Contribution to laboratory problems in the diagnosis of gonorrhea," by E. Geizer, et al. CESK DERM. 43:249-254, August, 1968.

"Contribution to the problem of ocular syphilis," by S. Merin, et al. CENT AFR J MED. 13:249-251, November, 1967.

"Contribution to problems of laboratory diagnostics of gonorrhoea," by E. Geizer, et al. CESK DERM. 43:249-254, August, 1968.

"Contribution to the problems of supplementing the conventional diagnosis of gonorrhea by the fluorescent antibody technic," by Z. Truksa, et al. CESK EPIDEM. 16:81-90, March, 1967.

"Contribution to the problem of supplementing the conventional diagnosis of gonorrhea by the fluorescent antibody technic. Reply to comments of graduate biologist A. Kabátová," by Z. Truksa. CESK EPIDEM. 17:64, January, 1968.

"Contribution to the prophylactic antibiotic treatment of syphilis with special consideration of questionable occupational infections," by K. Wulf. ARCH KLIN EXP DERM. 227:301-307, 1966.

"Contribution to the resistance of trichomonas vaginalis to metronidazole," by M. Valent, et al. BRATISL LEK LISTY. 52:58-61, July, 1969.

"A contribution to staining of Treponema pallidum in tissue. IV. Staining of Treponema pallidum in tissue of syphilid in test-rabbit and man," by M. Otani. BULL PHARM RES INST. 82:1-10, September, 1969.

"Contribution to the study of multiple pseudosclerosis of a syphilitic nature (7 cases)," by B. Pollingher, et al. NEUROLOGIA. 12:215-225, May-June, 1967.

"Contribution to the study of strains of pathogenic Treponema pallidum isolated in Rumania. II. Transmission of experimental syphilitic infection by intracorneal inoculation, in the rabbit, followed by symptoms of generalization," by D. I. Volosceanu, et al. ARCH ROUM PATH EXP MICROBIOL. 23:459-466, June, 1964.

"Contribution to the views on current therapy of gonorrhea by antibiotics," by M. Skencić. SRPSKI ARH CELOK LEK. 94:363-367, April, 1966.

"Control examinations in gonorrhea," by G. Brundin, et al. LAKARTIDNINGEN. 66:912-917, February 26, 1969.

"Control of blood donors. 3. Syphilis transmitted by blood transfusion," by E. Skog. LAKARTIDNINGEN. 64: 1970-1972, May 10, 1967.

"Control of concomitant vaginal moniliasis during metronidazole therapy for trichomonas vaginalis," by J. F. Clark. J NAT MED ASS. 58:464-465 Passim, November, 1966.

"The control of endemic syphilis of childhood," by T. Guthe, et al. DERM INT. 5:179-199, October-December, 1966.

"Control of infectious syphilis in Detroit," by B. Sch-Schwimmer. MICH MED. 65:837-838, October, 1966.

"Control of ophthalmia neonatorum. A position statement by the NSPB Committee on ophthalmia neonatorum." SIGHTSAV REV. 39:203-204, Winter, 1969.

"The control of venereal disease." LANCET. 2:1289-1290, December 10, 1966.

"The control of venereal diseases in British Columbia," by H. K. Kennedy. CANAD J PUBLIC HEALTH. 60:482-485, December, 1969.

"Controlled study of the prevalence of T-strain mycoplasmata in males with non-gonococcal urethritis," by H. R. Ingham, et al. BRIT J VENER DIS. 42:269-271, December, 1966.

"Controlling venereal disease through education," by P. E. Lenz. PUBLIC HEALTH REP. 81:996-998, November, 1966.

"Controls gonorrhea (doxycycline)." AM DRUGGIST. 160:50, October 6, 1969.

"Coombs' positive hemolytic anemia due to penicillin," by L. J. Lyon. J MOUNT SINAI HOSP NY. 35:258-264, May-June, 1968.

"Cooperation in venereal disease control," by S. L. Andelman. BULL MATERN CHILD HLTH. 4:17+, Summer, 1968.

"Cooperation of the gynecologist, dermato-venerologist and bacteriologist in the fight against gonorrhea in the woman," by J. Obrtel. CESK DERM. 42:351-356, October, 1967.

"Cooperation of the Military Health Service in the control of venereal diseases during 25-years of the Polish People's Republic," by K. Płoński, et al. PRZEGL DERM. 56:713-714, 1969.

"Co-operative evaluation of treatment for early syphilis. Preliminary report with special reference to spectinomycin sulphate (actinospectacin)," by J. B. Lucas, et al. BRIT J VENER DIS. 43:244-248, December, 1967.

"Cooperative studies on the serological tests for syphilis, especially the RPCF," by J. Tanaka. IRYO. 22:86-95, February, 1968.

"Correlation between fluorescent treponemal antibody absorption (FTA-ABS) results and the physicians' diagnoses," by S. S. Lindell, et al. J IOWA MED SOC. 58:1234-1239, December, 1968.

"Correlation between the quantitative F.T.A. test on serum and the qualitative F.T.A. test on dried blood. Preliminary note," by S. Sartoris, et al. MINERVA DERM. 42:14-15, January, 1967.

"A correlative immunologic, microbiologic and clinical approach to the diagnosis of acute and chronic infections in newborn infants," by C. A. Alford, et al. NEW ENG J MED. 277:437-449, August 31, 1967.

"Correspondence. Technique for iridocyclectomy," by M. Frenkel. AMER J OPHTHAL. 66:972-973, November, 1968.

"Course in a number of cases of serologic syphilis in blood donors (1962-1968)," by R. Andre, et al. REV FRANC TRANSFUS. 13:93-95, March, 1970.

"Credé's method for the prevention of gonorrheal blennorrhea in newborn infants," by I. van Doesschate. NEDERL T GENEESK. 112:1088-1090, June 8, 1968.

"Crede's prophylaxis after 85 years," by K. Znamenacek, et al. CESK PEDIAT. 22:46-54, January, 1967.

"Crede's prophylaxis after 85 years. Discussion," by K. Znamenacek, et al. CESK OFTAL. 22:335-338, September, 1966.

"Crisis in venereology," by R. D. Catterall, et al. BRIT MED J. 3:699-701, September 19, 1970.

"Critical evaluation of the current system of syphilis control in Poland," by T. Z. Capiński. FOLIA MED CRACOV. 9:521-581, 1967.

"Critical review of the Chediak test," by G. Moch, et al. DEUTSCH GESUNDH. 21:1719-1722, September 8, 1966.

"Cross-allergy caused by cephaloridine, cephalothin and

penicillin," by H. Vogt. HAUTARZT. 20:407-408, September, 1969.

"Cross reactivity between ampicillin and penicillin G," by R. H. Stewart. JAMA. 213:131, July 6, 1970.

"Cryoglobulinemia presenting as 'factitial ulceration'," by R. D. Baughman, et al. ARCH DERM. 94:725-731, December, 1966.

"Cryoglobulins and rheumatoid factor in sera from chronic false positive seroreactors for syphilis," by K. K. Mustakallio, et al. ACTA DERMATOVENER. 47:249-254, 1967.

"Cultivation of gonococci on selective media," by A. Wierer, et al. CESK DERM. 43:27-30, February, 1968.

"Culture and survival of treponema pallidum." WHO CHRON. 21:92-94, March, 1967.

"A culture method suitable in general practice for the diagnosis of gonorrhea," by H. A. Hirsch, et al. ARCH HYG BAKT. 153:473-477, October, 1969.

"Culture of gonococci. Advantages of culture in the diagnosis and treatment of gonorrhea," by K. Odegaard. T NORSK LAEGEFOREN. 86:791-793, May 15, 1966.

"Culture of gonococci from the rectum on Thayer and Martin's selective medium," by A. L. Heimans. DERMATOLOGICA. 133:319-324, 1966.

"Cure of syphilis," by U. Boncinelli, et al. MINERVA DERM. 42:247-258, July, 1967.

"Current approaches to the problem of 'prophylactic' therapy of syphilis," by F. Ormea. MINERVA MED. 58:1201-1205, April 7, 1967.

"Current aspect of syphilis in Belém o Pará," by D. Silva, et al. AN BRASIL DERM. 41:213-218, October-December, 1966.

"Current aspects in syphiligraphy," by M. J. Maleville. BORDEAUX MED. 3:1041-1042 passim, April, 1970.

"Current aspects of primo-secondary syphilis. I. Primary syphilis " PRESSE MED. 78:1848, October 10, 1970.

"Current aspects of primo-secondary syphilis. II. Secondary syphilis." PRESSE MED. 78:1945, October 24, 1970.

"Current aspects of prostitution. The moral aspects," by P. U. Rocco. MINERVA MED. 57:Varia 940+, July 21, 1966.

"Current aspects of vaginal trichomoniasis and candidiasis," by R. Bourg. BRUXELLES MED. 47:443-452, April 23, 1967.

"The current clinical aspect of recent syphilis in the navy. (3rd maritime region)," by J. Duluc, et al. REV CORPS SANTE ARMEES. 5:57-67, February, 1964.

"Current clinical aspects and statistics of early and late syphilis in Poland," by J. Towpik. POL TYG LEK. 22:1477-1480, September 25, 1967.

"The current clinical picture of gonorrhea in males and females," by V. Sedlácek. CESK DERM. 42:100-107, April, 1967.

"Current concepts in the serological diagnosis of syphilis," by M. J. Allison, et al. VIRGINIA MED MONTHLY. 94:186-187, March, 1967.

"Current etiological diversity of infectious urethritis," by A. Siboulet, et al. J UROL NEPHROL. 72:425-430, December, 1966.

"Current legislation concerning prostitution," by C. Rotta. MINERVA MED. 57:Varia 954+, July 21, 1966.

"Current methods in the serological diagnosis of syphilis," by J. Delacrétaz. THER UMSCH. 26:67-70, February, 1969.

"The current prevalence of gonococcal infections in children," by L. F. Nazarian. PEDIATRICS. 39:372-377, March, 1967.

"Current problems in the diagnosis and therapy of gonorrhea and syphilis," by O. Dietz, et al. MUNCHEN MED WSCHR. 107:2677-2678, December 31, 1965.

"Current problems in the diagnosis and therapy of gonorrhea and syphilis," by A. Meyer. MUNCHEN MED WSCHR. 107:2680-2681, December 31, 1965.

"Current problems in the diagnosis and therapy of gonorrhea and syphilis," by C. G. Schirren. MUNCHEN MED WSCHR. 107:2681-2683, December 31, 1965.

"Current problems in the treatment of gonorrhea," by H. Storck, et al. SCHWEIZ MED WSCHR. 96:1635-1641, December 10, 1966.

"Current problems of control of venereal diseases and spirochaeta infections in the light of world health organization data," by J. Towpik. POL TYG LEK. 21: 1513-1515, October 3, 1966.

"Current problems of the diagnosis and therapy of gonorrhea," by I. M. Porudominskii, et al. VESTN DERM VENER. 41:40-46, May, 1967.

"Current problems of syphilidology," by M. A. Rozentul, et al. VESTN DERM VENER. 41:3-7, April, 1967.

"Current problems of syphilis," by I. Károlyi. ORV HETIL. 110:225-236, February 2, 1969.

"Current problems of urogenital trichomoniasis in males," by S. Scultety, et al. ZUROL. 60:311-316, May, 1967.

"Current problems of venereal diseases in females," by A. Wiedmann. MUNCHEN MED WSCHR. 108:1837-1843, September 23, 1966.

"Current problems of venereal diseases in women," by A. Wiedmann. MINERVA MED. 57:3415-3419, October 20, 1966.

"Current problems of venereology," by R. Schuppli. PRAXIS. 57:1368-1372, October 8, 1968.

"Current problems of venereology abroad," by N. M. Turanov, et al. VESTN DERM VENER. 42:59-63, May, 1968.

"Current recrudescence of gonococcia," by A. Siboulet. J UROL NEPHROL. 75:Suppl 12:557+, December, 1969.

"Current serodiagnosis and treatment of syphilis," by S. Olansky, et al. JAMA. 198:165-168, October 10, 1966.

"Current serology of syphilis," by K. Király. ORV HETIL. 108:840-841, April 30, 1967.

"Current state of specific syphilis serology and its future perspectives," by L. Pospisil. CESK DERM. 44:

102-107, May, 1969.

"The current status and perspectives of development of Soviet dermatovenereology," by M. M. Zheltakov, et al. SOVET MED. 30:3-12, September, 1967.

"Current status of the in vitro sensitivity of gonococci to penicillin in Finland, by O. V. Renkonen, et al. ACTA DERMATOVENER. 50:151-153, 1970.

"The current status of ocular syphilis," by J. L. Smith. SURVEY OPHTHAL. 14:176-178, November, 1969.

"Current status of syphilis therapy," by A. Luger, et al. Z HAUT GESCHLECHTSKR. 43:875-886, November 1, 1968.

"Current status of tabes in Algeria," by F. G. Marill, et al. BULL SOC FRANC DERM SYPH. 77:245-248, 1970.

"Current status of venereal diseases," by K. Takeuchi, et al. SANFUJIN JISSAI. 17:131-137, February, 1968.

"Current therapy of gonorrhea and syphilis," by A. C. Kind. WISCONSIN MED J. 69:218-219, September, 1970.

"Current treatment of gonorrhea," by H. Szarmach. POL TYG LEK. 24:1250-1253, August 11, 1969.

"Current treatment of syphilis, particularly of early syphilis," by S. J. Ramos. REV BRASIL MED. 25:603-604, September, 1968.

"Current trends in the clinical diagnosis and therapy of syphilis," by K. Kubec, et al. CESK DERM. 42:306-317, October, 1967.

"Current trends in medical care of the pregnant woman," by D. Farina. POLICLINICO. 75:1579-1587, November 25, 1968.

"Current trends in the Reiter protein complement fixation test," by K. Nonaka, et al. NIPPON IKA DAIG Z 34:374-375, 1967.

"Current trends in venereology." UNIV NEWCASTLE TYNE MED GAZ. 63:34-39, October, 1968.

"Current venereal diseases. Transition in the diseases as seen from the microbiological aspect," by Y. Onoda. JAP J NURS ART. 8:87-96, August, 1969.

"Current venerealogic problems," by R. Staps. DEUTSCH GESUNDH. 21:503-508, March 17, 1966.

"Current views on vaginal trichomoniasis," by G. Leone. MINERVA MED. 61:913-918, March 7, 1970.

"Cutaneous gumma--a contemporary disease," by W. H. Eaglstein, et al. SOUTHERN MED J. 62:976-977, August, 1969.

"Cutaneous manifestations of recent luetic infection, their diagnosis and therapy," by V. Puccinelli. ATTI ACCAD MED LOMBARD. 22:Suppl:2779-2783, 1967.

"Cystoscopic changes and trichomoniasis," by B. Zivkovic, et al. LIJECN VJESN. 91:1175-1178, 1970.

"Cytological and histochemical study of the epithelium in trichomonas colpitis," by E. I. A. Brezhneva. AKUSH GINEK. 45:13-16, August, 1969.

"Cytological aspects of the adenogram in recent syphilis," by P. Morel, et al. LYON MED. 215:1363-1368, May 15, 1966.

"Cytological, colposcopic and histological changes of the uterine cervix associated with vaginal trichomoniasis," by B. Azocar. REV OBSTET GINEC VENEZ. 26:129-140, 1966.

"Cytomegaly, cirrhosis and cancer of the pancreas in a patient with gummatous visceral syphilis," by V. A. Samsonov. ARKH PAT. 28:59-62, 1966.

"Cytomorphologic analyses of smears from the male urethra in urethritis of gonococcal and non-gonococcal origin," by B. Lagerholm. ACTA DERMATOVENER. 46:457-459, 1966.

"Darkfield examination and causes of the most frequent errors," by F. Vosmik. CESK DERM. 43:334-337, October, 1968.

"Data concerning venereal diseases in metropolitan France for the year 1966," by G. Martin-Bouyer. BULL INST NAT SANTE. 22:1021-1055, September-October, 1967.

"Data on the clinical pathomorphological characteristics of post-trichomonas urethritis," by N. S. Liakhovitskii. UROL NEFROL. 32:40-43, January-February, 1967.

"Data on the incidence of syphilis among the population of Prikarpathia," by P. V. Parashchak. VESTN DERM VENER. 40:68-70, January, 1966.

"Data on the study of the clinical aspects, diagnosis, therapy and prevention of allergic reactions in dermatology," by BIu Sidaravichius, et al. VESTN DERM VENER. 43:3-7, July, 1969.

"Deafness and late congenital syphilis," by F. Baron, et al. REV LARYNG. 88:877-883, November-December, 1967.

"Deafness in congenital syphilis," by C. S. Karmody, et al. ARCH OTOLARYNG. 83:18-27, January, 1966.

"Decreased gonococcus sensitivity to penicillin and penicillin dosage, development and present situation," by E. Friedrich, et al. Z AERZTL FORTBILD. 63: 861-868, August 15, 1969.

"Definitive syphilis serology." S DAKOTA J MED. 20:31, February, 1967.

"Degranulation test of polynuclear basophils in rabbits: Shelley test. Clinical and experimental data," by J. Viallier, et al. ACTA ALLERG. 21:9-16, 1966.

"Delayed hypersensitivity to penicillin. Clinical significance and hyposensitization after therapy," by M. J. Fellner, et al. JAMA. 210:2061-2062, December 15, 1969.

"Delayed skin reactions to benzylpenicillin in man," by A. P. Redmond, et al. INT ARCH ALLERG. 33:193-206, 1968.

"Deliberate hypotension for the management of threatening hemorrhage," by M. R. Salem, et al. ANESTHESIOLOGY. 29:155-156, January-February, 1968.

"Demethylchlortetracycline compared with penicillin in the treatment of gonorrhoea in women," by W. Enfors, et al. BRIT J VENER DIS. 46:209-211, June, 1970.

"Demethlchlortetracycline in the treatment of gonorrhoea," by R. R. Willcox. BRIT J VENER DIS. 43:157-160, September, 1967.

"Demonstration, by cultures, of agents of the genus bedsonia in joint fluid in cases of fiessinger-leroy-Reiter rheumatism," by B. A'mor, et al. C R ACAD SCI. 264:1365-1367, March 6, 1967.

"Demonstration of antibodies by fluorescence in syphilis," by K. D. Gregorczyk. DERMATOLOGICA. 133:327-330, 1966.

"Demonstration of gonorrhea using the immunofluorescent technic. I. Methodical remarks," by V. Potuznik, et al. CESK EPIDEM. 16:163-167, May, 1967.

"Demonstration of treponema pallidum in smear preparations (fluorescence serologic examination)," by H. J. Heitmann, et al. Z HAUT GESCHLECHTSKR. 44:529-532, August 1, 1969.

"Demonstration of treponeme-like forms in cases of treated and untreated late syphilis and of treated early syphilis," by N. S. Rice, et al. BRIT J VENER DIS. 46:1-9, February, 1970.

"Dermatologic diseases observed at an assembly of nomads on the occasion of the salt cure of In Gall," by A. Basset, et al. BULL SOC FRANC DERM SYPH. 75:820-822, 1968.

"Dermatologic iconography. Donovanosis (granuloma venerum tropical). Treatment using doxicillin," by L. H. Paschoal, et al. AN BRASIL DERM. 43:Suppl:1-3, January-March, 1968.

"Dermatologic-venereologic service in the BSSR," by O. P. Komov. VESTN DERM VENER. 43:79-81, June, 1969.

"Dermatological don'ts," by K. Riley. J S CAROLINA MED ASS. 64:239, June, 1968.

"Dermato-venerologic education as reflected by records of the University of Halle at the end of the 18th century," by W. Kaiser. DERM MSCHR. 155:569-579, 1969.

"Dermato-venerological service in Tadzhikistan," by B. R. Rakhmatov, et al. VESTN DERM VENER. 42:63-66, April, 1968.

"Dermato-venereological trends," by L. Texier, et al. J MED BORDEAUX. 143:1621-1632, October, 1966.

"Detection of antibodies against myocardial constituents by means of the complement fixation test," by A. Ieri, et al. FOLIA ALLERG. 14:579-585, November-December, 1967.

"Detection of antitreponemal agglutinins in the routine serological tests for syphilis," by G. Lomuto. G ITAL DERM. 109:117-126, March-April, 1968.

"Detection of chlamydia (Bedsonia) in certain infections of man. II. Clinical study of genital tract, eye, rectum, and other sites of recovery of chlamydia," by E. M. Dunlop, et al. J INFECT DIS. 120:463-470, October, 1969.

"Detection of mycoplasma infection in routine laboratory testing," by R. Wik, et al. MUNCHEN MED WSCHR. 112: 888-889, May 8, 1970.

"Detection of mycoplasmas in upper parts of the urinary tract," by W. Witzleb, et al. ZBL BAKT. 208:427-430, 1968.

"Detection of Neisseria gonorrhoeae by means of fluorescent antibody technique. II. Clinical appraisal," by I. Saito. JAP J UROL. 58:1079-1091, October, 1967.

"Detection of Neisseria gonorrhoeae in clinical material by fluorescent antibodies," by L. Zelenkova, et al. CESK EPIDEM. 16:345-349, November, 1967.

"Detection of T. vaginalis in women. Comparison of 'wet smear' results with those of two cervical cytological methods," by R. N. Thin, et al. BRIT J VENER DIS. 45:332-333, December, 1969.

"The detection of treponema pallidum by a rapid, direct fluorescent antibody darkfield procedure," by D. S. Kellogg, Jr. HEALTH LAB SCI. 7:34-41, January, 1970.

"Detection of trichomonas vaginalis in chronic urethritis in men," by J. Darewicz, et al. WIAD PARAZYT. 15: 357-358, 1969.

"Determination of hyaluronidase in cultured pale treponema," by N. F. Kalashchnikova. LAB DELO. 2:94, 1969.

"Determination of therapeutic effects and therapeutic effects and therapeutic standards of anti-trichomonal agents," by S. Mizuno, et al. J JAP OBSTET GYNEC SOC. 21:198-203, February, 1969.

"Determination of trichomonads antigen in trichomoniasis," by L. M. Korik. VESTN DERM VENER. 40:50-55, January, 1966.

"Determining trichomonas antigen for diagnosing trichomonas infection of the accessory sexual organs," by L. M. Korik. VESTN DERM VENER. 43:48-50, May, 1969.

"Development of gonococcal sensitivity," by P. Durel, et al. PATH BIOL. 15:1197-1203, December, 1967.

"Development of immune haemolytic anaemia and thrombocytopenia in a chronic biologic false-positive reactor for syphilis," by K. Sievers, et al. SCAND J HAEMAT 5:264-270, 1968.

"Development of pinta in Mexico," by O. G. Gosset. SALUD PUBLICA MEX. 9:751-753, September-October, 1967.

"Development of resistance of gonococci to penicillin: An eight-year study," by C. R. Amies. CANAD MED ASS J. 96:33-35, January 7, 1967.

"Development of rheumatoid factor activity and cryoglobulins in primary and secondary syphilis," by A. Lassus. INT ARCH ALLERG. 36:515-522, 1969.

"Developmental trends in the occurrence of syphilis and gonorrhea in Czechoslovakia in the years 1948-1964," by J. Beniaková. CESK DERM. 42:263-270, August, 1967.

"Diagnosis and differential diagnosis of syphilitic diseases of the mouth mucosa," by K. W. Mach. OEST Z STOMAT. 65:350-357, September, 1968.

"The diagnosis and management of gonorrhea," by A. B. Greaves. MED ANN DC. 35:369-371, July, 1966.

"Diagnosis and therapy of chronic female gonorrhea," by J. Kvicera, et al. CESK DERM. 45:241-242, September, 1970.

"Diagnosis and therapy of luetic aneurysm of the thoracic aorta," by G. Heberer, et al. DEUTSCH MED WSCHR. 95:1707-1713 passim, August 21, 1970.

"Diagnosis and therapy of nongonorrheal urethritis and prostatitis," by G. Elste. Z AERZTL FORTBILD. 60:619-621, May 15, 1966.

"Diagnosis and therapy of trichmonal and monilial vaginitis," by F. Branger. PRAXIS. 57:1196-1198, September 3, 1968.

"Diagnosis and treatment of cardiovascular syphilis," by J. Pautrat, et al. PRESSE MED. 74:269-270, January 29, 1966.

"Diagnosis and treatment of gonorrhea in the female," by J. B. Lucas, et al. NEW ENG J MED. 276:1454-1459, June 29, 1967.

"Diagnosis and treatment of syphilis in pregnancy," by M. Kusumoto, et al. SANFUJIN JISSAI. 17:1082-1091, December, 1968.

"Diagnosis and treatment of vaginitis," by J. C. Hartgill. PRACTITIONER. 202:363-371, March, 1969.

"Diagnosis, control of course, and therapy of syphilis," by R. Schroter. THER UMSCH. 26:70-75, February, 1969.

"The diagnosis of borreliosis by immunofluorescence," by M. Allinne, et al. ANN INST PASTEUR. 111:Suppl 28-35, November, 1966.

"The diagnosis of early syphilis," by S. Olansky. MED ANN DC. 35:367-368, July, 1966.

"Diagnosis of early syphilis," by H. H. Volan. NEW YORK J MED. 66:2908-2912, November 15, 1966.

"Diagnosis of gonorrhea by a fluorescent antibody technique," by R. P. Mouton. DERMATOLOGICA. 132:343-352, 1966.

"Diagnosis of gonorrhea by the immunofluorescence technic. 3. Delayed immunofluorescence test and its comparison with cultivation on a selective medium," by V. Potuznik, et al. CESK DERM. 43:273-276, August, 1968.

"Diagnosis of gonorrhea in the asymptomatic female: comparison of slide and culture technics," by H. Pariser, et al. SOUTHERN MED J. 61:505-506, May, 1968.

"The diagnosis of gonorrhea in females," by O. I. Haavelsrud. T NORSK LAEGEFOREN. 90:1220-1222, June 1, 1970.

"Diagnosis of gonorrhea in women," by V. N. Aristova.

FELDSH AKUSH. 33:19-21, February, 1968.

"Diagnosis of gonorrhea with fluorescent antibodies," by D. Danielsson. NORD MED. 76:805-806, July 14, 1966.

"Diagnosis of intolerance to penicillin and other antibiotics," by G. Brehm. MED KLIN. 61:1180-1184, July 29, 1966.

"Diagnosis of skin changes caused by herpes simplex virus by means of fluorescence antibody technic," by O. P. Salo, et al. HAUTARZT. 20:112-113, March, 1969.

"Diagnosis of syphilis," by A. Perdrup. NORD MED. 75:483, April 28, 1966.

"The diagnosis of syphilis," by A. H. Wheeler. UNIV MICH MED CENT J. 32:67-76, March-April, 1966.

"Diagnosis of syphilis in the geriatric patient," by L. Nicholas, et al. GERIATRICS. 23:169-174, September, 1968.

"Diagnosis of vaginal discharge," by R. D. Catterall. BRIT J VENER DIS. 46:122-124, April, 1970.

"Diagnosis of vaginal discharges," by E. A. Shipton. MED J AUST. 1:1175-1176, June 6, 1970.

"Diagnosis of vaginal discharges. Another approach to an old problem," by G. J. Dennerstein. MED J AUST. 1:992-994, May 16, 1970.

"Diagnostic and therapeutic difficulties in late pulmonary syphilis in adults," by W. Kiesz, et al. WIAD LEK. 20:1181-1184, June 15, 1967.

"Diagnostic and therapeutic problems in gonorrhea," by K. Holzegel. DEUTSCH GESUNDH. 23:1172-1176, June 20, 1968.

"Diagnostic difficulties in a case of tabes dorsalis as a cause of several operative procedures," by M. Kozik. POL PRZEGL CHIR. 38:801-803, August, 1966.

"Diagnostic difficulties in tabetic arthropathy," by W. Kozina, et al. REUMATOLOGIA. 7:369:73, 1969.

"Diagnostic methods for trichomonas vaginitis. (Microscopic examination before and after staining, culture examination, examination by fluorescence microscopy," by G. Ortolani, et al. NUOVI ANN IG MICROBIOL. 17:539-549, November-December, 1966.

"Diagnostic methods in human trichomoniasis," by I. V. Boldescu. REV MEDICOCHIR IASI. 71:397-402, April-June, 1967.

"Diagnostic problems in gonorrhea," by L. O. Kallings, et al. NORD MED. 76:800-803, July 14, 1966.

"Diagnostic problems in a patient with habitual intrauterine fetal death," by A. M. Schellen, et al. BULL SOC ROY BELG GYNEC OBSTET. 36:187-194, 1966.

"Diagnostic significance of the fluorescent treponema antibody test (FTA)," by W. Manikowska-Lesinska. CESK DERM. 41:296-303, October, 1966.

"Diagnostic staining of dry smears for trichomonas," by R. G. Capet, et al. OBSTET GYNEC. 33:564-573, April, 1969.

"Did you protect the spread?," by E. C. Prather. J FLORIDA MED ASS. 54:1038-1039, November, 1967.

"Differential diagnostic problem: impetiginized eczematic scabies--luesII--psoriasis vulgaris," by V. Misgeld. MED KLIN. 64:2189-2192, November 21, 1969.

"Difficulties in the diagnosis of syphilis," by L. M. Toporovskii, et al. TER ARKH. 41:76-79, August, 1969.

"Difficulty in swallowing due to a large luetic aneurysm of the thoracic aorta," by H. Wehling. MED WELT. 2:106-108, January 8, 1966.

"Diffuse arteritis of aorta with a large aortic aneurysm. Report of a case in an African," by M. Gelfand. CENT AFR J MED. 13:179-181, August, 1967.

"Diffuse pseudo-angiomatous phlebectases," by J. Delacrétaz, et al. DERMATOLOGICA. 137:242-249, 1968.

"A diploma in venereology," by C. D. Alergant. BRIT J VENER DIS. 46:162-163, April, 1970.

"Direct microscopical examination of tube cultures for the detection of trichomonads," by G. I. Barrow, et al. J CLIN PATH. 23:91, February, 1970.

"Disappearance of chancroid in Algeria," by F. G. Marill, et al. BULL SOC FRANC DERM SYPH. 77:236-237, 1970.

"Disease dominant chronic inflammatory splenomegaly. Dysproteinanemic manifestations and lienal lues," by K. Bauch. MED KLIN. 62:47-50, January 13, 1967.

"Diseases of the ascending aorta with aortic insufficiency," by Y. Marquis, et al. UN MED CANADA. 97:1776-1786, December, 1968.

"Dislocation of the lens. A study of 166 hospitalized cases," by W. H. Jarrett, II. ARCH OPHTHAL. 78:289-296, September, 1967.

"Dissecting aneurysm in a 29-year old man with syphilis of main aorta," by H. Dzioba, et al. POL TYG LEK. 23:1148-1149, July 22, 1968.

"Dissecting aneurysm of the aorta in syphilitic mesaortitis," by S. G. Moisseev, et al. Z GES INN MED. 21:134-136, June 15, 1966.

"Do results of culture for gonococci vary with sampling phase of menstrual cycle?," by V. Falk, et al. ACTA DERMATOVENER. 47:190-193, 1967.

"Doctor Francisco Xavier Eugenio de Santa Cruz y Espejo," by N. H. de Huerta. REV ECUAT HIG. 26:55-58, January-April, 1969.

"A doctor speaks of college students and sex," by W. Dalrymple. J AMER COLL HEALTH ASS. 15:279-286, February, 1967.

"Does lues have a role in the intrauterine death today?," by I. Deml. ZBL GYNAEK. 90:240-242, February 17, 1968.

"Does syphilis still erode the spine?," by M. Baledent, et al. SEM HOP PARIS. 46:2354-2357, September 10, 1970.

"Domestic eradication of syphilis in Alabama," by W. H. Smith, et al. J MED ASS ALABAMA. 37:1364-1369, June, 1968.

"Donovanosis," by I. Sluis. DERMATOLOGICA. 133:325-326, 1966.

"Donovanosis and other venereal diseases in southern India.

3rd part of a travel report," by H. J. Weise. Z HAUT GESCHLECHTSKR. 43:425-428, May 15, 1968.

"Donovanosis (granuloma inguinale): a rare cause of osteolytic bone lesions," by D. J. Kirkpatrick. CLIN RADIOL. 21:101-105, January, 1970.

"'Double reaction' to penicillin. Anaphylactic and serum sickness-like reactions due to a single dose," by M. J. Fellner, et al. ARCH DERM. 96:687-688, December, 1967.

"Doxycycline treatment of gonorrhoea in cases with decreased penicillin susceptibility of gonococci," by A. Lassus. CHEMOTHERAPY. 15:125-128, 1970.

"Drug dependence among patients attending a Department of Venereology," by L. I. Ponting, et al. BRIT J VENER DIS. 46:111-113, April, 1970.

"Drug-induced hemolysis," by B. Dreyfus, et al. PRESSE MED. 76:1009-1012, April 27, 1968.

"Drug-induced nephropathies," by C. Huriet. SEM HOP PARIS. 43:1506-1507, May 8, 1967.

"Drug reactions. I. A protein contaminant causing penicillin hypersensitivity," by J. L. Turk, et al. BRIT J DERM. 80:199-201, March, 1968.

"Drug resistance of trichomonas vaginalis," by L. Slucki. WIAD LEK. 21:541-544, April 1, 1968; also in WIAD PARAZYT. 15:477-478, 1969.

"Drug-taking by patients with venereal disease," by D. C. Rawlins. BRIT J VENER DIS. 45:238-240, September, 1969.

"Drug toxicity in the human fetus and newborn child," by J. T. Litchfield, Jr. APPL THER. 9:922-926, November, 1967.

"Drug treatment of syphilis," by K. Wereide. T NORSK LAEGEFOREN. 86:865-866, June 1, 1966.

"Drugs and the Coombs antiglobulin test." NEW ENG J MED. 277:157-158, July 20, 1967.

"Dynamic changes in serum transaminases in patients with syphilis," by G. Spirov, et al. BRIT J VENER DIS. 42:129-131, June, 1966.

"Dysplasiasias caused by trichomonas infections and dyskaryoses," by P. D'Alessandro, et al. QUAD CLIN OSTET GINEC. 21:1318-1328, December, 1966.

"Early congenital syphilis," by C. Simao, et al. HOSPITAL. 75:1045-1057, March, 1969.

"Early congenital syphilis," by O. R. Turro, et al. ARCH ARGENT PEDIATR. 67:1-8, January-June, 1969.

"Early congenital syphilis and thrombocytopenia," by L. Juhlin. ACTA DERMATOVENER. 48:166-169, 1968.

"Early congenital syphilis in the newborn. (Clinicoradiological study)," by L. De Camillus, et al. UAD CLIN OSTET GINEC. 21:1134-1152, December, 1966.

"Early diagnosis and treatment of syphilis," by K. Higuchi. NAIKA. 23:1277-1284, June, 1969.

"Early diagnosis of neonatal syphilis. Evaluation of a gamma M-fluorescent treponemal antibody test," by P. Mamunes, et al. AMER J DIS CHILD. 120:17-21, July, 1970.

"Early history of syphilis: a reappraisal," by A. W. Crosby, Jr. AM ANTHROP. 71:218-227, April, 1969.

"Early malignant syphilis with a fatal course (anatomic examination)," by R. Degos, et al. BULL SOC FRANC DERM.SYPH. 77:10-15, July, 1970.

"Early primary syphilis--a fluorescent test to replace dark-ground examination of chancre exudate," by M. F. Garner. MED J AUST. 2:199-200, July 29, 1967.

"Early syphilis and homosexuality in the Berlin district from 1961 till 1966," by G. Elste, et al. DEUTSCH GESUNDH. 23:1510-1513, August 8, 1968.

"Early syphilis: immunoglobulins reactive in immunofluorescence and other serologic tests," by A. J. Julian, et al. J IMMUN. 102:1250-1259, May, 1969.

"Early syphilitic hepatitis," by H. E. Zellmann, et al. LAHEY CLIN FOUND BULL. 16:255-259, 1967.

"Early yaws," by L. Fry, et al. BRIT J VENER DIS. 42: 28-30, March, 1966.

"An easily prepared selective medium for the cultivation of Neisseria gonorrhoeae," by C. R. Amies, et al. BRIT J VENER DIS. 43:137-139, June, 1967.

"Educating teen-agers about venereal disease," by D. Rosenblatt, et al. J SCH HLTH. 37:432+, November, 1967.

"Education can help cure VD," by L. M. Garner. SCH & COM. 52:16-17, May, 1966.

"Education has vital role in correcting misconceptions about venereal diseases," by W. L. Porter, et al. DELAWARE MED J. 39:232-234, September, 1967.

"Education of the public about venereal diseases. Some views of venereologists," by R. S. Morton. BRIT J VENER DIS. 42:238-243, December, 1966.

"Education on venereal diseases in the school curriculum," by J. H. Milor, et al. J SEC ED. 42:135-139, March, 1967.

"Education vs. venereal disease," by S. Tolchin. FORECAST HOME ECON. 14:F30-1+, April, 1969.

"Effect of albothyl in trichomonas vaginalis infection on the changes in vaginal environment," by J. Fidler, et al. WIAD PARAZYT. 15:453-454, 1969.

"Effect of an antifungal agent, primaricin, on trichomonas vaginalis in vitro," by K. Asami, et al. J ANTIBIOT. 20:344-346, October, 1967.

"The effect of antisyphilitic treatment on the frequency of detection of antibrain autoantibodies in the blood and cerebrospinal fluid of patients with syphilis," by N. I. Tumasheva, et al. VESTN DERM VENER. 42: 43-47, 1968.

"Effect of cephalothin and cephaloridine against rabbit syphilis," by T. Ikeda, et al. ACTA DERM. 61:310-313, November, 1966.

"Effect of copper oxidase in the blood and cerebrospinal fluid of patients with syphilitic lesions of the central nervous system," by N. I. Tumasheva, et al. ZH NEVROPAT PSIKHIAT KORSAKOV. 66:391-393, 1966.

"Effect of debecycline on treponema pallidum," by J. Suchanek, et al. POL TYG LEK. 22:14-16, January 2, 1967.

"Effect of desiccation of the vaginal contents on the vitality of trichomonas vaginalis," by E. Grys. WIAD PARAZYT. 15:285-286, 1969.

"Effect of the development of social hygiene on the occurrence of gonorrhea," by A. Perdrup. ARCH KLIN EXP DERM. 227:640-644, 1966.

"Effect of dimethyl sulfoxide on skin. A macroscopic and microscopic investigation on human skin," by E. Skog, et al. ACTA DERMATOVENER. 47:426-434, 1967.

"Effect of encorton on the Lukasiewicz-Jarisch-Herxheimer reaction," by K. Bien, et al. 56:305-310, May-June, 1969.

"The effect of environmental temperature on the reactivity of the VDRL slide test," by J. F. D'Costa, et al. BULL WHO. 39:943-946, 1968.

"Effect of the fluorescein to protein ratio on anti-treponema pallidum conjugates," by S. M. Mothershed. APPL MICROBIOL. 18:806-809, November, 1969.

"Effect of gentamicin on the motility of treponema pallidum," by H. Holzmann, et al. HAUTARZT. 20:404-407, September, 1969.

"Effect of high doses of antibiotics on the course of trichomoniasis in women," by W. Jacyk, et al. WIAD PARAZYT. 15:423-424, 1969.

"The effect of lysozyme and temperature on acceleration of the treponema pallidum immobilization test," by N. M. Ovchinnikov, et al. VESTN DERM VENER. 42:67-69, November, 1968.

"The effect of metronidazole on the inflammatory changes in trichomonas vaginitis," by J. Mleziva, et al. ZBL GYNAEK. 90:425-431, March 23, 1968.

"The effect of metronidazole therapy on cervical histology in trichomoniasis," by B. Gray, et al. J OBSTET GYNAEC BRIT COMM. 74:98-103, February, 1967.

"Effect of new chlorosulfonamides on the female vagina. Considering trichomoniasis complicated by mycosis.

Experimental part," by A. Kurnatowska. WIAD PARAZYT. 15:19-33, 1969.

"Effect of a nitro-imidazole on primary experimental syphilis in rabbits," by A. R. Yobs, et al. BRIT J VENER DIS. 42:122-124, June, 1966.

"Effect of primaricin on vaginal trichomoniasis," by H. Wada, et al. J ANTIBIOT (B). 20:281-284, August, 1967.

"The effect of prednisolone on the Jarisch-Herxheimer reaction," by H. Gudjónsson, et al. ACTA DERMATOVENER. 48:15-18, 1968.

"The effect of specific treatment on the adrenal cortex function in patients with syphilis," by A. A. Shtein, et al. VESTN DERM VENER. 42:58-61, August, 1968.

"Effect of streptomycin on trepomena pallidum," by J. Suchanek, et al. POL TYG LEK. 22:89-91, January 16, 1967.

"Effect of temperature and environment on the vitality of the trichomonas vaginalis," by E. Grys. WIAD PARAZYT. 15:281-283, 1969.

"Effect of 2-mercaptoethanol treatment on anticardiolipin reactivity in sera from syphilitics and false positive reactors," by G. R. Tringali, et al. BRIT J VENER DIS. 45:202-204, September, 1969.

"Effect of V-cillin on trepomena pallidum," by J. Suchanek, et al. POL TYG LEK. 22:46-48, January 9, 1967.

"Effect of the vaginal microorganisms on the epithelium of the vaginal portion of the uterus. Further results," by A. Dzioba, et al. POL TYG LEK. 21:1556-1557, October 10, 1966.

"The effect of x-irradiation on the development of orchitis in rabbits and on the quality of antigen for the treponema pallidum immobilization test," by L. D. Butovetskii. ZH MIKROBIOL. 43:131-134, March, 1966.

"Effective drugs fail to stem VD rise." AM DRUGGIST. 154:35+, September 26, 1966.

"Effects of griseofulvin in experimental rabbit syphilis," by T. Hasegawa. BRIT J VENER DIS. 42:178-180, September, 1966.

"The effects of hypnotherapy on homosexuality," by P. Roper. CANAD MED ASS J. 96:319-327, February 11, 1967.

"Effects of 2-mercaptoethanol on treponemal antibodies in syphilis," by E. Csermely, et al. MINERVA DERM. 42:418-419, August, 1967.

"Effects on the public health of the incidence of venereal and skin diseases during the last quarter of the century," by C. Huriez. BULL ACAD NAT MED. 153:396-406, 1969.

"The efficiency of microscopic, culture and serological diagnostic methods in the different clinical forms of genito-urinary trichomonadosis," by J. Teras, et al. WIAD PARAZYT. 15:359-361, 1969.

"Efficiency of microscopic examination of fresh smears and cultures in diagnosis of trichomonas vaginalis," by I. De Carneri, et al. AMER J OBSTET GYNEC. 100:299-301, January 15, 1968.

"Ehrlich, his life and his work," by J. Montes, et al. ALERGIA. 15:29-42, November, 1967.

"Electrocardiographic and serum enzyme study with special reference to glutamic-oxalacetic and glutamic-pyruvic transaminase, lactate dehydrogenase and creatine phosphokinase in syphilis. Preliminary results," by M. Aricò. MINERVA DERM. 42:48-49, February, 1967.

"Electrocardiographic findings in syphilitic aortitis," by D. Knapikowá, et al. KARDIOL POL. 13:131-135, 1970.

"Electron microscopic observation of syphilid. I. The ultrastructure of treponema pallidum (Nicols strain)," by S. Abe. BULL PHARM RES INST. 60:1-6, January, 1966.

"Electron microscopic observation of syphilid. II. The ultrastructure of rabbit syphilitic orchitis," by S. Abe. BULL PHARM RES INST. 68:1-8, May, 1967.

"Electron microscopic observation of syphilid. 3. The ultrastructure of syphilitic chancre in man," by S. Abe. BULL PHARM RES INST. 79:6-22, March, 1969.

"Electron microscopic observations on the lesions of condyloma latum," by T. Hasegawa. BRIT J DERM. 81:367-374, May, 1969.

"Electron microscopic studies on secondary retinitis pigmentosa," by S. Nishida, et al. ACTA SOC OPHTHAL JAP. 71:1410-1417, September, 1967.

"An electron microscopic study of a syphilitic chancre. Engulfment of treponema pallidum by plasma cells," by H. A. Azar, et al. ARCH PATH. 90:143-150, August, 1970.

"Electron microscopic study of treponema pallidum in rabbit chancre tissue," by N. M. Ovchinnikov, et al. VESTN DERM VENER. 43:14-19, March, 1969.

"Electron microscopic study of treponema pallidum isolated from human syphilids," by V. V. Delektorskli. VESTN DERM VENER. 40:63-66, July, 1966.

"Electron microscopy of treponema pallidum occurring in a human primary lesion," by L. M. Drusin, et al. J BACT. 97:951-955, February, 1969.

"Embolico-toxic reaction following depot penicillin administration," by R. Kaufer. DEUTSCH GESUNDH. 24:1208-1211, June 26, 1969.

"Emotional problems of gonorrhoea," by S. E. Mbanefo. J ROY COLL GEN PRACT. 15:272-279, April, 1968.

"Emphysematous vaginitis," by E. F. Christensen, et al. JAMA. 200:1001-1002, June 12, 1967.

"Emphysematous vaginitis," by J. P. Whalen, et al. OBSTET GYNEC. 29:9-11, January, 1967.

"Encephalopathy from penicillin (Editorial)." BRIT MED J. 3:198, July 27, 1968.

"Encephalopathy with transitory amaurosis, visual agnosia and oculomotor apraxia following high-dose intravenous penicillin therapy," by B. Cagianut, et al. SCHWEIZ MED WSCHR. 100:42-43, January 3, 1970.

"Endemic pinta. Present situation in Mexico," by O. G. Gosset. SALUD PUBLICA MEX. 11:211-215, March-April, 1969.

"Endemic syphilis in the Karoo," by J. Du Toit. S AFR MED J. 43:355-358, March 29, 1969.

"Endemic treponematoses," by T. Guthe. ACTA DERMATOVENER. 44:169-179, 1964.

"Endogenous uveitis. V. Laboratory tests (W.R., G.R., E.S.R., S.A.T., HB Per cent)," by M. S. Norn. ACTA OPHTHAL. 47:848-864, 1969.

"Endometrial blastomycosis acquired by sexual contact," by E. R. Farber, et al. OBSTET GYNEC. 32:195-199, August, 1968.

"Enduracidin, a new antibiotic. 3. In vitro and in vivo anti-microbial activity," by K. Tsuchiya, et al. J ANTIBIOT. 21:147-153, February, 1968.

"Enforced legal regulations in venerology," by F. Novotny. CESK DERM. 42:58-68, February, 1967.

"Enlightened views on gonorrhoea," by D. Hill. NURSING TIMES. 62:566+, April 29, 1966.

"Environmental indicators and implications for control of infectious syphilis," by W. B. Neser. MISSOURI MED. 64:822-825, October, 1967.

"Enzymatic activity of ceruloplasmin in patients with syphilis and gonorrhea," by A. M. Borisenko, et al. VESTN DERM VENER. 41:66-69, September, 1967.

"Epidemic in rural Mississippi." SCI N. 94:362, October 12, 1968.

"Epidemic pediculosis and gonorrhea," by A. Altchek. OBSTET GYNEC. 35:638-641, April, 1970.

"Epidemiologic aspect of syphilis. City of Santa Maria, Rio Grande do Sul," by J. Fogliatto, et al. HOSPITAL. 76:739-746, August, 1969.

"Epidemiologic problems of venereal diseases," by K. Kalbarczyk. PRZEGL DERM. 54:655-658, November-December, 1967.

"Epidemiologic significance of the candida albicans infection of the vagina in pregnant women," by W. Mierzejewski, et al. GINEK POL. 37:501-506, May, 1966.

"Epidemiologic study of trichomoniasis in normal women," by G. W. Comstock, et al. OBSTET GYNEC. 27:607-616, May, 1966.

"Epidemiologic survey on Chagas' disease and syphilis in Ribeirao Préto," by N. Haddad. REV INST MED TROP S PAULO. 9:333-342, September-October, 1967.

"Epidemiological and statistical survey: ano-rectal localizations of venereal diseases," by J. Vilotte. ARCH FRANC MAL APPAR DIG. 59:Suppl 7-8: 3-8, July-August, 1970.

"Epidemiological situation of venereal diseases," by H. C. Sturde, et al. OEFF GESUNDHEITSWESEN. 31:348-353, July-August, 1969.

"Epidemiological study of vaginal trichomoniasis in the province of Udine," by G. C. Tosolini, et al. FRIULI MED. 23:723-744, September-October, 1968.

"Epidemiological study of yaws," by K. C. Sahu. INDIAN J DERM. 11:119-122, July 4, 1966.

"Epidemiology of cervical cancer: Study of a prison population," by K. S. Moghissi, et al. AMER J OBSTET GYNEC. 100:607-614, March 1, 1968.

"The epidemiology of infectious syphilis," by C. Lindman. J MAINE MED ASS. 60:237 passim, October, 1969.

"Epidemiology of lues and gonorrhea in Northrhine Westphalia from 1948 to 1968," by K. Gedicke. OEFF GESUNDHEITSWESEN. 32:218-226, May, 1970.

"The epidemiology of syphilis," by C. M. Barnes. J KANSAS MED SOC. 70:59-66, February, 1969.

"Epidemiology of syphilis," by E. Calas, et al. PROPHYL SANIT MORALE. 38:12-21, January, 1966.

"Epidemiology of syphilis," by N. J. Fiumara. MASSACHUSETTS GEN PRACT NEWS. 4pp, January-February, 1966.

"Epidemiology of syphilis in Brisbane, 1968-1969," by B. A. Smithurst. MED J AUST. 2:1143-1146, December 6, 1969.

"Epidemiology of syphilitic infection during the past 8 years (1958-1965) according to our clinical material," by R. Ruben, et al. GOD ZBORN MED FAK SKOPJE. 13: 185-193, 1966.

"Epidemiology of trichomoniasis in girls," by E. Gorzedowska. WIAD PARAZYT. 15:353-354, 1969.

"Epidemiology of venereal diseases in France from 1963 to 1967." BULL INST NATE SANTE RECH MED. 23:1477-1498, November-December, 1968.

"Epididymitis due to trichomonas vaginalis," by I. Fisher, et al. BRIT J VENER DIS. 45:252-253, September, 1969.

"Epilepsy and neurosyphilis," by E. Negulici-Baliff, et al. ACTA NEUROL BELG. 67:1138-1152, 1967.

"Equine coital exanthema," by K. Petzoldt. BERLIN MUNCHEN TIERAERZTI WSCHR. 83:93-95, March, 1970.

"Eradication of syphilis: the missing element," by W. J. Brown. ANN INTERN MED. 72:278-280, February, 1970.

"Errors in the diagnosis of syphillis in surgical practice," by L. M. Toporovskii, et al. SOVET MED. 29:132-135, May, 1966.

"Errors of dermatovenereologists in the diagnosis of syphilis," by N. A. Chaika, et al. VESTN DERM VENER. 42:86-89, January, 1968.

"Erythromycin," by R. S. Griffith, et al. MED CLIN NORTH AM. 54:1199-1215, September, 1970.

"Erythromycin and oleandomycin in therapy of fresh gonorrhea in women," by L. D. Kuntsevich. VESTN DERM VENER. 42:84-86, July, 1968.

"Erythromycin controls gonorrhea." AM DRUGGIST. 159:44, February 24, 1969.

"Erythromycin in the acqueous humour," by N. Shorr, et al. BRIT J OPHTHAL. 53:331-334, May, 1969.

"Erythromycin in early syphilis," by W. L. Fernando. BRIT J VENER DIS. 45:200-201, September, 1969.

"Erythromycin in the therapy of gonorrhea in women," by E. N. Turanova, et al. SOVET MED. 29:123-125, September, 1966.

"Erythromycin in the therapy of inguinal lymphogranuloma," by I. I. Il'in. VESTN DERM VENER. 40:69-70, August, 1966.

"Erythromycin in the treatment of acute gonococcal urethritis in males," by D. O. Smith, Jr., et al. CURR

THER RES. 11:1-4, January, 1969.

"Erythromycin in the treatment of gonorrhea in women," by B. A. Afanas'ev. VESTN DERM VENER. 41:83-86, April, 1967.

"Erythromycin in the treatment of non-gonococcal urethritis," by R. R. Willcox. BRIT J VENER DIS. 44: 157-159, June, 1968.

"Erythromycin stearate in 'single dose' in the treatment of acute masculine gonococcal urethritis," by R. Bialski. REV BRASIL MED. 26:256-258, April, 1969.

"Erythroplasia of queyrat as a consequence of arsenobenzene therapy," by F. Novotny, et al. CESK DERM. 42: 83-85, April, 1967.

"The essence of gonorrhoea control. III. The delineation of the male: female source ratio," by R. R. Willcox. ACTA DERMATOVENER. 46:250-256, 1966.

"The essence of gonorrhoea control. IV. The promiscuous female pool," by R. R. Willcox. ACTA DERMATOVENER. 46:460-465, 1966.

"The essence of gonorrhoea control. V. The influence of promiscuity," by R. R. Willcox. ACTA DERMATOVENER. 47:65-69, 1967.

"An estimate of the risk of men acquiring gonorrhea by sexual contact with infected females," by K. K. Holmes, et al. AMER J EPIDEM. 91:170-174, February, 1970.

"Etiological studies of atrio-ventricular blocks (clinical study of 573 cases)," by L. Prevosti, et al. FOLIA CARDIOL. 26:79-92, March-April, 1967.

"The etiology of non-gonococcal urethritis," by G. Furness. S DAKOTA J MED. 20:39-42, December, 1967.

"Etiology of painless, bilateral knee effusion," by P. M. Catalano. JAMA. 211:1190, February 16, 1970.

"Etiopathogenetic data concerning eczematous candidiasis of the genitals," by C. L. Meneghini, et al. DERM INT. 5:163-166, July-September, 1966.

"Evaluation of an automated fluorescent treponemal antibody test for syphilis," by E. M. Coffey, et al. BRIT J VENER DIS. 46:271-277, August, 1970.

"Evaluation of an automated serologic test for syphilis," by R. C. Bartlett, et al. AMER J CLIN PATH. 53:494-497, April, 1970.

"Evaluation of different therapeutic regimens in the treatment of acute urethritis (707 cases)," by P. L. Stebbins. MILIT MED. 132:535-538, July, 1967.

"An evaluation of the FTA-ABS test for syphilis," by W. E. Beam, Jr., et al. AMER J CLIN PATH. 47:404-407, March, 1967.

"An evaluation of gonorrhea case findings in the chronically infected female," by D. W. Johnson, et al. AMER J EPIDEM. 90:438-448, November, 1969.

"Evaluation of laboratory methods for detecting acute TRIC agent infection," by J. Schachter, et al. AMER J OPHTHAL. 70:375-380, September, 1970.

"Evaluation of a modified FTA-ABS test, multispot FTA-ABS," by P. O'Neill, et al. BRIT J VENER DIS. 46:278-283, August, 1970.

"Evaluation of the nitrimidazine activity in giardiasis and genital trichomoniasis," by J. M. Salles, et al. HOSPITAL. 77:1689-1697, May, 1970.

"Evaluation of a quantitative automated micro-hemagglutination assay for antibodies to treponema pallidum," by L. C. Logan, et al. AMER J CLIN PATH. 53:163-166, February, 1970.

"Evaluation of the plasmacrit test for use as a screen test for syphilis in the military," by C. E. Bushbee. MILIT MED. 132:262-264, April, 1967.

"Evaluation of quantitative reaction of immobilization of treponema pallidum by Nelson and Mayer (ITP) in the diagnosis of syphilis," by I. Orhel. MED GLAS. 22:157-160, May, 1968.

"Evaluation of RPCF and FTA in serological reactions of syphilis," by H. Ota, et al. J JAP ASS INFECT DIS. 42:131-135, August, 1968.

"Evaluation of the rapid plasma reagin card test (RPRCT) for serodiagnosis of syphilis," by G. P. Roxas, et al. MISSOURI MED. 66:37 passim, January, 1969.

"Evaluation of some new serological tests for diagnosis

of syphilis," by L. D. Butovetskii. VESTN DERM VENER. 40:68-75, September, 1966.

"Evaluation of the sorbents used in the FTA-ABS test," by T. Rathlev. BRIT J VENER DIS. 44:295-298, December, 1968.

"An evaluation of the Technicon Autoanalyzer for automating complement-fixation tests," by C. E. Taylor, et al. J CLIN PATH. 21:521-526, July, 1968.

"Evaluation of therapy for early syphilis," by J. Kvicera. CESK DERM. 45:218-221, September, 1970.

"An evaluation of the VDRL and FTA-ABS in a general hospital laboratory," by M. J. Allison, et al. TECHN BULL REGIST MED TECHN. 39:42-46, February, 1969.

"Evaluation of venereal disease information campaign for adolescents," by D. Rosenblatt, et al. AMER J PUBLIC HEALTH. 56:1104-1115, July, 1966.

"Evidence for the presence of circulating antibodies to an oral spirochete in the sera of clinic patients," by A. I. Steinberg. J PERIODONT. 41:213-214, April, 1970.

"Evolution of the 'problem of trichomoniasis in the past 5 years," by G. Chappaz, et al. BYNAECOLOGIA. 161:36-48, 1966.

"Evolution of syphilis in the region of Suceava in the years 1952 to 1966," by T. Costic. REV MEDICOCHIR IASI. 72:59-62, January-March, 1968.

"Evolution of vaginal trichomoniasis from 1957 to 1964. Statistical discussion," by M. Gaudefroy, et al. J SCI MED LILLE. 84:409-422, September-October, 1966.

"Excelsior." JAMA. 203:592, February 19, 1968.

"Experience in application of the elements of programmed instruction of students," by L. D. Butovetskii, et al. VESTN DERM VENER. 43:54-56, February, 1969.

"Experience in the dispensarization and treatment of trichomoniasis with flagyl," by I. I. Shkliar. VESTN DERM VENER. 41:67-70, May, 1967.

"Experience in gonorrhea treatment in an outpatient department," by L. Gip, et al. LAKARTIDNINGEN. 65:

1226-1230, March 20, 1968.

"Experience in raising the qualifications of dermatologists--venereologists in Leningrad," by I. G. Tsiura, et al. VESTN DERM VENER. 43:59-61, January, 1969.

"Experience in a shortened period of treatment of contagious forms of syphilis," by I. I. Pototskii, et al. VRACH DELO. 2:85-90, February, 1968.

"Experience in the treatment of gonorrhea in males with oletetrin," by I. I. Mavrov. VESTN DERM VENER. 43: 80-82, November, 1969.

"Experience in the treatment of trichomonas urogenital infections in males with flagyl," by M. M. Dadashzade. VESTN DERM VENER. 41:87-89, August, 1967.

"Experience in the treatment of trichomoniasis in women with flagyl," by A. M. Mezhebovskii, et al. AKUSH GINEK. 42:45-46, February, 1966.

"Experience of continuous treatment of early forms of syphilis with penicillin and bicillin," by L. A. Rozina. VESTN DERM VENER. 42:62-65, 1968.

"An experience of work of a dermato-venerologist in gynecological institutions of Riga," by N. N. Litvinova, et al. VESTN DERM VENER. 40:70-73, January, 1966.

"Experience with the diagnosis of trichomonas vaginitis," by L. Grunner, et al. BRATISL LEK LISTY. 53:578-580, May, 1970.

"Experience with a rapid immunofluorescent test for the gonococcus as a 'bench' procedure in venereal disease clinics," by R. A. Henderson, et al. BRIT J VENER DIS. 46:205-208, June, 1970.

"Experience with a selective medium in the routine diagnosis of gonorrhoae, with special regard to rectal gonorrhoae in women," by S. O. Roepstorff, et al. ACTA PATH MICROBIOL SCAND. 67:563-568, 1966.

"Experience with therapy of urogenital trichomoniasis in males with a new indigenous preparation, chlomizole," by F. B. Potapnev. VESTN DERM VENER. 42:41-46, December, 1968.

"Experience with the treatment of early forms of syphilis in the region of Eastern Slovakia in 1966," by E. Maly, et al. CESK DERM. 44:188-194, October, 1969.

"Experience with the treponema immunofluorescent absorption tests (FTA-ABS test)," by G. Palm. MED MSCHR. 24:58-60, February, 1970.

"Experience with the use of furadonin in trichomoniasis," by B. I. Il'In. UROL NEFROL. 32:40-43, March-April, 1967.

"Experiences of a doctor sexologist with youth," by Z. L. Starowicz. WIAD LEK. 23:1359-1362, August 1, 1970.

"Experiences with atricana in the treatment of trichomoniasis," by J. C. Aure, et al. T NORSK LAEGEFOREN. 89:1792-1794 passim, December 1, 1969.

"Experiences with the fluorescent treponema antibody absorption technic (FTA-ABS) as compared to other serological diagnostic methods for syphilis," by L. Krell, et al. DERM MSCHR. 155:545-553, 1969.

"Experiences with pimafucin in candida and trichomonas vaginitis," by T. Ozbay, et al. MED WELT. 50:2741-2743, December 13, 1969.

"Experiences with the use of sodium ampicillin in acute gonococcal infections in Vietnam," by R. G. Kercull. MILIT MED. 133:985-986, December, 1968.

"Experiment of study of immunofluorescent method in serodiagnosis of syphilis," by G. A. Zmechorovskaia, et al. LAB DELO. 1:22-25, 1968.

"Experimental method of differentiation between various treponematoses: venereal syphilis, endemic syphilis and pain," by A. Paris-Hamelin, et al. BULL SOC FRANC DERM SYPH. 75:547-549, 1968; also in BULL WHO. 38:808-809, 1968.

"Experimental ocular and neurosyphilis in the primate," by J. A. Wells, et al. BRIT J VENER DIS. 43:10-17, March, 1967.

"Experimental pinta in the chimpanzee," by G. Varela. SALUD PUBLICA MEX. 11:37-38, January-February, 1969; also in JAMA. 206:829, October 21, 1968.

"Experimental studies in vivo on the effect upon treponema pallidum of some antibiotics other than penicillin," by A. Jakubowski, et al. PRZEGL DERM. 55:

1-6, January-February, 1968.

"Experimental studies on the kinetics of the TPI-test. I. Effect of rabbit homologous antibodies on test-treponema in vivo," by F. Muller, et al. Z IMMUNITAETSFORSCH. 134:54-68, November, 1967.

"Experimental studies on the kinetics of the TPI-test (treponema pallidum immobilization test). II. Effect of rabbit-antibodies bound to the treponema in vivo on the result of the TPI-test and its reproducibility," by M. Pop-Aceva, et al. Z IMMUNITAETSFORSCH. 136: 208-217, August, September, 1968.

"Experimental studies on the kinetics of the TPI-test. 3. On the importance of the immobilizing complement activity for the TPI-test and attempts at their standardization," by F. Muller, et al. Z IMMUNITAETSFORSCH. 136:218-229, August-September, 1968.

"Experimental studies on the TPI tests (treponema pallidum immobilization test). IV. On a titrimetic procedure for the exact determination of the endpoint in the immobilization of problem serums," by F. Muller. Z IMMUNITAETSFORSCH. 136:340-346, November, 1968.

"Experimental studies on the kinetics of the TPI test (treponemal pallidum immobilization test). V. Differentiation between in vivo and in vitro presensitization by immobilizing antibodies from infected rabbits," by F. Muller, et al. Z IMMUNITAETSFORSCH. 138:264-272, July, 1969.

"Experimental studies on the masking effect of antibiotics on the course of treponemal infections," by R. Mielech, et al. PRZEGL DERM. Suppl:63-67, 1969.

"Experimental studies on the treatment of syphilis with various antibiotics," by A. Jakubowski, et al. PRZEGL DERM. Suppl:57-61, 1969.

"Experimental studies on trichomonas vaginalis and trichomonacidal agents," by M. Nakae. NIPPON IKA DAIG Z. 34:269-284, 1967.

"Experimental syphilis in the chimpanzee. Immunoglobulin class of early antibodies reactive with treponema pallidum," by W. J. Brown, et al. BRIT J VENER DIS. 46:198-200, June, 1970.

"Experimental under-treatment of early syphilis with probenecid and penicillin in anti-gonorrhoea dosages. A study to assess the best follow-up examination time for syphilis after gonorrhoea treatment in Greenland," by L. Hallinger. ACTA DERMATOVENER. 48:260-267, 1968.

"Experiments in accelerating the development of experimentally maintained specific orchitis in rabbits infected with the Nichols strain of treponema pallidum," by D. Naumova. VESTN DERM VENER. 43:40-44, May, 1969.

"Exploration of the possible allergic consequences of utilization of clemizole-penicillin," by J. Jubelin, et al. MARSEILLE MED. 105:189-192, 1968.

"Exploration of some cases of old syphilis by the study of treponema in the CSF, the response of the luo-test and the anamnestic serological reaction," by G. Tramier. BULL SOC FRANC DERM SYPH. 73:392-394, July-August, 1966.

"Extent and development of late syphilis according to autopsy statistics (1945-1965)," by G. Fromm, et al. DEUTSCH MED WSCHR. 92:1181-1185, June 30, 1967.

"Extra-and peri-genital chancre (2 cases)," by P. P. de Oliveira. AN BRASIL DERM. 43:273-276, December, 1968.

"Extremely severe hypersensitivity to antibiotics and its significance in the diagnosis of drug allery," by E. Hegyi. BRATISL LEK LISTY. 53:216-218, February, 1970.

"The FTA-ABS test," by C. H. Okey. J MAINE MED ASS. 57: 145-146, July, 1966.

"The FTA-ABS test for syphilis. Performance in 1,033 patients," by J. M. Knox, et al. BRIT J VENER DIS. 42:16-20, March, 1966.

"The F.T.A.-ABS test in the diagnosis of neurogenic bladder," by J. M. Harper, et al. J UROL. 97:862-863, May, 1967.

"The FTA-ABS test in late syphilis. A serological study in 1,985 cases," by R. E. Harner, et al. JAMA. 203: 545-548, February 19, 1968.

"FTA-ABS test in pregnancy. A probable false-positive reaction," by C. S. Buchanan, et al. ARCH DERM. 102:322-325, September, 1970.

"FTA and lysozyme," by A. Ribuffo, et al. MINERVA DERM. 42:433-434, August, 1967.

"F.T.A. in various stages of syphilis with the use of conjugated antigamma-globulin fractions," by P. Pagnes, et al. MINERVA DERM. 42:431-432, August, 1967.

"FTA test on dried blood. Quantitative evaluation," by S. Sartoris, et al. MINERVA DERM. 42:158-161, May, 1967.

"The FTA test on saliva," by S. Sartoris, et al. MINERVA DERM. 43:409-410, August, 1968.

"F.T.A. test with saliva in primo-secondary syphilis," by S. Sartoris, et al. MINERVA DERM. 43:23-26, January, 1968.

"Factors influencing the incidence of gonorrhoea and non-gonococcal urethritis in men in an industrial city," by L. Z. Oller, et al. BRIT J VENER DIS. 46:96-102, April, 1970.

"Factors influencing the spread of gonorrhea. I. Educational and social behavior," by L. Juhlin. ACTA DERMATOVENER. 48:75-81, 1968.

"Factors influencing the spread of gonorrhea. II. Sexual behavior at different ages," by L. Juhlin. ACTA DERMATOVENER. 48:82-89, 1968.

"Facts about venereal disease." BRIT MED J. 1:67-68, January, 1969.

"Failure of penicillin in a newborn with congenital syphilis," by J. B. Hardy, et al. JAMA. 212:1345-1349, May 25, 1970.

"Failure to control venereal disease." BRIT MED J. 1:447-448, February 21, 1970.

"Failure to control venereal disease," by A. King. BRIT MED J. 1:451-457, February 21, 1970.

"The false-negative treponema pallidum immobilization test in syphilis. Pseudobiologic false-positive syndrome," by J. L. Smith. JAMA. 199:128-129, January 9, 1967.

"False-positive reaction to VDRL test with prozone phenomena. Association with lymphosarcoma," by K. D. Wuepper, et al. JAMA. 195:868-869, March 7, 1966.

"False-positive reactions for syphilis. Serological abnormalities in relatives of chronic reactors," by D. L. Tuffanelli. ARCH DERM. 98:606-611, December, 1968.

"False positive reactions to the Reiter protein complement-fixation (RPCF) test," by L. Forstrom, et al. BRIT J VENER DIS. 45:126-128, June, 1969.

"False-positive serologic reactions induced by disinfectant," by R. W. Stevens, et al. AMER J CLIN PATH. 53:110, January, 1970.

"False-positive serological test for syphilis in pregnancy," by O. P. Salo, et al. ACTA DERMATOVENER. 49:332-335, 1969.

"False positive serology," by W. C. Peterson, Jr.. MINN MED. 52:1935-1936, December, 1969.

"False positive tests for syphilis." BRIT MED J. 2:394, May 13, 1967.

"Family physicians' role in the control of VD," by M. P. Vora. J INDIAN MED ASS. 46:370-373, April 1, 1966.

"The fate of gonococci in polymorphonuclear leucocytes," by P. J. Watt. J MED MICROBIOL. 3:501-509, August, 1970.

"Febrile Herxheimer reaction in different phases of primary and secondary syphilis," by T. Putkonen, et al. BRIT J VENER DIS. 42:181-184, September, 1966.

"Fetal infections with bacteria and protozoa," by H. Kraubig. MSCHR KINDERHEILK. 116:211-214, June, 1968.

"Fetal production of immunoglobulins in the course of congenital infections," by G. B. Serra, et al. MINERVA PEDIAT. 19:591-592, March 31, 1967.

"Fever following penicillin treatment as a symptom of syphilis," by K. Nordin, et al. LAKARTIDNINGEN. 63: 490-491, February 9, 1966.

"Fever therapy technique in syphilis and gonococcic infections," by H. W. Kendell, et al. ARCH PHYS MED.

50:603-608, October, 1969.

"Few notes on the prevention of venereal diseases," by F. Novotný. CESK DERM. 45:160-163, August, 1970.

"50 years of research work in the therapy of skin diseases and syphilis at the Faculty of Dermatology and Venereology of the I. M. Sechenov Moscow Medical Institute," by V. A. Rachmanov. CESK DERM. 42:361-367, December, 1967.

"Fifty years of V.D. service," BRIT MED J. 2:1344, December 3, 1966.

"Final report on the effectiveness of oxytetracycline in the treatment of gonorrhea in females," by L. H. Shapiro, et al. AMER J OBSTET GYNEC. 94:536-538, February 15, 1966.

"Findings and considerations on the behavior of C reactive protein in various stages of syphilitic infection," by M. De Luca, et al. G ITAL DERM. 109:109-116, March-April, 1968.

"Findings on changes in the complement activity of serums in dermatologic and syphilitic patients," by G. Cozza, et al. FOLIA ALLERG. 13:30-34, January-February, 1966.

"Findings on the management of syphilis in military personnel," by A. F. Giordano. REV SANID MILIT ARGENT. 67:38-44, January-June, 1968.

"Findings on trichomonas vaginitis--from the view of uterine cancer examination," by Y. Yokoyama, et al. SAISHIN IGAKU. 21:1585-1591, July, 1966.

"Fine structure of chromatic granules in trichomonas vaginalis Donne," by F. Filadoro. EXPERIENTIA. 26:213-214, 1970.

"First observations on the therapy of secondary syphilis with cephaloridine," by F. Flarer, et al. DIS NERV SYST. 27:271-277, September, 1966.

"The first venereologists," by R. S. Roberts. BRIT J VENER DIS. 45:58-60, March, 1969.

"5 years of mass serological examinations for syphilis in the province of Arezzo," by E. Ninu, et al. ANN SANIT PUBBLICA. 27:1071-1082, September-October, 1966.

"Five years of research on the treponematoses and venereal diseases," WHO CHRON. 24:53-60, February, 1970.

"5 years of studies on treponematoses and venereal diseases." PRENSA MED ARGENT. 57:585-591, May 22, 1970.

"Fixed eruption due to penicillin allergy," by W. L. Dennison, et al. ARCH DERM. 101:594-597, May, 1970.

"Flagyl in the therapy of trichomoniasis (results of a complex work)." VESTN DERM VENER. 40:88-92, November, 1966.

"Flocculation Venereal Diseases Research Laboratory reaction for lues after vaccination against variola," by S. Smálik, et al. VNITRNI LEK. 12:152-155, February, 1966.

"A fluorescence microscopic study of adsorption onto treponema pallidum of a heat-labile serum factor," by M. Metzger, et al. ARCH IMMUN THER EXP. 15:819-828, 1967.

"Fluorescence-serologic demonstration of an antibody against a heat-stable antigen of Reiter treponema, present in the sera of subjects with syphilis," by W. Bredt, et al. ARCH KLIN EXP DERM. 229:117-125, 1967.

"Fluorescence serologic differentiation of various antibodies directed against treponema pallidum," by F. Muller. KLIN WSCHR. 46:209-210, February 15, 1968.

"Fluorescence serological studies on the morphology of Reiter strain treponemas. 1. Demonstration of a heat unstable antigen in the terminal filaments," by W. Bredt. Z MED MIKROBIOL IMMUN. 153:116-121, 1967.

"Fluorescence serological studies on the morphology of Reiter strain treponemas. II. Demonstration of the cell membrane and localisation of group antigens," by W. Bredt. Z MED MIKROBIOL IMMUN. 153:122-128, 1967.

"Fluorescent antibody methods in the detection and control of venereal diseases. A bibliographical review of the literature," by Z. P. Mora. BRIT J VENER DIS. 45:23-32, March, 1969.

"Fluorescent antibody staining of treponemes in uveitis," by J. N. Goldman, et al. ARCH OPHTHAL. 79:716-722, June, 1968.

"Fluorescent-antibody techniques in the diagnosis of syphilis." LANCET. 2:327-328, August 6, 1966.

"Fluorescent antibody test for neonatal congenital syphilis: a progress report," by A. Scotti, et al. J PEDIAT. 75:1129-1134, December, 1969.

"The fluorescent antibody tissue stain in experimental ocular syphilis," by J. A. Wells, et al. ARCH OPHTHAL. 77:530-535, April, 1967.

"Fluorescent examinations of pupils and pupillary reactions in the early stages of syphilis," by A. V. Braitsev, et al. VESTN DERM VENER. 42:47-51, June, 1968.

"A fluorescent technique for demonstrating treponemes in films made from suspected chancres,"by M. F. Garner, et al. J CLIN PATH. 21:108-109, January, 1968.

"Fluorescent treponemal absorption and treponema pallidum immobilization tests in syphilitic patients and biologic false-positive reactors," by L. L. Bradford, et al. TECHN BULL REGIST MED TECHN. 37:59-66, March, 1967.

"Fluorescent treponemal antibodies in fractionated syphilitic sera. The immunoglobulin class," by W. G. Atwood, et al. ARCH DERM. 100:763-769, December, 1969.

"The fluorescent treponemal antibody-abosorption (FTA-ABS) test. Development, use and present status," by E. F. Hunter, et al. BULL WHO. 39:873-881, 1968.

"Fluorescent treponemal antibody-absorption (FTA-ABS) test for syphilis," by W. E. Deacon, et al. JAMA. 198: 624-628, November 7, 1966.

"Fluorescent treponemal antibody absorption (FTA-ABS) test in yaws," by M. F. Garner, et al. BRIT J VENER DIS. 46:284-286, August, 1970.

"The fluorescent treponemal antibody-absorption test (FTA-ABS) in treated latent and late syphilis," by L. Forstrom, et al. ACTA DERMATOVENER. 49:326-331, 1969.

"The fluorescent treponemal antibody absorption test for

syphilis: a comparison with the treponema pallidum immobilization test and the fluorescent treponemal antibody test," by M. F. Garner, et al. MED J AUST. 1:404-406, March 9, 1968.

"Fluorescent treponemal antibody-absorption test reactions in lupus erythematosus," by S. J. Kraus, et al. NEW ENG J MED. 282:1287-1290, June 4, 1970.

"Fluorescent treponemal-antibody absorption tests. Studies of false-positive reactions to tests for syphilis," by D. L. Tuffanelli, et al. NEW ENG J MED. 276:258-262, February 2, 1967.

"Fluorescent treponemal antibody (FTA) reaction in sera with antinuclear factors," by E. J. Jokinen, et al. ANN CLIN RES. 1:77-80, May, 1969.

"The fluorescent treponemal antibody (FTA-200) test in the serodiagnosis of syphilis," by M. F. Garner, et al. MED J AUST. 1:548-550, March 18, 1967.

"Fluorescent treponemal antibody inhibition test," by A. E. Wilkinson. BRIT J VENER DIS. 43:186-190, September, 1967.

"Fluorescent treponemal antibody test with antihuman immune sera of different specificity," by K. Király, et al. ACTA DERMATOVENER. 48:362-369, 1968.

"Fluorescent treponemal antibody tests. A summary and comparison," by J. Puffer, et al. CALIF MED. 104:166-167, March, 1966.

"Follicular papulopustular syphilid," by G. R. Mikhail, et al. ARCH DERM. 100:471-473, October, 1969.

"Follow-up of Reverin-treated patients in manifest, primary, secondary, tertiary and latent seropositive lues. IV," by V. Matanić. HAUTARZT. 17:121-123, March, 1966.

"For Syphilis Prevention Week," by T. Kawamura. J JAP MED ASS. 56:567-571, September 15, 1966.

"The formation of penicillin antigens," by A. L. De Weck. PROC ROY SOC MED. 61:894-897, September, 1968.

"40 years of dermato-venereological service in the Arkhangelsk region," by I. A. Lipskii, et al. VESTN DERM VENER. 40:63-66, November, 1966.

"Forward planning in the United Kingdom for anti-V.D. education," by A. J. Dalzell-Ward. BRIT J VENER DIS. 46:159-161, April, 1970.

"Four illustrious neuroluetics (Heinrich Heine, Jules De Goncourt, Alphonse Daudet, Guy de Maupassant)," by H. Heine, et al. PROC ROY SOC MED. 62:669-673, July 7, 1969.

"Frambesia in Indonesia (clinical manifestations and treatment)," by M. D. Tverskoi. VESTN DERM VENER. 43:59-67, September, 1969.

"Frequence of treponematosis in various populations in Bolivia," by P. Cirera, et al. BULL SOC PATH EXOT. 61:184-190, 1968.

"Frequency of human trichomoniasis in relation to the seasons," by M. J. Glewski. GYNEC PRAT. 15:227-238, 1964.

"From the dermatological literature of the USSR. II," by R. M. Bohnstedt. HAUTARZT. 17:481-484, November, 1966.

"From the diary of a regional ambulatory clinic for venereal diseases with special reference to the years 1956-1965," by W. DeWald. DEUTSCH GESUNDH. 21:1178-1181, June 23, 1966.

"From Ehrlich to Abraham," by P. Ehrlich, et al. HIPPOKRATES. 38:736-739, September 30, 1967.

"From the experience of the work of a dermatovenereologist in Yemen," by M. P. Vil'chinskii. VESTN DERM VENER. 40:82-85, July, 1966.

"Fructose in normal and pathological human semen," by G. Abelli, et al. ATTUALITA OSTET GINEC. 12:617-627, July-August, 1966.

"Fulminating meningitis with Waterhouse-Friderichsen syndrome due to Neisseria gonorrhoeae," by J. A. Swierczewski, et al. AMER J CLIN PATH. 54:202-204, August, 1970.

"Functional status of the liver in patients with congenital syphilis," by KhL Druian, et al. VRACH DELO. 1:145-146, January, 1966.

"Fundamental achievements of the Central Dermato-Venereal

Institute in the scientific study of venereal diseases," by A. A. Studnitsin, et al. VESTN DERM VENER. 45:3-8, December, 1969.

"Furazolidone in the therapy of trichomonas urethritis in men," by A. I. Poliakov, et al. VESTN DERM VENER. 40:70, July, 1966.

"Furazolidone in the therapy of trichomoniasis in men," by S. A. Artem'ev, et al. SOVIET MED. 29:128-130, October, 1966.

"Further experience with cephaloridine in gonorrhoea," by L. Z. Oller. POSTGRAD MED J. 43:Suppl 43:124-128, August, 1967.

"Further findings on the anti-treponemic action in vitro of cephalosporins," by F. Galla, et al. ANTIBIOTICA. 4:309-313, December, 1966.

"Further observations on the persistence of treponema pallidum after treatment in rabbits and humans," by A. R. Hobs, et al. BRIT J VENER DIS. 42:116-130, June, 1968.

"Further observations on strain sensitivity of trichomonas vaginalis to metronidazole," by J. A. McFadzean, et al. BRIT J VENER DIS. 45:161-162, June, 1969.

"Further statistical contribution on the relations between the Nelson-Mayer test and classical serological reactions (13000 cases)," by V. Resta, et al. MINERVA MED. 59:222-228, January 20, 1968.

"Further studies of an automated flocculation test for syphilis," by B. E. McGrew, et al. AMER J MED TECHN. 34:634-643, November, 1968.

"Further studies of the morphology of treponema pallidum under the electron microscope," by N. M. Ovcinnikov, et al. BRIT J VENER DIS. 45:87-116, June, 1969.

"Further studies of the sensitivity of gonococci to penicillin," by N. M. Ovcinnikov, et al. UROL NEFROL. 31:40-43, September-October, 1966.

"Further studies on the occurrence and treatment of trichomoniasis in connection with the problem of erosion of the cervix uteri," by J. Zawadzki. PRZEGL LEK. 22:689-694, 1966.

"Further study of ultrathin sections of treponema pallidum under the electron microscope," by N. M. Ovcinnikov, et al. BRIT J VENER DIS. 44:1-34, March, 1968.

"Gamma globulin and the treponema immobilization test," by A. K. Scherbakova, et al. VESTN DERM VENER. 40: 66-69, July, 1966.

"Gamma-M-fluorescent treponemal antibody in the diagnosis of congenital syphilis," by C. A. Alford, Jr., et al. NEW ENG J MED. 280:1086-1091, May 15, 1969.

"Gardner's syndrome with concomitant tertiary lues: report of case," by J. F. Welborn, et al. J ORAL SURG. 28: 131-133, February, 1970.

"Gastric syphilis: a case with pernicious anemia," by H. D. Frank, et al. CONN MED. 31:773-778, November, 1967.

"General paralysis and cerebral angiomatosis in a child. Apropos of a case," by H. Collomb, et al. BULL SOC MED AFR NOIRE LANG FRANC. 12:506-511, 1967.

"General paralysis in Victoria, Australia: historical study," by A. Stoller, et al. MED J AUST. 2:607-611, September 20, 1969.

"General paralysis of the insane with gumma of skull," by S. B. Mahapatra. BRIT J VENER DIS. 43:178-180, September, 1967.

"Genital and extragenital complications of trichomoniasis in men," by I. I. Iljin. DERM WSCHR. 154:294-300, March 30, 1968.

"Genital herpesvirus hominis infection: a venereal disease?," by S. Jeansson, et al. LANCET. 1:1064-1065, May 16, 1970.

"Genital infection in young delinquent girls," by E. Gallagher. BRIT J VENER DIS. 46:129-131, April, 1970.

"Genital infection with type 2 Herpes virus hominis. A commonly occurring venereal disease," by A. J. Nahmias, et al. BRIT J VENER DIS. 45:294-298,

December, 1969.

"Genital mycoplasma in pathology of the woman, fetus and neonate (literature review)," by M. A. Bashakova. VOP OKHR MATERIN DETS. 15:71-74, June, 1970.

"Genital mycoplasmosis in cattle and man," by R. S. Hirth, et al. J AMER VET MED ASS. 148:277-282, February 1, 1966.

"Genital trichomoniasis and conjugal sterility," by G. Nicora, et al. GYNEC PRAT. 19:309-327, 1968.

"Genital trichomoniasis in girls," by V. I. Rubnikov. VOP OKHR MATERIN DETS. 13:43-46, March, 1968.

"Genitourinary trichomoniasis," by F. Lillo. REV CHILE OBSTET GINEC. 33:367-374, 1968.

"Getting involved with V.D.," by J. A. Yacenda. J SCH HEALTH. 40:43-45, January, 1970.

"Glitisol in syphilis," by M. Spiezia. ANN MED NAV. 71: 247-252, March-April, 1966.

"Glossitis interstitialis luetica in the course of late congenital syphilis," by D. Niedzwiecka. PRZEGL DERM. 53:211-212, March-April, 1966.

"Gonoblenorrhea neonatorum in spite of Crede's preventive method," by P. Kober. MED KLIN. 62:424-426, March 17, 1967.

"Gonococcal arthritis," by A. H. Johnson. J S CAROLINA MED ASS. 66:74-76, March, 1970.

"Gonococcal arthritis," by A. B. Kirsner, et al. MOD TREATM. 6:1130-1139, September, 1969.

"Gonococcal arthritis," by I. Kushner. J INFECT DIS. 120:387-388, September, 1969; also in MED TIMES. 98:111-116, June, 1970.

"Gonococcal arthritis," by R. M. Poske, et al. GP. 39: 91-95, June, 1969.

"Gonococcal arthritis after treatment of gonorrhoea," by D. F. Marcus, et al. LANCET. 1:43-44, January 3, 1970.

"Gonococcal arthritis: a cause of monarticular disease,"

by J. H. Warner. J AMER COLL HEALTH ASS. 14:209-212, February, 1966.

"Gonococcal arthritis complicating gonorrheal pharyngitis," by A. L. Metzger. ANN INTERN MED. 73:267-269, August, 1970.

"Gonococcal arthritis in the newborn. Report of a case and review of the literature," by S. Glaser, et al. AMER J DIS CHILD. 112:185-188, September, 1966.

"Gonococcal arthritis in pregnancy," by J. H. Niles, et al. MED ANN DC. 35:69-70 passim, February, 1966.

"Gonococcal arthritis in pregnancy," by H. A. Taylor, et al. OBSTET GYNEC. 27:776-782, June, 1966.

"Gonococcal arthritis in pregnancy. Report of a case," by E. W. Parker, et al. N CAROLINA MED J. 28:433-436, October, 1967.

"Gonococcal arthritis in the young," by J. J. Calabro. NEW ENG J MED. 279:1002, October 31, 1968.

"Gonococcal arthritis with pericarditis," by W. M. Vietzke. ARCH INTERN MED. 117:270-272, February, 1966.

"Gonococcal bartholinitis," by E. Rees. BRIT J VENER DIS. 43:150-156, September, 1967.

"Gonococcal complement fixation reaction in patients with lung diseases in Greenland," by P. K. Lange, et al. UGESKR LAEG. 128:409-415, April 7, 1966.

"Gonococcal conjunctivitis of the newborn," by D. S. Friendly. CLIN PROC CHILD HOSP DC. 25:1-9, January, 1969.

"The gonococcal dermatitis syndrome. Demonstration of gonococci in skin lesions by immunofluorescence," by D. Danielsson, et al. ACTA DERMATOVENER. 46:256-261, 1966.

"Gonococcal diseases from the clinical and bacteriological viewpoint," by H. Modde, et al. SCHWEIZ MED WSCHR. 90:1242-1245, August 30, 1969.

"Gonococcal endocarditis with severe aortic regurgitation: Early valve replacement," by G. C. Voigt, et al. JOHNS HOPKINS MED J. 126:305-311, June, 1970.

"Gonococcal hemorrhagic bullae," by C. L. Roeth. NEW ENG J MED. 282:1105, May 7, 1970.

"Gonococcal infection in a prenatal clinic," by J. R. Waters, et al. AMER J OBSTET GYNEC. 103:532-536, February 15, 1969.

"Gonococcal infections," MED LETT DRUGS THER. 8:79-80, September 23, 1966.

"Gonococcal ophthalmia among newborn infants at Los Angeles County General Hospital, 1957-1963, by W. M. Brown, et al. PUBLIC HEALTH REP. 81:926-928, October, 1966.

"Gonococcal penile ulcer," by S. Haim, et al. BRIT J VENER DIS. 46:336-337, August, 1970.

"Gonococcal perihepatitis in a male. The Fitz-Hugh-Curtis syndrome," by M. W. Kimball, et al. NEW ENG J MED. 282:1082-1084, May 7, 1970.

"Gonococcal peritonitis in a prepubertal child," by G. L. Fuld. AMER J DIS CHILD. 115:621-622, May, 1968.

"Gonococcal resistance to penicillin," by H. Storck, et al. DERMATOLOGICA. 139:254-259, 1969.

"Gonococcal salpingitis," by E. Rees, et al. BRIT J VENER DIS. 45:205-215, September, 1969.

"Gonococcus sepsis," by M. Svanbom, et al. NORD MED. 84:988, July 30, 1970.

"Gonococcal skin lesions. Report of a case of gonococcal ecthyma," by J. M. Glicksman, et al. ARCH DERM. 96: 74-76, July, 1967.

"Gonococcal ulceration of the tongue in the gonococcal dermatitis syndrome," by L. Cowan. BRIT J VENER DIS. 45:228-231, September, 1969.

"Gonococcal urethritis in males in Vietnam: three penicillin regimens and one tetracycline regimen," by L. H. Maurer, et al. JAMA. 207:946-948, February 3, 1969.

"Gonococcal urethritis in Vietnam," by R. W. Dang. JAMA. 208:867, May 5, 1969.

"Gonococci in urethral exudates possess a virulence factor

lost on subculture," by M. E. Ward, et al. NATURE 227:382-384, July 25, 1970.

"Gonococcus sepsis," by M. Svanbom, et al. NORD MED. 84:988, July 30, 1970.

"Gonorrhoea." LANCET. 1:280-281, February, 1970.

"Gonorrhoea." LANCET. 1:675-676, March 30, 1968.

"Gonorrhoea," by R. S. Morton. LANCET. 1:824, April 13, 1968.

"Gonorrhoea," by E. Rees. LANCET. 1:572-573, March 14, 1970.

"Gonorrhea," by A. L. Schroeter, et al. ANN INTERN MED. 72:553-559, April, 1970.

"Gonorrhea-an alarming comeback." AM DRUGGIST. 157:37+, March 25, 1968.

"Gonorrhoea among prostitutes," by B. G. Wren. MED J AUST. 1:847-849, April 29, 1967.

"Gonorrhoea and the iceberg phenomenon," by W. J. Brown. BRIT J VENER DIS. 46:118-121, April, 1970.

"Gonorrhoea and the intrauterine contraceptive device," by R. Statham, et al. BRIT MED J. 4:623-625, December 7, 1968.

"Gonorrhoea and non-specific urethritis," by B. H. Hill. NEW ZEAL MED J. 69:198-204, April, 1969.

"Gonorrhea: arthritis, septicemia and cutaneous manifestations, a case report," by B. C. Frichot, 3d, et al. J OKLA MED ASS. 60:597-600, November, 1967.

"Gonorrhea during pregnancy," by G. W. Kraus, et al. OBSTET GYNEC. 31:258-260, February, 1968.

"Gonorrhea--frequently unrecognized reservoirs," by H. Pariser, et al. SOUTHERN MED J. 63:198-201, February, 1970.

"Gonorrhea getting out of control." AM DRUGGIST. 161: 49-50, April 6, 1970.

"Gonorrhea: growing menace to your students." SCH MGT. 12:36-42, August, 1968; also in PA SCH J. 117:414-

419, March, 1969.

"Gonorrhea in adult women," by V. Sebek. CESK GYNEK. 31:609-615, October, 1966.

"Gonorrhea in childhood," by R. Peter. CESK GYNEK. 31: 606-609, October, 1966.

"Gonorrhoea in a country town," by M J. Loughlin. NEW ZEAL MED J. 69:195-198, April, 1969.

"Gonorrhea in Czechoslovakia during the years 1960-1966," by K. Kopecký, et al. CESK EPIDEM. 17:356-363, October, 1968.

"Gonorrhoea in females treated with one oral dose of tetracycline," by D. G. McLone, et al. BRIT J VENER DIS. 44:218-219, September, 1968.

"Gonorrhoea in 1964. Cases treated at the Department of Dermatology, Karoliska Sjukhuset," by A. Lodin, et al. ACTA DERMATOVENER. 46:245-249, 1966.

"Gonorrhoea in 1966. Cases treated at the Department of Dermatology, Karolinska Sjukhuset, by L. Gip, et al. ACTA DERMATOVENER. 48:272-276, 1968.

"Gonorrhoea in 1968," by L. Molin. ACTA DERMATOVENER. 50:157-160, 1970.

"Gonorrhea in the obstetric and gynecologic clinic. Incidence in a voluntary hospital in an urban community," by V. G. Cave, et al. JAMA. 210:309-311, October 13, 1969.

"Gonorrhea in the obstetric clinic," by D. S. Friendly. JAMA. 211:124, January 5, 1970.

"Gonorrhea in recent years," by H. Okuma. JAP J UROL. 58:937, September, 1967.

"Gonorrhea-like urethritis due to Mima polymorpha var oxidens. Patient summary and bacteriological study," by W. R. Kozub, et al. ARCH INTERN MED. 122:514-516, December, 1968.

"Gonorrhea: the minimum effective dose," by R. H. Meade, 3d. NEW ENG J MED. 283:42-43, July 2, 1970.

"Gonorrhea--a new look at an old problem," by C. Lindman. J MAINE MED ASS. 61:162-163, August, 1970.

"Gonorrhea: not yet controllable," by W. J. Brown. ANN INTERN MED. 72:280-281, February, 1970.

"Gonorrhoea of a congenital duct in the raphe penis," by H. Diabalová, et al. ACTA DERMATOVENER. 49:202-205, 1969.

"Gonorrhea: the office management of acute infections," by L. Davis. CALIF MED. 107:4-7, July, 1967.

"The gonorrhea problem. 2-years data," by H. B. Svindland. T NORSK LAEGEFOREN. 24:2252-2255, December 15, 1968.

"Gonorrhea--a public-health problem." J IOWA MED SOC. 57:376-377, April, 1967.

"The gonorrhea situation in Greenland and the epidemiological control of this disease," by G. Lomholt. ARCH KLIN EXP DERM. 227:644-655, 1966.

"Gonorrhoea situation in South Greenland in the summer of 1964," by G. Lomholt, et al. BRIT J VENER DIS. 42: 1-7, March, 1966.

"Gonorrhoea study, 1966." BRIT J VENER DIS. 44:55-62, March, 1968.

"Gonorrhoea study, 1967," by British Cooperative Clinical Group. BRIT J VENER DIS. 44:299-306, December, 1968.

"Gonorrhoea study, 1968," by British Cooperative Clinical Group. BRIT J VENER DIS. 46:62-68, February, 1970.

"Gonorrhea therapy with a combination of probenecid and benzylsodiumpenicillin. A report from Greenland," by G. A. Olsen, et al. UGESKR LAEG. 130:1465-1468, September 5, 1968.

"Gonorrhoea treated by a combination of probenecid and sodium penicillin G," by G. A. Olsen, et al. BRIT J VENER DIS. 45:144-148, June, 1969.

"Gonorrhea. A treatment problem," by N. H. Dyer, et al. W VIRGINIA MED J. 64:182-183, May, 1968.

"Gonorrhoea, trichomoniasis and yeast infection in late pregnancy in an unselected series of gravidae," by E. Purola, et al. ANN CHIR GYNAEC FENN. 56:95-98, 1967.

"Gonorrhoea with skin and joint manifestations," by C.
B. Wolff, et al. BRIT MED J. 1:271-273, May 2,
1970.

"Gonorrheal abscess of preputium as a late complication
of gonorrheal urethritis," by M. Skencić SRPSKI ARH
CELOK LEK. 97:805-809, July-August, 1969.

"Gonorrheal and non-gonorrheal urethritis," by J. Bonelli,
et al. HOSPITAL. 70:921-935, October, 1966.

"Gonorrheal arthritis," by J. Grossman. NEW ENG J MED.
279:721, September 26, 1968.

"Gonorrheal arthritis. Report of a case in pregnancy
with negative GR in serum and positive GR in the synovial fluid," by A. Nielsen. UGESKR LAEG. 130:1867-1868, October 31, 1968.

"Gonorrheal conjunctivitis an old disease returned," by
T. Hansen, et al. JAMA. 195:1156, March 28, 1966.

"Gonorrhoeal frequency continues to increase. The importance of medical factors," by S. Liden. LAKARTIDNINGEN. 66:907-911, February 26, 1969.

"Gonorrheal pharyngitis," by N. J. Fiumara, et al. NEW
ENG J MED. 276:1248-1250, June 1, 1967.

"Gonorrheal reinfections among men treated at the dispensary of the Department of Dermatology in Cracow
in 1962-1967," by I. Prorok. PRZEGL DERM. 56:735-739, 1969.

"Gonorrheal urethritis in males treated with one oral
dose of ampicillin," by D. G. McLone, et al. SOUTHERN MED J. 61:278-280, March, 1968.

"Gonorrhoeal urethritis in males treated with one oral
dose of oxytetracycline," by D. G. McLone, et al.
BRIT J VENER DIS. 43:166-167, September, 1967.

"Gonorrheal urethritis in males treated with a single
oral dose of minocycline," by R. W. Thatcher, et al.
PUBLIC HEALTH REP. 85:160-162, February, 1970.

"Granuloma inguinale," by W. P. Hogarth, et al. CANAD
MED ASS J. 94:916-917, April 22, 1966.

"Granuloma inguinale," by S. Peck. ARCH DERM. 98:555-557, November, 1968.

"Granuloma inguinale. A clinical, histological and ultrastructural study," by C. M. Davis. JAMA. 211:632-636, January 26, 1970.

"Granuloma inguinale. Report of a case in California with notes on pathogenesis," by W. M. Gould, et al. CALIF MED. 104:392-395, May, 1966.

"Granuloma inguinale: an ultrastructural study of Calymmatobacterium granulomatis," by C. M. Davis, et al. J INVEST DERM. 53:315-321, November, 1969.

"Granuloma venereum," by O. I. Haavelsrud. T NORSK LAEGERFOREN. 88:2121-2122, November 15, 1968.

"Granuloma venereum in an 81-year-old man," by U. Brauer, et al. DERM WSCHR. 152:780-784, July 23, 1966.

"A graphic guide for clinical management of latent syphilis," by A. J. Pereyra, et al. ARIZONA MED. 27:13-18, May, 1970; also in: NORTHWEST MED. 69:Suppl:13-18, May, 1970.

"Grave form of trichomoniasis and lambliasis," by N. Mosora, et al. MED INTERN. 18:857-864, July, 1966.

"Group antibodies in fluorescent treponemal antibody (FTA) test," by K. Kiraly, et al. J INVEST DERM. 48:98-100, January, 1967.

"The growing menace of VD," by V. Block. PARENTS'. 45:86+, November, 1970.

"Guide to adequate treatment of gonorrhoea complicated by staphylococcus albus," by R. L. Tawes, Jr. BRIT J VENER DIS. 42:155-161, September, 1966.

"Guiding principles for the treatment of early syphilis," by K. Mach. WIEN KLIN WSCHR. 79:97-99, February 10, 1967.

"Gumma of the choroid," by F. Soukup. CESK OFTAL. 24:438-441, November, 1968.

"Gumma of the shoulder joint," by J. Singh, et al. J INDIAN MED ASS. 48:592-593, June 16, 1967.

"Gumma of the vocal cord. (Clinical record)," by H. K. Ismail. J LARYNG. 80:638-639, June, 1966.

"Gummata of tuberculous appearance in an 80-year-old syph-

ilitic woman. Syphilo-tuberculous hybrid?," by E.
Hadida, et al. BULL SOC FRANC DERM SYPH. 73:406-
407, July-August, 1966.

"Gummous syphilis of the penis refractory to penicillin
and bismuth preparations," by A. I. Levykin. VESTN
DERM VENER. 43:82-86, January, 1969.

"Gynecologists and cases of gonorrhea," by L. Nilsson.
LAKARTIDNINGEN. 65:1090-1091, March 13, 1968.

"Haemagglutination test utilizing pathogenic treponema
pallidum for the sero-diagnosis of syphilis," by T.
Rathlev. BRIT J VENER DIS. 43:181-185, September,
1967.

"Hair root status in secondary lues," by W. Kostanecki,
et al. Z HAUT GESCHLECHTSKR. 41:380-382, November 15,
1966.

"Hamburg dermatologic society. 3. Practice forum on 17-
9-1966 on board the motor boat 'Tom Kyle'," by A.
Wiskemann. DERM WSCHR. 153:1097-1101, September 30,
1967.

"Hanson's multineuritis in a syphilitic," by P. Warot,
et al. LILLE MED. 14:558-562, 1969.

"Has the clinical picture of tabes dorsalis changed due
to therapy," by H. Ley, et al. MUNCHEN MED WSCHR.
110:1924-1930, August 30, 1968.

"The hazards of Crede's prophylaxis of neonatal blennorrhea," by V. J. Mathesius. GYNAECOLOGIA. 164:274-
278, 1967.

"Health education and spreading of venereal diseases a-
mong youth," by L. Dyskin, et al. PRZEGL DERM. 55:
273-280, May-June, 1968.

"Health education and venereal disease." BRIT MED J.
1:493-494, February 25, 1967.

"Health education and venereal disease," by R. S. Morton.
NURSING TIMES. 63:957+, July 21, 1967.

"Health education by public health nurses as a preventive

measure against venereal diseases," by K. Imazu, et al. JAP J NURS ART. 8:21-25, August, 1969.

"Health in a rural hippie commune," by D. L. Palmer, et al. JAMA. 213:1307-1310, August 24, 1970.

"Health knowledge of prostitutes in Saigon, Vietnam. A study of health attitudes and habits relating to venereal diseases taken from a group of prostitutes," by R. S. Marcondes, et al. REV SAUDE PUBLICA. 1:18-23, June, 1967.

"Health of immigrants," by F. J. Kinsella. PROC ROY SOC MED. 61:23, January, 1968.

"Hemagglutinating anti-penicillin antibodies (HAPA). Incidence and significance in four groups of patients," by W. Q. Ascari, et al. TRANSFUSION. 9:35-39, January-February, 1969.

"Hemagglutination tests for diagnosis of syphilis. A preliminary report," by T. Tomizawa. JAP J MED SCI BIOL. 19:305-308, December, 1966.

"Hematuria in congenital lues," by J. Szabó, et al. SCHWEIZ MED WSCHR. 96:1446-1450, October 29, 1966.

"Hemiplegia following 1st injection of penicillin in a patient with secondary relapsing syphilis," by L. Ciecierski, et al. POL TYG LEK. 25:145-147, January 26, 1970.

"Hemodynamic study of aortic valvular cardiopathies by the isotope dilution curve," by J. Di Matteo, et al. ARCH MAL COEUR. 60:1061-1085, August, 1967.

"Hemolytic anemia caused by penicillin," JAMA. 204:635, May 13, 1968.

"Hemolytic anemia caused by penicillin. Report of a case by penicillin. Report of a case in which anti-penicillin antibodies crossreacted with cephalothin sodium," by L. W. Nesmith. JAMA. 203:27-30, January 1, 1968.

"Hemorrhagic bullae in gonococcemia," by A. B. Ackerman. NEW ENG J MED. 282:793-794, April 2, 1970.

"Hepatitis as a complication of early syphilis," by P. Davidoff. DAPIM REFUIIM. 24:530-533, December, 1965.

"Herpes genitalis," by D. C. Hutfield. BRIT J VENER DIS. 44:241-250, September, 1968.

"Herpes genitalis in Ibadan," by A. O. Osoba, et al. WEST AFR MED J. 19:117-119, August, 1970.

"Herpes progenitalis," by W. Minkin, et al. JAMA. 203:526, February 12, 1968.

"Herpesvirus cervicitis with gonorrhoea," by D. C. Hutfield. LANCET. 1311:1312, June 15, 1968.

"Herpesvirus hominis infection of the cervix associated with gonorrhoea," by J. O. Beilby, et al. LANCET. 1:1065-1066, May 18, 1968.

"Herxheimer-Lukasiewicz reaction after injection of debecillin in early acquired syphilis," by E. Peisert, et al. POL TYG LEK. 22:344-347, March 6, 1967.

"Herxheimer's reaction. Asymptomatic neurosyphilis treated with penicillin," by H. A. Podesta, et al. PRENSA MED ARGENT. 54:301-304, April 14, 1967.

"Herxheimer's reaction in maternal milk in early congenital syphilis," by R. Rollier, et al. BULL SOC FRANC DERM SYPH. 74:178-180, 1967.

"High dosage procaine penicillin combined with ampicillin in the treatment of gonorrhoea after failure with standard procaine penicillin dosage," by J. L. Fluker, et al. BRIT J VENER DIS. 45:317-320, December, 1969.

"High titer of Wassermann antibodies in a case of advanced myelomatosis," by A. B. Laurell, et al. ACTA DERMATOVENER. 46:406-411, 1966.

"Highest venereal disease rates for United States and Georgia in younger age groups," J MED ASS GEORGIA. 56:300-302, July, 1967.

"Higoumenakis's sign and its significance for the diagnosis of congenital syphilis," by K. G. Higoumenakis. DERM WSCHR. 154:697-705, July 27, 1968.

"Histochemical studies of syphilids during treatment with bicillin-4 and bicillin-6," by A. A. Akovbian, et al. VESTN DERM VENER. 42:38-41, December, 1968.

"Histologic structure of the lymph node of recent syphilis," by A. Bazex, et al. BULL SOC FRANC DERM SYPH. 75:140-143, 1968.

"Histopathologic demonstration of spirochetes in the human eye," by E. N. Montenegro, et al. AMER J OPHTHAL. 67:335-346, March, 1969.

"Histopathologic studies of the vaginal mucosa in chronic trichomoniasis," by J. Plonski, et al. GINEK POL. 38:887-892, August, 1967.

"Histopathology of serpiginous skin lesions in late syphilis (lues tubero-ulcero-serpiginosa)," by K. Lejman, et al. PRZEGL DERM. 53:419-423, July-August, 1966.

"History of herpes genitalis," by D. C. Hutfield. BRIT J VENER DIS. 42:263-268, December, 1966.

"History--venereal diseases." NEW ENGLAND NURS J. 61: 18+, April, 1968.

"Hoigne syndrome - nonallergic reaction to depot penicillin," by M. Ondrejicka, et al. BRATISL LEK LISTY. 52:703-708, 1969.

"Homosexual practice and venereal disease." BRIT MED J. 2:5-6, April 1, 1967.

"Homosexuality among syphilitic patients," by I. Rácz. BRIT J VENER DIS. 46:117, April, 1970.

"Homosexuality and its relation to venereal disease," by I. Rácz. ORV HETIL. 110:2146-2149, September 14, 1969.

"Homosexuality as seen in a New Zealand city practice," by E. Philipp. NEW ZEAL MED J. 67:397-401, March, 1968.

"Homosexuality--a current venereological problem?," by F. Schiller, et al. DERM WSCHR. 153:1161-1165, October,21, 1967.

"Homosexually-acquired venereal disease," by F. J. Jefferiss. BRIT J VENER DIS. 42:46-47, March, 1966.

"Homosexuals and venereal diseases," by D. F. Contreras. ACTAS DERMOSIF. 59:467-470, July-August, 1968.

"Hormonal function of the ovary in genitourinary trichomoniasis according to the urocytogram," by V. I.

Kleban. PEDIAT AKUSH GINEK. 5:49-51, September-October, 1966.

"How can venereal disease care be improved?," by V. Starck. LAKARTIDNINGEN. 65:2356-2359, June 5, 1968.

"How can we get doctors genuinely concerned about the VD problem," by W. L. Porter. MED TIMES. 94:1218-1219, October, 1966.

"How could this happen to our daughter?," by L. David. GOOD H. 169:86-87+, September, 1969.

"How is initial syphilis mistreated?," by G. Solente. PRESSE MED. 75:1656, July 1, 1967.

"How much does an inadequate syphilis control program cost a country?," by A. E. Callin. SALUD PUBLICA MEX. 10:611-614, September-October, 1968.

"How to interpret the serologic reactions to lipid antigens in syphilis and outside of it," by J. Delacrétaz. PRAXIS. 55:1497-1498, December 22, 1966.

"How to plan a program for VD education," by F. B. Benell. NATIONS SCH. 77:72-73+, February, 1966.

"Hutchinson's syndrome," OTOLARYNGOLOGY. 39:1299, December, 1967.

"Hutchinson's teeth," by B. J. Lawson. ORAL SURG. 24: 635-636, November, 1967.

"Hypeparathyreosis of syphilitic etiology in a patient with tertiary syphilis," by B. S. Pankov. VESTN DERM VENER. 40:51-54, April, 1966.

"Hypersensitivity and toxicity of the beta-lactam antibiotics," by G. T. Stewart. POSTGRAD MED J. 43:31-36, August, 1967.

"Hypokalaemia, metabolic alkalosis, and hypernatraemia due to 'massive' sodium penicillin therapy," by F. P. Brunner, et al. BRIT MED J. 4:550-552, November 30, 1968.

"Iatrogenic errors in the management of dermatovenereal diseases," by H. Rockl, et al. MUNCHEN MED WSCHR. 110:2010-2015, September 6, 1968.

"Iatrogenic infections and hazards in venerology," by Z. Somogyi. ORV HETIL. 107:2371-2373, December 11, 1966.

"Iatrogenic venereological complaints," by W. K. Bernfeld. BRIT J VENER DIS. 44:82, March, 1968.

"Identification of the asymptomatic female carrier of N. gonorrhoeae. Treatment with ampicillin," by E. S. Allen. BRIT J VENER DIS. 46:334-335, August, 1970.

"Identification of Neisseria gonorrhoeae by means of fluorescent antibody technique," by I. Lind. ACTA PATH MICROBIOL SCAND. 70:613-629, 1967.

"The identification of sarcoid granulomas in the nervous system," by W. J. Williams. PROC ROY SOC MED. 60: 1170-1172, November 1, 1967.

"The illness of Poliziano," by L. Szodoray. ORV HETIL. 109:771, April 7, 1968.

"Immediate and remote results of the treatment of male trichomonas infections with trichomonas vaccine," by L. M. Korik, et al. VESTN DERM VENER. 42:80-84, March, 1968.

"Immediate and remote results of the treatment of syphilis with antibiotics alone and in combination with bismuth," by G. B. Nesterenko, et al. VESTN DERM VENER. 43:37-40, May, 1969.

"Immediate and remote results of the treatment of urogenital trichomoniasis with flagyl (metronidazole)," by B. A. Teokharov, et al. VESTN DERM VENER. 41:52-58, April, 1967.

"Immediate reaction to penicillin. Association with penicilloyl-specific skin-sensitizing antibodies and low titers of blocking (IgG) antibodies," by M. J. Fellner, et al. JAMA. 202:909-911, November 27, 1967.

"Immediate results of treating patients with contagious forms of syphilis using simultaneously penicillin and bismuth preparations," by T. V. Vasil'ev, et al. VESTN DERM VENER. 44:50-55, April, 1970.

"Immigrants and venereal disease." BRIT MED J. 3:129-130, July 19, 1969.

"Immigration and venereal disease in Great Britain," by R. R. Willcox. BRIT J VENER DIS. 42:225-237, December, 1966.

"Immobilization of certain cultured treponemes in sera from syphilitic humans," by W. J. Guest, et al. J BACT. 93:1190-1191, March, 1967.

"Immobilizing antibodies to treponema pallidum in the cerebrospinal fluid in syphilis," by F. Muller. GERMAN MED MONTHLY. 12:120-124, March, 1967.

"Immunochemical mechanisms of penicillin induced Coombs positivity and hemolytic anemia in man," by B. Levine, et al. INT ARCH ALLERG. 31:594-606, 1967.

"Immunity in experimental syphilis. V. The immunogenicity of treponema pallidum attenuated by gamma-irradiation," by J. N. Miller. J IMMUN. 99:1012-1016, November, 1967.

"Immunization in the control of syphilis," BRIT MED J. 4:597, December 7, 1968.

"Immunobiological reactivity of chicks to treponema anserinum Sakharoff 1891," by I. Djankov, et al. ZBL VETERINAERMED. 14:677-681, November, 1967.

"Immunochemical characterization of aqueous ether extracted endotoxin from Neisseria gonorrhoeae," by J. A. Maeland. ACTA PATH MICROBIAL SCAND. 76:484-492, 1969.

"Immunochemical mechanisms in penicillin allergies," by M. Ledvina, et al. CAS LEK CESK. 109:138-146, February, 1970.

"Immunoelectrophoresis and simple radial immuno-diffusion tests of saliva of subjects with syphilis in the primary and secondary phases," by M. Pippione, et al. MINERVA DERM. 43:543, October, 1968.

"Immunoelectrophoretic pattern of Wassermann reagin and comparison of the appearance time between RPCF and FTA antibodies," by K. Kakusul. JAP J BACT. 24:28-36, January, 1969.

"Immunoelectrophoretic study of biological false positive

serum reactions for syphilis," by K. Kiraly, et al. ACTA DERMATOVENER. 46:506-510, 1966.

"Immunofluorescence anticomplement: Analysis of the antibodies reacting with treponema pallidum," by J. Pillot, et al. C R ACAD SCI. 265:1769-1772, November 27, 1967.

"Immunofluorescence demonstration of antibodies in urogenital trichomoniasis. A preliminary report," by J. Kramar, et al. J HYG EPIDEM. 10:85-88, November 1, 1966.

"Immunofluorescence in biological diagnosis. Its application to the serology of syphilis after adsorption of nonspecific antibodies by ultrasonicated Reiter treponema," by A. Fribourg-Blanc, et al. BIOL MED. 55:235-252, May-June, 1966.

"Immunofluorescence in tubes. Application to serologic study of syphilis," by P. Rimbaud, et al. BULL SOC FRANC DERM SYPH. 76:38-40, 1969.

"An immunofluorescence method for the diagnosis of primary syphilis using an absorption technique," by M. F. Garner, et al. J CLIN PATH. 21:576-577, September, 1968.

"The immunofluorescence reaction in syphilis," by N. M. Ovchinnikov, et al. VESTN DERM VENER. 40:59-63, July, 1966.

"The immunofluorescence reaction of the blood serum of syphilitic patients following therapy with various durable penicillin preparations," by T. V. Vasil'ev, et al. VESTN DERM VENER. 40:40-45, August, 1966.

"Immuno-fluorescence technic for treponema after adsorption of non-specific antibodies with Reiter's ultrasonicate in the diagnosis of syphilis. Apropos of 40000 sera," by A. Fribourg-Blanc, et al. BULL SOC FRANC DERM SYPH. 74:328-339, 1967.

"The immunofluorescence technic of gonococcus determination," by C. Simon, et al. MUNCHEN MED WSCHR. 109: 856-859, April 14, 1967.

"The immunofluorescence test (FTA-200) in the diagnosis of syphilis. Preliminary note," by A. Rocha, et al. HOSPITAL. 70:617-624, September, 1966.

"The immunofluorescence test for diagnosis of syphilis (FTA-200) performed with sera from lepromatous patients," by R. D. Azulay, et al. HOSPITAL. 71:79-85, January, 1967.

"The immunofluorescence test used in diagnosis of syphilis," by P. Latourelle, et al. MARSEILLE MED. 103:531-535, 1966.

"The immunofluorescence test with the blood serum of syphilitic patients after treatment with various durable preparations of penicillin," by T. V. Vasil'ev, et al. VESTN DERM VENER. 40:40-45, August, 1966.

"Immunofluorescent antibody technique in the diagnosis of gonorrhoea by direct smears from the female," by J. M. Gallwey, et al. BRIT J VENER DIS. 43:168-169, September, 1967.

"Immunofluorescent detection of treponema pallidum: a review," by D. S. Kellogg, Jr., et al. JAMA. 207:938-941, February 3, 1969.

"Immunofluorescent method for diagnosis of gonorrhoea in women," by R. N. Thin. BRIT J VENER DIS. 46:27-30, February, 1970.

"Immunofluorescent reaction in the diagnosis of syphilis," by L. A. D'iachenko. VESTN DERM VENER. 42:38-42, 1968.

"Immunogenic properties of the protein component of treponema pallidum," by M. Metzger, et al. BRIT J VENER DIS. 45:299-304, December, 1969.

"Immunoglobulin class and light chain type of human antibodies. Studies with anti-gammaG, -gammaM, -gammaA-globulin, -beta 1CA, E-globulins and anti-kappa, -lambda chains reagents," by T. Matuhasi, et al. JAP J EXP MED. 36:407-421, August, 1966.

"Immunoglobulins in congenital syphilis: analysis with fluorescein-labeled antigammaglobulin fractions," by M. Lospalluti, et al. G ITAL DERM. 45:184-185, March, 1970.

"Immunoglobulins in syphilis," by J. J. Delhanty, et al. LANCET. 2:1099-1103, November 22, 1969.

"Immunoglobulins of cerebrospinal fluid in syphilis," by V. A. Oxelius, et al. BRIT J VENER DIS. 45:121-125,

June, 1969.

"Immunohemolytic anemia following penicillin," by W. Straub. SCHWEIZ MED WSCHR. 97:1294, September 30, 1967.

"Immunologic aspects of congenital syphilis," by F. Aiuti, et al. HELV PAEDIAT ACTA. 21:66-71, April, 1966.

"Immunologic aspects of pinta," by A. P. Goncalves. DERMATOLOGICA. 135:199-204, 1967.

"Immunologic examinations for the diagnosis of fatal shock caused by penicillin," by A. Franchini, et al. MED LEG DOMM CORPOR. 3:160-168, April-June, 1970.

"Immunologic response of the fetus in congenital syphilis," by B. J. Fogel, et al. J FLORIDA MED ASS. 56:777-799, October, 1969.

"The immunologic response of goats to normal and syphilitic rabbit testicular tissue," by J. N. Miller, et al. J IMMUN. 97:184-188, August, 1966.

"Immunologic responses and 'altered reactivity' in syphilis," by D. H. Short, et al. ANN ALLERG. 24:430-436, August, 1966.

"Immunologic studies in a patient sensitive to tetracycline and penicillin," by M. J. Fellner, et al. ARCH KLIN EXP DERM. 224:157-167, February 3, 1966.

"Immunological and immunochemical investigations of patients suffering from general paralysis," by H. Schmidt, et al. BRIT J VENER DIS. 46:135-137, April, 1970.

"Immunological study on cardiolipin from Escherichia coli," by Y. Kanemasa. ACTA MED OKAYAMA. 22:241-249, October, 1968.

"Immunology, clinical features and therapy of penicillin allergy," by G. Filipp. MED WELT. 50:2763-2773, December 14, 1968.

"Immunology of syphilis," by G. R. Cannefax, et al. ANN REV MED. 18:471-482, 1967.

"Implications of spiral forms in the eye," by B. Golden, et al. SURVEY OPHTHAL. 14:179-183, November, 1969.

"Importance and epidemiological characteristics of venereal disease," by W. J. Brown. BOL OFIC SANIT PANAMER. 60:93-106, February, 1966.

"Importance of the anti-complement immunofluorescence technic in serodiagnosis of experimental treponomatoses in various animal species," by A. Vaisman, et al. BULL SOC FRANC DERM SYPH. 74:803-806, 1967.

"The importance of the fluorescent antibody technic (FAT) as a control of questionable Wassermann reactions in pregnancy," by I. Piacentini. FRACASTORO. 59:615-618, September-October, 1966.

"The importance of health education in the prevention of venereal diseases," by E. Sulutiu. MUNCA SANIT. 17:745-747, December, 1969.

"Importance of homosexuals and bisexuals in the epidemiology of syphilis," by W. B. Neser, et al. SOUTHERN MED J. 62:177-180, February, 1969.

"Importance of mass colpocytological examination in the diagnosis of uterine tumors in preclinical phases, of vaginal trichomoniasis and of prolonged pregnancy," by S. DeLeo, et al. MINERVA MED. 58:2821-2822, August 11, 1967.

"The importance of organized prophylaxis in the control of trichomoniasis," by J. Kiss. ORV HETIL. 107:2229-2231, November 20, 1966.

"Importance of serologically positive syphilis in Madagascar," by L. Mathurin, et al. MED TROP. 27:618-628, November-December, 1967.

"Importance of serology for the clinician," by J. Orfila. MAROC MED. 45:204-210, March, 1966.

"The importance of the treponema pallidum immobilization test in ophthalmology," by Z. Kumstat, et al. CESK OFTAL. 22:182-186, May, 1966.

"Improved medium selective for cultivation of N. gonorrhea and N. meningitidis," by J. D. Thayer, et al. PUBLIC HEALTH REP. 81:559-562, June, 1966.

"Improved methods for gonococcal sampling and examination on a large scale," by B. Gastrin, et al. ACTA PATH MICROBIOL SCAND. 74:362-370, 1968.

"Improved methods of contact tracing," by B. Muspratt, et al. BRIT J VENER DIS. 43:204-208, September, 1967; also in: CESK DERM. 45:184-186, August, 1970.

"Improvement of culture media of trichomonas for rapid diagnosis," by R. G. Capet. CANAD J PUBLIC HEALTH. 59:201-203, May, 1968.

"In memory of Professor Paruir Gavrilovich Oganesian." VESTN DERM VENER. 41:93, June, 1967.

"In relation to the article by V. N. Ivanov: 'Remote results of preventive treatment of children born of mothers suffering from or having sustained syphilis', (Vestn Derm Vener No. 1, 1969)," by I. G. Bal'barer. VESTN DERM VENER. 43:63-64, November, 1969.

"In a specialist's office," by A. Skriver. T SYGEPL. 67:217-221, May, 1967.

"In vitro activity of twelve antibacterial agents against Neisseria gonorrhoeae," by I. Phillips, et al. LANCET 1:263-265, February 7, 1970.

"In-vitro comparison of erythromycin, lincomycin, and clindamycin," by L. Phillips, et al. BRIT MED J. 2:89-90, April 11, 1970.

"In vitro susceptibility of Neisseria gonorrhoeae to different antibiotics," by C. W. Halverson, et al. MILIT MED. 134:1427-1429, November, 1969.

"In vitro susceptibility of Neisseria gonorrhoeae to nine antimicrobial agents," by J. E. Martin, Jr., et al. APPL MICROBIOL. 18:21-23, July, 1969.

"Inactivation of penicillins by carbohydrate solutions at alkaline pH," by M. S. Simberkoff, et al. NEW ENG J MED. 283:116-119, July 16, 1970.

"Incidence and pathomorphosis of congenital syphilis in the last 20 years," by D. Mazzacuva, et al. CLIN PEDIAT. 49:3-16, January, 1967.

"Incidence and role of mycoplasma in urogenital diseases," by A. Stangalini, et al. MINERVA GINEC. 21:1701-1706, December 31, 1969.

"Incidence of bacterial causes of ophthalmia neonatorum," by J. A. Kagwa-Nyanzi. E AFR MED J. 47:159-162,

March, 1970.

"Incidence of biologic false positive syphilis reactions among pregnant women," by K. Loe. T NORSK LAEGEFOREN. 86:1728-1731, December 15, 1966.

"Incidence of biological false-positive reactions in serological tests for syphilis in 6737 patients with various dermatoses," by E. A. Johansson, et al. ANN CLIN RES. 2:32-41, March, 1970.

"Incidence of cutaneous manifestations of syphilis," by S. B. Mandal. INDIAN J DERM. 11:123-124, July, 1966.

"Incidence of gonococci relatively resistant to penicillin occurring in the Southamptom area of England during 1958 to 1965," by R. M. Warren. BRIT J VENER DIS. 44:80-81, March, 1968.

"Incidence of immediate systemic penicillin reactions," by W. Minkin, et al. MILIT MED. 133:557-560, July, 1968.

"The incidence of lues," by C. H. Beek. NEDERL T GENEESK. 112:614-616, March 30, 1968.

"Incidence of neurosyphilis and its clinical forms in Sao Paulo," by E. Zukerman, et al. REV PAUL MED. 70:270-274, June, 1967.

"Incidence of reactive VDRL tests in the normal rabbit," by J. S. Pannu, et al. BRIT J VENER DIS. 43:114-116, June, 1967.

"The incidence of trichomonas vaginalis in cases of preinvasive and invasive cervical cancer. Relationship between cervical cancer and trichomonas vaginalis," by O. Berggren. LAKARTIDNINGEN. 64:3335-3340, August 31, 1967.

"Incidence of venereal and skin diseases among the population of the town of Stupino, Moscow region," by E. I. A. Filina. VESTN DERM VENER. 40:62-65, January, 1966.

"The incidence of venereal diseases in India and their control," by V. K. Tatochenko. VESTN DERM VENER. 41:72-77, September, 1967.

"Incidence of venereal diseases in the Netherlands," by H. Bijkerk. BRIT J VENER DIS. 46:247-261, June, 1970.

"Incomplete pachydermoperiostosis," by J. A. Savin. PROC ROY SOC MED. 61:239, March, 1968.

"Increase in gonorrhea in the Eastern Bohemian region and some problems of the antivenereal fight," by Z. Kraus. CESK DERM. 43:56-61, February, 1968

"The indirect basophil degranulation test for allergy to penicillin," by T. Feizi. TRANS ST JOHN HOSP DERM SOC. 53:162-164, 1967.

"Indirect immunofluorescent test for the diagnosis of syphilis in cerebrospinal fluid," by M. E. Camargo, et al. REV PAUL MED. 69:15-24, July, 1966.

"Individual prophylaxis in venereal diseases. Trial of a prophylactic silicon-terramycin ointment," by J. Duluc, et al. REV CORPS SANTE ARMEES. 8:91-98, February, 1967.

"Induction of anti-treponema pallidum antibodies in normal rabbits by RNA-immuno-carrier extraxcted from serum of syphilitic rabbits," by L. Michelazzi, et al. EXPERIENTIA. 23:207-208, March 15, 1967.

"Infection by Bedsoniae and the possibility of spurious isolation. 2. Genital infection, disease of the eye, Reiter's disease," by E. M. Dunlop, et al. AMER J OPHTHAL. 63:Suppl:1073-1081, May, 1967.

"Infection by TRIC agent and other members of the Bedsonia group, with a note on Reiter's disease. 1. Ocular disease in the adult," by B. R. Jones, et al. TRANS OPHTHAL SOC UK. 86:291-312, 1966.

--2. Ophthalmia neonatorum due to TRIC agent, by A. Freedman, et al. TRANS OPHTHAL SOC UK. 86:313-320, 1966.

--3. Genital infection and disease of the eye," by E. M. Dunlop, et al. TRANS OPHTHAL SOC UK. 86:321-324, 1966.

--4. Laboratory aspects," by I. A. Harper, et al. TRANS OPHTHAL SOC UK. 86:335-348, 1966.

"Infection of the sex organs in the years 1964-1966 and 1967-1969," by E. Zuber, et al. POL TYG LEK. 25: 1457-1458, September, 1970.

"Infections and first trimester losses: Possible role of

mycoplasmas," by S. G. Driscoll, et al. FERTIL STERIL. 20:1017-1019, November-December, 1969.

"Infections of the uterus and accessory organs," by H. Hirai. JAP J NURS ART. 7:39-50, July, 1970.

"Infectious and active yaws in a midland city," by F. M. Lanigan-O'Keeffe, et al. BRIT J DERM. 79:325-330, June, 1967.

"Infectious syphilis in South Carolina." J S CAROLINA MED ASS. 62:339, August, 1966.

"Infectious syphilis outbreak in Kentucky," by R. E. Teague. J KENTUCKY MED ASS. 67:22-23, January, 1969.

"Infectivity tests in syphilis," by T. B. Turner, et al. BRIT J VENER DIS. 45:183-196, September, 1969.

"The influence of chloroquine and related drugs on psoriasis and keratoderma blenorrhagicum," by H. Baker. BRIT J DERM. 78:161-166, March, 1966.

"Influence of contraceptive gestogen pills on sexual behaviour and the spread of gonorrhoea," by L. Juhlin, et al. BRIT J VENER DIS. 45:321-324, December, 1969.

"Influence of pH on vaginal discharges," by L. Cohen. BRIT J VENER DIS. 45:241-247, September, 1969.

"Influence of treatment of biologic false positive syphilis tests in leprosy," by H. G. Ruge. INT J LEPROSY. 36:328-332, July-September, 1968.

"Influence of trichomonas vaginalis on preinvasive nonradical treatment of carcinoma of the cervix uteri," by M. Wawrzkiewicz, et al. WIAD PARAZYT. 16:195-197, 1970.

"The influencing of syphilitic orchitis by different animal material," by G. Naumann, et al. Z MED MIKROBIOL IMMUN. 153:169-174, 1967.

"Information on venereal diseases in Los Angeles' county schools," by W. H. Smartt. BOL OFIC SANIT PANAMER. 66:226-230, March, 1969.

"Inhibition by acetazolamide of the growth of Neisseriae at increasing environmental concentration of CO_2," by A. Forkman. ACTA PATH MICROBIOL SCAND. 73:298-302, 1968.

"Inhibition of Neisseria gonorrhoeae by nifuratel," by G. M. Churcher, et al. BRIT J VENER DIS. 45:149-150, June, 1969.

"Inhibitory and toxic effect of various antibiotics on trichomonas and their practical use in the laboratory diagnosis of trichomoniasis," by B. Hoffmann, et al. WIAD PARAZYT. 15:425-428, 1969.

"Initial serological reactions in infectious syphilis," by S. Dandoy. BRIT J VENER DIS. 43:105-110, June, 1967.

"An instance of fatal reaction to the penicillin scratch-test," by M. Dogliotti. DERMATOLOGICA. 136:489-496, 1968.

"Instant syphilis screening: evaluation of the rapid plasma reagin teardrop card test," by J. Glicksman, et al. TEXAS MED. 63:46-48, January, 1967.

"Instant treatment ('traitement minute') of gonorrhea with a new oxytetracycline derivate--doxycycline (preliminary report)," by L. Sylvestre, et al. INT Z KLIN PHARMAKOL THER TOXIK. 1:401-403, July, 1968.

"The instruction of dermatovenereology in medical schools," by RKh Abudsametov, et al. VESTN DERM VENER. 43:71-72, April, 1969.

"Intercountry exchange of reports on sources of infection for prevention and control of venereal diseases in 1967," by G. Elste. DEUTSCH GESUNDH. 23:2489-2491, December 27, 1968.

"Intermediate report of the experiences of the collaborative study group 'Therapy of Syphilis'," by K. Grabner. Z HAUT GESCHLECHTSKR. 44:849-856, September 15, 1969.

"Interpretation of positive serological tests for syphilis in pregnancy," by A. Adeoba. BRIT J VENER DIS. 43:249-258, December, 1967.

"Interpretation of serologic reactions for syphilis," by J. E. Keilly. NEBRASKA MED J. 52:534-535, December, 1967.

"Interstitial keratitis and glaucoma," by P. R. Lichter, et al. AMER J OPHTHAL. 68:241-248, August, 1969.

"Interstitial keratitis associated with hidradenitis suppurativa," by J. R. Bergeron, et al. ARCH DERM. 95:473-475, May, 1967.

"The intimate evil," WORLD HLTH. 22:38+, July, 1969.

"Intracellular complement fixation by 'in vitro' stimulated lumphocytes (fluorescent serologic demonstration)," by H. J. Heitmann. Z HAUT GESCHLECHTSKR. 44:121-124, February 15, 1969.

"Intracerebral aneurysm of probably luetic origin," by S. Kopczynski, et al. POL TYG LEK. 25:1465-1466, September, 1970.

"Intradermal allergic reaction for the recognition of trichomoniasis," by L. M. Korik. UROL NEFROL. 31: 43-45, September-October, 1966.

"Intradermal allergic reaction in trichomonas infections in males," by L. K. Liubimova, et al. VESTN DERM VENER. 41:56-58, August, 1967.

"Intradermal treponemic color reaction (ITC) seen from the present immunologic standpoint," by G. Cocuzza, et al. DERM WSCHR. 152:699-702, July 2, 1966.

"The intradermal treponemal color reaction in neurosyphilis," by C. Lazzaro, et al. ACTA NEUROL. 21: 287-292, May-June, 1966.

"Intramuscular injection of procaine penicillin combined with oral administration of chloramphenicol in the treatment of gonorrhoea," by H. C. Gjessing, et al. BRIT J VENER DIS. 42:107-109, June, 1966.

"Intraocular penetration of cephalexin in man," by G. L. Boyle, et al. AMER J OPHTHAL. 69:868-872, January-June, 1970.

"Intraocular treponemes," by E. H. Christman, et al. ARCH OPHTHAL. 80:303-307, September, 1968.

"Intraocular treponemes in treated congenital syphilis," by J. N. Goldman, et al. ARCH OPHTHAL. 78:47-50, July, 1967.

"Intrauterine infection of the fetus with genital mycoplasma," by M. A. Bashmakova, et al. VOP OKHR MATERIN DETS. 14:69-73, November, 1969.

"Intravenous injection of reverin in syphilis," by Z. Matanić. MED GLAS. 20:193-198, May-June, 1966.

"Investigation into the sexual behavior of young men," by P. Hertoft. DANISH MED BULL SUPPL. 1:1-96, March, 1969.

"Investigation of neonatal conjunctivitis in the Gambia," by S. Sowa, et al. 2:243-247, August 3, 1968.

"An investigation of sorbing substances in the FTA-ABS test for syphilis," by G. R. Cannefax, et al. PUBLIC HEALTH REP. 83:411-416, May, 1968.

"Investigation of a specific IgM antibody test in neonatal congenital syphilis," by M. Sepetjian, et al. BRIT J VENER DIS. 46:18-20, February, 1970.

"Investigations on 21 PPLO strains isolated from urethral secretions," by A. Oner. TIP FAK MEC. 30:8-19, 1967.

"Involvement of the epididymis in secondary syphilis," by C. Korte, et al. HAUTARZT. 20:369-370, August, 1969.

"Iron metabolism in early symptomatic syphilis," by Z. Olszewska. POL MED J. 5:686-692, 1966; also in PRZEGL DERM. 53:15-20, January-February, 1966.

"Is education the answer to the venereal disease problem?," by H. Manser. J AMER OSTEOPATH ASS. 67:1031-1037, May, 1968.

"Is gonococcal sensitivity to antibiotics increasing in Norway," by K. Odegaard, et al. BRIT J VENER DIS. 43:284-286, December, 1967.

"Is it possible to control syphilis through treatment and epidemiologic measures?," by J. F. Donohue. SALUD PUBLICA MEX. 10:607-610, September-October, 1968.

"Is paromomycin appropriate for the treatment of trichomona infection in women. II. Clinical experiences," by H. Spitzbart, et al. ZBL GYNAEK. 88:563-566, April 30, 1966.

"Is there a penicillin resistance in gonorrhea?," by P. Wodniansky. ARCH KLIN EXP DERM. 227:650-652, 1966.

"Ischaemic heart disease due to syphilitic narrowing of

the coronary ostia," by K. K. Datey, et al. INDIAN HEART J. 21:253-258, July, 1969.

"Isolated lumbar tabetic arthropathy," by J. David-Chausse, et al. BULL SOC FRANC DERM SYPH. 77:105-107, July, 1970.

"Isolation and characterization of bacteriophages for Neisseria," by L. N. Phelps. J GEN VIROL. 1:529-536, October, 1967.

"The isolation and identification of the urinary oxidative metabolites of metronidazole in man," by J. E. Stambaugh, et al. J PHARMACOL EXP THER. 161:373-381, June, 1968.

"Isolation and propagation of mycoplasma," by A. C. Ruys, et al. ANN NY ACAD SCI. 143:390-393, July 28, 1967.

"Isolation, cultivation, low temperature preservation, and infectivity titration of trichomonas vaginalis," by W. H. Lunsden, et al. BRIT J VENER.DIS. 42:145-154, September, 1966.

"Isolation of the agent of lymphogranuloma venereum in Australia," by I. Cook, et al. MED J AUST 1:771-772, April 12, 1969.

"Isolation of an antigen of Neisseria gonorrhoeae involved in the human immune response to gonococcal infection," by J. D. Schmale, et al. J BACT. 99:469-471, August, 1969.

"Isolation of lymphogranuloma venereum agent in the Sudan," by A. R. Salim. J TROP MED HYG. 72:134-136, June, 1969.

"Isolation of mima polymorpha var. oxydans from 2 cases of urethritis and 1 of vaginitis," by L. Vergara. REV LAT AMER MICROBIOL. 11:141-144, July-September, 1969.

"Isolation of mycoplasmas and their significance in male urethritis," by G. Catalano, et al. G MAL INFETT. 20:1009-1013, December, 1968.

"Isolation of Neisseria gonorrhoeae in asymptomatic women," by R. V. Victoria, et al. REV INVEST SALUD PUBLICA. 28:119-126, April-June, 1968.

"Isolation of strains of treponema from endemic syphilis

during a survey made in Senegal," by J. Malgras, et al. BULL SOC FRANC DERM SYPH. 76:515-516, 1969.

"Isolation of TRIC agents and mycoplasma from the genitourinary tracts of patients of a venereal disease clinic," by S. Holt, et al. AMER J OPHTHAL. 63:Suppl: 1057-1064, May, 1967.

"Isolation of TRIC agents from the human genital tract," by D. K. Ford, et al. BRIT J VENER DIS. 45:44-46, March, 1969.

"It is time to clarify the results of serological reactions in syphilis," by A. I. Kartamyshev. LAB DELO. 2:82-83, 1969.

"Jackson's syndrome (hemiplegia infima alternans) of a leutic basis," by E. Lange, et al. PSYCHIAT NEUROL MED PSYCHOL. 19:32-34, January, 1967.

"Jarisch-Herxheimer reaction." BRIT MED J. 1:384, February 18, 1967.

"Jarisch-Herxheimer reaction and syphilitic aortitis," by G. R. Hughes. BRIT MED J. 1:360, February 10, 1968.

"Jarisch-Herxheimer reaction with interesting blood count," by R. B. Davis, et al. INDIAN MED ASS. 53:83-85, July 16, 1969.

"Jean Astruc (March 19, 1684 to May 5, 1766) and his work 'De morbis venereis' on the 200th anniversary of his death," by L. Mendel. DERM WSCHR. 153:105-111, February 4, 1967.

"Jonathan Hutchinson on vaccination syphilis," by C. T. Nelson. ARCH DERM. 99:529-535, May, 1969.

"Justification of serological examinations of lues during systematic examination," by R. Krunic, et al. VOJNOSANIT PREGL. 26:505-506, October, 1969.

"Juvenile GPI: a case study," by G. C. Kanjilal. NURS TIMES. 65:1066-1067, August 21, 1969.

"Kanamycin as treatment of acute gonorrhea in females," by L. H. Shapiro, et al. OBSTET GYNEC. 35:794-795, May, 1970.

"Kanamycin in non-gonococcal urethritis," by G. W. Csonka. POST GRAD MED J, London. 63-64, May, 1967.

"Kanamycin in the treatment of gonorrhoea in the female," by M. I. McGill, et al. SCOT MED J. 14:176-179, May, 1969.

"Kanamycin in the treatment of gonorrhoea in females," by W. F. Hooton, et al. POSTGRAD MED J. Suppl:68-71, May, 1967.

"Kanamycin in the treatment of gonorrhoea in males," by A. E. Wilkinson, et al. POSTGRAD MED J. Suppl:65-67, May, 1967.

"Kanamycin sulphate in the management of gonorrhoea failing to respond to penicillin," by L. Farrell. BRIT J VENER DIS. 45:232-234, September, 1969.

"Kanamycin sulfate in the treatment of acute gonorrheal urethritis in men," by J. E. Fischnaller, et al. JAMA. 203:909-912, March 11, 1968.

"Klion therapy of urogenital trichomoniasis," by M. Breier. ORV HETIL. 111:568-570, March 8, 1970.

"Kolmer's complement fixation and VDRL tests," by I. Tuna. TURK HIJ TECR BIYOL DERG. 27:78-106, 1967.

"Kolmer's test in the serodiagnosis of syphilis," by O. A. Stoinova, et al. VESTN DERM VENER. 43:53-57, September, 1969.

"Laboratory diagnosis of chronic forms of female gonorrhea," by K. L. Keburlia. VESTN DERM VENER. 41:50-53, March, 1967.

"The laboratory diagnosis of gonorrhoea in the female," by J. T. O'Brien, et al. NEW ZEAL MED J. 69:204-206, April, 1969.

"Laboratory diagnosis of gonorrhea in premenarchal females and in adults," by T. C. Gallanis, et al. OBSTET

GYNEC. 29:401-404, March, 1967.

"Laboratory diagnosis of syphilis," by L. Nicholas. INT J DERM. 9:64-68, January-March, 1970.

"The laboratory diagnosis of vaginal infections caused by trichomonas and candida (Monilia) species," by D. A. Eddie. J MED MICROBIOL. 1:153-159, August, 1968.

"Laboratory diagnosis of venereal disease," by G. W. Schepers. MED ANN DC. 35:357-366 passim, July, 1966.

"Laboratory experience in RPCF, latex, RA, ASO and latex tests," by H. H. Chen. J FORMOSAN MED ASS. 67: 134-141, April 28, 1968.

"Labyrinthitis luetica," by R. Haye. J OSLO CITY HOSP. 19:68-72, April, 1969.

"Large doses of penicillin for treatment of gonorrhea in women," by L. H. Shapiro, et al. OBSTET GENEC. 30: 89-92, July, 1967.

"Large-scale screening by the automated Wassermann reaction," by W. Wagstaff, et al. J CLIN PATH. 22: 236-239, March, 1969.

"Laryngeal edema following intramuscular administration of penicillin," by P. A. Kravchuk. ZH USHN NOS GORL BOLEZ. 28:94-95, November-December, 1968.

"Late atrophying syphilids," by B. Duperrat, et al. BULL SOC FRANC DERM SYPH. 76:798, 1969.

"Late complications of syphillis. A comparative epidemiological and serological study of cardiovascular syphilis and various forms of neurosyphilis," by K. Aho, et al. ACTA DERMATOVENER. 49:336-342, 1969.

"Late congenital syphilis in the 2nd generation," by E. N. Oganesian. VESTN DERM VENER. 42:91-92, May, 1968.

"Late ocular syphilis: transfer of infection from man to experimental animals," by J. L. Smith. TRANS AMER OPHTHAL SOC. 67:658-697, 1969.

"Late syphilis in experiment and clinic," by P. Collart, et al. MUNCHEN MED WSCHR. 109:1555-1564, July 21, 1967.

"Late syphilis in the primate," by F. J. Elsas, et al. BRIT J VENER DIS. 44:267-273, December, 1968.

"Late syphilis: a review of some of the recent literature," by L. Nicholas, et al. AMER J MED SCI. 254:549-569, October, 1967.

"Late yaws," by J. L. Fluker, et al. BRIT J VENER DIS. 46:264, June, 1970.

"Latent gonorrhea in women," by L. Clark. JAMA. 209:563, July 28, 1969.

"Latent syphilis," by J. A. Etcheverry, et al. PRENSA MED ARGENT. 54:777-785, June 23, 1967.

"Latent syphilis and cataract," by J. Sédan. BULL SOC OPHTHAL FRANC. 67:874-877, October, 1967.

"Latent trichomoniasis in men with gonorrhea," by M. A. Zelikman. VESTN DERM VENER. 40:55-58, January, 1966.

"Latex microreaction in syphilis, the Bordet-Wassermann cardiolipin test and Sachs-Witebski citochol test," by S. Kośmiderski, et al. POL TYG LEK. 24:721-722, May 12, 1969.

"Law, medicine and minors. I.," by D. H. Russell. NEW ENG J MED. 278:35-36, January 4, 1968.

--II. NEW ENG J MED. 278:265-266, February 1, 1968.

"Legal aspects of reporting and treating venereal disease," by G. E. Hall. JAMA. 195:309-310, March 28, 1966; also in ARCH ENVIRON HEALTH, Chicago. 13:388-392, September, 1966.

"The lesions of congenital syphilis," by B. J. Cremin, et al. BRIT J RADIOL. 43:333-341, May, 1970.

"Leucorrhoea due to trichomonas vaginalis--clinical trial with hamycin," by D. Ganju, et al. HINDUSTAN ANTIBIOT BULL. 9:69-75, November, 1966.

"Leukoplakia of the kidney pelvis; hydronephrosis and syphilis as a possible cause," by I. A. Rovinescu, et al. ACTA UROL BELG. 34:495-500, October, 1966.

"Leutic lymphadenitis: A clinical and histologic study of 20 cases," by R. J. Hartsock, et al. AMER J CLIN.

PATH. 53:304-314, March, 1970.

"Levorin in the therapy of trichomoniasis in men, and in post-trichomonas secondary infections," by L. M. Korik, et al. UROL NEFROL. 34:48-49, July-August, 1969.

"Levorin in the treatment of women with trichomoniasis and candidiasis of the sexual organs," by V. A. Lenartovich, et al. VESTN DERM VENER. 43:39-43, February, 1969.

"Liability for penicillin reactions," by A. R. Holder. JAMA. 212:2015-2016, June 15, 1970.

"A liberal education for the adolescent girl," by G. Browne. MED J AUST. 2:825-826, October 28, 1967.

"Life-threatening infection. Choice of alternate drugs when penicillin cannot be given," by G. O. Westenfielder, et al. JAMA. 210:845-848, November 3, 1969.

"Light microscopic observations on the pathology of endolymph," by H. F. Schuknecht, et al. J LARYNG. 80:1-10, January, 1966.

"Lincomycin: activity in vitro and absorption and excretion in normal young men," by C. E. McCall, et al. AMER J MED SCI. 254:144-155, August, 1967.

"Lincomycin, non-gonococcal urethritis, and mycoplasmata," by G. W. Csonka, et al. BRIT J VENER DIS. 45:52-54, March, 1969.

"Linear calcification of the ascending aorta without syphilis," by J. A. Cohen. JAMA. 214:375, October 12, 1970.

"Lipid composition of treponemal strains," by L. Vaczi, et al. ACT MICROBIOL ACAD SCI HUNG. 13:79-84, 1966.

"Liquor diagnosis of neurosyphilis," by G. Ritter, et al. DEUTSCH MED WSCHR. 93:1595-1596 passim, August 23, 1968.

"Little Miss Muffet sure is a tough-it," by N. B. Rawls. NORTHWEST MED. 69:352, May, 1970.

"Localization of treponema pallidum immobilizing antibody in human immunoglobulins," by G. Tringali, et al. RIV IST SIEROTER ITAL. 43:161-168, July-August, 1968.

"A localized arthus-type hypersensitivity reaction to penicillin," by A. Lupovitch, et al. ANN ALERG. 26: 206-210, April, 1968.

"Location of trichomonas vaginalis in the female genital tract," by E. Grys. POZNAN TWO PRZYJAC NAUK WYDZ LEK. 36:5-23, 1967.

"Locoregional complication after benzathine penicillin," by G. Vasiliu, et al. PEDIATRIA. 17:75-78, January-February, 1968.

"A logical notation of the degree of positivity of syphilitic sera by measuring the constant of the speed of complement fixation," by R. Vargues, et al. ANN BIOL CLIN. 26:621-631, May-June, 1968.

"Long-term cultivation of N. gonorrhoeae in tissue culture," by M. Gavrilescu, et al. BRIT J VENER DIS. 42:171-174, September, 1966.

"Long-term results in the use of modern therapeutic methods in recent syphilis," by C. L. Meneghini, et al. G ITAL DERM. 108:391-400, September-October, 1967.

"Long-term treatment of trichomonas infections with a diiodine derivative of oxyguinoline," by M. Arnold. PRAXIS. 57:1663-1666, November 26, 1968.

"Low frequency of chronic biological false positive reactors to serological tests for syphilis in rheumatoid arthritis and ankylosing spondylitis," by O. P. Salo, et al. ANN RHEUM DIS. 27:261-263, May, 1968.

"The lues curve in Switzerland since World War I," by W. Burckhardt, et al. DERMATOLOGICA. 135:341-344, 1967.

"Lues maligna. Presentation of a case and a review of the literature," by D. A. Fisher, et al. ARCH DERM. 99:70-73, January, 1969.

"Luetic aneurysms of the aortic valve, sinus of Valsalva, and aorta," by D. Sohn, et al. AMER J CLIN PATH. 46:99-102, July, 1966.

"Luetic lymphadenitis: a clinical and histologic study of 20 cases," by R. J. Hartsock, et al. AMER J CLIN PATH. 53:304-314, March, 1970.

"Luetic stenosis of the abdominal aorta and of the renal arteries," by H. Rykowski, et al. POL TYG LEK. 25: 694-695, May 11, 1970.

"A luminescent study of pupils and pupillary reactions in the early stages of syphilis," by A. V. Braitsev, et al. VESTN DERM VENER. 42:47-51, June, 1968.

"Lupoid hepatitis following administration of penicillin. Case report and immunological studies," by J. P. Girard, et al. HELV MED ACTA. 34:23-35, December, 1967.

"The lymph node biopsy in infectious diseases," by D. J. Winslow, et al. MARYLAND MED J. 15:55-58, February, 1966.

"Lymph-node, cutaneous and splenic tertiary syphilis with the aspects of sarcoidosis," by R. Cazzola. FRIULI MED. 21:1129-1141, November-December, 1966.

"The lymphocyte culture in penicillin allergy," by H. J. Heitmann, et al. HAUTARZT. 17:313-316, July, 1966.

"Lymphocyte stimulation in vitro in syphilitic subjects," by G. C. Chieregato, et al. MINERVA DERM. 42:406-407, August, 1967.

"Lymphocyte transformation test (LTT) for the diagnosis of drug allergy," by E. Schopf, et al. ARCH KLIN EXP DERM. 237:177-180, 1970.

"Lymphogranuloma inguinale," by W. F. Schoning, et al. MED WELT. 31:1713-1714, August 2, 1969.

"Lymphogranuloma venereum," by A. J. Abrams. JAMA. 205: 199-202, July 22, 1968.

"Lymphogranuloma venereum," by E. G. Weinstein, et al. J AMER GERIAT SOC. 14:80-84, January, 1966.

"Lymphogranuloma venereum. I. Comparison of the Frei test, complement fixation test, and isolation of the agent," by J. Schachter, et al. J INFECT DIS. 120: 372-375, September, 1969.

--II. Characterization of some recently isolated strains, J BACT. 99:636-638, September, 1969.

"Lymphographic findings in venereal diseases," by L. Kerk, et al. FORTSCHR ROENTGENSTR. 111:22-29, July, 1969.

"Lymphographic studies in lymphopathia venerea," by J. J. Herzberg. DERM WSCHR. 153:854-857, July 29, 1967.

"Lymphography and lymphoscintigraphy of the pelvis in venereal lymphopathy in the buboes condition," by K. Vessal, et al. HAUTARZT. 18:256-259, June, 1967.

"Lysozyme activity of serum in the course of experimental syphilis in rabbits. 1. Changing dynamics of lysozyme activity," by L. Sil, et al. Z IMMUNITAETSFORSCH. 131:444-448, December, 1966.

--2. Quantitative changes of lysozyme, by A. Jakubowski, et al. Z IMMUNITAETSFORSCH. 131:449-452, December, 1966.

"Lytic effect of trypsin, lysozyme, and complement on treponema pallidum," by R. H. Jones, et al. BRIT J VENER DIS. 44:193-200, September, 1968.

"Macmiror in the therapy of vaginal trichomoniasis," by A. Baron. MINERVA GINEC. 22:269-271, February 28, 1970.

"The main achievements of the Central Scientific-Research Dermatovenereological Institute (CDVI) in the field of scientific investigations in dermatology," by A. A. Studnitsin, et al. VESTN DERM VENER. 43:3-14, April, 1969.

"The main problems of public health organizations and institutions in the field of controlling venereal and fungous diseases from 1967 to 1970," by N. V. Nikitina. VESTN DERM VENER. 41:3-7, March, 1967.

"Main results of fulfilling plans for scientific studies on the problem 'scientific bases of dermatology and venereology' for 1968," by N. M. Turanov, et al. VESTN DERM VENER. 43:7-12, September, 1969.

"Main results of scientific studies on the problem of 'scientific principles of dermatology and venereology during 1967'," by N. M. Turanov, et al. VESTN DERM VENER. 42:3-9, August, 1968.

"Male-female ratios in the V.D. clinics of England and Wales," by R. S. Morton. BRIT J VENER DIS. 46:103-

105, April, 1970.

"Male urethritis caused by trichomonas," by R. Fioccardi. MINERVA MED. 57:3189-3191, October 3, 1966.

"Male urogenital trichomoniasis," by M. De Luca, et al. MINERVA DERM. 41:315-340, September, 1966.

"Man, monkeys, and treponemal disease (editorial)." LANCET. 1:562, March 15, 1969.

"Management of blennorrhagia using a dose of rimactan," by L. Migliano. HOSPITAL. 75:297-300, January, 1969.

"Management of chronic diseases and clinical judgment of cure--syphilis," by S. Okamoto. JAP J CLIN MED. 24: 2304-2308, December, 1966.

"Management of patients with a positive serologic screening test for syphilis," by M. E. Seay. J FLORIDA MED ASS. 54:457-459, May, 1967.

"Management of syphilitic patients allergic to penicillin," by J. Lebioda, et al. PRZEGL DERM. 55:311-316, May-June, 1968.

"Management of thoracic aneurysms," by J. Storer, et al. INT SURG. 47:344-355, April, 1967.

"Management of trichomonas vaginitis with pimaricin," by A. Papaloukas, et al. Z HAUT GESCHLECHTSKR. 43:343-348, April 15, 1968.

"Manifestations of early syphilis in the anoperineal region," by E. B. Molina Leguizamon. PRENSA MED ARGENT. 55:898-900, July 5, 1968.

"Manual use of punched cards in dermato-venereological dispensaries," by M. I. Arans. VESTN DERM VENER. 40:68-70, November, 1966.

"Martorell-Fabre syndrome of syphilitic etiology," by A. Bohorquez, et al. ANGIOLOGIA. 20:255-260, September-October, 1968.

"Meatoplasty," by J. P. Blandy, et al. BRIT J UROL. 39: 633, October, 1967.

"Mechanisms of clinical desensitization in urticarial hypersensitivity to penicillin," by M. J. Fellner, et al. J ALLERG. 45:55-61, January, 1970.

"Medical and legal problems in the treatment of delinquent girls in Scotland. I. Girls in custodial institutions," by D. H. Robertson. BRIT J VENER DIS. 45:129-139, June, 1969.

--II. Sexually transmitted disease in girls in custodial institutions. BRIT J VENER DIS. 46:46-53, February, 1970.

"Medical basis of the theory of abolition of the 'red light districts'," by T. Matsuda. JAP J NURS ART. 8:122-132, August, 1969.

"Medical grand rounds from the University of Alabama Medical Center." SOUTHERN MED J. 61:719-727, July, 1968.

"Medico-epidemiologic problems posed by masculine gonococcal urethritis (apropos of 10,000 cases)," by A. Siboulet, et al. BULL INST NAT SANTE. 21:737-780, July-August, 1966.

"Medicosocial background to gonococcal ophthalmia neonatorum," by C. B. Schofield. LANCET. 2:1182-1185, November 29, 1969.

"Meningoradiculitis, a disease misnamed atypical polyradiculoneuritis," by F. Thiebaut, et al. REV NEUROL. 115:1070-1075, December, 1966.

"Mental Health aspects of venereal disease in adolescents," by R. S. Lourie. J AMER MED WOM ASS. 23:167-168, February, 1968; also in ARCH ENVIRON HEALTH, Chicago. 12:684-685, June, 1966.

"Mesaortitis luica," by P. Ostendorf, et al. MED WELT. 11:419-422, March 14, 1970.

"Metabolic gas production by a variety of spirochetes." J DENT RES. 45:165-168, January-February, 1966.

"Methacycline in the management of donavanosis (granuloma inguinale)," by J. M. Santos, et al. HOSPITAL. 74:1661-1668, November, 1968.

"Methacycline (Rondomycin) in gonorrhoea," by R. S. Morton, et al. BRIT J VENER DIS. 42:175-177, September, 1966.

"Method for isolation and identification of corynebacterium vaginale (haemophilus vaginalis)," by W. E. Dunkelberg, Jr., et al. APPL MICROBIOL. 19:47-52,

January, 1970. ...

"Method for preparing Neisseria gonorrhoeae fluorescent antibody conjugate," by W. L. Peacock, Jr., PUBLIC HEALTH REP. 85:733-738, August, 1970.

"The method of antivenereal propaganda at the present time," by E. K. Reznikov. VESTN DERM VENER. 43:52-59, November, 1969.

"Methodic and immunologic aspects of current syphilis serodiagnosis," by F. Muller. MUNCHEN MED WSCHR. 109:1591-1595, July 28, 1967.

"Methodologic investigations and prevalence of genital mycoplasmas in preganancy," by P. Braun, et al. J INFECT DIS. 121:391-400, April, 1970.

"The methodology of serologic tests in experimental penicillin allergy," by H. P. Werner, et al. Z IMMUNITAETSFORSCH. 139:14-24, December, 1969.

"Methods of detection of immediate hypersensitivity to penicillin," by E. Maciejowska. PRZEGL DERM. 56:757-764, 1969.

"Methylenecycline in urology (rondomycin)," by R. Schilliro. J UROL NEPHROL. 74:498-501, June, 1968.

"Metronidazole and syphilis." BRIT MED J. 4:4-5, October 7, 1967.

"Metronidazole and treponema pallidum." BRIT J VENER DIS. 43:149, September, 1967.

"Metronidazole in human infections with syphilis," by A. H. Davies. BRIT J VENER DIS. 43:197-200, September, 1967.

"Metronidazole in pregnancy," by W. F. Peterson, et al. AMER J OBSTET GYNEC. 94:243-249, February 1, 1966.

"Metronidazole in the treatment of trichomoniasis in men," by A. I. Poliakov, et al. VESTN DERM VENER. 42:86-87, November, 1968.

"Metronidazole treatment of trichomonal vaginitis. A comparison of cure rates in 1961 and 1967," by J. C. Azure, et al. ACTA OBSTET GYNEC SCAND. 48:440-445, 1969.

"Metronidazole treatment of vaginal trichomoniasis. II. Oral vs. vaginal therapy," by S. Porapakkham. OBSTET GYNEC. 29:213-216, February, 1967.

"Microbiology of the Neisseria group," by H. Storck, et al. ARCH KLIN EXP DERM. 227:623-630, 1966.

"Microscopic studies on the placenta of a macerated fetus with important clinical implications," by J. C. Stut. NEDERL T VERLOSK. 66:56-64, February, 1966.

"Minute treatment of gonorrhea. Supplementary observations on the article by H. Biehler and E. Heinke: Single treatment of gonorrhea of the man with high doses of penicillins," by E. G. Jung, et al. MUNCHEN MED WSCHR. 109:296-300, 1967; also in MUNCHEN MED WSCHR. 110:152-153, January 19, 1968.

"Minute treatment of male gonococcal urethritis (600 cases)," by A. Siboulet. SEM THER. 41:307-309, May, 1965.

"Modern aspect of latent syphilis," by K. N. Suvorova. VESTN DERM VENER. 43:70-73, March, 1969.

"The modern management of venereal diseases," by A. Luger. WIEN KLIN WSCHR. 79:529-535, June 30, 1967.

"Modern methods of serological diagnosis of visceral syphilis," by L. D. Butovetskii. SOVET MED. 30:62-64, September, 1967.

"Modern serology of syphilis," by I. Orhel. RAD MED FAK ZAGREB. 17:103-110, 1969.

"Modifications to the automated Wassermann reaction," by V. W. Pugh, et al. J MED LAB TECHN. 23:126-128, April, 1966.

"Modified gram staining of smears in the diagnosis of gonorrhea," by M. K. Kuznetsova. LAB DELO. 9:554-555, 1966.

"Modified preparation of VDRL antigen suspensions," by L. R. Gorczyca. THE FILTER. 38:7-8, March, 1966.

"A modified technic for the complement deviation test in lues," by R. Bruno, et al. MINERVA DERM. 42:637-638. December, 1967.

"Molluscum contagiosum," by P. H. Jacobs. AEROSPACE MED.

41:1196-1197, October, 1970.

"Molluscum contagiosum as a sexually transmitted disease," by R. J. Cobbold, et al. PRACTITIONER. 204:416-419, March, 1970.

"Molluscum contagiosum of the adult. Probable venereal transmission," by P. J. Lynch, et al. ARCH DERM. 98:141-143, August, 1968.

"Morbidity and clinical symptoms of congenital syphilis in infancy," by K. Wechselberg, et al. DEUTSCH MED WSCHR. 95:1976-1981, September 25, 1970.

"Morphologic studies of mononuclear cells of human synovial fluid," by K. Takasugi, et al. ARTHRITIS RHEUM. 10:495-501, December, 1967.

"Morphological and biochemical differentiation of three types of small oral spirochetes," by S. S. Socransky, et al. J BACT. 98:878-882, June, 1969.

"Morphological study of vaginal trichomonas in cultures," by A. Noda. J JAP OBSTET GYNEC SOC. 20:1589-1598, December, 1968.

"Mouth mucosa findings in lues," by H. M. Hofmeier. HNO. 16:73-78, March, 1968.

"Multiple antigenic stimulation in vitro of lymphocytes of syphilis patients in various stages of the disease," by G. Chieregato, et al. MINERVA DERM. 43:264-269, June, 1968.

"Multiple aorto-cervical occlusions of syphilitic origin," by V. Maslenikov, et al. ACTA NEUROL LAT AMER. 12:48-55, 1966.

"Multiple cranial ostolysis associated with secondary syphilis (apropos of 2 cases)," by B. Duperrat, et al. BULL SOC FRANC DERM SYPH. 74:484-486, 1967.

"Multiple osteochondritis due to prenatal syphilis," by J. Mercadal-Peyri, et al. ACTAS DERMOSIF. 58:101-104, March-April, 1967.

"Multiple sensitization in experimental syphilis in rabbits (an investigation on the mechanism of gumma formation)," by T. Yano. JAP J BACT. 24:345-353, 1969.

"Multivalent antibiotic allergy with penicillin and tetra-

cycline anaphylaxis," by J. Zelger, et al. DERMATO-
LOGICA. 139:365-373, 1969.

"Muramidase from tissue fluid of syphilitic rabbit testes.
I. Purification and properties of the enzyme," by
W. Kopeć. ARCH IMMUN THER EXP. 15:161-175, 1967.

--II. Comparative study of the enzyme and hen egg white
muramidase. ARCH IMMUN THER EXP. 16:533-545, 1968.

"Mutilative syphilis at the prepuce with positive serologic reaction at an abnormally weak level," by M.
Renoux, et al. BULL SOC FRANC DERM SYPH. 75:749-
750, 1968.

"Mycoplasma hominis and abortion," by H. J. Harwick, et
al. J INFECT DIS. 121:260-268, March, 1970.

"Mycoplasma hominis in abortion," by D. M. Jones. BRIT
MED J. 1:338-340, February 11, 1967.

"Mycoplasma in clinical and experimental gynecology,"
by C. Trinka. CAS LEK CESK. 109:463-466, May, 1970.

"Mycoplasma in human urogenital pathology," by P. Altucci,
et al. G MAL INFETT. 19:487-497, August, 1967.

"Mycoplasma in urogenital tract," by M. E. Thomas, et al.
LANCET. 2:366-367, August 15, 1970.

"Mycoplasma recovery from the male genitourinary tract:
Voided urine versus the urethral swab," by J. E.
Gregory, et al. APPL MICROBIOL. 19:268-270, Febru-
ary, 1970.

"Mycoplasmas and arthritis," by J. T. Sharp. ARTHRITIS
RHEUM. 13:263-271, May-June, 1970.

"Mycoplasmas and diseases of the urogenital tract," by
I. Farber, et al. DEUTSCH GESUNDH. 24:2054-2057,
October 23, 1969.

"Mycoplasmas and human reproductive failure," by R. B.
Kundsin, et al. SURG GYNEC OBSTET. 131:89-92, July,
1970.

"Mycoplasmas and 'non-specific' genital infection. 1.
Previous studies and laboratory aspects," by D. Taylor-
Robinson, et al. BRIT J VENER DIS. 45:265-273, De-
cember, 1969.

--II. Clinical aspects, by E. M. Dunlop. et al. BRIT J VENER DIS. 45:274-281, December, 1969.

--III. Post-gonococcal urethritis. A prospective study, by M. J. Hare, et al. BRIT J VENER DIS. 45:282-286. December, 1969.

"Mycoplasmas in the female urogenital tract," by C. Del Bianco, et al. G MAL INFETT. 20:1006-1009, December, 1968.

"Mycoplasmas in human pathology," by P. L. Altucci. G MAL INFETT. 20:557-571, June, 1968.

"Mycoplasmas of the human urogenital tract and oropharynx and their possible role in disease: A review with some recent observations," by D. Taylor-Robinson, et al. PROC ROY SOC MED. 59:1112-1116, November, 1966.

"Mycotic diseases of the male genital organs with specific reference to non-gonorrheal or mycotic urethritis," by J. Rossberg. CESK DERM. 43:168-170, June, 1968.

"Mycocardial infarct in syphilitic aortitis," by J. M. Torre, et al. ARCH INST CARDIOL MEX. 36:300-307, May-June, 1966.

"Myocardial infarct on a background of syphilitic aortitis," by N. I. Ianushkevich, et al. KLIN MED. 45:119-120, February, 1967.

"Myocarditis in penicillin sensitivity," by D. Banerjee. INDIAN HEART J. 20:73-75, January, 1968.

"Narcotic addiction with false-positive reaction for syphilis. Immunologic studies," by D. L. Tuffanelli. ACTA DERMATOVENER. 48:542-546, 1968.

"Nasopharngeal syphilis with blindness," by W. E. Gager, et al. ARCH OTOLARYNG. 90:641-646, November, 1969.

"National survey of venereal disease treated by physicians in 1968," by W. L. Fleming, et al. JAMA. 211:1827-1830, March 16, 1970.

"National symposium on venereal disease control. Venereal disease and environmental health," by J. G. Telfer.

ARCH ENVIRON HEALTH, Chicago. 13:351-352, September, 1966.

"A nationwide serum survey of Colombian military recruits, 1966. I. Description of sample and antibody patterns with arboviruses, polioviruses, respiratory viruses, tetanus, and treponematosis," by A. S. Evans, et al. AMER J EPIDEM. 90:292-303, October, 1969.

"Natural and immune human antibodies reactive with antigens of virulent Neisseria gonorrhoeae: immunoglobulins G, M, and A.," by I. R. Cohen. J BACT. 94:141-148, July, 1967.

"Natural human antibodies to gram-negative bacteria: immunoglobulins G, A, and M," by I. R. Cohen, et al. SCIENCE. 152:1257-1259, May 27, 1966.

"Nature and extent of penicillin side effects with special reference to 151 fatal cases after anaphylactic shock," by O. Idsoe, et al. SCHWEIZ MED WSCHR. 99:1190-1197, August 16, 1969; also in BULL WHO. 38:159-188, 1968.

"Necessity for and technic of cultural diagnosis of gonococcus," by F. Fegeler. ARCH KLIN EXP DERM. 227:630-633, 1966.

"The necessity for heating sera for the VDRL slide test," by M. A. Lantz, et al. AMER J MED TECHN. 34:551-556, October, 1968.

"Necrotic cervicitis due to primary infection with the virus of herpes simplex," by R. R. Willcox. BRIT MED J. 1:610-612, March 9, 1968.

"Neisseria control," by S. E. Acres. MED SERV J CANADA 22:288-289, April, 1966.

"Neisseria gonorrhoeae. II. Colonial variation and pathogenicity during 35 months in vitro," by D. S. Kellogg, Jr., et al. J BACT. 96:596-605, September, 1968.

"Neisseria gonorrhoeae. A comparative study of the sensitivity of freshly isolated strains to antibiotics," by M. Hejzlar, et al. CESK DERM. 43:179-186, June, 1968.

"Neisseria gonorrhoeae strain showing an exceptional resistance to streptomycin and a considerable decreased susceptibility to some other antibiotics," by M. Pekowski, et al. PRZEGL DERM. 57:49-54, January-February, 1970.

"Neonatal ophthalmia." LANCET. 2:630, September 20, 1969.

"Nephrotic syndrome and acute hepatitis in secondary syphilis," by J. D. McCracken, et al. MILIT MED. 134: 682-686, September, 1969.

"Nephrotic syndrome associated with congenital syphilis," by P. Pollner. JAMA. 198:263-266, October 17, 1966.

"The nephrotic syndrome associated with secondary syphilis. An immune deposit disease," by G. D. Braunstein, et al. AMER J MED. 48:643-648, May, 1970.

"Nephrotic syndrome in secondary syphilis," by D. F. de Andrade, et al. REV ASS MED BRASIL. 13:97-98, March, 1967.

"Nerve compressions in tabetic arthropathy of the spine," by H. Serre, et al. BULL ACAD NAT MED. 154:212-216, March 17, 1970.

"Neurogenic arthropathies (Charcot's joints)," by P. C. Das, et al. J INDIAN MED ASSOC. 54:368-372, April 16, 1970.

"Neurologic disorders in the secondary stage of syphilis with the differential diagnosis of brain tumor," by G. Huffmann. MED WELT. 48:2614-2619, November 26, 1966.

"Neuropathic arthritis (Charcot's joint)," by R. Stien. T NORSK LAEGEFOREN. 88:1941-1943 passim, October 15, 1968.

"The neuro-radiology of carotid stenoses," by A. Tanzer. FRENCH REV NEUROL. 115:711-721, October, 1966.

"Neurosyphilis (letter to editor)," by K. W. Heathfield. BRIT MED J. 1:765-766, March 23, 1968.

"Neurosyphilis. Its current frequency in our medical clinic," by J. Garrachon, et al. REV CLIN ESP. 101: 279-282, May 31, 1966.

"Neurosyphilis associated with haematemesis: report of a case," by J. L. Verbov, et al. BRIT J CLIN PRACT. 21:515-517, October, 1967.

"Neurosyphilis in cases from the Departments of Neurology and Psychiatry of Medical Schools in Poland in 1956-1965 (clinical data)," by A. Dowzenko, et al. NEUROL NEUROCHIR POL. 3:559-566, September-October, 1969.

"Neurosyphilis in Uganda: A comparison of two five-year periods," by W. R. Billington. E AFR MED J. 43:469-473, November, 1966.

"Neurosyphilis lesions recorded in a group of 1,987 necropsies (statistical review and anatomical study)," by B. Rodriquez-Arias, et al. REV CLIN ESP. 108:153-156, January 31, 1968.

"Neurosyphilis, the search for adequate treatment. A review and report of a study using benzathine penicillin," by G. D. Short, et al. ARCH DERM. 93:87-91, January, 1966.

"The neurosyphilitic psychoses today. A survey of 91 cases," by K. Dewhurst. BRIT J PSYCHIAT. 115:31-38, January, 1969.

"Neurotoxic effects of large doses of penicillin administered intravenously (letter to editor)," by J. B. Borman, et al. ARCH SURG. 97:662-665, October, 1968.

"Neurotoxicity of penicillin," by M. I. Marks, et al. NEW ENG J MED. 279:1002-1003, October 31, 1968.

"New antibody in early syphilis," by D. J. Wright, et al. LANCET. 1:740-743, April 11, 1970.

"A new anti-trichomonal agent: negative clinical results," by U. Larsson-Cohn, et al. LAKARTIDNINGEN. 67:914-915, February 25, 1970.

"A new conception of the origin of syphilis in Europe," by A. Boneff. ANN DERM SYPH. 95:529-530, 1968.

"New data in the area of dermatology-venereology obtained at the chair of the Lvov Medical Institute," by A. A. Shtein. VESTN DERM VENER. 43:3-6, June, 1969.

"New developments in venereal disease research," by J. B. Lucas. MED ANN DC. 35:375-378 passim, July, 1966.

"A new fluid medium for cultivating gonococci," by M. Lazar, et al. RUM MED REV. 13:47-48, July-September, 1969.

"New forms of work of dermatovenereological institutions on the control of venereal diseases of the urogenital organs," by S. L. Kozin, et al. VESTN DERM VENER. 44:79-82, January, 1970.

"A new method of syphilis serodiagnosis by means of an 'in vivo' test," by P. Pophristov, et al. MAROC MED. 45:211-216, March, 1966.

"New methods in the therapy of gonorrhea," by J. Danda, et al. CESK DERM. 45:49-57, April, 1970.

"New methods of contact tracing in infectious venereal diseases," by A. M. Lamb. BRIT J VENER DIS. 42:276-279, December, 1966.

"New methods of diagnosis and treatment of vaginal trichomoniasis," by K. L. Keburlia, et al. VESTN DERM VENER. 43:55-57, January, 1969.

"New possibilities for the cultivation of trichomonas," by M. Valent, et al. CESK GYNEK. 32:414-416, August, 1967.

"New prospects in therapy of blennorrhagic urethritis," by R. Santini, et al. G ITAL DERMATOL. 45:590-594, October, 1970.

"A new rapid serologic screening test for syphilis," by J. E. Stauch, et al. MARYLAND MED J. 15:33-34 passim, June, 1966.

"A new serum reaction test of syphilis," by T. Iizuka. KANGO. 18:203, March, 1966.

"A new simple screening test for syphilis: the Portnoy reaction," by L. Surján, et al. ORV HETIL. 110:762-764, April 6, 1969.

"The new specialist education: Dermato-venereology," by K. Thomsen. YNG LAEG. 10:839-840, 1968.

"New statistical contribution on the relationships between the Nelson-Mayer test and classical serological reactions (13,000 cases)," by V. Resta, et al. MINERVA MED. 59:222-228, January 20, 1968.

"A new technic to control malariotherapy in syphilogenic psychoses," by J. A. Garcia, et al. REV BRASIL MED. 24:902-906, November, 1967.

"New therapeutic and diagnostic points of view in gynecology," by A. Stockli. THER UMSCH. 24:18-23, January, 1967.

"New trends in syphilogy," by V. G. Cave, J NAT MED ASS. 61:158-163 passim, March, 1969.

"A new trichomonicide. Experimental work done under Prof. Rosaldo Cavalcanti, gynecology clinic of F.M.U.F.P.," by N. P. De Almeida, et al. HOSPITAL. 77:1581-1585, May, 1970.

"New venereal disease; vibrio fetus infections," TIME. 87:62, February 25, 1966.

"New viewpoints in the management of vaginal discharge," by H. Spitzbart. Z AERZTL FORTBILD. 61:117-119, February 1, 1967.

"New views on the problem of allergy to penicillin," by E. Maciejowska. PRZEGL DERM. 55:299-306, May-June, 1968.

"New ways in the management of acute gonorrhea?," by W. Belda. HOSPITAL. 73:2001-2011, June, 1968.

"Newborn infection with herpesvirus hominis types 1 and 2," by A. J. Nahmias, et al. J PEDIAT. 75:1194-1203, December, 1969.

"Nicolas-Favre disease," by J. Duhamel, et al. ARCH FRANC MAL APPAR DIG. 59:Suppl 7-8:55+, July-August, 1970.

"Nicolas-Favre disease in Bordeaux," by P. Le Coulant, et al. BULL SOC FRANC DERM SYPH. 75:365-367, 1968.

"Nicolau syndrome following retacillin compositum injection," by A. Niedner, et al. Z AERZTL FORTBILD. 64:39-42, January 1, 1970.

"Nifuratel compared with metronidazole in the treatment of trichomonal vaginitis," by B. A. Evans, et al. BRIT MED J. 1:335-336, May 9, 1970.

"Nifuratel for trichomonal vaginitis," by M. Arnold. BRIT MED J. 2:792, June 27, 1970.

"Nifuratel for trichomonal vaginitis," by A. Grimble, et al. BRIT MED J. 2:542, May 30, 1970.

"Nifuratel for trichomonal vaginitis," by S. M. Laird. BRIT MED J. 2:731, June 20, 1970.

"Nifuratel for trichomonal vaginitis," by I. Sagone. BRIT MED J. 2:792, June 27, 1970.

"Nifuratel (Magmilor) in trichomonal vaginitis," by W. Fowler, et al. BRIT J VENER DIS. 44:331-333, December, 1968.

"1968 survey of treponematosis in the eastern highlands of New Guinea," by M. F. Garner, et al. BRIT J VENER DIS. 46:13-17, February, 1970.

"Nitrimidazone, a new systemic trichomonacide," by A. Cantone, et al. G MAL INFETT PARASSIT. 21:954-958, December, 1969.

"Nonallergic fatal incidents following depot penicillin. Pathogenesis and prevention," by G. Ernst, et al. DEUTSCH MED WSCHR. 95:618 passim, March 20, 1970.

"Non-gonococcal infections of the female genitalia," by B. A. Teokharov. BRIT J VENER DIS. 45:334-340, December, 1969.

"Non-gonococcal urethritis acquired concomitantly with gonorrhoea in males," by J. D. Mahoney. ULSTER MED J. 38:148-149, Summer, 1969.

"Non-gonococcal urethritis and Reiter's syndrome: personal experience with etiological studies during 15 years," by D. K. Ford. CANAD MED ASS J. 99:900-910, November 9, 1968.

"Nongonococcal urethritis associated with human strains of 'T' mycoplasmas," by M. C. Shepard. JAMA. 211: 1335-1340, February 23, 1970; also in US NAVAL MED FIELD RES LAB. 18:1-17, September, 1968.

"Non-gonorrheal urethritis," by C. H. Beek. NEDERL T GENEESK. 111:533-554, March 25, 1967.

"Non-gonorrheal urethritis in men'," by G. Rajka. LAKARTIDNINGEN. 63:4613-4620, November 30, 1966.

"Nonspecific positive results of serodiagnostic reactions for syphilis and the possibility of their recognition," by G. Ehrmann. WIEN KLIN WSCHR. 81:213-217, March 21, 1969.

"Non-specific reactions to the quantitative fluorescent antibody test (FTA) in the elderly," by E. I. Grin, et al. BRIT J VENER DIS. 44:216-217, September, 1968.

"Nonspecific urethritis in females," by S. Marshall, et al. NORTHWEST MED. 69:9-10, June, 1970.

"Non-specific urethritis treated with pyrrolidinomethyl tetracycline nitrate," by C. B. Schofield, et al. BRIT J VENER DIS. 45:47-49, March, 1969.

"Nonsyphilitic aortitis," by C. Restrepo, et al. ARCH PATH. 87:1-12, January, 1969.

"Non-tumor causes of the Foster Kennedy syndrome," by N. J. Schatz, et al. J NEUROSURG. 27:37-44, July, 1967.

"The nonvenereal genital diseases as an historical problem," by E. Seidler. HAUTARZT. 17:123-125, March, 1966.

"Nosological and nosographical aspects of syphilis in the province of Cuneo during a 5-year period. Statistical note," by E. Peirone. MINERVA MED. 57: 2777-2780, August 25, 1966.

"A note on the effect of metronidazole on the Nichols strain of treponema pallidum in vitro and in vivo," by A. E. Wilkinson, et al. BRIT J VENER DIS. 43: 201-203, September, 1967.

"A note on the fluorescent treponemal antibody-absorption (FTA-ABS) test," by R. W. Stevens, et al. AMER J CLIN PATH. 47:408-409, March, 1967.

"Note on the treatment of male gonococcic urethritis with vulcacycline," by F. Labouche, et al. BULL SOC FRANC DERM SYPH. 74:665-667, 1967.

"Notes on the treatment of gonorrhea with injectable thiophenicol," by H. Thiers, et al. LYON MED. 217:589-591, February 19, 1967.

"The nurse and venereal disease control," by F. A. Walsh. S CAROLINA NURS. 18:11-13, Winter, 1965-1966.

"The nurse's role in the control of venereal diseases," by J. Towpik. PIELEG POLOZ. 11:6-7, 1966.

"Nutritional requirements of anaerobic spirochetes. 1.

Demonstration of isobutyrate and bicarbonate as growth factors for a strain of treponema microdentium," by P. H. Hardy, et al. J BACT. 91:27-32, January, 1966.

"Objectivized diagnosis of acute pelvic inflammatory disease. Diagnostic and prognostic value of routine laparoscopy," by L. Jacobson, et al. AMER J OBSTET GYNEC. 105:1088-1098, December 1, 1969.

"Obliteration of the anterior cerebral artery by probable syphilitic arteritis," by G. Almard, et al. J MED LYON. 50:215-220, February 5, 1969.

"Observations and problems in the treatment of trichomonas vaginitis," by M. Arnold. THER UMSCH. 23:356-359, September, 1966.

"Observations in the Haight-Asbury Medical Clinic of San Francisco. Health problems in a 'hippie' subculture," by D. Smith, et al. CLIN PEDIAT. 7:313-316, June, 1968.

"Observations of the pathogenesis of syphilis in Aotus trivirgatus," by J. W. Clark, Jr., et al. BRIT J VENER DIS. 44:208-215, September, 1968.

"Observations on the bacteriology of penicillin-resistant gonococcal infections," by K. Kinda. REV MEDIOCOCHIR IASI. 73:967-970, October-December, 1969.

"Observations on a case of Lilliputian hallucinations in the course of a delirious episode in a patient with an ocular disease," by L. Tremelloni. G PSYCHIAT NEUROPAT. 94:625-636, 1966.

"Observations on the culture diagnosis of gonorrhea in women," by J. D. Schmale, et al. JAMA. 210:312-314, October 13, 1969.

"Observations on the development in dermatovenereology in the period from 1912 to 1956," by J. Gate-Lyon. HAUTARZT. 17:81-83, February, 1966.

"Observations on the nature of the F wave in man," by R. F. Mayer, et al. NEUROLOGY. 17:147-156, February, 1967.

"Observations on the occurrence of venereal diseases in Berlin 1933-1939," by M. Sturzbecher. MED MSCHR. 23:259-264, June, 1969.

"Observations on the problem of trichomoniasis and its systemic treatment with nitrimidazine," by I. Signorelli, et al. MINERVA GINEC. 21:1649-1654, December 15, 1969.

"Observations on the use of Rifampicinin dermatovenereology," by G. Bonu, et al. MINERVA MED. 60:4840-4844, December 1, 1969.

"Observations on the versatile symptomatology of trichomonas infections in women in gynecological practice," by H. Deis. MED WELT. 39:2095-2099, September 28, 1968.

"The observed incompatibility of viruses, bacteria and treponema pallidum in the syphilitic patient. Verified by a new in vitro technique for propagating the human pathogen, treponema pallidum," by G. Di Virgilio. GYNAECOLOGIA. 165:338-348, 1968.

"Occurrence of agranulocytic reaction in connection with the use of biomycin and penicillin," by M. L. Aviosor, et al. KLIN MED. 46:139-140, May, 1968.

"Occurrence of biologic false positive reactions with RPR (circle) card test on leprosy patients," by A. Achimastos, et al. PUBLIC HEALTH REP. 85:66-68, January, 1970.

"Occurrence of congenital syphilis in its dependence on the treatment of syphilitic mothers. I. Serologic evaluation of the prevention of congenital syphilis by means of the Nelson-Mayer test," by E. Maly, et al. CESK DERM. 44:108-117, May, 1969.

--II. Comparison of classical reagin seroreactions with the Nelsem-Mayer test in 612 children of syphilitic mothers," by E. Stammová, et al. CESK DERM. 45:164-170, August, 1970.

"Occurrence of gonorrhea in the last 10 years," by J. Obrtel, et al. CESK DERM. 43:22-26, February, 1968.

"Occurrence of gonorrhea in our material during the past 10 years," by V. Plintovic, et al. CESK GYNEK. 35:269-271, 1970.

"The occurrence of gonorrhoeal ophthalmia neonatorum and the efficiency of prophylaxis," by K. Osterlund, et al. ANN PAEDIAT FENN. 14:23-25, 1968.

"The occurrence of Neisseria gonorrhoeae in 'routine' genital cultures," by P. D. Ellner. AMER J CLIN PATH. 52:174-175, August, 1969.

"The occurrence of oxidase-positive nongonococcal strains on Thayer-Martin selective media used in the laboratory diagnosis of N. gonorrhoeae," by E. Geizer. ZBL BAKT. 214:75-78, 1970.

"Occurrence of T-strains and other mycoplasmata in nongonococcal urethritis," by F. T. Black, et al. BRIT J VENER DIS. 44:324-330, December, 1968.

"Occurrence of trichomonas in the male urethra," by M. L. Antunes. REV ASS MED BRASIL. 11:213-214, May, 1965.

"Occurrence of vaginal trichomoniasis and mycosis in our material," by M. Valent, et al. BRATISL LEK LISTY. 53:573-577, May, 1970.

"Occurrence of venereal diseases in the Central Bohemian Region," by J. Obrtel. CESK DERM. 43:48-50, February, 1968.

"Ocular manifestations of polyarteritis nodosa," by M. R. Nanjiani. BRIT J OPHTHAL. 51:696-697, October, 1967.

"The office management of acute infections," by L. Davis. CALIF MED. 107:4-7, July, 1967.

"The oldest department for skin and venereal diseases in Russia," by V. A. Rakhmanov, et al. VESTN DERM VENER. 44:51-58, May, 1970.

"Oletetrin in the therapy of gonorrhea," by A. I. Poliakov, et al. VESTN DERM VENER. 41:71-73, June, 1967.

"Oletetrine in the therapy of patients with gonorrhea," by Z. V. Ermol'eva, et al. VESTN DERM VENER. 42:81-86, April, 1968.

"Oletetrine in the treatment of fresh gonorrhea in men," by T. A. Kislova, et al. ANTIBIOTIKI. 14:467-469, May, 1969.

"On the acquired lung syphilis," by H. Stanulla. ZBL

CHIR. 93:1503-1514, October 26, 1968.

"On the allergic origin of the Jarisch-Herxheimer reaction," by E. Skog, et al. ACTA DERMATOVENER. 46: 136-143, 1966.

"On a case of parafemoral ossification in a patient with Tabes dorsalis," by G. Rava. ARCH SCI MED. 121:228-234, April, 1966.

"On the antigenic properties of a protein-polysaccharide complex of cultured treponema pallidum studies in experiments on rabbits," by S. A. Ugrimov. LAB DELO. 3:173-175, 1968.

"On the antitreponemic action of cephaloridine," by F. Flarer. POSTGRAD MED J. 43:Suppl 43:133-134, August, 1967.

"On the autoinhibition in classical syphilis reactions in neurologic-psychiatric patients," by J. Berndt, et al. ARCH PSYCHIAT NERVENKR. 210:198-210, 1967.

"On a case of congenital syphilis," by M. Passoni, et al. G MAL INFETT. 19:672-674, October, 1967.

"On a case of congenital syphilitic pemphigus," by G. Reynaud. MINERVA PEDIAT. 19:778-780, April 21, 1967.

"On a case of syphilitic pemphigus in a newborn infant with multiple osteochondritic lesions," by G. Sciafani. MINERVA PEDIAT. 22:902-903, April 28, 1970.

"On certain difficulties in the diagnosis of syphilitic aortitis," by S. V. Shestakov. KLIN MED. 45:117-122, June, 1967.

"On certain properties and behavior of so-called luetic reagins: the problem of biologically false reactions," by M. Miklaszewska, et al. POL TYG LEK. 23:104-106, January 15, 1968.

"On certain properties and behavior of the so-called syphilitic reagins (the problem of seroresistance)," by M. Miklaszewska, et al. POL TYG LEK. 22:1867-1869, November 27, 1967.

"On the clinical aspects and treatment of syphilis," by M. M. Zheltakov, et al. SOVET MED. 31:65-68, August, 1968.

"On the clinical early diagnosis of venereal lymphopathy," by H. Roder, et al. Z HAUT GESCHLECHTSKR. 40:158-164, March 1, 1966.

"On the clinical use of a new antibiotic, pimaricin, in the therapy of vaginitis caused by candida albicans and by trichomonas," by B. Ferrari, et al. QUAD CLIN OSTET GINEC. 21:929-945, November, 1966.

"On the current picture of early syphilis," by H. Kresbach. Z HAUT GESHLECHTSKR. 43:109-118, February 1, 1968.

"On the demonstration of immobilizing antibodies against treponema pallidum in the cerebrospinal fluid in syphilis," by F. Muller. DEUTSCH MED WSCHR. 91:2292-2297, December 23, 1966.

"On the determination of treponeme immobilizing potency of weakly reactive sera and its suggested interpretation," BULL WHO. 33:705-720, November 5, 1966.

"On the diagnosis of pulmonary syphilis," by F. Mersch. THORAXCHIRURGIE. 15:456-460, August, 1967.

"On the diagnosis of trichomonas infection," by V. Grunberger. WIEN KLIN WSCHR. 79:551-553, June 30, 1967.

"On the diagnosis of trichomonas invasion on dry smears by the method of luminescent microscopy," by I. A. Fridman, et al. LAB DELO. 1:14-16, 1968.

"On the diagnostic value of serum phosphohexose isomerase in some liver diseases in childhood," by C. M. Berni, et al. BOLL SOX ITAL BIOL SPER. 42:1765-1768, December 15, 1966.

"On the distribution, incidence and laboratory diagnosis of trichomoniasis in Bulgaria," by N. Iankov, et al. AKUSH GINEK. 5:188-191, 1966.

"On the effectiveness of low doses of thiamphenicol in the treatment of urethritis," by A. Riboldi. MINERVA DERM. 41:35-37, January, 1966.

"On the epidemiologic situation in the sector of venereal disease in the Western Slovakia region," by E. Hegyi, et al. CESK DERM. 43:65-71, February, 1968.

"On epidemiology and control of venereal disease in the German Democratic Republic," by H. D. Jung. DERM

WSCHR. 152:793-800, July 30, 1966.

"On the epidemiology of syphilis and gonorrhea in Nordhein-Westfalia," by K. Gedicke. OEFF GESUNDHEITS-WESEN. 29:28-33, January, 1967.

"On the etiologic relationship between leukoplakia syphilis and cancer of the oral cavity," by K. Anastassov, et al. REV FRANC ODONTOSTOMAT. 14:1530-1536, November, 1967.

"On the etiology of the urethrooculosynovial syndrome," by I. A. Zhodzishskii. UROL NEFROL. 31:36-40, January-February, 1966.

"On the evaluation of results of serologic reactions. II. Qualitative demostration of antibodies," by J. Morenz. Z IMMUNITAETSFORSCH. 131:376-389, October, 1966.

"On evaluation of systemic trichomonacide activity," by R. Giannone. MINERVA GINEC. 18:900-906, August 31, 1966.

"On the FTA test," by K. Mizuoka, et al. JAP J CLIN PATH. 16:354-359, April, 1968.

"On the foundling of the Syphilis Therapy work team," by H. Weitgasser. Z HAUT GESCHLECHTSKR. 43:887-888, November 1, 1968.

"On the frequency of positive unspecific syphilis reactions in mononucleosis infectiosa," by G. Tauchnitz, et al. Z GES INN MED. 23:404-406, July 1, 1968.

"On the frequency of syphilis in various populations in the Caribbean area," by P. Cirera, et al. BULL SOC PATH EXOT. 61:169-176, 1968.

"On gonorrhea and moniliasis in Finnish battalion 8 on Cyprus in winter 1967-1968," by E. E. Vuori, et al. SOTILASLAAK AIKAK. 43:126-129, 1968.

"On a granuloma of the vulva by trichomonads. (Case history contribution to the differential diagnosis of primary syphilitic lesion," by N. Sonnichsen, et al. Z HAUT GESCHLECHTSKR. 41:202-204, September 1, 1966.

"On the hemagglutination reaction using treponema pallidum as an antigen (TPHA)," by T. Tomizawa. JAP J CLIN

PATH. 16:360-364, April, 1968.

"On the history of the All-Union Scientific-Medici Dermatovenerologic Society," by A. A. Studnitsin, et al. VESTN DERM VENER. 41:3-13, August, 1967.

"On the history of the development of serological help in the prevention of syphilis in Uzebekistan," by T. U. Usmanov. LAB DELO. 10:633-634, 1968.

"On the ideological history of the early period of chemotherapy," by P. Klein. DEUTSCH MED WSCHR. 91:2281-2284, December 23, 1966.

"On the immunological diagnosis of trichomoniasis," by L. M. Korik. LAB DELO. 4:230-233, 1967.

"On the immunological reactivity of penicillin, cephalosporin and tetracycline antibiotics," by J. Lochmannova, et al. J HYG EPIDEM. 14:201-210, 1970.

"On an 'in vitro' stimulation of lymphocytes by treponema pallidum. Fluorescence-serological detection of gamma globulins," by H. J. Heitmann. HAUTARZT. 19:556-558, December, 1968.

"On an incomplete luetic cerebrospinal fluid syndrome in connection with a skull-brain trauma," by G. Ehrmann, et al. WIEN Z NERVENHEILK. 25:68-75, 1967.

"On the investigation of uncertainties in the effect and treatment of venereal diseases and other ailments in the 19th century," by R. Brachwitz. Z HAUT GESCHLECHTSKR. 44:513-516, 1969.

"On the level of immobilisin in the blood of patients treated for syphilis," by I. Orhel. RAD MED FAK ZAGREB. 14:193-209, 1966.

"On the method of arrangement of the reaction of immobilization of weak treponema," by MIa. Goldberg. LAB DELO. 12:735-736, 1967.

"On methods of control of cure of female gonorrhea," by IuN. Dobrovol'skii. VESTN DERM VENER. 40:73-75, January, 1966.

"On methods of lymphocyte culture as an allergy test," by H. J. Heitmann. HAUTARZT. 18:152-156, April, 1967.

"On the morbidity of gonorrhea in railway workers," by M. M. Vilenskii, et al. VESTN DERM VENER. 43:61-62, January, 1969.

"On my initial experiences with the immunofluorescence method for detection of gonococci," by H. Medebach. MED WELT. 39:2100-2105, September 28, 1968.

"On the participation of Soviet dermato-venereologists in the development of international scientific relations," by N. M. Turanov, et al. VESTN DERM VENER. 41:3-10, June, 1967.

"On the pathogenicity of L-form bacteria and mycoplasmataceae and their role in infectious pathology. II. The significance of mycoplasmataceae (PPLO) in infectious pathology," by V. D. Timakov, et al. ZH MIKROBIOL. 43:1-7, January, 1966.

"On postgonorrheo-posttrichomonas urethritis in men," by A. I. Lopatin. SOVET MED. 30:113-117, September, 1967.

"On the practical value of Nelson's test," by U. Boncinelli. MINERVA DERM. 42:618-620, December, 1967.

"On the present status of our knowledge of lymphogranuloma venereum," by W. Schmidt. THER UMSCH. 26:81-88, February, 1969.

"On the prevention of congenital syphilis," by C. Simon, et al. THER GEGENW. 105:1430-1435, November, 1966; also in MUNCHEN MED WSCHR. 107:1813-1815, September 17, 1965.

"On the prevention of venereal diseases in a city," by J. Kvicera. CESK DERM. 42:404-410, December, 1967.

"On the problem of allergic reactions of the immediate type during treatment with penicillin and streptomycin," by I. I. Dantsig, et al. PROBL TUBERK. 44:70-71, 1966.

"On the problem of credeization in newborn infants," by V. Dvorak. CESK OFTAL. 22:329-330, September, 1966.

"On the problem of gonorrheal and postgonorrheal urethritis," by J. Soltz-Szots, et al. WIEN MED WSCHR. 117:1030-1033, November 18, 1967.

"On the problem of isolated involvement of the paraurethral

passages in gonorrheal infection," by A. V. Klimenko, et al. VESTN DERM VENER. 42:56-57, May, 1968.

"On the problem of reinfection in early syphilis," by J. Bowszyc. PRZEGL DERM. 54:659-664, November-December, 1967.

"On the problem of re-infection in syphilis," by P. Fritsch, et al. DERM WSCHR. 154:387-395, April 27, 1968.

"On the problems of evaluation of 2 reactive tests in otherwise non-reactive spectrum in routine serology of syphilis," by A. Kern. HAUTARZT. 19:520-525, November, 1968.

"On the protective effect of blood sera of persons infested with trichomonas vaginalis Donne," by J. Teras, et al. WIAD PARAZYT. 15:481-483, 1969.

"On the provocative effect of the T.P.I. Test Nelson-Mayer and a possibility of the therapeutic modification of the so-called seroresistant lues," by G. Ehrmann. ARCH KLIN EXP DERM. 227:993-1004, 1966.

"On the question of penicillin resistance in gonorrhea," by P. Wodniansky. Z HAUT GESCHLECHTSKR. 41:16-21, July 1, 1966.

"On the question of sterility and infertility," by H. Muth. HIPPOKRATES. 37:501-509, July 15, 1966.

"On the recurrence of interstitial keratitis," by J. Sédan. BULL SOC OPHTHAL FRANC. 66:432-435, April, 1966.

"On the removal from the register of patients with seroresistant syphilis," by E. K. Reznikov. SOVET MED. 31:117-120, January, 1968.

"On the results, principles, methods and problems of the venereal diseases control in the USSR," by V. A. Rakhmanov, et al. VESTN AKAD MED NAUK SSSR. 22:64-71, 1967.

"On the role of trichomonas infection of the sperm in sterility," by E. B. Bank. ZBL GYNAEK. 88:566-569, April 30, 1966.

"On the routine serology for detection of syphilis in pregnant women treated by the ONMI from 1956-1967," by A. Marcozzi. G ITAL DERM. 45:185-186, March, 1970.

"On sensitivity of the treponema pallidum immobilization test in late forms of syphilis," by M. V. Milich. VESTN DERM VENER. 42:62-65, July, 1968.

"On the sensitivity of trichomonas vaginalis strains to metronidazole," by E. Kovacs, et al. ORV HETIL. 110:66-68, January 12, 1969.

"On sensitivity to penicillin of the gonococcus and the clinical dosage effect of penicillin," by G. Ludwig. DERM WSCHR. 152:1-4, January 8, 1966.

"On the serologic diagnosis of syphilis," by H. Bornemann. LEBENSVERSICHERUNGSMEDIZIN. 19:16-20, January, 1967.

"On the side effects of bicillin-1 and bicillin-3," by B. P. Skokh, et al. VOP OKHR MATERIN DETS. 11:53-56, June, 1966.

"On some organizational measures necessary for further reduction of gonorrhea incidence," by Z. P. Poliakova. VESTN DERM VENER. 40:84-87, September, 1966.

"On specific trochanteritis," by G. Rava, et al. MINERVA ORTOP. 18:143-147, March, 1967.

"On the status of gonorrhea in women," by B. Holzegel, et al. Z AERZTI FORTBILD. 60:82-88, January 15, 1966.

"On syphilis serodiagnosis using treponema pallidum," by T. Tomizawa, et al. JAP J CLIN MED. 26:1003-1007, April, 1968.

"On the therapeutic value of flagyl in trichomoniasis in the male," by L. M. Rozhinskii. VESTN DERM VENER. 40:59-60, April, 1966.

"On the therapy of cerebrospinal positive late syphilis," by H. H. Wiek, et al. MED WELT. 35:1883, August 31, 1968.

"On the therapy of gonorrhea in males," by V. I. Zhukov. VOENNOMED ZH. 3:70-72, March, 1966.

"On the therapy of skin and venereal diseases. Review of the literature 1965-1966," by H. Walther. DEUTSCH

MED J. 19:171-176. March 5, 1968.

"On the therapy of venereal diseases according to the current status," by W. Undeutsch. HIPPOKRATES. 39: 89-97, February 15, 1968.

"On the timing of penicillin treatment of syphilis during pregnancy," by H. Walther. ARCH KLIN EXP DERM. 227:307-308, 1966.

"On the transmission of trichomoniasis by thermal water," by G. Catar, et al. BRATISL LEK LISTY. 47:196-204, February 28, 1967.

"On the treatment of bacterial skin infections and venereal diseases," by A. Steppert. WIEN MED WSCHR. 118:599-602, June 22, 1968.

"On the treatment of fluor vaginalis," by A. Bradenburg. MED KLIN. 61:307-308, February 25, 1966.

"On the use of benzathine penicillin 'penduran' for the long term therapy of syphilis," by A. Kern. DEUTSCH GESUNDH. 21:1739-1750, September 15, 1966.

"On the use of a new drug in the treatment of vaginal trichomona infections," by A. Segre. HOSPITAL. 75: 1483-1492, April, 1969.

"On the use of protein-polysaccharide complex of cultures of treponema pallidum as an antigen in the complement fixation test," by S. A. Ugrimov. LAB DELO. 10:618-620, 1968.

"On the usefulness of a new agglutination test (S.p.A.) in the diagnosis of syphilis," by L. Caldera, et al. FRACASTORO. 61:293-297, May-June, 1968.

"On the value of the complement fixation test in the laboratory diagnosis of trichomoniasis," by N. Iankov, et al. AKUSH GINEK. 7:187-189, 1968.

"On the value of routinely conducted swab examinations of the urethra and cervix of all clinical admissions in gynecology to discover all formerly unknown cases of gonorrhea," by C. Zwahr. ZBL GYNAEK. 90:1192-1196, August 31, 1968.

"On the venereal ulcer of the vulva," by G. Adinolfi, et al. ARCH OSTET GINEC. 72:173-181, March-April, 1967.

"One hundred teenagers in Copenhagen infected with gonorrhoea. A socio-psychiatric study," by K. Ekstrom. BRIT J VENER DIS. 42:162-166, September, 1966.

"The 100th anniversary of the Department of Skin and Venereal Diseases of the Military Medical Academy," by O. K. Shaposhnikov. VESTN DERM VENER. 43:54-60, July, 1969.

"One minute treatment of gonococcal urethritis by spiramycin," by L. Sylvestre, et al. UN MED CANADA. 96:199-201, February, 1967.

"One-session treatment of gonorrhoea in males with procaine penicillin plus probenecid," by R. J. Cobbold, et al. POSTGRAD MED J. 46:142-145, March, 1970.

"Ophthalmia neonatorum. Prevention with 5-nitro-2-furaldehyde semicarbazone (Furacin)," by O. R. Baptista. HOSPITAL. 71:187-193, January, 1967.

"Ophthalmia neonatorum in Glasgow," by J. A. Smith. SCOT MED J. 14:272-276, August, 1969.

"Oral administration of new drugs in the treatment of recent syphilis," by G. Argenziano, et al. MINERVA DERM. 42:396-399, August, 1967.

"Oral administration of a single dosage of ampicillin K in the treatment of gonorrhea," by J. M. de Barros, et al. REV SAUDE PUBLICA. 4:31-34, June, 1970.

"Oral ampicillin in gonorrhoea. Clinical evaluation," by O. Groth, et al. BRIT J VENER DIS. 46:21-26, February, 1970.

"Oral chloramphenicol alone and with intramuscular procaine penicillin in the treatment of gonorrhoea," by H. C. Gjessing, et al. BRIT J VENER DIS. 43:133-136, June, 1967.

"Oral contraception among special clinic patients. With particular reference to the diagnosis of gonorrhoea," by A. B. Hewitt. BRIT J VENER DIS. 46:106-107, April, 1970.

"Oral disorders associated with ocular disease. II. Disorders affecting dentition," by B. Harcourt. BRIT J OPHTHAL. 51:284-285, April, 1967.

"The oral manifestations of acquired syphilis. A study

eighty-one cases," by I. Meyer, et al. ORAL SURG. 23:45-57, January, 1967.

"Oral penicillin and anaphylactoid reactions," by J. H. Dunn. JAMA. 202:552-553, November 6, 1967.

"Oral tetracycline phosphate complex (tetrex) in the treatment of non-specific urethritis," by E. B. Wijetunga, et al. BRIT J VENER DIS. 45:50-51, March, 1969.

"Orally administered erythromycin level in body fluids," by J. Bowszyc, et al. POL TYG LEK. 25:241-243, February 16, 1970.

"The order of appearance of reactivity to treponemal and lipoidal tests in early syphilis," by A. Lassus, et al. ACTA PATH MICROBIOL SCAND. 69:612-613, 1967.

"Organization of continuing education for dermato-venereologists," by A. I. Kartamyshev, et al. VESTN DERM VENER. 42:58-62, 1968.

"Osteoarthropathia tabetica of the ankle joint following a fracture," by T. Krezel. CHIR NARZAD RUCHU ORTOP POL. 31:757-761, 1966.

"Osteolytic lesions in early syphillis," by M. F. Bauer, et al. BRIT J VENER DIS. 43:175-177, September, 1967.

"Ounce of prevention: new interest in syphilis research." NEWSWEEK. 70:54, August 28, 1967.

"Our experiences with the use of indirect fluorescence test in the serodiagnosis of syphilis," by P. Schneiderka, et al. CESK EPIDEM. 16:193-198, July, 1967.

"Outbreak of non-specific urethritis associated with the presence of complement-fixing antibodies to the LB4 strain of TRIC agent," by T. Pasieczny, et al. BRIT J VENER DIS. 42:191-194, September, 1966.

"Outbreak of syphilis," by J. C. Hedden, et al. J S CAROLINA MED ASS. 62:471-473, December, 1966.

"Outline of the history of syphilis," by K. Lejman. ARCH HIST MED. 32:125-145, 1969.

"Overcoming teacher reluctancy toward VD education," by F. B. Benell. J SCH HEALTH. 40:483-486, November, 1970.

"Overtreatment in cases with positive serological syphilis reactions," by C. Gjessing, et al. T NORSK LAEGEFOREN. 87:1981-1982, December 1, 1967.

"Palmar lesions in lupus erythematosus," by L. C. Parish, et al. ARCH DERM. 96:273-276, September, 1967.

"Parallel studies on modifications of the behavior of Reiter's treponema (in vitro) and treponema pallidum (in vivo)," by P. Collart, et al. PATH BIOL. 15:470-479, May, 1967.

"Parallelism of the pathologic changes in the spinal fluid, nonspecific, in patients with neurosyphilis and cerebral cysticercosis. Importance of the Weinberg test," by N. S. Filho. HOSPITAL. 69:317-322, February, 1966.

"Parenteral cephaloridine treatment of patients with early syphilis," by J. M. Glicksman, et al. ARCH INTERN MED. 121:342-344, April, 1968.

"Paresis of the recurrent nerve as the first symptom of luetic aortic aneurysm," by Z. Jina. CESK OTOLARYNG. 16:247-251, August, 1967.

"Paroxysmal cold haemoblobinuria in Jamaica. A case report," by J. K. Wood. W INDIAN MED J. 17:175-179, September, 1968.

"Participation of health education in prevention of gonorrhea in the age categories 15-24 years," by M. Beniak. CESK ZDRAV. 15:249-254, May, 1967.

"Pasomycin treatment of women with gonorrhea," by B. S. Kaliner. VESTN DERM VENER. 42:57-58, May, 1968.

"Passive cutaneous anaphylaxis with guinea-pig and rabbit antibodies to penicillin derivatives," by A. E. Cronin. AUST J DERM. 9:65-69, June, 1967.

"Past and future of the evaluation of syphilis serodiagnosis," by T. Ogata. JAP J CLIN PATH. 16:336-337, April, 1968.

"Pathogenesis of pupillary disorders in various forms of syphilis of the nervous system," by V. D. Kochetkov, et al. VESTN DERM VENER. 44:53-58, March, 1970.

"Pathogenicity of fresh isolates of trichomonas vaginalis, 'the mouse assay' versus clinical and pathologic findings," by B. M. Honigberg, et al. ACTA CYTOL. 10:353-361, September-October, 1966.

"Pathologic-anatomical ocular findings in fetal lues," by H. J. Thiel, et al. KLIN MBL AUGENHEILK. 154:712-716, May, 1969.

"Patients with venereal disease or a health education problem," by T. Z. Capinski, et al. PRZEGL DERM. 53:87-94, January-February, 1966.

"Patterns of sexual behaviour in relation to venereal disease," by K. Ekstrom. BRIT J VENER DIS. 46:93-95, April, 1970.

"Patterns of venereal disease morbidity in recent years." STATIST BULL METROP LIFE INSUR CO. 50:5-7, April, 1969.

"Paul Ehrlich (1854-1915)," by D. Kirchheim. INVEST UROL. 7:257-259, November, 1969.

"Pavilion 8. Dr. Carlos Seminario syphilis and skin services," by O. Dodero. PRENSA MED ARGENT. 55:1980-1983, December 6-13, 1968.

"Peculiarities in dermatology. A case of granuloma inguinale (donovanosis)," by H. J. Kingsley. CENT AFR J MED. 13:145-146, June, 1967.

"Peculiarities of skin and venereal morbidity of the population of some countries of Asia, Africa and Latin America," by R. S. Babaiants. VESTN DERM VENER. 41:49-54, February, 1967.

"Pedagogic considerations on a lecture on syphilis," by J. Danda. CESK DERM. 41:189-190, July, 1966.

"Pedagogical false-positive test for syphilis?," by A. L. Metzger. ANN INTERN MED. 69:1075-1076, November, 1968.

"Pediatric use of the rapid plasma reagin (circle) card test," by J. C. Herweg, et al. PEDIATRICS. 40:440-443, September, 1967.

"Penetrating keratoplasty in interstitial keratitis," by M. F. Rabb, et al. AMER J OPHTHAL. 67:907-917, June, 1969.

"The penetration of bicillin-6 into the cerebrospinal fluid," by O. K. Loseva. VESTN DERM VENER. 41:47-51, August, 1967.

"The penetration of penicillin and other antimicrobials into joint fluid. Three case reports with a reappraisal of the literature," by D. J. Drutz, et al. J BONE JOINT SURG. 49:1415-1421, October, 1967.

"Penicillin allergy." MED LETT DRUGS THER. 10:101-103, December 13, 1968.

"Penicillin allergy," by J. Charpin, et al. MARSEILLE MED. 103:577-578, 1966.

"Penicillin allergy," by J. Jouglard, et al. MED LEG DOMM CORPOR. 2:252-273, July-September, 1969.

"Penicillin allergy (Commentary)," by G. T. Stewart. CLIN PHARMACOL THER. 11:307-311, May-June, 1970.

"Penicillin allergy. A report of thirteen cases of severe reactions," by A. H. Rosenblum. J ALLERG. 42:309-318, December, 1968.

"Penicillin allergy in the light of clinical investigations and results of skin tests with crystalline penicillin, novocaine and trichophytin," by Z. Starzycki. PRZEGL DERM. 57:203-209, March-April, 1970.

"Penicillin and urethritis," by H. N. De Carvalho. HOSPITAL. 76:763-768, August, 1969.

"Penicillin-bicillin treatment of patients with infectious forms of syphilis," by G. I. Egorov. VESTN DERM VENER. 41:42-46, February, 1967.

"Penicillin dosage in fresh gonorrhea in men," by T. Putkonen, et al. DUODECIM. 84:512-516, 1968.

"Penicillin dosage in treatment of gonorrhea," by I. Juhlin. NORD MED. 76:806-808, July 14, 1966.

"Penicillin encephalopathy in children," by S. R. Ullal. J INDIAN MED ASSOC. 54:513-515, July 1, 1970.

"Penicillin hypersensitivity," by M. G. Maheras. MINN MED. 52:1811-1817, November, 1969.

"Penicillin-induced granulopenia, by J. Forshaw. BRIT MED J. 3:184, July 20, 1968.

"Penicillin-induced haemolytic anaemia." BRIT MED J. 3:4, July 6, 1968.

"Penicillin-induced haemolytic anaemia," by H. E. Amos, et al. BRIT MED J. 2:436, August 17, 1968.

"Penicillin-induced haemolytic anaemia," by M. A. Rossiter, et al. BRIT MED J. 3:616-617, September 7, 1968

"Penicillin-induced haemolytic anaemia," by J. M. White, et al. BRIT MED J. 3:26-29, July 6, 1968.

"Penicillin-induced seizures during cardiopulmonary bypass. A clinical and electroencephalographic study," by K. B. Seamans, et al. NEW ENG J MED. 278:861-868, April 18, 1968.

"Penicillin is losing effect on gonorrheal infections." AM DRUGGIST. 159:57, May 5, 1969.

"Penicillin-resistant gonorrhea," by N. Blumberg. J UROL. 101:106, January, 1969.

"Penicillin-resistant gonorrhoea and post-gonococcal urethritis," MED J AUST. 1:275-276, February 17, 1968.

"Penicillin resistant syphilis," by M. A. Rozentul, et al. VESTN DERM VENER. 40:55-58, April, 1966.

"Penicillin sensitivity of gonococci and its significance in the clinic and treatment of gonorrhea in women," by A. V. Chastikova, et al. ANTIBIOTIKI. 15:561-564, June, 1970.

"Penicillin skin tests as predictive and diagnostic aids in penicillin allergy," by R. G. Van Dellen, et al. MED CLIN N AMER. 54:997-1007, July, 1970.

"Penicillin treatment in neurosyphilis," by W. Schubert. MED KLIN. 63:806-810, May 17, 1968.

"Penicillinase-producing staphylococci in the male urethra and their effect on penicillin treatment of gonorrhoea," by B. Lagerholm, et al. ACTA DERMATO-VENER. 46:345-347, 1966.

"Penicillins and aqueous humor," by E. E. Goldman, et al. AMER J OPHTHAL. 65:717-721, May, 1968.

"Performance and use of the Reiter protein complement-fixation (RPCF) test," by J. H. Bekker, et al. BRIT

J VENER DIS. 42:42-43, March, 1966.

"Pericarditis. Anatomoclinical study," by E. Salazar, et al. ARCH INST CARDIOL MEX. 36:624-650, September-October, 1966.

"Perinatal mastocytosis. Gonococcal infection in the mother," by C. Grupper, et al. BULL SOC FRANC DERM SYPH. 73:847-849, December, 1966.

"Perinuclear halo versus koilocytotic atypia," by E. De Girolami. OBSTET GYNEC. 29:479-487, April, 1967.

"Persistence of particular forms of treponema pallidum in syphilitic patients detected in the late stages of their infection and not treated in time," by S. G. Nicolau, et al. ANN DERM SYPH. 96:253-264, 1969.

"Persistence of syphilis antibodies in the immunofluorescence reaction of treponema," by M. Hanczakowska, et al. PRZEGL DERM. 56:301-304, May-June, 1969.

"Persistence of treponemes after treatment of syphilis." LANCET. 2:718-719, September 28, 1968.

"Persistence of treponemes and the infectivity test in syphilis." LANCET. 1:130-131, January 17, 1970.

"Personal experience in surgical treatment of thoracic aortic aneurysms. Observations on 16 cases," by R. Donatelli, et al. ANN ITAL CHIR. 43:987-1027, December, 1967.

"Personality characteristics of V.D. patients," by B. W. Wells. BRIT J SOC CLIN PSYCHOL. 8:246-252, September, 1969.

"Perspectives in venereology-1965," by R. R. Willcox. BULL HYG. 41:1033-1056, October, 1966.

--1966. BULL HYG. 42:1169-1200, November, 1967.

"Phagocytic capability of the vaginal trichomonas and its role in female infertility," by A. P. Kolesov. UKRANIAN PEDIAT AKUSH GINEK. 2:63, March-April, 1966.

"Philippe Ricord (1800-1889), syphilographer." JAMA. 211:115-116, January 5, 1970.

"Physician breaks chain of infectious syphilis," N CAROLINA MED J. 28:107, March, 1967.

"Physician reporting of venereal disease in the USA," by J. S. McKenzie-Pollock. BRIT J VENER DIS. 46:114-116, April, 1970.

"Physicians' attitudes toward venereal disease reporting. A survey by the national opinion research center," by R. L. Cleere, et al. JAMA. 202:941-946, December 4, 1967.

"Physician's responsibility in venereal disease control," by C. W. Freeman. MED ANN DC. 35:382, July, 1966.

"The 'pill' promiscuity, and venereal disease," by L. Cohen. BRIT J VENER DIS. 46:108-110, April, 1970.

"A pilot survey of venereal disease in general practice," by B. W. Christmas. NEW ZEAL MED J. 67:188-191, February, 1968.

"Pimaricin," by J. Bret. SEM THER. 41:427-428, October, 1965.

"Pimaricin, an antibiotic towards fungi and trichomonads by W. Raab. ARZNEIMITTELFORSCHUNG. 17:538-543, May, 1967.

"Pimaricin in the treatment of trichomoniasis and vaginal moniliasis," by H. Zorn. Z ALLGEMEINMED. 45:1640-1643, December 10, 1969.

"Pinta in Puerto Rico," by A. L. Carrion. BOLL ASOC MED P RICO. 60:456-461, October, 1968.

"Pitfalls in the diagnosis of trichomonas vaginalis by the Papanicolaou smear," by G. Perl. MT SINAI J MED. 37:632-634, September-October, 1970.

"Pitfalls of the treponema pallidum immobilization test," by L. Pospisil, et al. CESK DERM. 45:187-191, August, 1970.

"The pitfalls of trichomonas," by A. Lieveaux. REV FRANC GYNEC OBSTET. 65:433-436, July-August, 1970.

"Plan of scientific research during 1968 on the problem: 'scientific foundations of dermatology and venereology'," by N. M. Turanov, et al. VESTN DERM VENER. 42:3-6, March, 1968.

"Planning and construction of dermato-venereological dispensaries," by N. M. Turanov, et al. VESTN DERM VENER.

43:56-59, February, 1969.

"Pleuro-pulmonary localization of trichomonas," by L. Abed, et al. BULL SOC PATH EXOT. 59:962-964, November-December, 1966.

"Polish dermatology and venerology for 25 years in the Polish People's Republic," by B. Michalowski, et al. PRZEGL DERM. 56:437-440, July-August, 1969.

"Polymyalgia rheumatica," by G. G. Hunder, et al. MAYO CLIN PROC. 44:849-875, December, 1969.

"A polyvalent latex slide test for rapid screening of syphilis in blood donors," by K. Lou, et al. BIBI HAEMAT. 29:1029-1032, 1968.

"Positive fluorescent treponemal antibody reactions in diabetes," by M. K. Hughes, et al. APPL MICROBIOL. 19:425-528, March, 1970.

"Possible advantages of highly purified penicillin in avoiding penicilloyl-specific sensitization and allergic reactions," by J. Pedersen-Bjergaard. ACTA ALLERG. 24:303-325, November, 1969.

"Possible mycoplasma hominis urethritis revealed by differing responses of 'abacterial urethritis' to treatment with tetracycline and erythromycin," by A. S. Grimble. BRIT J VENER DIS. 44:230-231, September, 1968.

"The possible scope of trimethoprim-sulphonamide treatment," by L. P. Garrod. POSTGRAD MED J SUPPL, London. 45:52-55, November, 1969.

"Post-gonorrhoeal urethral stricture and hypertension in Nigeria," by E. A. Elebute. TRANS ROY SOC TROP MED HYG. 60:678-680, 1966.

"The post-treatment disappearance of reactivity to treponemal and lipoidal tests in early syphilis," by A. Lassus, et al. ACTA DERMATOVENER. 50:148-150, 1970.

"The pox," by S. E. Acres. CANAD J PUBLIC HEALTH. 60:457-458, December, 1969.

"Practical aspects of gonorrhea treatment," by G. Krook. NORD MED. 76:809-810, July 14, 1966.

"Practical possibilities of the use of immunological phenomena in syphilis," by J. Towpik. POL TYG LEK. 22: 360-363, March 6, 1967.

"Practical use of the auto-analyzer for the serodiagnosis of syphilis (study of 1,009 sera) using a cardiolipid antigen," by R. Gaillon, et al. PATH BIOL. 14:952-954, October, 1966.

"Practical value of cytological and cytochemical diagnosis in trichomoniasis," by A. Marconato, et al. MINERVA GINEC. 18:954-955, September 15, 1966.

"The practical value of the immunofluorescence (FTA) test in the diagnosis and prognosis of syphilis," by A. Midana. MINERVA MED. 57:4438-4440, December 22, 1966; also in PANMINERVA MED. 9:181-183, May, 1967.

"The practical value of the Melangeur method of the treponema immobilization test," by S. G. Alieva, et al. VESTN DERM VENER. 42:46-50, January, 1968.

"Prediction of penicillin allergy by immunological test," by B. B. Levine, et al. J ALLERG. 43:231-244, April, 1969.

"Pregnancy, trichomoniasis, and metronidazole. A novel dose schedule," by R. X. Sands. AMER J OBSTET GYNEC. 94:350-353, February 1, 1966.

"Preliminary clinical findings using Nifuratel in vaginal trichomoniasis," by C.G. de Netto, et al. REV BRASIL MED. 26:190-192, March, 1969.

"Preliminary observations on the use of pimaricin in vaginitis due to candida albicans, trichomonas vaginalis and in aspecific vaginitis," by B. I. De Luca. MINERVA GINEC. 18:840-846, August 15, 1967.

"Preliminary report on a mass program for detection of gonorrhea," by J. Zackler, et al. PUBLIC HEALTH REP. 85:681-684, August, 1970.

"Preliminary research on the classes of immunoglobulins which are responsible for syphilitic positive serologic reactions," by F. P. Merklen, et al. BULL SOC FRANC DERM SYPH. 75:57-61, 1968.

"Preliminary results of penicillin treatment in symptomatic early syphilis in 1959-1963," by J. Towpik. PRZEGL DERM. 53:29-32, January-February, 1966.

"Preliminary studies of the kinin-forming properties of the blood in certain skin diseases," by Z. Onisk, et al. PRZEGL DERM. 54:557-564, September-October, 1967.

"Preliminary study on the epidemiology of venereal diseases in Turin from 1958 to 1968," by B. Erber, et al. G BATT VIROL IMMUN. 62:3-15, January-February, 1969.

"Premarital pregnancy and status before and after marriage," by L. C. Coombs, et al. AM J SOCIOL. 75:800-820, March, 1970.

"Pre-or post-Columbian? 1st appearance of syphilis in Europe," by T. Mildner. MED KLIN. 63:1392-1395, August 30, 1968.

"Preparation and standardization of the sorbent used in the fluorescent treponemal antibody-absorption (FTA-ABS) test," by G. W. Stout, et al. HEALTH LAB SCI. 4:5-8, January, 1967.

"Preparation of fluorescein-labelled immune glubulin for the identification of treponema pallidum," by S. M. Mothershed, et al. BRIT J VENER DIS. 44:201-207, September, 1968.

"Prescribing contraception for teen-agers--a moral compromise," by R. J. Pion. OBSTET GYNEC. 30:752-755. November, 1967.

"The presence of spirochetes in late seronegative syphilis," by J. L. Smith, et al. JAMA. 199:126-130, March 27, 1967.

"Presence of spirochaetes in paresis despite penicillin therapy," by W. E. Gager, et al. BRIT J VENER DIS. 44:277-282, December, 1968.

"Present aspects of urogenital trichomoniasis," by L. Scarpellini, et al. MINERVA GINEC. 19:668-681, July 15, 1967.

"Present clinical and serological aspects of syphilis," by G. B. Cottini, et al. HAUTARZT. 17:74-79, February, 1966.

"Present-day situation regarding venereal diseases in Mexico," by S. A. Campos, et al. SALUD PUBLICA MEX. 8:553-560, July-August, 1966.

"Present panorama of syphilis. Basic measurements to control it," by C. Bopp. AN BRASIL DERM. 41:157-164, July-September, 1966.

"Present problems of the epidemiology and diagnosis of gonorrhea," by J. Bartunek, et al. CESK DERM. 43: 31-38, February, 1968.

"Present problems of venereal diseases in women," by A. Wiedmann. REV CLIN ESP. 103:429-435, December 31, 1966.

"Present sensitivity to antibiotics of 65 strains of Neisseria gonorrhoeae isolated in Marseille region," by P. Le Noc, et al. MARSEILLE MED. 107:43-46, 1970.

"Present state of experimental studies on the effect of antibiotics other than penicillin on treponema pallidum in vitro," by A. Jakubowski. PRZEGL DERM. Suppl: 7-12, 1969.

"Present status and variation in syphilis patients," by H. Tsugami. JAP J NURS ART. 8:11-20, August, 1969.

"Present status of the control of venereal diseases in Mexico," by S. A. Campos. SALUD PUBLICA MEX. 7: 371-380, May-June, 1965.

"Present status of female trichomoniasis in Okinawa," by T. Okawa, et al. SANFUJIN JISSAL. 19:201-203, February, 1970.

"Present status of gonorrhea therapy with special reference to penicillin-sensitivity loss of specific gonococci strains," by J. Meyer-Rohn. Z HAUT GESCHLECHTSKR. 45:533-534, July 15, 1970.

"Present status of serological examinations of syphilis," by K. Mizuoka. 24:13-18, July, 1969.

"Present status of trichomoniasis in women in Fukushima prefecture," by T. Okawa, et al. J JAP OBSTET GYNEC SOC. 21:1360-1363, November, 1969.

"The present status of urogenital trichomoniasis. A general review of the literature," by Z. Gallai, et al. APPL THER. 8:773-778, September, 1966.

"Present status of venereal disease," by S. Mizuno. J JAP OBSTET GYNEC SOC. 18:871-872, August, 1966.

"Present status of venereal diseases," by Y. Onoda. J JAP MED ASS. 60:1081-1095, December 1, 1968.

"Present tasks and possibilities of the Polish health services in the field of venereal disease control," by T. Z. Capiński. PRZEGL DERM. Suppl:85-91, 1969.

"Preservation of serum antibodies in syphilis," by A. Vaisman, et al. BULL WHO. 34:461-466, 1966.

"The preservation of syphilis serum antibodies subjected to different temperatures," by A. Vaisman, et al. BULL WHO. 40:153-157, 1969.

"The prevalence of infectious syphilis in patients with acute gonorrhea," by R. C. Brown. SOUTHERN MED J. 61:98-100, January, 1968.

"Prevention and disinfection of syphilis," by Y. Shimizu. JAP J NURS ART. 8:81-86, August, 1969.

"Prevention of cancer of the cervix uteri in patients with chronic gonorrhea," by A. D. Tselischeva. VESTN DERM VENER. 40:57-62, March, 1966.

"Prevention of complications after gynecological operations in cases with trichomonas vaginalis," by J. Starzyk, et al. PRZEGL LEK. 23:446-448, 1967.

"Prevention of post-metronidazole candidosis with amphotericin B pessaries," by L. Z. Oller, BRIT J VENER DIS. 45:163-166, June, 1969.

"The prevention of syphilis," by C. W. Freeman. J NAT MED ASS. 59:189-192, May, 1967.

"The prevention of venereal disease in the Royal Navy," by S. Dudley. J ROY NAV MED SERV. 53:36-42, Spring, 1967.

"Prevention of venereal disease 'quackery'?," by G. Lomholt. LAKARTIDNINGEN. 65:2156-2158, May 22, 1968.

"Prickle-cell carcinoma of the supra-and infra-clavicular fossa resembling the pancoast-tobias syndrome in a patient with syphilis of the nervous system," by S. Zelazny, et al. PRZEGLAD LEK. 22:514-515, 1966.

"Primary and secondary syphilis. Country of origin study, 1965," by British Cooperative Clinical Group. BRIT J VENER DIS. 43:89-95, June, 1967.

--1966. BRIT J VENER DIS. 42:167-173, June, 1968.

--1967. BRIT J VENER DIS. 44:307-314, December, 1968.

--1968. BRIT J VENER DIS. 46:69-75, February, 1970.

"Primary chancre of cervix uteri," by V. Tchertkoff, et al. NEW YORK J MED. 66:1921-1924, July 15, 1966.

"Primary isolation of N. gonorrhoeae with a new commercial medium," by J. E. Martin, Jr, et al. PUBLIC HEALTH REP. 82:361-363, April, 1967.

"Primary isolation of Neisseria gonorrhoeae on hemoglobin-free Thayer-Martin medium," by D. M. Pariser, et al. PUBLIC HEALTH REP. 85:532-534, June, 1970.

"Primary, secondary, and congenital syphilis from 1938 to 1965 on the basis of statistics of the dermosyphilopathic clinic of Genoa and the 'Giannina Gaslini' Pediatric Hospital of Genoa," by E. Rampini, et al. MINERVA DERM. 41:442-444, December, 1966.

"Primary syphilis of the anorectal region," by B. Samenius. DIS COLON RECTUM. 11:462-466, November, 1968; also in PROC ROY SOC MED. 59:629-631, July, 1966.

"Primary syphilis of the gingiva. Report of two cases," by M. Steiner, et al. ORAL SURG. 21:530-535, April, 1966.

"Primo-secondary syphilis; digital chancre with unusual localization," by F. Labouche, et al. BULL SOC FRANC DERM SYPH. 74:154-155, 1967.

"Principles and technique of a simple method to automate the complement fixation reactions," by R. Vargues. BIBL HAEMAT. 29:958-967, 1968.

"Principles for treating gonorrhea," by L. Molin. LAKARTIDNINGEN. 66:1008-1010, March 5, 1969.

"Principles for treatment of gonorrhea. Comments and alternatives," by I. Juhlin. LAKARTIDNINGEN. 66:2078-2081, May 14, 1969.

"The private physician and venereal disease control in the Western Pacific Region," by R. R. Willcox. BRIT J CLIN PRACT. 24:97-99, March, 1970.

"Probable trichomonas vaginalis epididymitis," by A. D.

Amar. JAMA. 200:417-418, May 1, 1967.

"The problem of cure in syphilis," by F. Flarer. MINERVA DERM. 42:235-236, July, 1967.

"The problem of failures in the treatment of gonorrhea," by F. Miedziński, et al. POL MED J. 5:206-211, 1966.

"The problem of Jarish-Herxheimer-Lukasiewicz reaction in congenital syphilis in infants," by K. Lejman, et al. POL MED J. 6:1069-1073, 1967; also in PRZEGL DERM. 54:51-56, January-February, 1967.

"The problem of penicillin resistant gonococci," by C. S. Nicol, et al. BRIT J VENER DIS. 44:315-318, December, 1968.

"The problem of syphilis and gonorrhea today," by W. L. Fleming. ARCH ENVIRON HEALTH, Chicago. 13:357-366, September, 1966.

"Problem of syphilis in blood donors in the light of data of the Provinc Blood Service Center in Gdańsk," by J. Kozakiewicz, et al. WIAD LEK. 21:645-648, April 15, 1968.

"Problem of venereal diseases in the area of Stalowa Wola," by K. Wojas. ZDROW PUBLICZNE. 4:493-499, April, 1967.

"The problem of venereal diseases in the capital Prague," by J. Konopik. CESK DERM. 43:46-47, February, 1968.

"Problems caused by complications of penicillin therapy in antivenereal dispensaries," by F. X. Carton. BULL SOC FRANC DERM SYPH. 74:189-190, 1967.

"Problems in the evaluation of syphilis serodiagnosis," by K. Jo. JAP J CLIN PATH. 16:373, April, 1968.

"Problems in the management of patients with gonorrhea," by W. L. Porter. DELAWARE MED J. 41:157-158, May, 1969.

"The problems of the antivenereal fight in the Northern Bohemian Region," by V. Seycek. CESK DERM. 43:51-55, February, 1968.

"Problems of diagnosis and therapy of acute and chronic nonspecific urethritis," by H. D. Jung. Z UROL. 59:865-871, December, 1966.

"Problems of obstetrics and gynecology in an African developing country (Ethiopia)," by A. Huber, et al. BIBL GYNAEC. 47:1-128, 1968.

"Problems of postgonorrhea urethritides," by V. Semrádová. CESK DERM. 45:181-183, August, 1970.

"Problems of public health resulting from migration of workers," by A. Roussel. BULL INST NAT SANTE. 21: 1121-1138, November-December, 1966.

"The problems of urogenital trichomonasis in pre-puberal girls," by B. Beric, et al. GYNEC PRAT. 21:217-222, 1970.

"Problems with gonorrhea in the Southern Moravian region," by J. Horácek. CESK DERM. 43:62-64, February, 1968.

"Problems with venereal diseases in the Eastern Slovakian region in 1966 according to districts," by E. Malý. CESK DERM. 43:72-76, February, 1968.

"Prodigiozane in the therapy of skin and venereal diseases," by M. A. Rozentul, et al. VESTN DERM VENER. 40:46-47, October, 1966.

"Prognosis in syphilis," by F. E. Rabello. AN BRASIL DERM. 43:243-260, December, 1968.

"The prognosis of syphilitic infection. (Clinical, serological and statistical data)," by U. Boncinelli, et al. G ITAL DERM. 107:463-512, September-December, 1966.

"Programmed instruction and prospects of its application in teaching of dermato-venereology," by V. A. Rakhmanov, et al. VESTN DERM VENER. 42:52-57, 1968.

"Programmed text gives students facts about VD." OHIO SCH. 44:15+, March, 1966.

"Progress in the diagnosis and management of venereal disease," by B. A. Smithurst. MED J AUST. 1:308-310, February 8, 1969.

"Progressive paralysis--Past and present," by S. Stojiljkovic, et al. SRPSKI ARH CELOK LEK. 94:211-218, March, 1966.

"Proliferation of pigmented cells in the corneal endothelium," by M. L. Restivo-Manfridi, et al. ANN OTTAL.

92:1007-1011, November, 1966.

"Promiscuity and contraception in a sample of patients attending a clinic for venereal diseases," by A. Linken, et al. BRIT J VENER DIS. 46:243-246, June, 1970.

"Proof of gonorrhea by the immunofluorescent technic. II. Comparison of the cultivation and immunofluorescent technics," by V. Potuznik, et al. CESK DERM. 42:86-90, April, 1967.

"Proper interpretation of serologic tests for syphilis in the aged," by L. Nicholas. J AMER GERIAT SOC. 15:224-229, March, 1967.

"Properties of fragments of human Wassermann antibodies," by K. Amiraian, et al. IMMUNOLOGY. 10:349-353, April, 1966.

"Prophylactic treatment of syphilis in human carriers of a recent blenorrhagic urethritis," by C. Grupper. SEM THER. 42:239-241, April, 1966.

"Prophylaxis against gonorrhoeal ophthalmia," by V. G. Cave. JAMA. 212:630, April 27, 1970.

"Prophylaxis in congenital syphilis," by A. Chmielecki. WIAD LEK. 23:1487-1490, September 1, 1970.

"Protein fractions of blood serum in patients with syphilis during Ecmonovocillin therapy," by T. A. Malygina, et al. VRACH DELO. 11:132-133, November, 1968.

"Provocation of the Nelson-Mayer TPI test and a possibility of therapeutic effect on the so-called seroresistant syphilis. II. Theoretical bases, further results of investigation and treatment," by G. Ehrmann. ARCH KLIN EXP DERM. 230:13-33, 1967.

"Pseudoanaphylactic reactions to procaine penicillin G," by R. Tompsett. ARCH INTERN MED. 120:565-567, November, 1967.

"Pseudogonococcal ophthalmia infection with herellea vaginicola," by J. P. Canby. MED J AUST. 2:1104-1105, December 14, 1968.

"Pseudo-gummatous scrotal pyodermitis associated with isolated pyodermitis of the right leg," by M. Bolgert, et al. BULL SOC FRANC DERM SYPH. 73:14-15, January-

February, 1966.

"Pseudo-neoplastic aspects of syphilis of the cervix," by D. Rossi, et al. RIV ITAL GINEC. 51:480-491, June-July, 1967.

"Pseudo-retinopathy pigmentosa caused by acquired syphilis," by U. Volpi. ANN OTTAL. 92:408-414, June, 1966.

"Pseudo-retinopathy pigmentosa in congenital syphilis. Description of a case," by M. Santori. MINERVA OFTAL. 8:89-92, May-June, 1966.

"Psuedo-syphilis papulosa naevoides. (Differential diagnostic problems with nevi resembling condylomata lata in the genital region)," by L. Szego, et al. DERM MSCHR. 155:580-595, 1969.

"Pseudosyphilitic pneumonia," by V. I. Pokrovskii, et al. KLIN MED. 47:119-121, June, 1969.

"Psychiatric differences in Ashkenazim and Sephardim," by F. Grewel. PSYCHIAT NEUROL NEUROCHIR. 70:339-347, September-October, 1967.

"Psychiatric drugs and trends. The alarming comeback of gonorrhea," by E. L. Dembicki. J PSYCHIAT NURS. 6:176-177, May-June, 1968.

"Psychiatric referral of patients in a venereal diseases clinic," by J. R. Pedder. BRIT J VENER DIS. 46:54-57, February, 1970.

"Psychosocial background of servicemen contracting venereal diseases," by K. Singh, et al. J INDIAN MED ASS. 46:270-274, March 1, 1966.

"Psychosomatic aspects of female genital trichomoniasis," by G. Pinoli, et al. MINERVA GINEC. 21:508-511, April 30, 1969.

"Psychotic reaction to penicillin," by S. Jacobson. AMER J PSYCHIAT. 124:999, January, 1968.

"Public education in venereal disease," by F. S. Rowntree. BRIT J VENER DIS. 42:246-250, December, 1966.

"Public health and the Vietnam returnee," by D. L. Nathan. JAMA. 208:154, April 7, 1969.

"Public health aspects of syphilis," by W. J. Brown. SOUTHERN MED J. 59:639-642, June, 1966.

"Public health problems relating to the Vietnam returnee," by J. H. Greenberg. JAMA. 207:697-702, January 27, 1969

"Public health report," by L. Breslow. CALIF MED. 106: 429-430, May, 1967.

"The public health service venereal disease program," by W. J Brown. ARCH ENVIRON HEALTH, Chicago. 13:372-375, September, 1966.

"Publicity material on VD." HEALTH BULL. 28:6, January, 1970.

"Purification of ampicillin," by G. T. Stewart, et al. BRIT MED J. 1:295, May 2, 1970.

"Purple permanganate." JAMA. 195:214-215, January 17, 1966.

"Purulent vulvovaginitis in a newborn girl as a rare form of a trichomonas vaginalis infection and its treatment," by C. Sander. Z KINDERHEILK. 98:364-369, 1967.

"Pyrogenal in the therapy of nongonococcal urethritis and its complications," by A. M. Kukushkin. VESTN DERMATOL VENEROL. 44:80-83, March, 1970.

"Quantitative automated reagin test for syphilis," by B. E. McGrew, et al. AMER J MED TECHN. 36:1-7, January, 1970.

"Quantitative determination of immunoglobulins in cerebrospinal fluid," by S. Takase, et al. TOHOKU J EXP MED. 98:189-198, June, 1969.

"Quantitative F.T.A. test made with fluorescent fractionated anti-gamma globulin. I. Primary and secondary syphilis," by S. Sartoris, et al. MINERVA DERM. 43:219-223, May, 1968.

"Quantitative fluorescent treponemal antibody (FTA) studies with balanitis and 'problem' sera," by K. Kiraly. PATH MICROBIOL. 29:75-83, 1966.

"Quantitative fluorescent treponemal antibody test, using fluorescent fractionated antigammaglobulins," by S. Sartoris, et al. G ITAL DERM. 110:18-22, January, 1969.

"A quantitative method for the treponema pallidum immobilization test," by L. V. Sazonova, et al. VESTN DERM VENER. 44:63-66, January, 1970.

"Quantitative Reiter protein complement-fixation test," by O. P. Salo, et al. BRIT J VENER DIS. 43:264-266, December, 1967.

"Quick cytochrome oxidase test for the detection of gonococcal urethritis," by G. C. Fuga, et al. MINERVA DERM. 42:647-648, December, 1967.

"A quick reagin reaction and the TPIT," by L. Pospisil. CESK DERM. 41:102, April, 1966.

"RPC of the month from the AFIP," by R. F. Kilcoyne, et al. RADIOLOGY. 94:687-690, March, 1970.

"RPCF test", by F. Osada. JAP J CLIN PATH. 16:348-353, April, 1968.

"Radicular and medullary complications of tabetic vertebral osteoarthropathies," by R. Thurel, et al. REV NEUROL. 114:62-65, January, 1966.

"Radicular compression due to tabetic arthropathies of the spine," by H. Serre, et al. REV RHUM MAL OSTEO-ARTIC. 37:525-533, August-September, 1970.

"The radiologic aspects of the osseous lesions of yaws," by R. P. Delahaye, et al. J RADIOL ELECTR. 49:41-48, January-February, 1968.

"Radiological case of the month. Congenital syphilis with Parrot's pseudoparalysis," by J. L. Gwinn, et al. AMER J DIS CHILD. 120:243-244, September, 1970.

"Radiological notes. Case No. 340," by C. Bloch, et al. MOUNT SINAI J MED NY. 37:156-158, March-April, 1970.

"Rapid biochemical presumptive test for gonorrheal urethritis in the male," by A. H. Pedersen, et al. PUB-

LIC HEALTH REP. 81:318-322, April, 1966.

"Rapid card test for syphilis diagnosis", by P. Muller. SCHWEIZ MED WSCHR. 97:1196, September 9, 1967.

"The rapid detection of metronidazole in urine," by P. Durel, et al. BRIT J VENER DIS. 43:111-113, June, 1967.

"A rapid macroscopic screening test for syphilis. II. Further evaluation," by F. M. Lucatorto, et al. J AMER DENT ASS. 73:100-101, July, 1966.

"Rapid panorama of the most frequent dermato-venerological diseases. Their importance for the public health," by C. Huriez. BULL SOC FRANC DERM SYPH. 76:803-813, 1969.

"The rapid plasma reagin card test for the diagnosis of syphilis," by S. Nolting, et al. MUNCHEN MED WSCHR. 108:845-847, April 15, 1966.

"Rapid staining of treponema pallidum in tissue," by K. Ito, et al. BULL PHARM RES INST. 72:1-6, January, 1968.

"A rapid syphilis test (RPRC-test)," by P. Muller. DERMATOLOGICA. 135:238-242, 1967.

"Rapid technic for the Bordet-Wasserman sero-reaction with hemolytic complex," by P. Cirera. ANN BIOL CLIN. 24:709-714, May-June, 1966.

"Rapid test for the diagnosis of syphilis with a treponema antigen," by E. Engelbrecht. PATH MICROBIOL. 29:553-557, 1966.

"Rapid test for syphilis in medical practice," by K. H. Simon. MED MSCHR. 23:466-468, October, 1969.

"Rapidly progressive cases of neurosyphilitic psychosis," by K. Dewhurst. PSYCHIAT CLIN. 1:320-326, 1968.

"Rapidly progressive deafness caused by syphilitic neurolabyrinthitis," by G. Pellegrini, et al. REV OTO-NEUROOPHTAL. 41:203-211, May-June, 1969.

"A rare case of aneurysm of the ascending aorta," by Z. Zaborowski, et al. WIAD LEK. 22:655-656, April 1, 1969.

"Rare case of Simmonds' disease possibly caused by syphilitic lesion. Clinical diagnosis: adrenal cortical insufficiency and autopsy study. Severe atrophy of pituitary gland," by T. Oda, et al. CLIN ENDOCR. 14:479-486, June, 1966.

"A rare case of tabetic arthropathy of the hip," by G. Sgarbi, et al. OSPED ITAL CHIR. 16:615-625, June, 1967.

"Rare complication after plastic operation in the oral cavity vestibule," by W. Rytlowa, et al. CZAS STOMAT. 19:525-528, May, 1966.

"Reaction of cardiolipin antigen," by T. Suzuta. JAP J CLIN PATH. 16:341-347, April, 1968.

"Reactions of treponema pallidum, especially to TPI, FTA, TPHA," by T. Tomizawa. JAP J CLIN MED. 26:304-309, February, 1968.

"Reactions to penicillins." LANCET. 2:673, September 21, 1968.

"Reactivations of immunofluorescence in certain cases of old syphilis," by G. Tramier, et al. BULL SOC FRANC DERM SYPH. 73:522-523, September-November, 1966.

"Reactivity in the FTA-ABS test of rabbits hyperimmunized with nonpathogenic treponemes," by G. R. Tringali, et al. BRIT J VENER DIS. 46:313-317, August, 1970.

"Reactivity of two selected antigens of Neisseria gonorrhoeae," by G. Reising, et al. APPL MICROBIOL. 18:337-339, September, 1969.

"Reappearance of gonorrhea and its diagnosis using the gonorrhea reaction," by E. Russo. HOSPITAL. 76:1693-1713, November, 1969.

"Recapitulation of data received during the year 1965, concerning statistics for venereal disease in metropolitan France," by P. Chassagne. BULL INST NAT SANTE. 21:709-736, July-August, 1966.

"Recent cases of congenital syphilis in infants," by M. Hoir, et al. JAP J NURS ART. 8:60-69, August, 1969.

"Recent clinical experience in the management of gonococcal arthritis," by R. D. Altman. J FLORIDA MED ASS. 56:318-322, May, 1969.

"Recent clinicolaboratory observations in the treatment of acute gonococcal urethritis in men," by G. Ashamalla, et al. JAMA. 195:1115-1119, March 28, 1966.

"Recent developments in the laboratory diagnosis of gonococcal infections," by A. Reyn. BULL WHO. 40:245-255, 1969.

"Recent developments in the treatment of gonorrhoea," by R. R. Willcox. BRIT J VENER DIS. 46:141-144, April, 1970.

"Recent observations on the treatment of late ocular syphilis and neurosyphilis," by J. L. Smith. TRANS AMER ACAD OPHTHAL OTOLARYNG. 73:1113-1132, November-December, 1969.

"Recent progress in the serology of syphilis. Lues: selective rapid tests," by R. Martins, et al. REV BRASIL MED. 23:354-357, May, 1966.

"Recent progress in syphilis serodiagnosis--the complement fixation system (including cardiolipin reaction and RPCF)," by F. Osada. JAP J CLIN MED. 26:293-298, February, 1968.

"Recent progress in syphilis serodiagnosis--precipitation and agglutination tests," by K. Mizuoka. JAP J CLIN MED. 26:299-303, February, 1968.'

"Recent studies on late experimental and human syphilis," by P. Collart, et al. MINERVA MED. 57:4478-4486, December 26, 1966.

"Recent studies on latent syphilis, experimental and human," by P. Collart, et al. REV CLIN ESP. 103:456-465, December 31, 1966.

"Recent syphilis in pregnancy and early congenital syphilis in the province of Milan. Statistico-epidemiological findings for 1967 and 1968 (through November 1968). Considerations and proposals," by C. Ducrey. G ITAL DERM. 45:156-163, March, 1970.

"Recent trends in homosexuality in West London," by J. L. Fluker. BRIT J VENER DIS. 42:48-49, March, 1966.

"Recent trends in syphilis," by K. Minami. JAP J CLIN PATH. 16:338-340, April, 1968.

"Recent trends of syphilis incidence in Korea," by J. Lew,

et al. YONSEI MED J. 9:74-80, 1968.

"Recognition of infectious pregnancy disorders," by O. Fenner. LANDARZT. 42:1430-1432, November 20, 1966.

"Recovery of the gonococcus from exudates dried on filter paper," by C. F. Pait, et al. HEALTH LAB SCI. 7:30-33, January, 1970.

"Recovery of spirochaetes in the monkey by passive transfer from human late sero-negative syphilis," by J. L. Smith, et al. BRIT J VENER DIS. 42:109-115, June, 1968.

"Recovery of treponema pallidum from aqueous humor removed at cataract surgery in man by passive transfer to rabbit testis," by J. L. Smith, et al. AMER J OPHTHAL. 65:242-247, February, 1968.

"Recurrent lymphogranuloma venereum. Report of a case," by L. Z. Oller. BRIT J VENER DIS. 44:154-156, June, 1968.

"Recurrent parenchymatous keratitis in 2d generation congenital syphilis," by A. Ullmo. BULL SOC FRANC DERM SYPH. 75:654-656, 1968.

"'Red eye' as the presenting sign of syphilis d'emblée," by K. D. Wuepper. CALIF MED. 107:518-520, December, 1967.

"Reduced lymphocyte transformation due to a plasma factor in patients with active syphilis," by G. M. Levene, et al. LANCET. 2:246-247, August 2, 1969.

"Reduction of nonspecific background staining in the fluorescent treponemal antibody-abosrption test," by M. E. Roberts, et al. J BACT. 96:1500-1506, November, 1968.

"A reevaluation of the chronic biological false positive-phenomenon with the fluorescent treponemal antibody absorption test," by A. Lassus, et al. ACTA PATH MICROBIOL SCAND. 69:159-160, 1967.

"Referrals from VD to family planning. An obvious oversight," by O. J. Sikes, 3d. AMER J PUBLIC HEALTH. 58:1586-1587, September, 1968.

"Reflections on 8 cases of early congenital syphilis recently observed," by M. Bethenod, et al. J MED LYON.

46:1743-1757, November 5, 1965.

"Reinfection with early syphilis in homosexuals," by G. Elste, et al. DERM WSCHR. 154:985-994, October 19, 1968.

"Reiter Protein Complement-Fixation (RPCF) test as a serological test for syphilis. A clinical study," by L. Forstrom. ACTA DERMATOVENER. 47:Suppl. 59:1-65, 1967.

"The Reiter protein complement-fixation test using the Auto-Analyzer," by V. W. Pugh, et al. J CLIN PATH. 19:595-599, November, 1966.

"Reiter treponeme. A review of the literature," by A. L. Wallace, et al. BULL WHO. 36:Supplement No. 2, 1-103, 1967.

"Reiter's disease in two brothers," by A. G. Mowat. BRIT J VENER DIS. 44:334-336, December, 1968.

"Reiter's spirochete agglutination reaction (Roemer's test). Correlation with the FTA test and with the classic serologic tests in different stages of lues," by G. F. Strani, et al. MINERVA DERM. 43:329-333, July, 1968.

"Reiter's spirochete agglutination test, Romer and Schilpkoter modification, in syphilis serodiagnosis (clinico-serological contribution)," by T. Cainelli. G ITAL DERM. 108:317-324, July-August, 1967.

"Reiter's syndrome," by E. P. Engleman, et al. CLIN ORTHOP. 57:19-29, March-April, 1968.

"Reiter's syndrome - an infection-induced defect in inflammation," by O. J. Stone. DERM INT. 7:137-140, July-September, 1968.

"Reiter's treponema," by M. DeLuca. RASS INT CLIN TER. 48:643-644, May 31, 1968.

"Relapse of gonorrhoea after treatment with penicillin or streptomycin," by A. J. Evans. BRIT J VENER DIS. 42:251-262, December, 1966.

"Relapse of interstitial keratisis," by J. Sedan. BULL SOC OPHTAL FRANC. 66:432-435, April, 1966.

"Relapses in the cerebrospinal fluid and acquired resistance to penicillin in cases of neurosyphilis," by A. Dowzenko, et al. J NEUROL SCI. 2:197-202, March-April, 1965.

"Relation of TRIC agent to 'non-specific genital infection'," by E. M. Dunlop, et al. BRIT J VENER DIS. 42:77-87, June, 1966.

"Relation of various epidemiologic factors to cervical cancer as determined by a screening program," by S. M. Naguib, et al. OBSTET GYNEC. 28:451-459, October, 1966.

"Relations between hepatic cirrhosis and microcythemia," by A. Garagnani, et al. ARCH ITAL MAL APPAR DIG. 33:529-546, November-December, 1966.

"Relations between trichomoniasis and male infertility. Preliminary note," by G. Argenziano, et al. MINERVA DERM. 42:388-391, August, 1967.

"The relationship between complete and incomplete antibodies in various manifestations of gonorrhea," by N. I. Tumasheva, et al. VESTN DERM VENER. 42:69-73, November, 1968.

"Relationship between in vitro treponema immobilizing action of antibiotics and rabbit immunity against treponema," by T. Ikeda, et al. ACTA DERM. 62:9-13, February, 1967.

"Relationship between skin allergy tests and Boyden's test in syphilis," by N. I. Tumasheva, et al. VRACH DELO. 3:152, March, 1967.

"The relationship of propagation of trichomonas vaginalis to the amount of inoculating material," by E. Grys. WIAD PARAZYT. 15:275-276, 1969.

"Relationships between mycoplasma and the etiology of nongonococcal urethritis and Reiter's syndrome," by D. K. Ford. ANN NY ACAD SCI. 143:501-504, July 28, 1967.

"Relationships between the sensitivities in vitro of Neisseria gonorrhoeae to spiramycin, penicillin, streptomycin, tetracycline, and erythromycin," by A. Reyn, et al. BRIT J VENER DIS. 45:223-227, September, 1969.

"Relative incidence of corynebacterium vaginale (haemophilus vaginalis), Neisseria gonorrhoeae, and trichomonas spp. among women attending a venereal disease clinic," by W. E. Dunkelberg, Jr., et al. BRIT J VENER DIS. 46:187-190, June, 1970.

"Reliable and practical procedure for the diagnosis of gonorrhea," by H. A. Hirsch, et al. MED KLIN. 64: 2193-2196, November 21, 1969.

"Remarks apropos of a case of early congenital syphilis," by P. Combe, et al. PEDIATRIE. 21:603-604, July-August, 1966.

"Remarks apropos of 5 cases of syphilis of the testis," by F. G. Marill, et al. BULL SOC FRANC DERM SYPH. 77:241-245, 1970.

"Remarks on lues serology of today. Si duo faciunt idem, non est idem," by H. Ruge. MED WELT. 19:1132-1135, May, 10, 1969.

"Remarks on the reports of regional dermatovenerologists," by J. Obrtel. CESK DERM. 43:39-42, February, 1968.

"Remission possibilities in early seropositive syphilis using high doses of penicillin," by E. Malý, et al. CESK DERM. 45:63-69, April, 1970.

"Remote results of bicillin-3 therapy of patients with active forms of syphilis," by V. A. Rakhmanov, et al. VESTN DERM VENER. 40:43-45, October, 1966.

"Remote results of the continuous treatment of fresh forms of syphilis with penicillin and bicillin," by S. T. Pavlov, et al. VESTN DERM VENER. 41:8-11, April, 1967.

"Remote results of metallo-chemotherapy treatment of recent syphilis," by M. Lancellotti. MINERVA DERM. 42:260-261, July, 1967.

"Remote results of prophylactic treatment of children born to mothers with syphilis or with a history of syphilis," by V. N. Ivanov. VESTN DERM VENER. 43:86-90, January, 1969.

"Remote results of pyro-penicillin therapy of syphilis," by I. I. Pototskii. VESTN DERM VENER. 42:60-62, April, 1968.

"Remote results of the treatment of gonorrhea in girls

with sulfanilamide preparations and antibiotics," by V. N. Matveev, et al. VESTN DERM VENER. 41:81-83, April, 1967.

"Remote results of the treatment of patients with various forms of syphilitic aortitis," by M. P. Frishman. VESTN DERM VENER. 41:76-80, January, 1967.

"Remote results of treatment of syphilis patients with bicillin-I and bicillin-3," by E. P. Nikol'skaia, et al. VESTN DERM VENER. 41:46-48, February, 1967.

"Remote results of the treatment of syphilitic patients with ecmonovocillin and heavy metal salts," by T. V. Vasil'ev. VESTN DERM VENER. 40:52-57, March, 1966.

"Remote results of treatment with metal-chemotherapy in recent syphilis," by M. Lancellotti. MINERVA DERM. 42:28-34, January, 1967.

"Renal damage associated with prolonged administration of ampicillin, cephaloridine, and cephalothin," by E. J Benner. ANTIMICROB AGENTS CHEMOTHER. 9:417-420, 1969.

"Renal failure and interstitial nephritis due to penicillin and methicillin," by D. S. Baldwin, et al. NEW ENG J MED. 279:1245-1252, December 5, 1968.

"Replacement of ascitic fluid or rabbit serum requirement of treponema dentium by alphaglobulin," by S. S. Socransky, et al. J BACT. 94:1795-1796, November, 1967.

"Report of a serological survey of Cape Verdeans living on the island of Sao Nicolau and in New England, U.S.A. treponematosis, yellow fever and tetanus antibodies," by C. V. Du Florey, et al. AN ESC NAC SAUDE PUBLICA MED TROP. 2:3-9, January-December, 1968.

"Report on a phantom epidemic of gonorrhea," by J. S. Mausner, et al. AMER J EPIDEM. 85:320-331, March, 1967.

"Report on a study of cerebral biopsy in general paretics," by R. A. Venkoba, et al. NEUROL INDIA. 17:26-27, January-March, 1969.

"The reported and actual morbidity of syphilis and gonorrhea," by A. C. Curtis. ARCH ENVIRON HEALTH, Chicago. 13:381-384, September, 1966.

"Reported patterns of venereal diseases in adolescents," by H. C. Faigel. CLIN PEDIAT. 8:620, November, 1969.

"Reporting venereal disease," by W. J. Brown. JAMA. 202: 981-982, December 4, 1967.

"Repositivation of Nelson's test in a syphilitic, induced by a nonspecific antigenic influence," by A. Bazex, et al. BULL SOC FRANC DERM SYPH. 73:113-116, January-February, 1966.

"Research on lues in children and juveniles," by L. Pospísil. CESK PEDIAT. 25:462-463, September, 1970.

"Research on Mimeae-Herellae in venereal diseases," by F. Caprilli, et al. MINERVA DERM. 42:663-664, December, 1967.

"Research on syphilitic spondylitis," by F. G. Marill, et al. BULL SOC FRANC DERM SYPH. 75:311-314, 1968.

"Research on treponema in lymph glands of treated serum- and Nelson-negative syphilitics," by U. Boncinelli, et al. MINERVA DERM. 42:259-260, July, 1967.

"Resistance of human Neisseria species against desiccation," by U. Berger, et al. ARCH HYG BAKT. 153:556-559, December, 1969.

"Resistance of the manifestations of syphilis to the action of penicillin," by M. N. Bukharovich. SOVET MED. 31:137-138, March, 1968.

"Resistant monilial vaginitis. The male aspect," by C. A. Gilpin. J FLORIDA MED ASS. 54:337-338, April, 1967.

"Resource guide on venereal disease control," by New York (city) Board of Education. N Y C BD ED CURRIC BUL. No.9:18 p, 1967-1968.

"The results of catamnestic examination of 138 patients with neurosyphilis," by M. P. Frishman, et al. VESTN DERM VENER. 40:57-61, February, 1966.

"Results of complex treatment and clinical-laboratory examinations of men with trichomoniasis," by E. R. Gordon. VESTN DERM VENER. 42:46-49, December, 1968.

"Results of the control of contagious forms of syphilis in the Chelyabinsk region," by MIa Trofimova. VESTN DERM VENER. 40:76-78, October, 1966.

"The results of control of venereal and communicable skin diseases in the USSR," by N. M. Turanov, et al. VESTN DERM VENER. 41:21-27, October, 1967.

"Results of discussions on the treatment of syphilis," by A. A. Studnitsin, et al. VESTN DERM VENER. 42:48-51, 1968

"Results of inoculation of rabbits from biopsies of primo-secondary syphilitic lesions taken from untreated patients," by P. Collart, et al. ANN DERM SYPH. 95: 285-292, 1968.

"Results of investigation of the nature of syphilitic reagins by means of thin layer ion exchange and paper chromatography," by L. S. Reznikova, et al. VESTN DERM VENER. 41:46-51, May, 1967.

"Results of scientific research work of the Uzbek Dermatologic-Venereologic Institute for the period 1962-1968," by N. T. Tursunov, et al. VESTN DERM VENER. 43:6-7, June, 1969.

"Results of scientific studies at the Faculty of Skin and Venereal Diseases of the I. M. Sechenov I Moscow Medical Institute," by V. A. Rakhmanov, et al. VESTN DERM VENER. 44:8-13, April, 1970.

"Results of serologic studies in endogenous ocular inflammations," by W. Paul, et al. KLIN MBL AUGENHEILK. 151:332-344, 1967.

"Results of studies of a new local antitrichomonal agent 'tricho-kolpicortin'," by L. Kiss. PRAXIS. 58:58-59, January 14, 1969.

"Results of studies of the sensitivity of Neisseria gonorrheae to penicillin in soldiers ill with gonorrhea," by J. Rodovský, et al. CESK DERM. 43:9-14, February, 1968.

"Results of syphilis therapy at the dermatologic clinic in Erfurt," by F. Schiller, et al. Z HAUT GESCHLECHTSKR. 43:691-696, September 1, 1968.

"Results of a study on the occurrence of trichomoniasis in the Ostrava region," by J. Asmera, et al. CESK EPIDEM. 19:199-205, July, 1970.

"Results of syphilis therapy at the dermatologic clinic in Erfurt," by F. Schiller, et al. Z HAUT GESCHLECHT-

SKR. 43:691-696, September 1, 1968.

"Results of 3 years of activity (1964-1966) at the Centro di Medicina Preventiva del Comune di Novara," by C. Meloni, et al. ANN SANIT PUBBLICA. 29:43-59, January-February, 1968.

"The results of treatment of gonorrhea," by J. Forssell, et al. LAKARTIDNINGEN. 66:4198+, October 8, 1969.

"Results of treatment of gonorrhoea with tetraverin," by E. Chodyń, et al. PRZEGL DERM. Suppl:69-73, 1969.

"Results of the treatment of recent syphilids with bizmuth alone," by G. Falchi. G ITAL DERM. 107:683-689, September-December, 1966.

"Results of the use of the treponema pallidum immobilization test and standard serological tests in syphilis," by G. A. Zmechorovskaia, et al. VESTN DERM VENER. 40:23-27, December, 1966.

"Resuscitation in embolic and toxic complication caused by intravascular administration of a depot-penicillin," by G. Clauberg. ANAESTHESIST. 15:284-285, August, 1966.

"Retino-choroidal pigmented paravenous degeneration," by M. Ardouin, et al. BULL SOC OPHTAL FRANC. 67:742-744, September, 1967.

"Reversed passive hemagglutination for serodiagnosis of syphilis," by J. M. Biasco-Zuasti, et al. J LAB CLIN MED. 72:670-673, October, 1968.

"A review of the activities of the Kuibyshev branch of the All-Russia Society of Dermatologists and Venereologists," by A. S. Zenin. VESTN DERM VENER. 41:77-79, October, 1967.

"Review of current methods for the detection of trichomonas in clinical material," by J. Hess. J CLIN PATH. 22:269-272, May, 1969.

"A review of the Hungarian Journal of Dermatology and Venereology for the year 1967," by K. Kirai, et al. VESTN DERM VENER. 43:60-62, February, 1969.

"Revision of the concept of venereal vaginal infection," by R. Peter. CESK GYNEK. 31:290-293, May, 1966.

"Rheumatoid factor in syphilitics," by Z. Hrncir, et al. CESK DERM. 43:190-198, June, 1968.

"Rifampicin in dermatology. Clinical trial," by E. Cappelli. ARCH MARAGLIANO PAT CLIN. 25:397-401, September-October, 1969.

"Rifampicin in dermatology and venereology," by L. Ayala. G ITAL DERM. 44:665-672, December, 1969.

"Rifampicin (rimactane) in the treatment of gonorrhoea," by R. R. Willcox, et al. BRIT J VENER DIS. 46:145-148, April, 1970.

"The rise and fall of the treponematoses. I. Ecological aspects and international trends in venereal syphilis," by O. Idsoe, et al. BRIT J VENER DIS. 43:227-243, December, 1967.

--II. Endemic treponematoses of childhood. BRIT J VENER DIS. 44:35-48, March, 1968.

"The rise in venereal disease: epidemiology and prevention," by R. H. Kampmeier. MED CLIN N AMER. 51:735-751, May, 1967.

"The risk of penicillin reactions (Editorial)," by P. P. Van Arsdel, Jr. ANN INTERN MED. 69:1071-1073, November, 1968.

"Roentgenographic diagnosis of congenital syphilis in the newborn," by D. R. Coblentz, et al. JAMA. 212:1061-1064, May 11, 1970.

"Role and functions in the prevention and control of congenital syphilis," by M. Oros, et al. MUNCA SANIT. 17:241-245, April, 1969.

"Role of acquired immunity to T. pallidum in the control of syphilis," by J. F. Jekel. PUBLIC HEALTH REP. 83:627-632, August, 1968.

"The role of the bursa of Fabricius in immunity against spirochetosis in fowls," by I. Soumrov, et al. ZBL VETERINAERMED. 14:672-676, November, 1967.

"The role of colonic-rectal adenomas as a precarcinomatous condition," by M. Reifferscheid. ERGEBN CHIR ORTHOP. 50:83-105, 1967.

"The role of the general practitioner in the prevention

and treatment of venereal diseases," by E. Perti. MED GLAS. 22:121-125, May, 1968.

"Role of the male in reinfestation of the female with trichomonas vaginalis," by L. Dao. GYNEC PRAT. 15: 25-28, 1964.

"Role of mycoplasma in nongonococcal urethritis," by J. Thivolet, et al. PRESSE MED. 76:1755-1776, October 5, 1968.

"Role of mycoplasma in urethritis. I. Mycoplasma hominis type I," by M. Sepetjian, et al. PATH BIOL. 17:953-959, November, 1969.

"The role of the nurse in venereal disease control," by J. Towpik. PIELEG POLOZ. 2:13-15, 1967.

"Role of penicilloyl-polylysin in the detection of delayed hypersensitivity to penicillin," by E. Maciejowska. PRZEGL DERM. 57:55-59, January-February, 1970.

"The role of penicilloyl-polylysins for the diagnosis of penicillin allergy," by E. Maciejowska. DERM MSCHR. 155:751-760, 1969.

"The role of penicilloylated protein impurities, penicillin polymers and dimers in penicillin allergy," by A. I. DeWeck. INT ARCH ALLERG. 33:535-567, 1968.

"The role of public health laboratories in the diagnosis of venereal diseases," by A. M. Vilches. BOL OFIC SANIT PANAMER. 60:328-334, April, 1966.

"The role of serum protein fractions on serologic tests in syphilis," by L. D. Butovetskii. VESTN DERM VENER. 41:67-70, July, 1967.

"The role of trichomonas and candida albicans as the principal cause of rupture of some perineorrhaphies after delivery," by D. Maroudi, et al. GYNEC OBSTET. 65: 651-654, November-December, 1966.

"The role of trichomonas urogenitalis in the development of adnexitis and its treatment," by B. Pejtsik, et al. Z GEBURTSH GYNAEK. 170:68-72, 1969.

"The role of trichomonas vaginalis in sterility," by P. Kostic. GYNEC PRAT. 15:467-469, 1964.

"The role of trichomoniasis in the development of portio

uteri preblastomoses," by I. Szell, et al. ZBL GYNAEK. 89:312-323, March 4, 1967.

"The role of trichomoniasis in the development of precancerous state of the uterine cervix," by I. Szell, et al. ORV HETIL. 108:150-156, January 22, 1967.

"The role of urogenital trichomonas in the genesis of changes in the portio epithelium," by B. Toth, et al. ZBL GYNAEK. 91:547-551, April 26, 1969.

"The role of urogenital trichomonas infections in the incidence of changes in the cervix epithelium," by B. Toth, et al. ORV HETIL. 108:924-926, May 14, 1967.

"Rolitetracycline by injection and tetracycline phosphate complex by mouth given in a single session in the treatment of gonorrhoea in males," by R. R. Wilcox. ACTA DERMATOVENER. 50:154-156, 1970.

"Room temperature storage of treponema pallidum on microscope slides for use in the FTA-ABS test," by R. M. Wood, et al. APPL MICROBIOL. 17:335-336, February, 1969.

"Rosette-like variety of trichomonadosis granulocytica," by M. Z. Kwoczynski. POL TYG LEK. 21:744-745, May 16, 1966.

"Round table on chemotherapy of venereal diseases," ANTIMICROB AGENTS CHEMOTHER. 5:1115-1119, 1965.

"Rovamycin in the treatment of gonorrhea," by B. Raszeja-Kotelba. PRZEGL DERM. Suppl:75-78, 1969.

"Rubber latex in the slide microserological test of syphilis," by S. Kośmiderski. POL TYG LEK. 23:1639-1641, October 21, 1968.

"Runting syndrome in neonatal rabbits infected with treponema pallidum," by H. Festenstein, et al. CLIN EXP.IMMUN. 2:311-320, May, 1967.

"Rupture of the aortic aneurysm into the superior vena cava," by A. Kropfl, et al. LIJECN VJESN. 89:233-239, 1967.

"Rural health in northern Nigeria: some recent developments and problems," by K. D. Thomson. TRANS ROY SOC TROP MED HYG. 61:277-302, 1967.

"Sarcoid granuloma in secondary syphilis," by L. R. Lantis, et al. ARCH DERM. 99:748-752, June, 1969.

"The school nurse and VD education," by E. W. Collum. S CAROLINA NURS. 20:7, 30-33, Spring, 1968.

"The school nurse-teacher's role in controlling venereal disease," by D. E. Barlow. J NY SCH NURSE-TEACH ASS. 1:16-19, June, 1970.

"Scientific activity of the Department of Dermatology and Venereal Diseases of the Leningrad Sanitary-Hygiene Medical Institute for the period 1963-1968," by S. E. Gorbovitskii, et al. VESTN DERM VENER. 43:3-8, March, 1969.

"Scientific organization of the work of physicians of dermatovenerological institutions," by A. I. Sul'zhenko, et al. SOVET ZDRAVOOKHR. 27:31-35, 1968.

"Scientific research of the department of dermatology and venereology at the Kiev Medical Institute in 1961-1969," by I. I. Pototskii. VESTN DERM VENER. 44:3-8, May, 1970.

"Screening test for gonorrhea in male suspects," by D. S. Kwalick. JAMA. 213:626, July 27, 1970.

"Search for treponemes in lymph nodes of treated serum- and TPI-negative syphilitics," by U. Boncinelli, et al. MINERVA DERM. 42:259-260, July, 1967.

"The search for a vaccine for syphilis. An epidemiological approach," by R. W. Thatcher. BRIT J VENER DIS. 45:10-12, March, 1969.

"A search for viruses in smegma, premalignant and early malignant cervical tissues. The isolation of herpesviruses with distinct antigenic properties," by W. E. Rawls, et al. AMER J EPIDEM. 87:647-655, May, 1968.

"Secondary oral and laryngeal syphilis," by R. W. Dodd. VIRGINIA MED MONTHLY. 94:229-231, April, 1967.

"Secondary syphilis. Report of 2 cases," by P. H. Nexmand. UGESKR LAEG. 132:1157-1158, June 11, 1970.

"Secondary syphilis after 1 injection of 2,400,000 units of penicillin for primary preserologic syphilis," by R. Degos, et al. BULL SOC FRANC DERM SYPH. 75:289-

290, 1968.

"Secondary syphilis misdiagnosed as infectious mononucleosis," by M. A. Conant, et al. CALIF MED. 109:462-464, December, 1968.

"Secondary syphilis misdiagnosed as lymphoma," by D. R. Goffinet, et al. NORTHWEST MED. 69:Suppl:22-23, May, 1970; also in ARIZONA MED. 27:22-23, May, 1970.

"Secondary syphilis with negative serology," by F. Blez, et al. LYON MED. 223:860-861, April 19, 1970; also in BULL SOC FRANC DERM SYPH. 77:261-262, 1970.

"Secondary syphilis with osteolysis of skull bones," by P. Franceschini, et al. BULL SOC FRANC DERM SYPH. 76:763-764, 1969.

"Secondary syphilis with unusual clinical and laboratory findings," by L. Biro, et al. ARCH DERM. 99:240-243, February, 1969; also in JAMA. 206:889-891, October 21, 1968.

"Sectorial pigmented retinopathy secondary to acquired syphilis," by R. Cristiani. ANN OTTAL. 93:1099-1108, October, 1967.

"Segmental exzema reaction in a tabetic patient in the area of lancinating back pains," by G. W. Korting, et al. MED WELT. 45:2440, November 5, 1966.

"Selected aspects of penicillin allergy," by R. L. Baer, et al. BRIT J DERM. 83:Suppl:37-47, 1970.

"Selected aspects of syphilis and gonorrhoea. Research in the United States, 1967," by L. C. Norins. BRIT J VENER DIS. 42:103-108, June, 1968.

"Selective culture media in the microbiologic diagnosis of gonorrhea," by V. Potuznik. CESK DERM. 42:173-174, June, 1967.

"Selective inhibition in vitro of mycoplasma hominis by lincomycin," by G. Csonka, et al. BRIT J VENER DIS. 46:203-204, June, 1970.

"Self-medication by patients attending a venereal diseases clinic," by K. Anderson. BRIT J VENER DIS. 42:44-45, March, 1966.

"A semester experience at the Bari University obstetric

and gynecologic clinic on the incidence and therapy of trichomonas vaginalis (in 3313 patients examined)," by G. Giocoli, et al. MINERVA GINEC. 19:740-745, July 31, 1967.

"Senile hypophyseal syndromes," by E. Herman. J NEUROL SCI. 4:101-110, January-February, 1966.

"Sensitivity of gonococci to antibiotics in strains isolated from 'prostitutes' in Copenhagen," by R. Nielsen. BRIT J VENER DIS. 46:153-155, April, 1970.

"Sensitivity of gonococcus to penicillin in patients with gonorrhea," by L. D. Kuntsevich, et al. VESTN DERM VENER. 43:44-45, February, 1969.

"Sensitivity of Neisseria gonorrhoeae to penicillin and other antibiotics. Studies carried out in Toronto during the period 1961 to 1968," by C. R. Amies. BRIT J VENER DIS. 45:216-222, September, 1969.

"Sensitivity of Neisseria gonorrhoeae to penicillin and other drugs," by V. G. Cave, et al. NEW YORK J MED. 70:844-847, April 1, 1970.

"Sensitivity of strains of N. gonorrhoeae to some antibiotics," by S. Hausnerova, et al. CESK DERM. 44:91-94, May, 1969.

"Sensitivity to penicillin of Neisseria gonorrhoeae. Relationship to the results of treatment," by D. A. Leigh, et al. BRIT J VENER DIS. 45:151-153, June, 1969.

"Sensitivity to 2-mercaptoethanol of reagins in human syphilis, in B.F.P. reactors and in 'normal' rabbits. The macroglobulin nature of B.F.P. reagins," by G. Tringali, et al. RIV IST SIEROTER ITAL. 41:291-298, September-October. 1966.

"Septic gonococcal dermatitis. Demonstration of gonococci and gonococcal antigens in skin lesions by immunofluorescence," by G. Kahn, et al. ARCH DERM. 99:421-425, April, 1969.

"Septicaemia caused by Neisseria flavescens," by P. T. Wertlake, et al. J CLIN PATH. 21:437-439, July, 1968.

"Sequential therapy and trichomoniasis," by A. Calugi, et al. QUAD CLIN OSTET GINEC. 22:551-556, August, 1967

"Sergei Timofeevich Pavlov." VESTN DERM VENER. 41:89, June, 1967.

"Sero-diagnosis of gonorrhoea with a microprecipitin test using a lipopolysaccharide antigen from N. gonorrhoeae," by C. W. Chacko, et al. BRIT J VENER DIS. 45:33-39, March, 1969.

"Serodiagnosis of syphilis," by W. J. Brown. JAMA. 205: 800, September 9, 1968.

"Serodiagnosis of syphilis," by M. F. Garner. MED J AUST. 2:328-331, August 13, 1966.

"Serodiagnosis of syphilis," by L. Nicholas. ARCH DERM. 96:324-328, September, 1967.

"The serodiagnosis of syphilis and automation," by L. C. Norins. SALUD PUBLICA MEX. 10:601-606, September-October, 1968.

"Serodiagnosis of syphilis by fluorescent treponemal antibody-absorption tests (FTA-ABS)," by K. Oikawa, et al. JAP J CLIN PATH. 17:538-544, July, 1969.

"Serologic control of Hungarian-made VDRL antigens," by L. Surján, et al. ORV HETIL. 109:1755-1757, August 11, 1968.

"Serologic detection of gonorrhea," by E. V. Hess, et al. ANN INTERN MED. 73:340-341, August, 1970.

"Serologic detection of gonorrhea," by J. D. Schmale. ANN INTERN MED. 72:593-595, April, 1970.

"Serologic investigations in narcotic addicts. I. Syphilis, lymphogranuloma venereum, herpes simplex, and Q fever," by C. E. Cherubin, et al. ANN INTERN MED. 69:739-742, October, 1968.

"Serologic reactions to specific complement-fixing antigens from micro-organisms of the psittacosis-lymphogranuloma venereum-trachoma (PLT) group," by R. N. Philip, et al. AMER J OPTHAL. 63:1499-1504, May, 1967.

"Serologic reactivity in consecutive patients admitted to a general hospital. A comparison of the FTA-ABS, VDRL, and automated reagin tests," by P. Cohen, et al. ARCH INTERN MED. 124:364-367, September, 1969.

"Serologic study after inoculation of treponema pallidum in normal mice and mice thymectomized at birth," by J. Thivolet, et al. EXPERIENTIA. 25:304-305, March 15, 1969.

"The serologic syphilis test required for marriage in other states," by R. L. Cavenaugh. MARYLAND MED J. 18:33, May, 1969.

"Serologic testing for syphilis. Report from the Subcommittee on Serology of the Standards Committee of the College of American Pathologists," by M. F. Beeler, et al. AMER J CLIN PATH. 52:300-302, September, 1969.

"Serologic tests for syphilis among narcotic addicts," by W. D. Harris, et al. NEW YORK J MED. 67:2967-2974, November 15, 1967.

"Serologic tests for syphilis and the false-positive reactor," by K. D. Wuepper, et al. ARCH DERM. 94:152-155, August, 1966.

"Serologic tests with sera from patients with lepromatous leprosy during the periods of exacerbation," by G. V. Mertslin, et al. VESTN DERM VENER. 40:41-43, October, 1966.

"Serologic yaws in Paris," by G. Solente. PRESSE MED. 74:1681-1682, June 25, 1966.

"Serological activity of mycobacterial cardiolipin in comparison with cardiolipin from the cardiac muscle," by M. Sasaki, et al. SCI REP RES INST TOHOKU UNIV (MED). 16:68-71, October, 1969.

"Serological and epidemiological evaluation of the present methods of examination of blood donors," by S. Jasser, et al. POL TYG LEK. 22:1237-1239, August 14, 1967.

"Serological and experimental studies in the field of syphilis and gonorrhea in the USSR," by N. M. Ovchinnikov. VESTN DERM VENER. 41:23-37, September, 1967.

"Serological cross-reactions of aqueous ether extracted endotoxin from Neisseria gonorrhoeae strains," by J. A. Maeland. ACTA PATH MICROBIOL SCAND. 77:505-517, 1969.

"Serological diagnosis of syphilis," by B. Hederstedt.

NORD MED. 77:217-218, February 16, 1967.

"Serological diagnosis of syphilis," by F. Knierim, et al. BOL CHILE PARASIT. 22:21-26, January-March, 1967.

"The serological diagnosis of syphilis in dental patients," by M. Harris. BRIT J ORAL SURG. 4:235-239, March, 1967.

"Serological fluorescence studies on syphilitic veinous changes in animals," by H. J. Heitmann. DERMATOLOGICA. 137:129-132, 1968.

"Serological properties of aqueous ether extracted endotoxin from Neisseria gonorrhoeae," by J. A. Maeland. ACTA PATH MICROBIOL SCAND. 77:495-504, 1969.

"Serological resistance in syphilis and its causes," by M. N. Bucharowicz. PRZEGL DERMATOL. 57:621-630, September-October, 1970.

"A serological review of 156 patients presenting with primary chancres," by M. F. Garner. MED J AUST. 1:672-673, April 20, 1968.

"Serological studies on trichomonads," by E. Mannweiler, et al. Z TROPENMED PARASIT. 19:308-316, September, 1968.

"Serological techniques," by C. E. Taylor. J CLIN PATH. 3:Suppl3:14-19, 1969.

"Serological tests for syphilis." LANCET. 1:1187-1188, June 1, 1968.

"Serological tests for syphilis," by H. R. Cayton. BRISTOL MEDICOCHIR J. 81:32-34, April, 1966.

"Serological tests for syphilis in diseases of the thyroid," by F. S. Ashkar, et al. JAMA. 213:872, August 3, 1970.

"Serological tests for syphilis in the elderly," by E. A. Johansson, et al. ANN CLIN RES. 2:47-50, March, 1970.

"Serological tests for syphilis in healthy rabbits," by J. W. Clark, Jr. BRIT J VENER DIS. 46:191-197, June, 1970.

"Serological tests for treponemal disease in adults in two Jamaican communities," by M. T. Ashcroft, et al. BRIT J VENER DIS. 43:96-104, June, 1967.

"Serological tests for treponemal infection in leprosy patients. An evaluation of the fluorescent treponemal antibody absorption (FTA-ABS) test," by M. F. Garner, et al. BRIT J VENER DIS. 45:19-22, March, 1969.

"Serology in control of venereal diseases," by N. C. Bhattacharyya. INDIAN J DERM. 14:129-132, April, 1969.

"Serology in gyneco-obstetrics," by Y. Fukuoka. REV CHILE PEDIAT. 37:633-648, July, 1966.

"Serology in leprosy," by H. Schmidt, et al. DERM INT. 7:43-45, January-March, 1968.

"Serology of normal primates," by B. M. Levine, et al. BRIT J VENER DIS. 46:307-310, August, 1970.

"Serology of syphilis," by L. Rouquès. PRESSE MED. 74:1263-1264, May 14, 1966.

"Serology of syphilis and related aspects," by N. Ulker, TURK TIP CEM MEC. 34:277-284, 1968.

"Serology of syphilis in blood transfusion service," by F. Kail. BIBL HAEMAT. 32:247-249, 1969.

"Serology of syphilis in Tassill n'Ajjer (Central Sahara)," by P. Cirera, et al. BULL SOC PATH EXOT. 60:33-43, January-February, 1967.

"Sero-negative maternal syphilis. Report of a case," by A. E. Tinkler. BRIT J VENER DIS. 42:136-139, June, 1968.

"Sero-negative polyarthritis. The Bedsonia (chlamydia) group of agents and Reiter's disease. A progress report," by E. M. Dunlop, et al. ANN RHEUM DIS. 27:234-239, May, 1968.

"Sero-positive syphilitic aorto-myocarditis in a woman treated during 20 years and after several years of negative serology," by R. Degos, et al. BULL SOC FRANC DERM SYPH. 77:32-33, July, 1970.

"Serum antibody response in experimental human gonorrhoea.

Immunoglobulins G, A, and M," by I. R. Cohen, et al. BRIT J VENER DIS. 45:325-327, December, 1969.

"Serum immuncelectrophoretic pattern in primary and secondary syphilis," by M. Pippione, et al. G ITAL DERM. 45:193-194, March, 1970.

"Serum immunoglobulin levels in syphilis," by A. B. Laurell, et al. ACTA DERMATOVENER. 48:268-271, 1968.

"Serum mucoproteins in the course of certain skin diseases and in early syphilis," by Z. Cygan, et al. POL MED J. 8:682-686, 1969.

"Serum proteinogram in the course of the febrile reaction of Jarish-Herxheimer-Lukasiewicz," by W. Powrozny, et al. PRZEGL DERM. 55:677-680, September-October, 1968.

"The serum reaction to choroid melanin. Henry's reaction. Trenz's technique. 3. Physiopathological significance and practical value," by F. Trensz, et al. ANN BIOL CLIN. 24:1081-1096, October-December, 1966.

"Severe anaphylactic reaction to penicillin," by L. I. Geller, et al. KLIN MED. 44:138, January, 1966.

"Sex and the medical student," by W. M. Sheppe, Jr., et al. J MED EDUC. 41:457-464, May, 1966.

"Sex and the practicing physician," by W. F. Sheeley. JAMA. 195:195-196, January 17, 1966.

"Sex and V.D. education in Central Newfoundland schools." CANAD J PUBL HLTH. 58:265+, June, 1967.

"Sex attitudes of young people; London, England," by M. Holmes, et al. ED RES. 11:38-42, November, 1968.

"Sex behavior of adolescent patients," by U. Sprafke. DERM MSCHR. 155:554-568, 1969.

"Sexual and reproductive correlates of chronic cervicitis," by H. J. Osofsky, et al. OBSTET GYNEC. 30:481-485, October, 1967.

"Sexual assault on women and girls in the District of Columbia," by C. R. Hayman, et al. SOUTHERN MED J. 62:1227-1231, October, 1969.

"The sexual behavior of young people. Practical implications of the C.C.H.E. report," by A. J Dalzell-Ward.

ROY SOC HEALTH J. 86:167-170, May-June, 1966.

"Sexual morality: Campus dilemna," by D. L. Farnsworth. INT PSYCHIAT CLIN. 7:133-151, 1970.

"Sexually acquired gonorrhoeal urethritis in a 6-year-old boy," by N. J. Fiumara, et al. BRIT J VENER DIS. 45:254, September, 1969.

"Sexually deviant behavior in expectant fathers," by A. A. Hartmen, et al. J ABNORM PSYCHOL. 71:232-234, June, 1966.

"Sexually transmitted disease in antenatal patients," by R. N. Thin, et al. BRIT J VENER DIS. 46:126-128, April, 1970.

"Sexually transmitted disease in gynaecological out-patients with vaginal discharge," by A. M. Driscoll, et al. BRIT J VENER DIS. 46:125, April, 1970.

"Sexually transmitted diseases. Part 1," by J. Ribeiro. DISTRICT NURS. 12:201+, January, 1970.

--Part 2. DISTRICT NURS. 12:225+, February, 1970.

"The sexually transmitted diseases. Part 1. History and epidemiology," by J. K. Oates. NURS MIRROR. 128:17-19, January 31, 1969.

--Part 2. Syphilis. NURS MIRROR. 128:24+, February 7, 1969.

--Part 3. Infectious urethritis. NURS MIRROR. 128:24+, February 14, 1969.

--Part 4. Minor infections. NURS MIRROR. 128:38-39, February 21, 1969.

"The sexually-transmitted diseases and marriage," by J. R. Seale. BRIT J VENER DIS. 42:31-36, March, 1966.

"Shall our schools teach about venereal disease?," by S. Podair. SAT R. 49:72-73+, March 19, 1966.

"Shelf life of fluorescent treponemal antibody-absorption test reagents," by M. E. Roberts, et al. J BACT. 96:1507-1511, November, 1968.

"Shock death after oral penicillin administration," by H. Bankl, et al. WIEN KLIN WSCHR. 80:43-44, January 19, 1968.

"Shocking facts about VD," by P. Deutsch, et al. PARENTS MAG. 42:44-45, January, 1967.

"A shortened and simplified treponema test in diagnostic practice," by J. Weberschinke, et al. J HYG EPIDEM. 10:483-487, 1966.

"Should cases of gonorrhea in men be treated by urologists?," by L. Andersson, et al. LAKARTIDNINGEN. 65:1381, April 3, 1968.

"Side-effects of chemotherapeutic agents," by O. Mustala. DUODECIM. 86:192-202, 1970.

"The significance of the complement fixation test with protein fraction of treponema pallidum (TPCF) for serodiagnosis of syphilis," by L. D. Butovetskii, et al. VESTN DERM VENER. 40:52-57, November, 1966.

"Significance of the 'defaulter' in the assessment of efficiency of treatment in gonorrhoea," by A. B. Hewitt. BRIT J VENER DIS. 45:40-41, March, 1969.

"Significance of the FTA-ABS test in diagnosis of lues. Comparison with the classical TPI test," by P. Schneiderka, et al. CESK EPIDEMIOL MIKROBIOL IMUNOL. 19:225-229, September, 1970.

"Significance of the FTA-test for primary syphilis," by J. Meyer-Rohn. Z HAUT GESCHLECHTSKR. 42:309-312, May 1, 1967.

"Significance of a low-titre V.D.R.L.," by D. G. McLone. J MED ASS GEORGIA. 56:60, February, 1967.

"Significance of mycoplasma (PPLO) in diseases of men," by G. Schabinski, et al. Z AERZTL FORTBILD. 63:1076-1081, October 15, 1969.

"Significance of a positive serological reaction in a subject originating from a tropical region," by P. Limbos. ACTA ORTHOP BELG. 32:755-764, September-October, 1966.

"Significance of S. T. S. in skin diseases and syphilis," by N. C. Bhattacharyya. INDIAN J DERM. 14:12-18, October, 1968.

"The significance of serum penicillin levels in syphilis therapy," by K. Mach, et al. Z HAUT GESCHLECHTSKR. 44:81-86, February 1, 1969.

"Significance of the treatment of trichomoniasis in gynecology and obstetrics," by J. Zawadzki, et al. WIAD PARAZYT. 15:473-475, 1969.

"Silent limb contracture as a diagnostic indicator of tertiary syphilis," by K. Dawson-Butterworth. BRIT J CLIN PRACT. 22:471-473, November 11, 1968.

"Silent limb contracture in syphilitic geriatric patients," by K. Dawson-Butterworth. PRACTITIONER. 199:68-70, July, 1967.

"Simple anaerobic technique for the treponema pallidum immobilization test," by V. Bokkenheuser, et al. HEALTH LAB SCI. 6:162-163, July, 1969.

"A simple diagnostic method in uro-genital trichomoniasis," by A. Pandele, et al. RUM MED REV. 12:70-73, April-June, 1968.

"A simple procedure for the preparation of diagnostic antigens from culture treponemes," by K. Kiraly, et al. Z IMMUNITAETSFORSCH. 134:32-44, November, 1967.

"Simplified complex of serological syphilis reactions in mass donor examination," by A. M. Chistiakov. LAB DELO. 2:83-86, 1969.

"Simplified laboratory technique for diagnosis of chanchroid," by K. A. Borchardt, et al. ARCH DERM. 102:188-192, August, 1970.

"Simplified method for the preparation of selective culture media used in microbiological diagnosis of gonorrhea," by V. Potuznik. CESK DERM. 43:321-322, October, 1968.

"A simplified method of performing the treponema pallidum immobilization test," by S. Stoianov, et al. VESTN DERM VENER. 41:11-14, April, 1967.

"Simplified method of serum dilutions for performance of the quantitative VDRL test useful for mass examinations," by A. Garlacz. PRZEGL DERM. 56:589-591, September-October, 1969.

"Simplified TPI test. Preliminary report," by T. Ikeda, et al. ACTA DERM. 63:323-327, November, 1968.

"Simultaneous isolation of trichomonas vaginalis and collection of vaginal exudate," by D. H. Robertson, et al. BRIT J VENER DIS. 45:42-43, March, 1969.

"Simultaneous occurrence of toxic hepatitis and Stevens-Johnson syndrome following therapy with sulfisoxazole and sulfamethoxazole," by D. J. Shaw, et al. JOHNS HOPKINS MED J. 126:130-133, March, 1970.

"Single-dose antibiotic treatment of asymptomatic gonorrhea in hospitalized women," by D. W. Johnson, et al. NEW ENG J MED. 283:1-6, July 2, 1970.

"Single dose therapy of gonorrhea with rovamycin," by P. Schmid. DERMATOLOGICA. 134:279-282, 1967.

"Single-dose treatment of gonorrhea with selected antibiotic agents," by T. F. Keys, et al. JAMA. 210:857-861, November 3, 1969.

"Single doses of cephaloridine in the treatment of gonococcal urethritis in males," by M. J. Marshall, et al. POSTGRAD MED J. 43:Suppl 43:121-122, August, 1967.

"Single treatment of gonorrhea in males with high doses of penicillin," by H. Biehler, et al. MUNCHEN MED WSCHR. 109:296-300, February 10, 1967.

"The sins of the fathers," by A. D. G. Gunn. NM. 122:221, June 10, 1966.

"Six-city study of treatment of gonorrhoea in men using single oral doses of 1.5 or 3 G tetracycline hydrochloride," by C. E. Cornelius, 3d. BRIT J VENER DIS. 46:330-333, August, 1970.

"625 cases of trichomoniasis treated with metronidazole (statistical discussion)," by M. Gaudefroy, et al. GYNEC PRAT. 19:339-362, 1968.

"The sixtieth year of the Wassermann Reaction," by T. A. Demchenko. LAB DELO. 1:3-7, 1966.

"Skin diseases and venereal diseases in Cracow during the 2d World War," by K. Capińska. PRZEGL LEK. 26:34-39, 1970.

"Skin granuloma in the Nile Valley," by A. M. Mofty, et al. INT J DERM. 9:33-40, January-March, 1970.

"Skin-sensitizing antibodies in serum from patients with penicillin allergy studied by passive transfer to monkey skin and compared with results obtained on human skin,(Prausnitz-Kuster technique)," by J. Pedersen-Bjergaard. ACTA ALLERG. 24:57-72, March, 1969.

"Skin testing in urticarial penicillin hypersensitivity," by T. Matner, et al. ARCH KLIN EXP DERM. 227:349-352, 1966.

"Skull changes in early syphilis. A contribution to the differential diagnosis of localized clearings in the x-ray film of the skull," by E. Nagele, et al. RADIOLOGE, 6:242-245, June, 1966.

"Skull lacunae during secondary syphilis," by C. Bénichou, et al. REV RHUM. 37:330-333, April, 1970.

"Social behaviour and the use of medical services," by J. A. Savin. BRIT J PREV SOC MED. 23:53-55, February, 1969.

"Social board of the dermato-venereologic institution," by I. A. L. Iudin. VESTN DERM VENER. 40:59-61, January, 1966.

"Social diseases and the structure of society," by S. Gorbovitskii. VESTN DERM VENER. 44:5-8, January, 1970.

"Social problems of venereal diseases among New York youth," by W. Curth. ARCH KLIN EXP DERM. 227:637-640, 1966.

"Sociomedical study of young gonorrhea patients," by B. H. Hatt. NORD MED. 76:816, July, 1966.

"Sociopsychiatric investigation of teenage girls with gonorrhea," by L. Palmgren. ACTA PSYCHIAT SCAND. 42:295-314, 1966.

"Somatopsychic aspect of hypopituitarism in a congenital syphilitic. Report of a case," by G. J. Taylor. NEW ZEAL MED J. 66:77-78, February, 1967.

"Some aspects of the field work of the ancillary staff in the dermato-venereologic department in the family," by E. Sulutiu, et al. MUNCA SANIT. 16:357-360, June, 1968.

"Some aspects of the management of venereal disease," by S. Olansky. ARCH ENVIRON HEALTH, Chicago. 13:376-380, September, 1966.

"Some aspects of penicillin allergy," by F. R. Batchelor, et al. PROC ROY SOC MED. 61:897-899, September, 1968.

"Some basic trends, results and prospectives of scientific-research at the Chair of Dermatologic and Venereal Diseases of the Patrice Lumumba University of Friendship of Peoples," by R. S. Babaiants. VESTN DERM VENER. 43:3-7, November, 1969.

"Some changing aspects of aortic regurgitation," by J. A. Barondess, et al. ARCH INTERN MED. 124:600-605, November, 1969.

--An autopsy study. TRANS AMER CLIN CLIMAT ASS. 80: 23-36, 1969.

"Some comments on the cooperation of microbiologists and dermatovenerologists in the prevention of gonorrhea," by V. Potuznik. CESK DERM. 42:217-223, August, 1967.

"Some current problems of syphilis immunology," by L. Pospisil. CESK DERM. 44:95-101, May, 1969.

"Some current problems of the treatment of syphilis (based on data of the inquiry session of the Donets District Scientific Society Dermatovenerologists," by N. A. Torsuev, et al. VESTN DERM VENER. 41:65-69, August, 1967.

"Some data on change in the electric activity of the brain in neurosyphilis," by L. A. Brozgol'd. VESTN DERM VENER. 43:58-70, April, 1969.

"Some data on evaluation of treponema pallidum immobilization test in syphilis (TIR)," by KhN. Khidyrov. VESTN DERM VENER. 42:66-68, July, 1968.

"Some data on the serodiagnosis of syphilis in Surinam. II," by P. Kooy, et al. BULL SOC PATH EXOT. 59:65-70, January-February, 1966.

"Some epidemiological and administrative aspects of venereal disease control," by C. L. Gonzalez. BOL SANIT PANAMER. 60:107-114, February, 1966.

"Some features of clinical picture and course of secondary syphilis nowadays," by V. A. Rakhmanov, et al. VESTN DERM VENER. 42:56-60, April, 1968.

"Some legal problems in venereal disease control," by

Golebiowska-Podgórczyk. PRZEGL DERM. Suppl:101-105, 1969.

"Some methods of serological proof of trichomonas infections in women," by J. Krupova. CESK EPIDEM. 17:162-168, May, 1968.

"Some observations of the effectiveness of monomycin in the treatment of gonorrhea in men," by V. E. Grigor'ev, et al. VESTN DERM VENER. 44:59-62, April, 1970.

"Some observations on the diagnosis of rectal gonorrhoea in both sexes using a selective culture medium," by J. Scott, et al. BRIT J VENER DIS. 42:103-106, June, 1966.

"Some observations on the sorbing agent used in the absorbed fluorescent treponemal antibody (FTA-ABS) test," by A. E. Wilkinson, et al. BRIT J VENER DIS. 44:291-298, December, 1968.

"Some observations on syphilis and pregnancy," by P. C. Brochery, et al. BULL FED GYNEC OBSTET FRANC. 20:45-49, January-March, 1968.

"Some of the problems in the control of syphilis in the United States," by W. J. Brown. SALUD PUBLICA MEX. 10:615-618, September-October, 1968.

"Some problems of organizing programmed instruction at the Department of Dermatology and Venereal Diseases," by A. N. Torsuev, et al. VESTN DERM VENER. 42:49-52, February, 1968.

"Some problems of the treatment of syphilis," by S. S. Gorbulev. VESTN DERM VENER. 40:75-77, September, 1966.

"Some remote results of the treatment of syphilis with bicillin-1, bicillin-3 and bicillin-4," by KhN Khidyrov, et al. VESTN DERM VENER. 41:47-50, June, 1967.

"Some results and perspectives of scientific investigations at the Faculty of Skin and Venereal Diseases of the N.I. Pirogov II Moscow Medical Institute," by IuK Shripkin, et al. VESTN DERM VENER. 43:3-6, September, 1969.

"Some results and prospects of research work of the Chair of Skin and Venereal Diseases of the Donetsk Medical Institute," by N. A. Torsuev, et al. VESTN DERM VENER.

43:11-16, January, 1969.

"Some results and prospects of scientific work of the Chair of Skin and Venereal diseases of the Leningrad Institute of Physician Training for 1962-1967," by P. V. Kozhevnikov. VESTN DERM VENER. 43:5-11, January, 1969.

"A special case of congenital lues," by P. M. Bakker. NEDERL T GENEESK. 110:1721-1722, September 24, 1966.

"The special clinic," by J. F. Foulkes. NM. 131:22+, July 3, 1970.

"Specific and aspecific cervico-vaginitis. Diagnostic aspects and new therapeutic trends," by A. Aluigi. MINERVA GINEC. 18:913-918, August 31, 1966.

"Specific antiluetic antibody production in a newborn with congenital lues with hypergamma M globulinemia," by F. Aiuti, et al. G MAL INFETT. 19:332-333, May, 1967.

"Specific hyposensitization of patients with penicillin allergy," by J. Pedersen-Bjergaard. ACTA ALLERG. 24:333-361, November, 1969.

"A specific IgM antibody test in neonatal congenital syphilis," by A. T. Scotti, et al. J PEDIAT. 73:242-243, August, 1968.

"Specific prophylaxis of gonorrheal ophthalmia neonatorum. A review," by P. C. Barsam. NEW ENGL J MED. 274:731-734, March 31, 1966.

"Specificity for benzyl-penicillin, penicilloyl compounds, and benzyl-penciloate in human allergy to penicillin," by J. Pedersen-Bjergaard. ACTA ALLERG. 24:87-106, May, 1969.

"Specificity of FTA-ABS and TPHA," by Y. Sasagawa, et al. JAP J CLIN PATH. 16:907-910, December, 1968.

"Specificity of the FTA-ABS test for syphilis," by D. M. Mackey, et al. JAMA. 207:1683-1685, March 3, 1969.

"The specificity of various serological tests for syphilis. Further observations on the reactivity of leprosy sera," by H. G. Ruge. GERMAN MED MONTHLY. 12:337-338, July, 1967.

"Spectinomycin hydrochloride in the treatment of uncomplicated gonorrhoea," by C. E. Cornelius, 3d, et al. BRIT J VENER DIS. 46:212-213, June, 1970.

"Spermatogenic transmission of the 'Marburg virus'. (Causes of "Marburg simian disease')," by G. A. Martini, et al. KLIN WSCHR. 46:398-400, April 1, 1968.

"Spinal fluid findings five years or more after infection in patients with early symptomatic syphilis treated with neo-arsphenamine bismuth," by F. M. Haagsma, et al. DERMATOLOGICA. 135:115-120, 1967.

"Spinal puncture and cerebrospinal fluid diagnosis," by A. Bischoff. SCHWEIZ MED WSCHR. 99:1381-1388, September 27, 1969.

"Spiramycin the 'minute treatment' of gonorrhoea," by E. Heinke, et al. GERMAN MED MONTHLY. 14:479-482, October, 1969.

"Spiramycin in the therapy of gonococcal infection," by V. Terminello. MINERVA MED. 61:1423-1425, April 11, 1970.

"Spiramycin in the treatment of gonorrhoea." BRIT MED J. 2:129, April 18, 1970.

"Spirochaeta antigens," by G. Siefert. ERGEBN MIKROBIOL IMMUNITAETSFORSCH. 39:14-42, 1966.

"Spirochetes in the aqueous humor in seronegative ocular syphilis. Persistence after penicillin therapy," by J. L. Smith, et al. ARCH OPHTHAL. 77:474-477, April, 1967.

"Spirochetes in late seronegative syphili, despite penicillin therapy," by J. L. Smith. MED TIMES. 96:611-623, June, 1968.

"Spontaneous deaths among rabbits inoculated with treponema pallidum less than 2 weeks before. Abnormal susceptibility in apparently normal laboratory rabbits indicated by serological tests for human syphilis," by B. B. Jorgensen. Z VERSUCHSTIERK. 10:46-54, 1968.

"Spontaneous fecal contamination of cerebrospinal fluid: An unusual complication of lymphogranuloma venereum," by E. Lozada, et al. AMER J DIG DIS. 14:30-34, January, 1969.

"Spontaneous rupture of aortic aneurysm into the esophagus," by J. Komorowski, et al. BULL POL MED SCI HIST. 9:24-25, January, 1966.

"Statistical considerations on the pathogenesis of epithelioma of the lip," by L. Tobia. MINERVA CHIR. 21:966-968, November 15, 1966.

"Statistical data on venereal diseases in Czechoslavakia in 1965," by J. Obrtel. CESK DERM. 42:72, February, 1967.

"Statistical evaluation of syphilis serodiagnosis," by S. Yamamoto, et al. JAP J CLIN PATH. 16:374, April, 1968.

"Statistical findings on the curability of syphilis," by G. Argenziano, et al. MINERVA DERM. 42:630-632, December, 1967.

"The status of cold reception of the skin (cold spots) in patients with syphilis," by A. A. Shtein. VESTN DERM VENER. 40:44-47, December, 1966.

"Status of serological testing for congenital syphilis," by F. D. Hoffmann, et al. J PEDIAT. 71:686-690, November, 1967.

"The status of the sexual organs of women whose husbands have nongonorrheal inflammatory diseases of the urogenital system," by S. N. Kheifets, et al. VESTN DERM VENER. 43:51-55, May, 1969.

"Status of trichomonas vaginalis among 15,000 women in Fukushima prefecture," by T. Okawa, et al. J JAP OBSTET GYNEC SOC. 19:93-96, January, 1967.

"Steroid treatment in congenital syphilitic deafness," by R. S. Dawkins, et al. J LARYNG. 82:1095-1107, December, 1968.

"Stevens-Johnson syndrome caused by allergy to sulfonamides and penicillin. Histological study with the electronic microscope," by T. J. Guillen. ALLERGIA. 15:8-18, August, 1967.

"Streptomycin in the treatment of gonorrhoea in London in 1966," by R. J. Spitzer, et al. ACTA DERMATO-VENER. 48:537-541, 1968.

"Stresses role of MD in VD control," by J. A. Cowan.

MICH MED. 65:552, July, 1966.

"Students as special clinic patients," by R. S. Morton. BRIT J VENER DIS. 42:280-282, December, 1966.

"Studies in syphilis epidemiology," by W. J. Brown. BRIT J VENER DIS. 42:110-115, June, 1966.

"Studies of the education of young people concerning venereal diseases," by P. Many, et al. BULL SOC FRANC DERM SYPH. 74:772-780, 1967.

"Studies of false positive serological tests for syphilis following smallpox vaccination," by O. P. Salo, et al. ANN MED EXP FENN. 44:304-306, 1966.

"Studies of patients with penicillin allergy with a review of literature," by H. Strassmann. HAUTARZT. 20:323-329, July, 1969.

"Studies of syphilitic antibodies. I. Anti-lipoidal antibodies in various stages of syphilis," by K. Aho. BRIT J VENER DIS. 43:259-263, December, 1967.

--II. Substances responsible for biological false positive sero-reactions. BRIT J VENER DIS. 44:49-54, March, 1968.

--III. Anamnestic reactions and 19S predominance of the anti-lipoidal antibodies in aged persons. BRIT J VENER DIS. 44:283-286, December, 1968.

--IV. Evidence of reactant partner common for C-reactive protein and certain anti-lipoidal antibodies. BRIT J VENER DIS. 45:13-18, March, 1969.

"Studies of the value of erythromycin and oxytetracycline in treatment of early syphilis," by J. Bowszyc, et al. POL TYG LEK. 25:1394-1396, September, 1970.

"Studies of venereal disease. I. Probenecid-procaine penicillin G combination and tetracycline hydrochloride in the treatment of 'penicillin-resistant' gonorrhea in men," by K. K. Holmes, et al. JAMA. 202:461-473, November 6, 1967.

--II. Observations on the incidence, etiology, and treatment of the postgonococcal urethritis syndrome. JAMA. 202:467-473, November 6, 1967.

"Studies on the bone marrow and lymph nodes in primary

syphilis," by W. Rasiewicz, et al. Z HAUT GESCHLECHTSKR. 43:351-358, May 1, 1968.

"Studies on carcinoma of the urinary bladder. I. Statistical and epidemiological studies on cancer of the bladder in Japanese," by O. Yoshida. ACTA UROL JAP. 12:1040-1064, October, 1966.

"Studies on the diagnosis of syphilis using the fluorescent antibody technic (absorption method)-FTA-ABS," by M. Murata, et al. JAP J CLIN MED. 26:466-474, February, 1968.

"Studies on the disappearance of treponema pallidum from the eruption of early syphilis under the effect of various antibiotics. Effect of oxyterracine on treponema pallidum," by J. Suchanek, et al. POL TYG LEK. 22:1103-1106, July 17, 1967.

"Studies on durable long term preservation of stained preparations of treponema pallidum. Experiment I. Detection of treponema pallidum in testes of syphilitic rabbits by fluorescent antibody reaction," by H. Furukawa. BULL PHARM RES INST. 61:1-12, March, 1966.

"Studies on the effect of most frequently used antibiotics on the course of syphilitic infection," by R. Mielech, et al. PRZEGL DERM. 55:143-149, March-April, 1968.

"Studies on fluorescence-microscopy differentiation of antibodies in syphilis," by F. Muller, et al. ARCH HYG BAKT. 152:76-78, January, 1968.

"Studies on the fluorescent treponemal antibody (FTA) test," by A. E. Wilkinson, et al. BRIT J VENER DIS. 42:8-15, March, 1966.

"Studies on the fluorescent treponemal antibody test using fluorescent anti-gamma, anti-alpha, anti-mu, anti-lambda, anti-kappa chains and beta-1CA, E globulin reagents," by T. Matuhasi, et al. BULL WHO. 34: 466-472, 1966.

"Studies on granuloma inguinale. 8. Serological reactivity of sera from patients with carcinoma of penis when tested with Donovania antigens," by J. Goldberg, et al. BRIT J VENER DIS. 42:205-209, September, 1966.

"Studies on immunity and allergy in ectopic infections

with trichomonas vaginalis," by A. Westphal, et al. Z TROPENMED PARASIT. 19:60-73, March, 1968.

"Studies on immunity in experimental syphilis. 2. Transfer of antibodies to the fetus in rabbits," by T. Tomizawa, et al. JAP J BACT. 21:222-225, April, 1966.

"Studies on immunofluorescence test for syphilis," by V. K. Gokhale, et al. J POSTGRAD MED. 12:13-25, January, 1966.

"Studies on non-inflammatory lesions in neurosyphilis. I. An autopsy case of tabes dorsalis combined with status dysraphicus and Alzheimer's fibrillary changes in the horn of Ammon," by T. Matsuoka, et al. BRAIN NERVE. 20:27-32, January, 1968.

"Studies on the occurrence and the frequency of various microorganisms (anaerobic bacteria, trichomonads, mycoplasms and yeasts) in the human vagina in vaginitis," by W. A. Muller, et al. ARCH HYG BAKT. 151: 609-621, November, 1967.

"Studies on the pathogenic significance of female urogenital trichomoniasis with special reference to its effects of fertility," by D. Hofmann, et al. ARCH GYNAEK. 203:1-19, 1966.

"Studies on reagin formation in rabbits immunized with pallidum and Reiter treponeme," by G. Tringali, et al. RIV IST SIEROTER ITAL. 43:144-149, May-June, 1968.

"Studies on the risk of trichomonas infection in swimming pools," by J. Sarosiek. WIAD PARAZYT. 13:37-39, 1967.

"Studies on the trichomonacidal effects of various nitrofuran preparations," by H. Birnbaum. ZBL GYNAEK. 89:1303-1313, September 9, 1967.

"Studies on trichomonas vaginalis," by M. S. Grewal. INDIAN PRACT. 19:403-410, June, 1966.

"Studies on trichomonas vaginalis donne. IV. Size of the population of trichomonads in the vaginal secretions of women," by A. Kurnatowska. ACTA MED POL. 9:175-182, 1968.

"Studies on trichomonas vaginalis in the urological field. I.," by N. Kawamura. JAP J UROL. 60:15-24, January, 1969.

--2. JAP J UROL. 60:25-28, January, 1969.

"Studies on the value of atrican (TC 109) in the treatment of trichomonal and monilial infections," by W. Kilczewski, et al. PRZEGL DERM. 55:531-535, July-September, 1968.

"Studies with an intradermal test of infections caused by viruses of the psittacosis-ornithosis-venereal lymphogranulomatosis type," by S. D'Agostino, et al. G MAL INFETT. 18:777-779, November, 1966.

"A study and new description of corynebacterium vaginale (Haemophilus vaginalis)," by W. E. Dunkelberg, Jr., et al. AMER J CLIN PATH. 53:370-377, March, 1970.

"A study in New Zealand mortality. 7. Infectious diseases (concluded)," by J. W. Donovan. NEW ZEAL MED J. 71:143-147, March, 1970.

"Study of the antigenic relationships between treponema pallidum and Borrelia hispancia," by J. Ranque, et al. MED TROP. 27:519-524, September-October, 1967.

"A study of the causes of diagnostic discrepancies in the examination of women who are sources of gonorrhea infection," by E. N. Turanova, et al. VESTN DERM VENER. 41:69-71, September, 1967.

"Study of the concentration of oletetrine in the blood serum from patients with gonorrhea," by Z. V. Ermol'eva, et al. VESTN DERM VENER. 40:77-79, September, 1966.

"A study of drug-taking among young patients attending a clinic for venereal diseases," by A. Linken. BRIT J VENER DIS. 44:337-341, December, 1968.

"Study of the existence of treponemic antibodies in dry blood," by A. Utrilla. ACTAS DERMOSIF. 58:167-170, May-June, 1967.

"Study of a glycolipidic antigen of treponema reiteri and of the corresponding antibody contained in a human serum," by P. Dupouey, et al. ANN INST PASTEUR. 117:395-407, September, 1969.

"A study of the heat-labile antigen of treponema pallidum," by M. Metzger, et al. ARCH IMMUN THER EXP. 16:888-894, 1968.

"Study of the identification of Neisseria gonorrhoeae by fluorescent antibody technic," by N. Bansho. J JAP OBSTET GYNEC SOC. 20:1437-1445, November, 1968.

"Study of the increase of primary-secondary and early congenital syphilis from 1938 to 1965 based on the statistics of the Clinical Dermosifilopatica of the University of Genoa and of the Ospedale Pediatrico 'Giannina Gaslini' of Genoa," by E. Rampini, et al. MINERVA DERM. 41:442-444, December, 1966.

"Study of late ocular syphilis. Demonstration of treponemes in aqueous humour and cerebrospinal fluid. I. Methods of demonstration of treponemes," by A. E. Wilkinson. TRANS OPHTHAL SOC UK. 88:251-256, 1969.

--II. Ocular findings, by N. S. Rice, et al. TRANS OPHTHAL SOC UK. 88:257-273, 1969.

--III. General and serological findings, by E. M. Dunlop, et al. TRANS OPHTHAL SOC UK. 88:275-294, 1969.

"Study of 1,929 cases of primo-secondary syphilis observed in the Clinique des Maladies Cutanées et Syphilitiques of the Faculté de Médecine de Paris," by R. Degos, et al. BULL INST NAT SANTE. 23:549-585, May-June, 1968.

"Study of the non-inflammatory lesions of neurosyphilis. 3. Case of progressive paralysis association with Huntington's chorea," by T. Matsuoka, et al. BRAIN NERVE. 20:925-930, 1968.

"A study of 183 cases of leucorrhea: Incidence of trichomonas vaginalis, candida spp., and hemophilus vaginalis," by Z. D. Desai, et al. J POSTGRAD MED. 12:91-98, April, 1966.

"A study of the relationships between the sensitivities of Neisseria gonorrhoeae to sodium penicillin G, four semi-synthetic penicillins, spiramycin, and fusidic acid," by A. Reyn, et al. BRIT J VENER DIS. 44:140-150, June, 1968.

"Study of seasonal variations and general development of trichomonas vaginitis from 1957 to 1966," by M. Gaudefroy, et al. GYNEC PRAT. 18:355-379, 1967.

"A study of sensitivity induced by certain drugs by intradermal skin tests," by B. Raj, et al. INDIAN

J MED RES. 57:1769-1775, September, 1969.

"Study of the therapeutic effectiveness of bicillin-6 in patients with communicable forms of syphilis," by O. K. Loseva. VESTN DERM VENER. 41:59-62, May, 1967.

"A study of the trichomonicidal activity of the association of chloramphenicol and 1-hydroxyethyl-2methyl-5nitro-imidazole," by F. Filadoro. ANTIBIOTICA. 5: 105-113, June, 1967.

"Study on doxycycline in the treatment of acute infections of the respiratory system and lymphogranuloma venereum," by J. Neves, et al. REV ASS MED BRASIL. 14:65-70, June, 1968.

"Study on the persistance of treponema pallidum in the lymph nodes of treated luetics," by U. Boncinelli, et al. G ITAL DERM. 107:1-14, January-February, 1966.

"Study on the serological diagnosis of syphilis using the TPHA-test," by T. Kawai, et al. SAISHIN IGAKU. 23: 1929-1932, September 10, 1968.

"A study on the serological diagnostic techniques for syphilis," by B. Cacciapuoti, et al. ANN SCLAVO. 8:97-119, February 1, 1966.

"A study on the Wassermann and TPI antibodies in relation to histopathological findings in T. pallidum infected animals and man," by T. Fredriksson, et al. ACTA PATH MICROBIOL SCAND. 72:125-138, 1968.

"Study with an intradermal test of infections caused by viruses of the psittacosis-ornithosis-lymphogranuloma venereum group," by S. D'Agostino, et al. G MAL INFETT. 18:777-779, November, 1966.

"Subacute inflammatory rheumatism due to secondary syphilis," by M. F. Kahn, et al. PRESSE MED. 78:750, March 28, 1970.

"Subacute inflammatory rheumatism in secondary syphilis. 4 cases," by M. F. Kahn, et al. REV RHUM. 37:431-436, June-July, 1970.

"Substrates usable for absorption in the reaction of FTA-ABS," by M. Sepetjian, et al. PATH BIOL. 18:393-397, April, 1970.

"Sudden death occurring during 'massive-dose' potassium penicillin G therapy. An argument implicating potassium intoxication," by G. L. Tullett. WISCONSIN MED J. 69:216-217, September, 1970.

"Sulphamethoxazole combined with 2-4-diamino-pyrimidines in the treatment of gonorrhoea," by D. J. Wright, et al. BRIT J VENER DIS. 46:34-36, February, 1970.

"Supplementary findings on methods for the serodiagnosis of syphilis. 1. Serological specificity of the antigen of treponema pallidum Reiter strain," by T. Tomizawa, et al. JAP J BACT. 21:251-255, May, 1966.

--2. On the specificity of the hemagglutination test and fluorescent antibody technic. JAP J BACT. 22: 607-611, December, 1967.

"Surgical problems associated with tabes dorsalis," by M. T. Hoerner. INDUSTR MED SURG. 35:483-488, June, 1966.

"A survey by questionnaire of psychiatric disturbance in patients attending a venereal diseases clinic," by J. R. Pedder, et al. BRIT J VENER DIS. 46:58-61, February, 1970.

"A survey of problems in the antibiotic treatment of gonorrhoea. With special reference to South-East Asia," by R. R. Willcox. BRIT J VENER DIS. 46:217-242, June, 1970.

"A survey of the range of sensitivity in vitro of N. gonorrhoea to penicillin," by C. W. Chacko, et al. INDIAN J MED RES. 54:823-838, September, 1966.

"Survey of recent developments in some fields of serologic diagnosis of disease," by K. F. Petersen. HIPPOKRATES. 38:714-719, September 30, 1967.

"Survey of serologic evidence for syphilis among the Masai of Tanzania," by G. V. Mann, et al. PUBLIC HEALTH REP. 81:513-518, June, 1968.

"A survey of trichomonal and neisserian infection in antenatal patients," by R. Gaal, et al. MED J AUST. 1: 634-635, April 13, 1968.

"A survey of trichomonal and neisserian infection in antenatal patients," by R. A. Osborn, et al. MED J AUST. 2:92, July 13, 1968.

"Survey on information on health among citizens of a large city with special reference to cancer and venereal disease." J JAP MED ASS. 59:117-121, January 1, 1968.

"Susceptibility of common pathogenic bacteria to seven tetracycline antibiotics in vitro," by N. H. Steigbigel, et al. AMER J MED SCI. 255:179-195, March, 1968.

"Susceptibility of Neisseria gonorrhoeae to penicillin and tetracycline," by A. R. Ronald, et al. ANTIMICROB AGENTS CHEMOTHER. 8:431-434, 1968.

"Swallowing disorders due to a large luetic aneurysm of the thoracic aorta," by H. Wehling. MED WELT. 2: 106-108, January 8, 1966.

"Swelling in the lower abdomen of the patients with cervix cancer is not necessarily an indication of metastasis," by M. Jin, et al. SANFULIN JISSAI. 15:1102-1105, December, 1966.

"Swelling of the inguinal lymph nodes in syphilis of the anus," by A. H. Schmid. MED KLIN. 61:914-915, June 10, 1966.

"Symmetrical synovitis of the knee in hereditary syphilis," by H. H. Clutton. CLIN ORTHOP. 57:5-8, March-April, 1968.

"Symposium on certain forms of infective kerato-uveitis or uveitis: 1. An approach to the problem, and the technique of anterior chamber tap," by B. R. Jones, et al. TRANS OPHTHAL SOC UK. 88:235-242, 1969.

"Symptomatic gonorrhea during pregnancy," by P. M. Sarrel, et al. OBSTET GYNEC. 32:670-673, November, 1968.

"Symptomatic 'migrating' phlebitis," by R. Verjat. PHLEBOLOGIC. 19:159-160, April-June, 1966.

"Symptomatology and therapy of female and male trichomoniasis," by H. Walther. THER GEGENW. 105:886-889, July, 1966.

"Symptoms 20 years after treatment of secondary syphilis," by S. Olansky. JAMA. 207:961, February 3, 1969.

"Syphilis," LYON MED. 215:69-117, January 9, 1966.

"Syphilis--an ancient enemy grows weaker. (Editorial),"
by W. H. Kaufman. VIRGINIA MED MONTHLY. 96:499-
500, August, 1969.

"Syphilis and biologic false positive reactors among leprosy patients," by A. T. Scotti, et al. ARCH DERM. 101:328-330, March, 1970.

"Syphilis and the eye," by W. E. Gager. WISCONSIN MED J. 68:38, May, 1969; also in SIGHT SAVING R. 39:137-143, Fall, 1969.

"Syphilis and gonorrhea in general practice," by R. Schmitz. MED WELT. 11:434-437, March 14, 1970.

"Syphilis and guidance of expectant mothers," by M. Sumudi. JAP J NURS ART. 8:77-80, August, 1969.

"Syphilis and hepatic cirrhosis." LANCET. 1:28-29, January 3, 1970.

"Syphilis and hepatic cirrhosis," by I. A. Kellock, et al. LANCET. 1:369, February 14, 1970.

"Syphilis and homosexuality," by I. Kirjakov, et al. CESK DERM. 41:25-27, February, 1966.

"Syphilis and iridocyclitis," by Z. Kumstát, et al. CESK OFTAL. 23:103-108, March, 1967.

"Syphilis and serology," by E. E. Vella. MILIT MED. 132:243-251, April, 1967.

"Syphilis as a differential diagnosis of neck masses," by C. T. Yarington, Jr., et al. ARCH OTOLARYNG. 86:219-221, August, 1967.

"Syphilis as an unusual cause of aches and pains," by A. Beardwell, et al. PROC ROY SOC MED. 62:197, February, 1969.

"Syphilis casefinding through the laboratory reporting system," by G. Pickett. MICH MED. 66:1416-1468, November, 1967.

"Syphilis control in a southern state," by R. W. Ball. MED TIMES. 94:520-530, May, 1966.

"Syphilis control: joint responsibility of private medicine and public health," by T. J. Friddell, et al. J TENN MED ASS. 59:141-143, February, 1966.

"The syphilis control program in North Carolina," N CAROLINA MED J. 28:32-33, January, 1967.

"Syphilis: current disease," by J. Grandbois. UN MED CANADA. 95:728-733, June, 1966.

"Syphilis: a difficult diagnosis?," by J. Smoler, et al. LARYNGOSCOPE. 78:404-410, March, 1968.

"Syphilis epidemic in South Greenland 1965," by G. A. Olsen. UGESKR LAEG. 128:1071-1076, September 15, 1966.

"Syphilis: evaluation of blood tests," by V. M. Torres Rodriguez. BOL ASOC MED P RICO. 60:414-421, September, 1968.

"Syphilis in current neurology. 1," by G. Moya, et al. ARCH NEUROBIOL. 30:138-166, April-June, 1967+.

"Syphilis in the new-born in La Paz, Bolivia," BY G. G. de Murillo. J AMER MED WOM ASS. 24:420-422, May, 1969.

"Syphilis in pregnancy. Diagnosis through VDRL and FTA-200 tests," by C. Krahe, et al. HOSPITAL. 74:975-978, September, 1968+.

"Syphilis latex microreaction, the Bourdet-Wassermann cardiolipin test and the Sachs-Witebsky test," by S. Kośmiderski, et al. PRZEGL DERM. Suppl:107-110, 1969.

"Syphilis maligna praecox. Syphilis of the great epidemic? An historical review," by D. J. Cripps, et al. ARCH INTERN MED. 119:411-418, April, 1967.

"Syphilis of the brain based on data from a psychiatric hospital," by A. P. Tikhonova, et al. VESTN DERM VENER. 40:31-35, December, 1966.

"Syphilis of the lung. A case report and discussion of its clinical diagnosis," by S. Haim, et al. ACTA DERMATOVENER. 49:97-102, 1969.

"Syphilis of the lungs," by I. I. Pototskii. VRACH DELO. 8:81-84, August, 1967.

"Syphilis of the nervous system. (The problem as it stands today.)," by M. V. Milich. SOVET MED. 31:94-99, January, 1968.

"Syphilis of nose and paranasal sinus," by H. Y. Lee. OHIO MED J. 64:1264-1267, November, 1968.

"Syphilis of the parents as a cause of several neuropsychic disorders in children," by L. V. Sazonova, et al. VESTN DERM VENER. 43:57-59, September, 1969.

"The syphilis of Ulrich von Hutten. Sensational studies of a group of experts of the medical school of the University of Zurich," by H. Jung. HAUTARZT. 20:334-336, July, 1969.

"Syphilis of the uterine cervix," by L. Gostin, et al. REV CHILE OBSTET GINEC. 30:95-98, January-February, 1965.

"Syphilis past and present." LANCET. 2:503-504, September,2, 1967.

"Syphilis--the persistent problem." EYE EAR NOSE THROAT MONTHLY. 45:88 passim, November, 1966.

"Syphilis reactions in leprosy sera. Mass screening tests," by H. Ruge. MED WELT. 48:2620-2627, November 26, 1966.

"Syphilis--rediscovered," by S. Olansky. DM. 3-30, May, 1967.

"Syphilis screening using the multi-channel blood-grouping machine," by J. W. Lockyer. BRIT J VENER DIS. 46:290-294, August, 1970.

"Syphilis serodiagnosis: introduction," by N. Matsuhashi, et al. JAP J CLIN PATH. 16:335, April, 1968.

"Syphilis serodiagnostic findings during the course of disease," by J. Meyer-Rohn. DEUTSCH MED WSCHR. 94:1037, May 9, 1969.

"Syphilis serology today," by A. F. Disalvo. J S CAROLINA MED ASS. 64:503-505, December, 1968.

"Syphilis therapy 1967," by W. T. Linton. APPL THER. 9:529, June, 1967.

"Syphilis under our noses," by D. R. Richardson, et al. VIRGINIA MED MONTHLY. 95:607-609 passim, October, 1968.

"Syphilis: was it endemic in pre-Columbian America or was

it brought here from Europe?," by A. I. Weisman. BULL NY ACAD MED. 42:284-300, April, 1966.

"Syphilis with macroglobulinemia," by R. Francois, et al. PEDIATRIC. 21:47-59, January-February, 1966.

"Syphilis yesterday and today," by M. G. Achten. J MED LYON. 49:685-702, April 20, 1968.

"Syphilitic amyotrophy," by A. Datta, et al. J INDIAN MED ASS. 47:287-290, September 16, 1966.

"Syphilitic amyotrophy. A case occurring after apparently successful treatment in primary syphilis," by A. B. Hewitt. BRIT J VENER DIS. 43:272-274, December, 1967.

"Syphilitic aneurysm of the ascending aorta producing pulmonic stenosis by compression," by T. Watanabe, et al. AMER J CARDIOL. 20:575-578, October, 1967.

"Syphilitic aortic insufficiency. Its increased incidence in the elderly," by T. A. Prewitt. JAMA. 211:637-639, January 26, 1970.

"Syphilitic aortic insufficiency. Some observations on a vanishing disorder," by B. Friedman. ALABAMA J MED SCI. 6:8-17, January, 1969.

"Syphilitic aortitis," by D. B. Reddy, et al. INDIAN HEART J. 19:86-95, April, 1967.

"Syphilitic aortitis. 56 cases followed-up for 10 years after treatment with penicillin," by S. E. Vivas. ARCH INST CARDIOL MEX. 36:316-321, May-June, 1966.

"Syphilitic arthropathy," by M. Makuch, et al. CHIR NARZAD RUCHU ORTOP POL. 33:673-677, 1968.

"Syphilitic chancre complicated by fusospirochaetal infection from the same partner. Development of necrotizing ulcer perforating the prepuce," by K. Lejman, et al. BRIT J VENER DIS. 45:313-316, December, 1969.

"Syphilitic chorioretinitis. A histologic study," by F. C. Blodi, et al. ARCH OPHTHAL. 79:294-296, March, 1968.

"Syphilitic coronary ostial occlusion," by V. Schrive, et al. S AFR MED J. 40:553-555, July 2, 1966.

"Syphilitic coronary ostial sclerosis," by R. W. Frater, et al. ANN THORAC SURG. 6:463-468, November, 1968.

"Syphilitic disease of the stomach," by W. Lindheimer. MUNCHEN MED WSCHR. 109:638-643, March 24, 1967.

"Syphilitic gumma of the tongue," by F. G. Marill, et al. BULL SOC FRANC DERM SYPH. 74:216-217, 1967.

"Syphilitic keratitis," by G. M. de Weisenberg, et al. REV FAC CIENC MED CORDOBA. 27:27-35, January-March, 1969.

"Syphilitic lesions of the kidney," by K. S. Reddy. INDIAN J MED SCI. 20:424-426, June, 1966.

"Syphilitic ocular manifestations in our clinical experience," by Z. Pavisič, et al. RAD MED FAK ZAGREB. 14:241-252, 1966.

"Syphilitic optic neuritis. A case report," by S. E. Lorentzen. ACTA OPHTHAL. 45:769-772, 1967.

"Syphilitic osteoarthritis of the hip joint," by A. Sobbe, et al. FORTSCHR ROENTGENSTR. 110:249-253, February, 1969.

"Syphilitic osteochondritis in congenital late syphilis," by H. Wendler. ARCH KINDERHEILK. 176:184-190, 1967.

"Syphilitic osteomyelitis of the mandible," by I. H. Heslop, BRIT J ORAL SURG. 6:59-63, July, 1968.

"Syphilitic osteoperiostitis of the orbital apex," by P. Cernea, et al. ANN OCULIST. 201:436-462, April, 1968.

"Syphilitic ostial coronaritis: 5 cases of surgical disobstruction, 2 of which including a valve replacement for aortic insufficiency," by P. Michaud, et al. ARCH MAL COEUR. 63:674-693, May, 1970; also in LYON CHIR. 66:3-9, January-February, 1970.

"Syphilitic temporal arteritis," by J. L. Smith, et al. ARCH OPHTHAL. 78:284-288, September, 1967.

"Syphilization," by J. R. Prakken. NEDERL T GENEESK. 114:1019-1023, June 13, 1970.

"Syphilophobia in the practice of the dermatovenereologist by V. D. Kochetkov, et al. VESTN DERM VENER. 42:62-67, November, 1968.

"Systemic lupus erythematosus with oscillating syphilitic serology," by C. Grupper, et al. BULL SOC FRANC DERM SYPH. 76:497-502, 1969.

"T-strain mycoplasma. Selective inhibition by erythromycin in vitro," by M. C. Shepard, et al. BRIT J VENER DIS. 42:21-24, March, 1966.

"T-strain mycoplasma in nongonococcal urethritis," by G. W. Csonka, et al. ANN NY ACAD SCI. 143:794-798, July 28, 1967.

"T-strain mycoplasma in nongonococcal urethritis. Pathogen or commensal?," by W. Fowler, et al. BRIT J VENER DIS. 45:287-293, December, 1969.

"T-strain mycoplasmas in non-specific urethritis," by A. Shipley, et al. MED J AUST. 1:794-796, May 11, 1968.

"The TPI and FTA-ABS tests in treated late syphilis," by W. G. Atwood, et al. JAMA. 203:549-561, February 19, 1968.

"TPI and FTA tests in the evaluation of effectiveness of the oral treatment of early symptomatic syphilis with detreomycin, erythromycin and oxytetracycline with consideration of the clinical picture," by J. Lebioda, et al. PRZEGL DERM. Suppl:39-51, 1969.

"T.P.I. test and blastic transformation of lymphocytes in vitro," by A. Sapuppo, et al. MINERVA DERM. 42:12-13, January, 1967.

"Tabes dorsalis," by C. L. Gerard. PROC MINE MED OFFICERS ASS. 46:23-26, May-July, 1966.

"Tabes dorsalis of sudden onset associated with possible transverse myelitis," by A. S. Wigfield. BRIT J VENER DIS. 46:262-263, June, 1970.

"Tabetic arthropathies," by E. Delvecchio. OSPED ITAL CHIR. 18:481-493, May, 1968.

"Tabetic arthropathy," by M. L. Livshits. VRACH DELO. 11:147-149, November, 1967.

"Tabetic arthropathy and secondary neurological manifestations," by M. Cardas, et al. NEUROLOGIA. 12:341-353, July-August, 1967.

"The tabetic spine," by A. Passerini, et al. RADIO MED. 52:23-29, January, 1966.

"Takayasau's syndrome and disease," by A. Zuch. WIAD LEK. 20:1271-1273, July 1, 1967.

"A tale of two cities," by G. S. Hayes. QUEENSLAND NURSES J. 8:29+, June, 1966.

"'Target' sites for anti-V.D. propaganda," by B. P. Wells, et al. HEALTH BULL. 28:75-77, January, 1970.

"Tasks of the journal 'Vestnik dermatologil i venereologil' in 1969," by B. M. Pashkov. VESTN DERM VENER. 43:3-5, January, 1969.

"Teaching about venereal disease and its control," by B. Webster. ARCH ENVIRON HEALTH, Chicago. 13:367-371, September, 1966.

"Teaching of the clinical, epidemiological, public health, and social aspects of the venereal diseases in the medical schools throughout the world. Interim report of the continuing cooperative study between WHO and the IUVDT," by B. Webster. BRIT J VENER DIS. 46:156-158, April, 1970.

"Teaching of dermatovenerology in the school of medicine. Goals and methods," by J. Obrtel, et al. CESK DERM. 44:37-40, February, 1969.

"Teaching of venereal disease in medical schools throughout the world. Preliminary report," by B. Webster. BRIT J VENER DIS. 42:132-133, January, 1966.

"A technique for detecting treponema pallidum through the use of membrane filters and immunofluorescence staining," by F. W. Chandler, Jr. BRIT J VENER DIS. 45:305-307, December, 1969.

"Technic for the fluorescent treponemal antibody-absorption (FTA-ABS) test." HEALTH LAB SCI. 5:23-30, January, 1968.

"The teenager and VD." AMER J PUBLIC HEALTH. 59:898-899, June, 1969.

"Tegretol, a new therapy of tabetic lightning pains. Preliminary report," by K. Ekbom. ACTA MED SCAND. 179: 251-252. Fasc. 2., February 2, 1966.

"Temporal bone treponemes," by L. W. Mack, Jr., et al. ARCH OTOLARYNG. 90:11-14, July, 1969.

"Ten-year study of Neisseria gonorrhoeae sensitivity to antibiotics in Czechoslovakia," by M. Hejzlar, et al. J HYG EPIDEM. 12:296-305, 1968.

"The terrain favorable for trichomoniasis," by G. Chappaz. GYNEC PRAT. 17:391-396, 1966.

"Tertiary form of frambesia with localization in the spine," by V. Benes. ACTA CHIR ORTHOP TRAUM CECH. 33:440-442, October, 1966.

"The tesa-film patch test for the demonstration of penicillin allergy in practice," by M. Reichenberger. Z HAUT GESCHLECHTSKR. 40:293-300, April 15, 1966.

"Tests for syphilis in children for adoption," by C. E. Cooper. LANCET. 2:261, August 1, 1970.

"Tests for syphilis in children for adoption," by O. P. Gray. LANCET. 2:673, September 26, 1970.

"Tests for syphilis in children for adoption," by D. H. Robertson. LANCET. 2:568, September 12, 1970.

"Tests for syphilis in young males. An analysis of a seven-year series from a Central Military Hospital," by O. P. Salo, et al. MILIT MED. 132:258-261, April, 1967.

"Theoretic and practical aspects of the scientific activity of the Gor'kii Institute of Dermatology and Venereology," by O. D. Kochura, et al. VESTN DERM VENER. 44:9-14, January, 1970.

"Therapeutic and diagnostic problems of vaginal trichomoniasis treated with imidazole," by B. Toth, et al. ORV HETIL. 108:452-455, March 5, 1967.

"Therapeutic effects of bicillin-6 in treatment of gonorrhea in men," by S. L. Kozin, et al. VESTN DERM VENER. 44:75-79, May, 1970.

"Therapeutic experiences with aureocort," by F. Von Fischer. PRAXIS. 55:1240-1242, October 27, 1966.

"Therapeutic failures in gonorrhea. Discussion on symposium II," by H. Biehler. ARCH KLIN EXP DERM. 227: 656-662, 1966.

"Therapeutic problems of trichomoniasis of the urogenital apparatus in men," by J. Darewicz, et al. POL PRZEGL CHIR. 42:Suppl:6A:969+, 1970.

"Therapeutic trial of some genital infections with trimethoprim-sulphamethoxazole," by G. W. Csonka. POSTGRAD MED J. 45:Suppl:77-80, November, 1969.

"Therapeutic trial of trimethoprim as a potentiator of sulphonamides in gonorrhoea," by G. W. Csonka, et al. BRIT J VENER DIS. 43:161-165, September, 1967.

"Therapy of early syphilis," by O. Braun-Falco. DEUTSCH MED WSCHR. 95:1611-1613, July 31, 1970.

"Therapy of early syphilis during the last 21 years at the dermatologic clinic of Wiesbaden," by F. Nemec. Z HAUT GESCHLECHTSKR. 45:561-575, August 1, 1970.

"Therapy of early syphilis--review of the literature," by M. Pacenovská, et al. CESK DERM. 45:171-180, August, 1970.

"Therapy of early syphilis with cephaloridine," by O. A. Gonzalez, et al. REV INVEST SALUD PUBLICA. 27: 201-214, July-September, 1967.

"Therapy of fluor vaginalis," by S. Iversen. T NORSK LAEGEFOREN. 88:769-773, May 1, 1968.

"Therapy of gonococcal infection with rifamycin in a 'single dose'," by A. Califano, et al. MINERVA DERM. 43:516-519, October, 1968.

"Therapy of neurosyphilis," REV CLIN ESP. 104:425-426, March 15, 1967.

"Therapy of neurosyphilis," by H. Bammer. DEUTSCH MED WSCHR. 1280-1283, June 14, 1967.

"Therapy of skin and venereal diseases. Review of the literature of 1967-1968," by H. Walther. DEUTSCH MED J. 20:480-485, August, 1969.

"Therapy of syphilis," by J. Obrtel. CESK DERM. 45:154-159, August, 1970.

"Therapy of syphilis with penicillin with special consideration of the time factor," by A. Kern, et al. Z AERZTL FORTBILD. 60:1201-1206, November 15, 1966.

"Therapy of trichomonas and thrush colpitis using nifuratel," by A. Weidenbach, et al. MUNCHEN MED WSCHR. 110:343-345, February 9, 1968.

"Therapy of trichomoniasis," by R. M. Baker, et al. WISCONSIN MED J. 66:370-371, August, 1967.

"3 cases of congenital syphilis in infants," by E. Majima. SAISHIN IGAKU. 22:1260-1265, June, 1967.

"Three incidents after intracutaneous tests with penicilloyl-polylysine," by I. Luckerath, et al. HAUTARZT. 18:183-185, April, 1967.

"Three lipoidal tests in screening for syphilis and biological false-positive reactions in a dermatological series," by E. A. Johansson, et al. ANN CLIN RES. 2:42-46, March, 1970.

"Thrombocytopenia and congenital syphilis in South African Bantu infants," by I. Freiman, et al. ARCH DIS CHILD. 41:87-90, February, 1966.

"The thyroid and phospho-calcic metabolism. IV. The behavior of the specific radioactivity of plasmatic calcium during infusion of swine thyrocalcitonin (TCT) in man," by C. Scandellari, et al. ACTA ISOTOP. 7:153-161, December 15, 1967.

"Tietze's syndrome and syphilis," by J. Vachtenheim. DEUTSCH GESUNDH. 21:1387-1388, July 21, 1966.

"Time saving method for staining treponema pallidum in tissue," by K. Ito, et al. HAUTARZT. 20:85-88, February, 1969.

"Time to put an end to venereal disease care," by H. Moller. LAKARTIDNINGEN. 65:987-990, March 6, 1968.

"Timely serodiagnosis of lues and its evaluation with special reference to quantitative methods," by H. Roser. DEUTSCH MED WSCHR. 93:2017-2019, October 18, 1968.

"Tinidazole and metronidazole pharmacokinetics in man and mouse," by J. A. Taylor, Jr., et al. ANTIMICROB AGENTS CHEMOTHER. 9:267-270, 1969.

"Tinidazole, a new antiprotozoal agent: Effect on trichomonas and other protozoa," by H. L. Howes, Jr., et al. ANTIMICROB AGENTS CHEMOTHER. 9:261-222, 1969.

"Titration of complement by 50 percent hemolysis in patients with skin and venereal diseases," by L. S. Reznikova, et al. VESTN DERM VENER. 40:64-69, October, 1966.

"Tonsillectomy--a bloody mess," by H. Faigel. CLIN PEDIAT. 5:652-653, November, 1966.

"Toward a syphilis vaccine," by F. Marley. SCI N. 92:356, October 7, 1967.

"Town and country in the spreading of venereal diseases," by J. Kolankowski. PRZEGL DERM. 54:651-653, November-December, 1967.

"Toxic reactions from depot-penicillin," by R. Kiesewetter, et al. DEUTSCH GESUNDH. 23:631-634, April 4, 1968.

"Transformation of antibody from IgM to IgG in experimental syphylitic rabbits. I. Syphylitic serum reaction," by M. Ogata, et al. ACTA MED OKAYAMA. 24:93-99, February, 1970.

"Transmissible venereal tumour in a boxer bitch," by J. B. Tutt. VET REC. 84:13, January 4, 1969.

"Transmission of syphilis by fresh blood components," by R. W. Chambers, et al. TRANSFUSION. 9:32-34, January-February, 1969.

"Transmission of trichomonas," by R. D. Catterall, et al. BRIT MED J. 1:765, June 21, 1969.

"Traumatic ectopia lentis. Some relationships to syphilis and glaucoma," by L. J. Rosenbaum, et al. AMER J OPHTHAL. 64:1095-1098, December, 1967.

"Treated late syphilis: immunoglobulin class of antibodies reactive with treponema pallidum," by L. C. Logan, et al. J INVEST DERM. 53:300-301, October, 1969.

"Treatment of acute gonococcal urethritis," by L. A. Blanco Gutierrez. REV VENEZ. UROL. 21:93-100, January-June, 1969.

"Treatment of acute male gonococcal urethritis with a single dose of erythromycin-stearate," by J. Martini, et al. REV MED CHILE. 96:525-527, August, 1968.

"The treatment of Bartholin abscesses and Bartholin cysts," by H. G. Mayer. MED KLIN. 65:200-203, January 30, 1970.

"Treatment of chancroid. A comparison of tetracycline and sulfisoxazole," by R. E. Kerber, et al. ARCH DERM. 100:604-607, November, 1969.

"Treatment of dermato-venereal diseases with chlorocide injections," by G. Maramarosi. THER HUNG. 14:11-15, 1966.

"Treatment of early and latent syphilis," by A. Steppert. THER GEGENW. 105:314-322, March, 1966.

"The treatment of early lues with oxytetracycline," by K. Bosse. HAUTARZT. 17:306-309, July, 1966.

"Treatment of early symptomatic syphilis with tetraverin 'Polfa'," by D. Janicka. PRZEGL DERM. Suppl:53-55, 1969.

"The treatment of early syphilis with cephaloridine," by O. A. Gonzalez, et al. POSTGRAD MED J. 43:Suppl: 43:134-135, August, 1967.

"The treatment of early syphilis with vibramycin. Preliminary communication," by P. Wodniansky, et al. Z HAUT GESCHLECHTSKR. 44:571-574, September 1, 1969.

"Treatment of female and male trichomoniasis with metronidazol," by W. Lapuszek. POL TYG LEK. 24;533-534, April, 1969.

"Treatment of genital trichomonas using a new drug: nitrimidazine," by M. A. Fonngera, et al. REV COLOMBIA OBSTET GINEC. 21:141-146, March-April, 1970.

"Treatment of gonococcal urethritis with single injections of 2-4 mega units of aqueous procaine penicillin," by G. D. Morrison, et al. BRIT J VENER DIS. 44:319-323, December, 1968.

"Treatment of gonococcia with Tetroid Lactic," by H. Thiers, et al. LYON MED. 222:1172-1173, December 14, 1969.

"Treatment of gonorrhoea." BRIT MED J. 1:398-399, February 17, 1968.

"Treatment of gonorrhea," by V. Kaupas. JAMA. 213:2272, September 28, 1970.

"Treatment of gonorrhea," by W. Minkin. JAMA. 208:535, April 21, 1969.

"Treatment of gonorrhea," by P. Muller, et al. THER UMSCH. 26:75-80, February, 1969.

"The treatment of gonorrhea and nongonorrheal urethral diseases," by H. Kresbach, et al. Z HAUT GESCHLECHT-SKR. 43:865-873, November 1, 1968.

"Treatment of gonorrhoea by one oral dose of ampicillin and probenecid combined," by T. Gundersen, et al. BRIT J VENER DIS. 45:235-237, September, 1969.

"Treatment of gonorrhoea by penicillin and a renal blocking agent (probenecid)," by G. Hatos. MED J AUST. 1:1096-1099, May 30, 1970.

"Treatment of gonorrhea by penicillin in a single large dose," by M. Minkin. MILIT MED. 133:382-386, May, 1968.

"Treatment of gonorrhea in males with cephaloridine," by J. B. Lucas, et al. JAMA. 195:919-921, March 14, 1966.

"The treatment of gonorrhoea in women with sulphamethoxazole-trimethoprim," by C. B. Schofield, et al. POSTGRAD MED J. 45:Suppl:81-86, November, 1969.

"Treatment of gonorrhoea patients with intolerance to penicillin," by G. Rajka. ACTA DERMATOVENER. 48: 532-536, 1968.

"Treatment of gonorrhoea today." BRIT MED J. 2:391-392, August 17, 1968.

"Treatment of gonorrhea with bicilein," by I. I. Shkliar. VESTN DERM VENER. 40:84-85, January, 1966.

"The treatment of gonorrhea with cephaloridine intramuscularly," by H. Pariser, et al. SOUTHERN MED J. 63: 384-386, April, 1970.

"Treatment of gonorrhoea with double doses of demethyl-chlortetracycline," by R. R. Willcox. ACTA DERMATOVENER. 49:103-105, 1969.

"The treatment of gonorrhoea with doxycycline as a single dose," by A. Lassus. CHEMOTHERAPY. 13:366-368, 1968.

"Treatment of gonorrhea with semisynthetic penicillin," by J. Kozerski. PRZEGL DERM. 55:551-555, July-September, 1968.

"The treatment of gonorrhea with a single high-dosed penicillin injection (so-called 'one-shot' treatment)," by F. Nemec. Z HAUT GESCHLECHTSKR. 44:507-512, 1969.

"Treatment of gonorrhoea with single oral doses of refampicin," by R. J. Cobbold, et al. BRIT MED J. 4:681-682, December 14, 1968.

"Treatment of gonorrhoea with trimethoprim-sulphamethoxazole in Uganda," by O. P. Arya, et al. BRIT J VENER DIS. 46:214-216, June, 1970.

"Treatment of gonorrheal urethritis evaluated in 230 men," by E. B. Berry. JAMA. 202:657-659, November 13, 1967.

"Treatment of infectious granulomas of the liver and infectious mononucleosis. Treatment of hepatic schistosomiasis, tuberculosis, syphilis and echinococcus cyst," by M. A. Spellberg. AMER J GASTROENT. 52:203-212, September, 1969.

"Treatment of latent syphilis with jasomycin," by R. Osako, et al. J JAP ASS INFECT DIS. 43:44-48, May, 1969.

"Treatment of male homosexuals in groups," by S. B. Hadden. INT J GROUP PSYCHOTHER. 16:13-22, January, 1966.

"Treatment of the neurosyphilitic psychoses," by K. Dewhurst. ACTA PSYCHIAT SCAND. 45:62-74, 1969.

"Treatment of ophthalmic syphilis, with special reference to cephaloridine therapy," by M. Mikuni, et al. OPHTHALMOLOGY. 12:724-731, September, 1970.

"Treatment of penicillin anaphylaxis with injection of the same antigen (penicillin) in high doses," by L. Katsilabors. REV MED MOYEN ORIENT. 24:346-348, July-August, 1967.

"Treatment of penicillin-resistant gonococcal conjunctivitis with ampicillin," by G. L. Spaeth. AMER J OPH-

THAL. 66:427-429, September, 1968.

"Treatment of 'penicillin-resistant' gonorrhea in military personnel in S.E. Asia: a cooperative evaluation of tetracycline and of penicillin plus probenecid in 1263 men," by K. K. Holmes, et al. MILIT MED. 133:642-646, August, 1968.

"Treatment of pregnant syphilitic as full protection against congenital syphilis," by T. Iwanowska, et al. PRZEGL DERM. 56:753-756, 1969.

"Treatment of recent syphilis in the adult," by W. M. Stewart. SEM THER. 41:156-158, March, 1965.

"Treatment of syphilis," by G. Garnier. MAROC MED. 45: 199-203, March, 1966.

"The treatment of syphilis," by D. H. Rasmussen. SURVEY OPHTHAL. 14:184-197, November, 1969.

"Treatment of syphilis," by E. Skog. NORD MED. 76:814-815, July 14, 1966.

"Treatment of syphilis," by T. H. Sternberg. WESTERN MED. Suppl:1:32-33, February, 1967.

"Treatment of syphilis," by V. A. Tomari. REV CORPS SANTE ARMEES. 7:533-553, August, 1966.

"The treatment of syphilis and gonorrhea," by E. J. Gillespie. MED ANN DC. 35:372-374, July, 1966.

"Treatment of syphilis in 1967," by G. Leclerc. UN MED CANADA. 96:833-836, July, 1967.

"Treatment of syphilis with antibiotics other than penicillin," by J. Towpik. POL TYG LEK. 25:1033-1036, July 13, 1970.

"Treatment of syphilis with demethyltetracycline (ledermycin)," by S. Nolting. MED KLIN. 61:2043-2044, December 23, 1966.

"Treatment of syphilitic patients with a single course of penicillin," by G. I. Egorov. VESTN DERM VENER. 40:68-71, May, 1966.

"Treatment of trichomonas colpitis," by G. Zwerenz. Z ALLGEMEINMED. 45:1590-1591, November 30, 1969.

"Treatment of trichomonas colpitis with thyadione," by E. Vartiainen, et al. DUODECIM. 82:755-757, 1966.

"Treatment of trichomonas infection," by W. Raab. THER GEGENW. 108:967-974, July, 1969.

"Treatment of trichomonas infection in males with metronidazole," by M. E. Babichenko. VESTN DERM VENER. 41:86, August, 1967.

"The treatment of trichomonas infestations with klion," by P. Salacz, et al. Z AERZTL FORTBILD. 60:805-808, July 1, 1966.

"Treatment of trichomonas vaginitis," by T. Okawa. SAN-FUJIN JISSAI. 19:623-631, June, 1970.

"Treatment of trichomonas vaginitis in the pregnant woman with metronidazole (8823 RP). Absence of teratogenic effects," by P. Magnin, et al. REV FRANC OBSTET. 61:861-867, December, 1966.

"Treatment of trichomonas vaginitis with nifuratel," by H. Gjonnaess, et al. ACTA OBSTET GYNEC SCAND. 48: 85-94, 1969.

"Treatment of trichomonas vaginitis with paromomycin," by M. Dumont, et al. GYNEC PRAT. 15:247-251, 1964.

"Treatment of trichomoniasis during puerperium," by R. Wawryk, et al. WIAD PARAZYT. 15:467-468, 1969.

"Treatment of trichomoniasis in men with antibiotics-sodium salt of usnic acid," by I. I. Shkliar. VESTN DERM VENER. 42:89-91, April, 1968.

"Treatment of trichomoniasis in women with flagyl," by J. Zawadzki, et al. PRZEGL LEK. 22:367-369, 1966.

"Treatment of trichomoniasis in women with macmiror," by A. Baron. WIAD PARAZYT. 15:379-380, 1969.

"Treatment of trichomoniasis of the urogenital organs with the 2nd fraction of ASD preparation," by E. P. Eganov, et al. VESTN DERM VENER. 44:71-73, January, 1970.

"Treatment of trichomoniasis with citral," by V. I. Danilin. SOVET MED. 31:139-140, May, 1968.

"Treatment of trichomoniasis with complications," by E.

Szule. THER HUNG. 14:30-33, 1966.

"Treatment of urethritis in males," by R. L. Dougherty, Jr. MED TIMES. 98:171-173, July, 1970.

"Treatment of urogenital trichomoniasis," by V. I. Zhukov. VESTN DERM VENER. 42:51-55, June, 1968.

"Treatment of urogenital trichomoniasis with flagyl," by L. Slucki. WIAD LEK. 19:855-858, June 1, 1966.

"Treatment of vaginal trichomoniasis using a new drug. Results using naxogin (K-1900)," by F. V. Rodrigues, et al. HOSPITAL. 77:417-424, February, 1970.

"Treatment of vaginal trichomoniasis with metronidazole flagyl in gel form. Preliminary results," by C. G. de Netto, et al. HOSPITAL. 70:447-449, August, 1966.

"Treatment of vaginal trichomonadosis with nifuratel," by H. Schmidt, et al. WIAD PARAZYT. 15:373-376, 1969.

"Treatment of vaginal trichomoniasis with nitrofurazone," by Z. Malachowski, et al. POL TYG LEK. 24:1823-1824, October 24, 1969.

"Treatment of venereal diseases in The Royal Navy," by F. E. Willmott. J ROY NAV MED SERV. 54:254-257, Winter, 1968.

"Treatment of venereal sarcoma in a bitch by vulvo-vagino-ovario-hysterectomy with perineal urethrostomy. (A case report)," by P. J. Philip. INDIAN VET J. 45: 874-877, October, 1968.

"Trends in the incidence and sociology of venereal diseases," by G. Wagner. THER UMSCH. 26:60-66, February, 1969.

"Treponema immobilization and immunofluorescence tests in the cerebrospinal fluid," by L. A. D'iachenko. VESTN DERM VENER. 43:48-53, July, 1969.

"The treponema immunofluorescence absorption test (FTA-ABS). Studies on the technic of quantitative absorption and its significance for the specificity," by G. Schierz, et al. Z HAUT GESCHLECHTSKR. 43:9-16, January 1, 1968.

"Treponema pallidum immobilization reaction with fresh

blood," by T. I. Milonova. VESTN DERM VENER. 44:56-58, April, 1970.

"The treponema pallidum immobilization test in oncological diseases," by S. G. Alieva, et al. LAB DELO. 8:484-487, 1966.

"The treponema pallidum immobilization test of cerebrospinal fluid in syphilis patients treated with various delayed-action penicillin preparations," by T. V. Vasil'ev, et al. VESTN DERM VENER. 41:40-45, March, 1967.

"Treponema reactions of syphilis," by K. Aho, et al. DUODECIM. 83:57-59, 1967.

"Treponemal and lipoidal tests in old treated syphilis, A clinical evaluation of 367 cases with special reference to the fluorescent treponemal antibody-absorption (FTA-ABS) test," by A. Lassus. ACTA DERMATOVENER. 48:Suppl:60:1-43, 1968.

"Treponemal antibodies in non-syphilitic, positive antinuclear factor sera," by T. R. Neblett, et al. J INVEST DERM. 46:84-90, January, 1966.

"Treponemal immobilization tests in leprosy," by H. G. Ruge. BRIT J VENER DIS. 43:191-196, September, 1967.

"Treponemal infection and arthritis," by C. J. Goodwill, et al. PROC ROY SOC MED. 62:198-199, February, 1969.

"Treponemal-like organisms in the aqueous of nonsyphilitic patients. An immunologic study," by B. Golden, et al. ARCH OPHTHAL. 80:727-731, December, 1968.

"Treponematosis and man's social evolution," by E. H. Hudson. AM ANTHROP. 67:835-901, August, 1965.

"--Reply," by J. B. Ford. AM ANTHROP. 68:1507-1508, December, 1966.

"Treponematosis in the eastern highlands of New Guinea," by M. F. Garner, et al. BULL WHO. 38:189-195, 1968.

"Treponematoses in Ethiopia," by K. F. Schaller. Z HAUT GESCHLECHTSKR. 43:17-28, January 1, 1968.

"Treponemes in aqueous humor in late seronegative syphilis," by J. L. Smith, et al. TRANS AMER ACAD OPHTHAL OTOLARYNG. 72:63-75, January-February, 1968.

"Trial of a terramycin foam for local usage in treatment of vaginitis of bacterial and parasitic (trichomonas) origin," by M. Levrier, et al. GYNEC PRAT. 18:381-389, 1967.

"Trial treatment of primo-secondary syphilis with intravenous perfusion of penicillin. Long persistence of seropositivity in favor of actual clinical penicillin resistance of treponema," by M. Bolgert, et al. BULL SOC FRANC DERM SYPH. 74:325-328, 1967.

"Trials of treatment of primary and secondary syphilis by intravenous perfusion of penicillin. Long persistence of a seroreactivity in view of the presence of clinical penicillin resistance of the treponeme," by M. Bolgert, et al. BULL SOC FRANC DERM SYPH. 74:325-328, 1967.

"Tric agent. Characteristics and detection by laboratory methods," by I. A. Harper. BRIT J VENER DIS. 42:71-76, June, 1966.

"Tric agent as a cause of neonatal eye sepsis," by P. G. Watson, et al. BRIT MED J. 3:527-528, August 31, 1968.

"The trichomonacidal action of flagyl," by G. A. Voskresenskaia. VESTN DERM VENER. 39:54-58, October, 1965.

"Trichomonads and other flagellates from the vaginal secretion," by E. Dyner. WIAD PARAZYT. 15:309, 1969.

"Trichomonal erosive-ulcerative balanoposthitis," by A. A. Avanesov. VESTN DERM VENER. 42:84-85, June, 1968.

"Trichomonal vaginitis: Epidemiology and therapy," by W. F. Peterson, et al. AMER J OBSTET GYNEC. 97:472-478, February 15, 1967.

"Trichomonas and candida albicans as a cause of conjugal sterility. Proposal of a new fundic test," by S. Gaffuri, et al. MINERVA GINEC. 20:1260-1268, July 31, 1968.

"Trichomonas and haematospermia," by H. C. Walton. BRIT MED J. 1:514, May 24, 1969.

"Trichomonas infection and its importance to the cytological smear diagnosis," by J. A. Ruiz-Moreno, et al. GEBURTSH FRAUENHEILK. 26:231-243, February, 1966.

"Trichomonas infection in an infant," by E. Grys, et al. PEDIAT POL. 41:969-971, August, 1966.

"Trichomonas infections in children," by A. Stolyhwo-Suchanek, et al. PEDIAT POL. 45:319-322, March, 1970.

"Trichomonas infections in the province of Verona, social implications of their diffusion," by L. Caldera, et al. FRACASTORO. 61:289-292, May-June, 1968.

"Trichomonas invasion and intraepithelial cancer of the cervix uteri," by R. M. Sokolovskii, et al. VOP ONKOL. 12:37-43, 1966.

"Trichomonas vaginalis. A pathogen of prostatis," by P. H. Van Laarhoven. ARCH CHIR NEERL. 19:263-273, 1967.

"Trichomonas vaginalis and accompanying microflora," by C. Zwierz. WIAD PARAZYT. 15:305-306, 1969.

"Trichomonas vaginalis and trichomoniasis," by O. Jirovec, et al. ADVANCES PARASIT. 6:117-188, 1968.

"Trichomonas vaginalis in general practice," by F. Bruhn-Petersen. UGESKR LAEG. 130:648-650, April 11, 1968.

"Trichomonas vaginalis in gram-stained smears," by G. E. Cree. BRIT J VENER DIS. 44:226-227, September, 1968.

"Trichomonas vaginalis infection in a newborn infant," by R. J. Blattner. J PEDIAT. 71:608-610, October, 1967.

"Trichomonas vaginalis: resistance to metronidazole," by A. W. Diddle. AMER J OBSTET GYNEC. 98:583-585, June 15, 1967.

"Trichomonas vaginalis, a review," by J. F. O'Sullivan. IRISH J MED SCI. 6:207-212, May, 1967.

"Trichomonas vaginalis: Urinary infection in a boy," by J. R. Harper. PROC ROY SOC MED. 60:897, September, 1967.

"Trichomonas vaginitis and accompanying microflora," by H. Walecki, et al. WIAD PARAZYT. 15:307-308, 1969.

"Trichomonas vaginitis and sex circles," by T. Morita, et al. J JAP OBSTET GYNEC SOC. 21:1417-1423,

December, 1969.

"Trichomonas vaginitis in young girls," by O. Jirovec, et al. GYNEC PRAT. 18:351-353, 1967.

"Trichomonas vaginitis, its treatment and colposcopic findings before and after treatment," by W. Konopada. POL TYG LEK. 22:2020-2021, December 25, 1967.

"Trichomoniasis and gonorrhea," by D. F. Hawkins. BRIT MED J. 2:116, April 12, 1969.

"Trichomoniasis and gonorrhoea," by W. Tsao. BRIT MED J. 1:642-643, March 8, 1969.

"Trichomoniasis - genitourinary disease and urological problem," by A. Drazancic. LIJECN VJESN. 91:1203-1207, 1970.

"Trichomoniasis in pregnant women and its treatment with RP 8823," by M. Glowinski, et al. GYNEC PRAT. 15:239-246, 1964.

"Trichomoniasis in women. A personal method of treatment," by A. Senra. HOSPITAL. 76:245-283, July, 1969.

"Trichomoniasis in women treated at the Ciechocinek Resort," by D. Kozlowska, et al. GINEK POL. 40:407-412, 1969.

"Trichomoniasis, sterility and abortion," by G. Carvalho, et al. VIRGINIA MED MONTHLY. 96:444-448, August, 1969.

"Trichomoniasis urogenitalis and metronidazol therapy in dermato-venerologic practice," by G. Elste. DERM WSCHR. 152:263-266, March 12, 1966.

"Trichopol in the treatment of trichomoniasis in women," by F. V. Potapnev, et al. AKUSH GINEK. 45:66-68, August, 1969.

"Trichopol in trichomoniasis infections," by F. V. Potapnev. VESTN DERM VENER. 42:55-60, June, 1968.

"Trimethoprim mixture," by D. J. Wright, et al. BRIT MED J. 1:637, March 8, 1969.

"Trimethoprim-sulphamethoxazole in the treatment of nongonococcal urethritis and gonorrhoea," by B. R. Carroll, et al. BRIT J VENER DIS. 46:31-33, February, 1970.

"Tropical gynaecology. Pelvic inflammatory disease," by R. R. Trussell. PROC ROY SOC MED. 61:365-368, April, 1968.

"Tropical gynaecology. Ulcerative and hypertrophic lesions of the vulva," by D. B. Stewart. PROC ROY SOC MED. 61:363-365, April, 1968.

"Tropical treponematoses," by K. F. Schaller. ARCH KLIN EXP DERM. 237:332-340, 1970.

"Truth can stop VD," by P. Deutsch, et al. READ DIGEST. 90:55-59, January, 1967.

"Tubal and cervical cultures in acute salpingitis with special reference to mycoplasma hominis and T-strain mycoplasmas," by P. A. Mardh, et al. BRIT J VENER DIS. 46:179-186, June, 1970.

"Tuberculosis-syphilis correlations. (Clinical and experimental study)," by P. Cornea, et al. MED INTERN. 20:1387-1398, November, 1968.

"Tuberous mucinosis in a syphilitic," by P. Franceschini, et al. BULL SOC FRANC DERM SYPH. 76:860-861, 1969.

"Tumoral form of syphilis of the cheek," by A. Tarel, et al. REV STOMATOODONT NORD FRANCE. 23:179-184, October-December, 1968.

"Twenty-five years of dermatovenereology in India. A review," by S. C. Desai. J ASSOC PHYSICIANS INDIA. 18:135-153, January, 1970.

"Twenty-five years of penicillin in the service of venereology," by R. R. Willcox. BRIT J CLIN PRACT. 21: 165-170, April, 1967.

"A 20 years persisting tubero serpiginous syphilis treated as psoriasis," by W. G. Roth. DERM WSCHR. 154: 459-463, May 18, 1968.

"2 cases of cerebral gummata," by A. Kunicki, et al. MEUROL MEUROCHIR POL. 4:251-254, March-April, 1970.

"2 cases of dissecting aneurysm of the aorta in syphilitic mesaortitis diagnosed during life," by S. G. Moiseev, et al. TER ARKH. 38:108-111, June, 1966.

"2 cases of nonspecific serologic reactions with high titers in patients with toxicodermia," by S. N. Dmitriev. VESTN DERM VENER. 43:85-86, September, 1969.

"2 cases of seronegativity in secondary syphilis," by M. F. Roitburd. VESTN DERM VENER. 42:82-83, August, 1968.

"2 cases of spinal disease due to tabes dorsalis," by K. Fuse, et al. ORTHOP SURG. 19:518-523, June, 1968.

"2 cases of syphilitic aortic aneurysm of a very prolonged development (15 and 30 years), 1 a juvenile form," by G. Plauchu, et al. LYON MED. 215:1575-1601, June 5, 1966.

"2 cases of tertiary syphilis diagnosed in dental field practice," by J. Bukový. CESK STOMAT. 68:297-301, July, 1968.

"2 cases of tertiary cutaneous syphilis in a 63-year-old man and in a 22-year-old man," by M. Bolgert, et al. BULL SOC FRANC DERM SYPH. 76:794-796, 1969.

"Two darkfield-positive reinfections in treated congenital syphilis," by B. Schwimmer, et al. JAMA. 208:1705, June 2, 1969.

"Two interesting case reports," by K. D. Lahiri. INDIAN J DERM. 15:31-32, October, 1969.

"Two observations of gummatous disease of the liver, diagnosed during surgery," by M. P. Serdiuk. KHIRURGIIA. 41:126-128, December, 1965.

"Typing the gonococcus (Letter to Ed.)," by R. I. Hutchinson. BRIT MED J. 3:107, July 11, 1970.

"A U.S. youngster is infected with VD every two minutes," by N. Keifetz. N Y TIMES MAG. p85+, March 9, 1969.

"Ultrafine structure of te cell elements in hard chancres of the rabbit and their interrelationship with treponema pallidum," by N. M. Ovcinnikov, et al. BULL WHO. 42:437-444, 1970.

"Unique course focuses on the VD interview," by L. Alexander. RN. 29:47-52, April, 1966.

"The unlabeled antibody enzyme method of immuno-histochemistry: Preparation and properties of soluble antigen-antibody complex (horseradish peroxidase-antihorseradish peroxidase) and its use in identification of spirochetes," by L. A. Sternberger, et al. J HISTOCHEM CYTOCHEM. 18:315-333, May, 1970.

"Unusual bullous dermatitis of the fingers and face in a newborn with very important monocytosis," by F. Gianotti. ANN DERM SYPH. 96:395-398, 1969.

"An unusual case of congenital syphilis," by P. M. Bakker. DERMATOLOGICA. 133:430-432, 1966.

"Unusual case of morbid association of parenchymatous keratitis, diffuse choroiditis and Jensen's chorioretinitis in a patient with syphilis," by E. Preste. ANN OTTAL. 92:539-547, July, 1966.

"Unusual case of nephrotic syndrome," by K. Fujita, et al. JAP J CLIN MED. 26:1220-1224, May, 1968.

"An unusual case of tabetic polyarthropathy," by A. Osti. MINERVA ORTOP. 19:637-643, November, 1968.

"Unusual complications of an aortic aneurysm of syphilitic origin," by E. Kodlová. VNITRNI LEK. 13:1015-1017, October, 1967.

"Unusual electrophoretic aspects of the blood of newborn infants with cytomegalic disease and congenital syphilis," by G. Turbessi, et al. MINERVA PEDIAT. 19:590-591, March 31, 1967.

"Unusual jaundice during primary syphilis," by J. Duverne, et al. BULL SOC FRANC DERM SYPH. 74:57-58, 1967.

"An unusual picture of congenital syphilitic dysproteinemia: cryoglobulinemia. Report of a case)," by A. G. Marchi, et al. MINERVA PEDIAT. 18:1155-1157, July 28, 1966.

"An unusual solitary lesion of secondary syphilis," by W. Minkin, et al. ARCH DERM. 95:217, February, 1967.

"Upgrading V.D. departments," by A. King. BRIT MED J. 3:46, July 4, 1970.

"Urethral stricture in African men in Dakar (clinical

and radiologic study)," by X. Serafino, et al. J UROL NEPHROL. 75:141-165, March, 1969.

"Urethritis in infection with germs of the Miamae group as a contribution to the differential diagnosis of gonorrhea," by U. Heyl, et al. HAUTARZT. 19:463-465, October, 1968.

"Uridine nucleotide synthesis in cells infected by the agent of benign inguinal lymphogranulomatosis," by G. A. Galegov, et al. VOP MED KHIM. 15:201-203, March-April, 1969.

"Urinary tract infection by trichomonas vaginalis in a newborn baby," by J. M. Littlewood, et al. ARCH DIS CHILD. 41:693-695, December, 1966.

"'Urinary tract infection' in women caused by gonococci," by V. Starck. LAKARTIDNINGEN. 67:3206-3210, July 8, 1970.

"Urogenital trichomoniasis in the daily consultation of the dermato-venereologist," by A. Kraus. DERM WSCHR. 152:97-103, June 29, 1966.

"Urogenital trichomoniasis in dermatologic practice," by H. Walther. DERM MSCHR. 155:988-989, 1969.

"Usability of Boroviczeny's rapid hematological staining method for routine protozoological diagnosis," by W. Granz, et al. Z TROPENMED PARASITOL. 21:261-266, September, 1970.

"Use of the Auto-Analyzer to perform serological tests for syphilis. Study of 1,009 sera using a complement fixation test with the cardiolipidic antigen," by R. Gaillon, et al. INT ARCH ALLERG. 32:278-281, 1967.

"Use of the automatic kinetic technic of complement fixation in the problems of syphilis serology," by R. Vargues, et al. ANN DERM SYPH. 94:265-272, 1967.

"Use of behavioral research in venereal disease control," by W. J. Brown, et al. PUBLIC HEALTH REP. 83:583-586, July, 1968.

"Use of doxycycline in the treatment of syphilis," by L. H. Paschoal, et al. HOSPITAL. 75:1965-1967, June, 1969.

"Use of the F.T.A. test as a method of mass screening,"

by S. Sartoris, et al. MINERVA DERM. 43:18-22, January, 1968.

"Use of hetacillin in urogenital infections," by L. H. Rodriguez Diaz, et al. REV VENEZ UROL. 19:163-180, January-June, 1967.

"Use of immunofluorescent antibody technic in the diagnosis of bacterial and viral diseases," by B. Babudieri. G MAL INFETT. 20:35-49, January, 1968.

"Use of methacycline in blennorrhagic infection," by E. Ferrea, et al. MINERVA DERM. 43:285-287, June, 1968.

"Use of metronidazole in trichomonas vaginitis," by R. J. Moreno. REV OBSTET GINEC VENEZ. 28:275-290, 1968.

"Use of metronidazole in vaginal trichomoniasis," by R. J. Moreno. REV OBSTET GINEC VENEZ. 29:275-290, 1968.

"Use of Nelson's test in the diagnosis of specific diseases of the cornea," by F. Beauchamp, et al. MED TROP. 27:679-681, November-December, 1967.

"The use of a new drug (deflamon) in the treatment of vaginal trichomoniasis," by A. Segre. MINERVA GINEC. 20:52-59, January 15, 1968.

"Use of the plate micromethod for performance of the Bordet-Wassermann test with blood serum obtained from the finger-tip," by A. Garlacz. PRZEGL DERM. 56:773-777, 1969.

"Use of plate micromethod for studies in Bordet-Wassermann Test," by A. Garlacz. PRZEGL DERM. 56:51-55, January-February, 1969.

"The use of pyrogenal in the treatment of late forms of syphilis," by A. K. Shcherbakova. VESTN DERM VENER. 41:43-47, June, 1967.

"Use of a single dose of doxycycline monohydrate for treating gonorrheal urethritis in men," by G. Domescik, et al. PUBLIC HEALTH REP. 84:182-183, February, 1969.

"Use of slide technics in the mass screening for Bordet-Wasserman test," by A. Garlacz. PRZEGL DERM. 54:483-487, July-August, 1967.

"Use of testing and teaching devices at the Department

of Dermatology and Venereal Diseases," by I. I. Il'in. VESTN DERM VENER. 43:49-53, February, 1969.

"The use of urotropin for artificial activation of trichomonas infection in men," by V. I. Zhukov. VESTN DERM VENER. 40:45-52, August, 1966.

"Use of vancomycin, colistimethate, nystatin medium to transport gonococcal specimens," by M. H. Robinson, et al. PUBLIC HEALTH REP. 85:390-392, May, 1970.

"Use of the venereal disease clinic of San Mateo County, California," by D. L. White, et al. PUBLIC HEALTH REP. 83:954-956, November, 1968.

"Usefulness of the addition of an antimycotic agent in the culture medium for trichomonas vaginalis," by D. Patrono, et al. NUOVI ANN IG MICROBIOL. 19:361-363, September-October, 1968.

"Usefulness of the fluorescent antibody method for the demonstration of gonococci in routine work," by K. L. Wendland, et al. ARCH HYG BAKT. 151:118-123, May, 1967.

"Usefulness of the hemagglutination test using treponema pallidum antigen (TPHA) for the serodiagnosis of syphilis," by T. Tomizawa, et al. JAP J MED SCI BIOL. 22:341-350, December, 1969.

"The usefulness of the isotope labelled lymphocyte-stimulation test in the diagnosis of syphilis," by N. Simon, et al. ARCH KLIN EXP DERM. 236:1-7, 1969.

"Usefulness of long-acting penicillin in combination with short-acting preparations for treatment of gonorrhea," by E. Fowinkle, et al. J TENN MED ASS. 59:1115-1118, November, 1966.

"The usefulness of a modification of the fluorescent complement fixation test in syphilis diagnosis," by W. Zajac, et al. DERM MSCHR. 155:531-534, 1969.

"The utility of Reiter's complement fixation test in the prognosis of treated syphilis," by J. Lochmannová, et al. DERMATOLOGICA. 139:115-122, 1969.

"Uveitis and intraocular treponemes," by R. Whitfield, et al. ARCH OPHTHAL. 84:12-15, July, 1970.

"Uveitis as a presenting sign of acquired syphilis. Report of three cases," by D. H. Pendergrast. J NAT MED ASS. 59:41-42, January, 1967.

"VD and the teenager," by A. Stitt. EMERGENCY MED. 1:60+, October, 1969.

"VD and vision." J MED SOC NEW JERSEY. 66:266, June, 1969.

"'V.D.' as a diagnosis." BRIT MED J. 3:630-631, September 14, 1968.

"VD clinic," by D. Bashforth. DIST NURS. 8:285-286, February, 1966.

"VD clinic, James Pringle house, the Middlesex hospital," by H. Elliott, et al. NURS TIMES. 64:827-828, June 21, 1968.

"VD: consent for care," by D. A. Dukelow. TODAYS HEALTH. 47:88, February, 1969.

"VD detectives; doctors and nurses in Boston." TIME. 90:32, September 1, 1967.

"V.D. a disease with a sorry stigma." J W AUST NURSES. 35:20+, August, 1969.

"VD: the greatest threat to teen-age health," by A. Lake. SEVENTEEN. 28:146-147+, May, 1969.

"VD in D.C. health department notes," by M. Grant. MED ANN DC. 35:388-389, July, 1966.

"VD in Vietnam," by R. S. Cooperman. NEW ENG J MED. 283:546, September 3, 1970.

"VD is more than a dirty word," by F. Field. FAMILY HLTH. 2:43+, June, 1970.

"VD is on the increase--social aspects." NEW ZEALAND NURS J. 61:12+, April, 1968.

"VD: a major health problem," by S. D. Furst, Jr. PARENTS MAG. 42:104, November, 1967.

"VD menace alarming," by P. McBroom. SCI N. 90:402,

November 12, 1966.

"VD, a military-civilian problem," by W. J. Brown. MILIT MED. 132:316-317, April, 1967.

"VD must be reported," by M. I. Shanholtz. VIRGINIA MED MONTHLY. 94:188-190, March, 1967.

"VD: a national problem that can no longer be ignored." SR SCHOL. 88:11-14, February 25, 1966.

"VD on the increase: gonorrhea cases climb as promiscuity rises and drugs lose effect," by R. R. Leger. WALL ST J. 171:1+, June 18, 1968.

"VD--protect children against venereal disease," by F. H. Richardson. LIFE AND HLTH. 83:18+, August, 1968.

"V.D., the unconquered menace," by S. Golub. RN. 33:38+, March, 1970.

"VD: wages of ignorance; excerpt from address," by W. F. Schwartz. PTA MAG. 61:14-17, September, 1966.

"VDRL reaction after vaccination against smallpox," by S. Smalik, et al. VNITRNI LEK. 12:152-155, February, 1966.

"The V.D.R.L. test. Significance of 'rough' results," by M. F. Garner, et al. BRIT J VENER DIS. 42:131-133, June, 1968.

"VDRL test in normal albino and pigmented rabbits," by B. M. Levine, et al. BRIT J VENER DIS. 45:197-199, September, 1969.

"VDRL tests in representative communities of Guyanese adults," by M. T. Ashcroft, et al. BRIT J VENER DIS 45:140-143, June, 1969.

"Vaginal corynebacteria with distinctive properties," by B. Brzin. ZBL BAKT. 210:202-206, June, 1969.

"Vaginal discharge in puberty. A survey of 1000 adolescents," by J. Orley, et al. GYNAECOLOGIA. 168:191-202, 1969.

"Vaginal diseases," by W. R. Lang. J AMER COLL HEALTH ASS. 15:Suppl:22-25, May, 1967.

"Vaginal implantation of flagellates of trichomonas

strains from the intestine and the effects on these flagellates to adapt," by P. Georges, et al. ANN PARASIT HUM COMP. 43:121-130, March-April, 1968.

"Vaginal trichomonas infections and sensitization of small laboratory animals," by A. Westphal, et al. Z TROPENMED PARASIT. 20:60-66, March, 1969.

"Vaginal trichomoniasis and cervix uteri changes," by A. Drazancic, et al. GEBURTSH FRAUENHEILK. 29:914-919, October, 1969.

"Vaginal trichomoniasis and lesions of cervical epithelium," by E. Guerresi. RIV ITAL GINEC. 52:819-837, December, 1968.

"Vaginal trichomoniasis as a cause of false cytologic positivity," by G. C. Tosolini, et al. FRIULI MED. 23:807-817, November-December, 1968.

"Vaginitis: diagnosis and treatment," by R. E. Burmeister, et al. POSTGRAD MED, Minneapolis. 48:159-163, August, 1970.

"Vaginitis in general practice," by J. H. Kelley. J MED ASS GEORGIA. 57:339-341, July, 1968.

"Vaginostic diagnostic kit." MED LETT DRUGS THER. 10:19-20, March 8, 1968.

"Value and possibility of long-lasting penicillin therapy in early syphilis," by A. Kern. PRZEGL DERM. 54:95-101, January-February, 1967.

"Value and security of a weekly injection interval in dispensing doses of 1.8 mega units of benzathine penicillin (penduran-AWD) during long-term therapy of early syphilis," by A. Kern. DERM WSCHR. 154:608-616, June 29, 1968.

"Value of the cardiolipin antigen prepared by the Institute 'Dr. I. Cantacuzino' for the flocculation microreaction of VDRL type," by M. Soresco, et al. ARCH ROUM PATH EXP MICROBIOL. 26:573-578, September, 1967.

"The value of the fluorescent treponemal antibody inhibition test for the diagnosis of syphilis," by J. Ruczkowska, et al. POL MED J. 8:497-508, 1969.

"Value of the fluorescent treponemal antibody inhibition

test for the diagnosis of syphilitic infection," by J. Ruczkowska, et al. PRZEGL DERM. 55:287-298, May-June, 1968.

"The value of the immunofluorescence reaction in the control of syphilis cures. Reproducibility of the FTA test in dubious cases," by G. Leigheb, et al. MINERVA DERM. 42:261-263, July, 1967.

"Value of the immunofluorescent reaction after absorption of sera by Reiter's treponeme for serodiagnosis of syphilis," by A. Betz. BULL WHO. 34:154-160, 1966,

"Value of the intradermal test and scarification test in the determination of penicillin sensitivity," by A. R. Tuszkiewicz, et al. POL TYG LEK. 22:1197-1199, August 7, 1967.

"Value of medical diagnostic screening tests for dental patients," by W. R. Sabes, et al. J AMER DENT ASS. 80:133-136, January, 1970.

"The value of penicilloyl-polylysine (PPL) in the detection of penicillin allergy in man," by H. Prochacki, et al. PRZEGL DERM. 57:325-329, May-June, 1970.

"Value of positive serologic reactions in systematic examinations of Africans," by H. Van Wymeersch, et al. PRESSE MED. 76:1774, October 5, 1968.

"Value of re-interviewing in contact tracing," by T. Z. Capiński, et al. BRIT J VENER DIS. 46:138-140, April, 1970.

"The value of routine serological testing for syphilis in a mental hospital," by G. D. Banks. BRIT J PSYCHIAT. 114:113-114, January, 1968.

"Value of serology for the clinician," by J. Orfila. MAROC MED. 45:204-210, March, 1966.

"The value of the Shelley test in complications to intolerance of antibiotics," by G. Despierres, et al. J MED LYON. 48:1097-1104, July 5, 1967.

"The value of the treponema pallidum immobilization test (T.P.I.) in anomalous syphilis serology," by M. F. Garner, et al. MED J AUST. 2:1101-1103, December 3, 1966.

"The value of treponemic agglutination test (TAT)," by

A. Galliera. FRIULI MED. 23:1-91, January-February, 1968.

"Various experimemtal studies on the behavior of 3 strains of treponema pallidum (Nichols strain, cortisone treated Nichols strain and Gand strain)," by P. Collart, et al. ANN DERM SYPH. 95:59-68, 1968.

"Various stages of syphilis and its diagnosis," by T. Tomizawa. JAP J NURS ART. 8:97-104, August, 1969.

"Various therapeutic aspects of bacterial, mycotic and protozoan cervico-vaginitis," by G. Candela, et al. MINERVA GINEC. 20:1626-1629, October 31, 1968.

"Vascular erythematous reaction by administration of vitamin PP (nicotinic acid). Demonstration of a pre and post-clinical luetic roseola," by E. Ionescu. DERM WSCHR. 152:184-187, February 19, 1966.

"Vascular involvement in congenital syphilis--an autopsied case with aortic arch syndrome and coarctation of the aorta," by S. Kimata, et al. NAIKA. 22:1431-1436, December, 1968.

"Vascular manifestations in some forms of neurosyphilis," by V. F. Aliferova. VRACH DELO. 6:131-132, June, 1966.

"Venereal disease." LANCET. 2:250-251, August 1, 1970.

"Venereal disease," by T. H. Bierre. OCCUP HEALTH. 4:3-4, December, 1970.

"Venereal disease," by N. J. Fiumara. PEDIAT CLIN N AMER. 16:333-345, May, 1969.

"Venereal disease," by J. Jefferiss. LANCET. 2:673, September 26, 1970.

"Venereal disease," by Z. Sternadel. PIELEG POLOZ. 9:9-10, September, 1969+.

"Venereal disease," by L. Watt. LANCET. 2:364, August 15, 1970.

"Venereal disease among seafarers on board of Polish ships," by S. Tomaszunas. BULL INST MAR MED GDANSK. 18:67-72, 1967.

"Venereal disease and treponematosis in African countries,"

by A. P. Shchepin. VESTN DERM VENER. 42:71-75, June, 1968.

"Venereal disease and the young woman. Part 1," by J. L. Fluker. NM. 121:633+, March 4, 1966.

--Part 2. NM. 121:663+, March 11, 1966.

"Venereal disease books available in schools." SCI N L. 89:56, January 22, 1966.

"Venereal disease control," by W. J. Brown. BOL OFIC SANIT PANAMER. 68:288-296, April, 1970.

"Venereal disease control in Australia," by G. S. Hayes. MED J AUST. 1:1151-1152, May 31, 1969.

"Venereal disease control in the 2nd Marine Division, Camp Lejeune, North Carolina," by P. C. White, Jr., et al. MILIT MED. 132:252-257, April, 1967.

"Venereal disease education in schools of the state of New Jersey," by W. E. Ferinden, Jr. J SCH HEALTH. 38:611-614, November, 1968.

"Venereal disease in adolescence," by J. A. Knowles. MED ARTS SCI. 22:45-48, 1968.

"Venereal disease in an Australian metropolis," by A. Adams. MED J AUST. 1:145-151, January 28, 1967.

"Venereal disease in an elite group (university students) in east Africa," by O. P. Arya, et al. BRIT J VENER DIS. 43:275-279, December, 1967.

"Venereal disease in New Zealand," by W. M. Platts. BRIT J VENER DIS. 45:61-66, March, 1969.

"Venereal disease in public health practice today," by O. Ravenholt. ARCH ENVIRON HEALTH, Chicago. 13:397-398, September, 1966.

"The venereal disease problem facing the private physician and his patient," by A. N. Johnson. ARCH ENVIRON HEALTH, Chicago. 13:393-396, September, 1966.

"The venereal disease problem in schools, rural areas, and among juveniles," by J. L. Logan. ARCH ENVIRON HEALTH, Chicago. 13:385-387, September, 1966.

"Venereal disease problems and adolescent health," by

A. King. CLIN PEDIAT. 5:597-603, October, 1966.

"Venereal disease program." J ARKANSAS MED SOC. 67:75-76, July, 1970.

"Venereal disease rates and student attitudes," by I. E. Robinson, et al. J MED ASS GEORGIA. 56:298-299, July, 1967.

"Venereal disease; society's stigma," by M. Kamp. AM COUNTY GOVT. 32:44-45+, May, 1967.

"Venereal disease: this hazard to public health could be eliminated; instead, it grows worse." CONSUMER REPTS. 35:118-123, February, 1970.

"Venereal disease today," by H. Shryock. LIFE AND HLTH. 83:16+, July, 1968.

"Venereal disease today," by J. R. Spencer. LIFE AND HLTH. 85:18+, October, 1970.

"Venereal disease: the unmentionable menace," SR SCHOL. 90:10-11, May 12, 1967.

"Venereal diseases." LYON MED. 223:287-317, February 1, 1970.

"Venereal diseases." MONTHLY BULL MINIST HEALTH. 25:170, August, 1966.

"Venereal diseases." MONTHLY BULL MINIST HEALTH. 26:31, February, 1967.

"Venereal diseases." NEW ZEAL MED J. 69:234-235, April, 1969.

"Venereal diseases." WORLD HLTH. 22:26. June, 1969.

"The venereal diseases," by J. L. Breen. J AMER COLL HEALTH ASS. 15:Suppl:26-34, May, 1967.

"Venereal diseases," by P. J. De Amorim. HOSPITAL. 70:1739-1745, December, 1966.

"Venereal diseases. Extract from the Annual Report of the Chief Medical Officer for the Department of Health and Social Security for the year 1968." BRIT J VENER DIS. 46:76-83, February, 1970.

"Venereal diseases. Introduction," by S. Hellerstrom.

NORD MED. 76:797-799, July 14, 1966.

"Venereal diseases. Social aspects," by M. Tottie. NORD MED. 76:817-818, July 14, 1966.

"Venereal diseases among adolescents in the agrarian district Neubrandenburg sociological study," by G. G. Bartschies, et al. DEUTSCH GESUNDH. 25:455-460, March 13, 1970.

"Venereal diseases and homosexuality (considerations apropos of 2 cases recorded in minors," by A. Serena. ARCH ITAL DERM VENER. 34:159-168, 1966.

"Venereal diseases and their significance in obstetrics," by K. Grabner. OEST HEBAMMENZEITUNG. 15:13-14 passim, February, 1968.

"Venereal diseases are reappearing," by C. D. Carrillo. ACTAS DERMOSIF. 59:487-489, July-August, 1968.

"Venereal diseases campaign," by W. J. Brown. BOL OFIC SANIT PANAMER. 68:288-296, April, 1970.

"Venereal diseases educational project," by E. M. Andrews. HUTT HEALTH DISTRICT. September, 1967; also in OCCUP HEALTH NURSE. 1:11, December, 1967.

"Venereal diseases--environmental changes," by T. Guthe, et al. T NORSK LAEGEFOREN. 89:1784-1789 passim, December 1, 1969.

"Venereal diseases in adolescents," by P. Baribeau. INFIRM CANAD. 11:17-21, July, 1969.

"Venereal diseases in Dresden 1946 to 1965," by H. Roder. DEUTSCH GESUNDH. 22:313-317, February 16, 1967.

"Venereal diseases in England and Wales. Extract from the Annual Report of the Chief Medical Officer for the year 1964." BRIT J VENER DIS. 42:50-57, March, 1966.

--Extract from the annual report of the Chief Medical Officer for the year 1966." BRIT J VENER DIS. 44:83-91, March, 1968.

--Extract from the annual report of the Chief Medical Officer for the year 1967." BRIT J VENER DIS. 45:67-75, March, 1969.

"Venereal diseases in Finland," by A. Lassus. SAIRAAN-HOITAJA. 45:520-521, August 11, 1969.

"Venereal diseases in N.Z." NEW ZEALAND NURS J. 61:20+, November, 1968.

"Venereal diseases in Vojvodina," by S. Cvejić, et al. MED PREGL. 22:229-241, 1969.

"Venereal diseases in women," by K. S. Krishna. INDIAN PRACT. 19:173-176, February, 1966.

"Venereal diseases to date," by E. Mach. DEUTSCH ZBL KRANKENPFI. 12:624-626, November, 1968.

"Venereal infection in the elderly," by M. U. Krishnan, et al. GERONT CLIN. 12:76-79, 1970.

"Venereal infection in elderly people," by A. M. Mechie, et al. GERONT CLIN. 8:207-214, 1966.

"Venereal infection in old age: an autopsy study," by A. M. Mechie, et al. GERIATRICS. 22:176-179, September, 1967.

"The venereal nature of inclusion conjunctivitis," by J. Schachter, et al. AMER J EPIDEM. 85:445-452, May, 1967.

"The venereological scene," by A. S. Grimble. BRIT J CLIN PRACT. 22:243-247, June 6, 1968.

"Venereology and the sexually transmitted diseases in Denmark, Sweden and Holland. Part 1," by N. O. J. Hallis. NT. 66:105, July 23, 1970.

--Part 2. NT. 66:109+, July 30, 1970.

"Venereology in midwifery. Part 1," by E. Gourlay. NT. 62:242+, February 25, 1966.

--Part 2. NT. 62:298+, March 4, 1966.

"Venereology ought to be a subspecialty," by M. Skogh. LAKARTIDNINGEN. 65:1296-1297, March 27, 1968.

"Venereology today. Part 1," by W. V. Macfarlane. NM. 124:229+, June 9, 1967.

--Part 2. NM. 124:261+, June 16, 1967.

"Vertebro-basilar arterial insufficiency (subclavian steal syndrome) (6 cases)," by J. Caron, et al. J RADIOL ELECTR. 49:157-162, January-February, 1968.

"Very grave pustular psoriasis probably caused by penicillin. Presentation of 6 fatal cases observed in black Africa," by Y. Privat, et al. BULL SOC FRANC DERM.SYPH. 76:505-509, 1969.

"Preventive medicine orientation," by D. N. Gilbert, et al. MILIT MED. 132:769-790, October, 1967.

"Viewpoints on the clinical aspects and therapy of venereal diseases," by J. Soltz-Szots. WIEN KLIN WSCHR. 77:1001-1003, December 24, 1965.

"Violent Herxheimer-Lukasiewicz reaction in the course of congenital syphilis," by A. Garlicka, et al. WIAD LEK. 21:1261-1264, July 15, 1968.

"Viral and virus-like infections of the female genital tract," by W. E. Josey, et al. CLIN OBSTET GYNEC. 12:161-178, March, 1969.

"Viral urethritis of a venereal origin," by I. I. Il'in. UROL NEFROL. 35:41-44, May-June, 1970.

"Virulence of gonococci," by D. S. Kellogg, Jr, et al. ANN REV MED. 20:323-328, 1969.

"Virus diseases of the external female genitalia. 1. Herpes (simplex) genitalis (Herpes progenitalis, herpes venereus, vulvitis or vulvovaginitis herpetica)," by H. Grimmer. Z HAUT GESCHLECHTSKR. 45:23-28, March 1, 1970.

"Visceral syphilis based on the data of the Moscow District Scientific-Research Institute," by A. R. Zlatkina. VESTN DERM VENER. 40:27-31, December, 1966.

"Visit to a clinic: Northwest Washington, D.C. venereal disease clinic," by D. Sanford. NEW REPUB. 159:12-13, December 7, 1968.

"The vitamin C concentration in the cervical mucus in women with and without trichomonas vaginitis," by B. Hoffmann, et al. GINEK POL. 40:773-778, July, 1969.

"Vladimir Nikolaevich Dobronravov," VESTN DERM VENER. 41:90, June, 1967.

"Vulvitis and vaginitis," by E. Landes. MED WELT. 27: 1450-1453, July 2, 1966.

"Vulvovaginitis in the premenarcheal child," by R. H. Heller, et al. J PEDIAT. 74:370-377, March, 1969.

"WHO meeting on Neisseria research." MED SERV J CANADA. 22:298-302, April, 1966.

"Wassermann". BRIT MED J. 5485:436-437, February 19, 1966.

"We who treat but don't report are responsible for the rising venereal disease incidence. Editorial," by A. C. Curtis. UNIV MICH MED CENT J. 32:215-216, September-October, 1966.

"What does the Nelson test tell us," by G. Ehrmann. WEIN KLIN WSCHR. 78:6-10, January 7, 1966.

"What information may and may not be provided by the Nelson test?," by J. Langer, et al. CESK DERM. 41:31-32, February, 1966.

"What is the significance of a positive Wasserman or VDRL?," by D. G. Walker. J ORAL SURG. 27:748, September, 1969.

"What our kids don't know about health," by T. Irwin. TODAY'S HLTH. 44:19+, May, 1966.

"What would be the cost to a country of an inadequate syphilis control program?," by A. E. Callin. SALUD PUBLICA MEX. 10:611-614, September-October, 1968.

"What you should know about VD-and why," by B. Webster. SR SCHOL. 91:Suppl:27, November 30, 1967.

"What's new in venereal disease?," by V. G. Cave. RHODE ISLAND MED J. 52:519-522, September, 1969.

"Which diagnosis would you make?." MED KLIN. 64:2311 passim, December 5, 1969.

"Who discovered the causative agent of syphilis? (Fritz Schaudinn)," by J. Kenéz. ORV HETIL. 107:1477-1480, July 31, 1966.

"Who ought to take care of the gonorrhea cases?," by H. Moller. LAKARTIDNINGEN. 65:2628-2629, June 5, 1968.

"Why prophylaxis for ophthalmia neonatorum?," by R. H. Dennis. J MAINE MED ASS. 57:27-28, February, 1966.

"Why South Carolina's high VD rate," by R. W. Ball. J S CAROLINA MED ASS. 62:175-176, April, 1966.

"Why sulphonamides when combined with 2-4-diamino-pyrimidines, are effective in sulphonamide-resistant gonorrhoea," by D. J. Wright. GUY HOSP REP. 118:287-291, 1969.

"Work disability due to dermatologic and venereal diseases in Czechoslovakia during 1955-1964," by J. Stach. CESK DERM. 41:343-349, October, 1966.

"Work experience of a dermatologist--venereologist in a screening room," by G. I. Filatov. VESTN DERM VENER. 43:57-59, January, 1969.

"The work of a screening nurse in venerology," by F. Novotny. CESK DERM. 41:84-91, April, 1966.

"Work on mycoplasma at the Rackham Arthritis Research Unit," by L. E. Bartholomew. UNIV MICH MED CENT J. 229:30, 1968.

"The x-ray picture of bone changes in yaws," by K. Chmel. CESK RADIOL. 21:185-192, May, 1967.

"Yaws--incidence and epidemiology (study in Dudhi Tehsil of district Mirzapur, Uttar Pradesh, India)," by B. L. Taneja. J TROP MED HYG. 70:215-223, September, 1967.

"You and VD. (Editorial)," by C. B. Kanterman. DENT STUD MAG. 44:379-380, February, 1966.

"Young should know more about V.D.," by M. Binyon. TIMES ED SUPPL. 2792:1154, November 22, 1968.

"Zosteriform late cutaneous syphilide," by C. Kodanda-pani. BRIT MED J. 1:685, March 16, 1968.

SUBJECT INDEX

ACD PREPARATIONS
"Comparative assessment of the treatment of trichomonad urethritis in males with iodinol and ACD preparations," by L. M. Korik, et al. VESTN DERM VENER. 40:62-65, March, 1966.

ACTH
"ACTH as a prophylactic against the Jarisch-Herxheimer reaction," by E. Sylvester. Z HAUT GESCHLECHTSKR. 44:125-126, February 15, 1969.

ACETAZOLAMIDE
"Inhibition by acetazolamide of the growth of Neisseriae at increasing environmental concentration of CO_2," by A. Forkman. ACTA PATH MICROBIOL SCAND. 73:298-302, 1968.

ADOLESCENTS & VENEREAL DISEASE
SEE: YOUTH

ADOPTION
"Tests for syphilis in children for adoption," by C. E. Cooper. LANCET. 2:261, August, 1970.

"Tests for syphilis in children for adoption," by O. P. Gray. LANCET. 2:673, September, 1970.

ALBOTHYL
"Effect of albothyl in trichomonas vaginalis infection on the changes in vaginal environment," by J. Fidler, et al. WIAD PARAZYT. 15:453-454, 1969.

ALLERGY
SEE: REACTIONS

ALPACHLOROMETHYL-2-METHLY-5-NITRO-1-IMIDAZOLE ETHANOL
"Alpha-chloromethyl 2-methyl-5-nitro-1-imidazole (RO 7-2-7), a substance exhibiting antiparasitic activity against amoebae, trichomonads, and pinworms," by E. Grunberg, et al. PROC SOC EXP BIOL MED. 133:490-492, February, 1970.

AMPHOTERICIN B
"Prevention of post-metronidazole candidosis with ampho-

AMPHOTERICIN B

tericin B pessaries," by L. Z. Oller. BRIT J VENER DIS. 45:163-166, June, 1969.

AMPICILLIN

"Agranulocytosis with monohistiocytosis associated with ampicillin therapy," by M. Graf, et al. ANN INTERN MED. 69:91-95, July, 1968.

"Ampicillin in the treatment of gonorrhoea," by A. Finger. MED J AUST. 2:250-251, August 1, 1970.

"Ampicillin in the treatment of granuloma inguinale," by M. A. Thew, et al. JAMA. 210:866-867, November 3, 1969.

"Ampicillin in the treatment of penicillin-resistant gonorrhea," by E. B. Smith. MILIT MED. 131:345-347, April, 1966.

"Clinical experience with ampicillin and probenecid in the management of treponeme-associated uveitis," by J. N. Goldman. TRANS AMER ADAD OPHTHAL OTOLARYNG. 74:509-514, May-June, 1970.

"Comparative study of the therapeutic effect of a single dose of hetacillin and ampicillin in gonococcal urethritis," by D. C. Rodriguez, et al. REV VENEZ UROL. 21:143-151, January-June, 1969; also in HOSPITAL. 75:979-986, March, 1969.

"Experiences with the use of sodium ampicillin in acute gonococcal infections in Vietnam," by R. G. Kercull. MILIT MED. 133:985-986, December, 1968.

"Gonorrheal urethritis in males treated with one oral dose of ampicillin," by D. G. McLone, et al. SOUTHERN MED J. 61:278-280, March, 1968.

"High dosage procaine penicillin combined with ampicillin in the treatment of gonorrhoea after failure with standard procaine penicillin dosage," by J. L. Fluker, et al. BRIT J VENER DIS. 45:317-320, December, 1969.

"Oral administration of a single dosage of ampicillin K in the treatment of gonorrhea," by J. M. de Barros, et al. REV SAUDE PUBLICA. 4:31-34, June, 1970.

"Oral ampicillin in gonorrhoea. Clinical evaluation,"

AMPICILLIN

by O. Groth, et al. BRIT J VENER DIS. 46:21-26, February, 1970.

"Purification of ampicillin," by G. T. Stewart, et al. BRIT MED J. 1:295, May 2, 1970.

"Treatment of gonorrhoea by one oral dose of ampicillin and probenecid combined," by T. Gundersen, et al. BRIT J VENER DIS. 45:235-237, September, 1969.

ANO-RECTAL
"Anorectal venereal diseases," by J. Lentini. REV ESP ENFERM APAR DIG. 30:339-355, February 1, 1970.

"Epidemiological and statistical survey: ano-rectal localizations of venereal diseases," by J. Vilotte. ARCH FRANC MAL APPAR DIG. 59:Suppl:7-8, 3-8, July-August, 1970.

ANTIMICROBIAL TREATMENT
"Antimicrobial poly-peptide synthesized by mucor pusillus NRRL 2543," by G. A. Somkuti, et al. PROC SOC EXP BIOL MED. 133:780-785, March, 1970.

"Antimicrobial therapy in patients allergic to penicillin," by P. A. Bunn. NEW YORK J MED. 69:1859-1865, July 1, 1969.

"Cefazolin, a new semisynthetic cephalosporin antibiotic. II. In vitro and in vivo antimicrobial activity," by M. Nishida, et al. J ANTIBIOT. 23:137-148, March, 1970.

AORTITIS
SEE: Syphilis, Cardiovascular

ARSENOBENZENE
"Erythroplasia of queyrat as a consequence of arsenobenzene therapy," by F. Novotny, et al. CESK DERM. 42:83-85, April, 1967.

ARTHRITIS
"Arthritis and gonococcal infection," NEW ENG J MED. 279:268, August 1, 1968.

"Arthritis associated with gonorrhoea," by J. O. Partain, et al. ANN RHEUM DIS. 27:156-162, March, 1968.

"Arthritis gonorrhoea. Report of a case in pregnancy

ARTHRITIS
> with negative GR in serum and positive GR in the synovial fluid," by A. Nielsen. UGESKR LAEG. 130:1867-1868, October 31, 1968.

> "A complex diagnostic problem: the differentiation among gonococcal arthritis, Reiter's syndrome, and rheumatoid arthritis," by J. C. Brooks, Jr. J MED ASS. 56:291-296, July, 1967.

> "Mycoplasmas and arthritis," by J. T. Sharp. ARTHRITIS RHEUM. 13:263-271, May-June, 1970.

> "Sero-negative polyarthritis. The Bedsonia (chlamydia) group of agents and Reiter's disease. A progress report," by E. M. Dunlop, et al. ANN RHEUM DIS. 27:234-239, May, 1968.

ATRICANA
> "Experiences with atricana in the treatment of trichomoniasis," by J. C. Aure, et al. T NORSK LAEGEFOREN. 89:1792-1794 passim, December 1, 1969.

> "Studies on the value of atrican (TC 109) in the treatment of trichomonal and monilial infections," by W. Kilczewski, et al. PRZEGL DERM. 55:531-535, July-September, 1968.

BALANOPOSTHITIS
> SEE: Minor Venereal Disease and Infections.

BEDSONIAE
> SEE ALSO: Trichomoniasis
>   Minor Venereal Disease and Infections.

> "A Bedsonia isolated from a patient with clinical lymphogranuloma venereum," by J. Schachter. AMER J OPHTHAL. 63:1049-1053, May, 1967.

> "Bedsoniae inclusions in two newborn infants in Lebanon," by N. A. Haddad. AMER J OPHTHAL. 64:124-128, July, 1967.

> "Clinical studies on gonococcal arthritis and Reiter's syndrome and measurement of gonococcal and Bedsonia antibodies," by J. T. Sharp, et al. ARTHRITIS RHEUM. 11:569-578, August, 1968.

> "Complement-fixing antibodies to Bedsonia organisms in Reiter's syndrome and ankylosing spondylitis," by

BEDSONIAE

T. D. Kinsella, et al. ANN RHEUM DIS. 27:241-244, May, 1968.

"Demonstration, by cultures, of agents of the genus bedsonia in joint fluid in cases of fiessinger-leroy-Reiter rheumatism," by B. A'mor, et al. C R ACAD SCI. 264:1365-1367, March 6, 1967.

"Detection of chlamydia (Bedsonia) in certain infections of man. II. Clinical study of genital tract, eye, rectum, and other sites of recovery of chlamydia," by E. M. Dunlop, et al. J INFECT DIS. 120:463-470, October, 1969.

"Infection by Bedsoniae and the possibility of spurious isolation. 2. Genital infection, disease of the eye, Reiter's disease," by E. M. Dunlop, et al. AMER J OPHTHAL. 63:Suppl:1073-1081, May, 1967.

"Infection by TRIC agent and other member of the Bedsonia group, with a note on Reiter's disease. 1. Ocular disease in the adult," by B. R. Jones, et al. TRANS OPHTHAL SOC UK. 86:291-312, 1966.

--2. Ophthalmia neonatorum due to TRIC agent," by A. Freedman, et al. TRANS OPHTHAL SOC UK. 86:313-320, 1966.

--3. Genital infection and disease of the eye," by E. M. Dunlop, et al. TRANS OPHTHAL SOC UK. 86:321-334, 1966.

--4. Laboratory aspects," by I. A. Harper, et al. TRANS OPHTHAL SOC UK. 86:335-348, 1966.

"Sero-negative polyarthritis. The Bedsonia (chlamydia) group of agents and Reiter's disease. A progress report," by E. M. Dunlop, et al. ANN RHEUM DIS. 27:234-239, May, 1968.

BEJEL
SEE: MINOR AND VENEREAL DISEASES & INFECTIONS

BIBLIOGRAPHY
"The Argyll Robertson pupil, 1868-1969. A critical survey of the literature," by I. E. Loewenfeld. SURVEY OPHTHAL. 14:199-200, November, 1969.

"The association of syphilis with hepatic cirrhosis: a

report of six cases and a review of the literature," by G. Karmi, et al. POSTGRAD MED J. 45:675-579, October, 1969.

"Congenital luetic macroglobulinemia and cryoglobulinemia. Literature review and personal contribution," by A. G. Marchi, et al. G MAL INFETT. 20:249-251, March, 1968.

"Fluorescent antibody methods in the detection and control of venereal diseases. A bibliographical review of the literature," by Z. P. Mora. BRIT J VENER DIS. 45:23-32, March, 1969.

"From the dermatological literature of the USSR. II.," by R. M. Bohnstedt. HAUTARZT. 17:481-484, November, 1966.

"Genital mycoplasma in pathology of the woman fetus and neonate (Literature review)," by M. A. Bashakova. VOP OKHR MATERIN DETS. 15:71-74, June, 1970.

"Gonococcal arthritis in the newborn. Report of a case and review of the literature," by S. Glaser, et al. AMER J DIS CHILD. 112:185-188, September, 1966.

"Lues maligna. Presentation of a case and a review of the literature," by D. A. Fisher, et al. ARCH DERM. 99:70-73, January, 1969.

"On the therapy of skin and venereal diseases. Review of the literature 1965-1966," by H. Walther. DEUTSCH MED J. 19:171-176, March 5, 1968+.

"The present status of urogenital trichomoniasis. A general review of the literature," by Z. Gallai, et al. APPL THER. 8:773-778, September, 1966.

"Reiter treponeme. A review of the literature," by A. L. Wallace, et al. BULL WHO. 36:Supplement No. 2, 101-103, 1967.

"Resource guide on venereal disease control," by New York City Board of Education. CURRIC BULL. 1967-1968, No. 9:18p.

"A review of the Hungarian Journal of Dermatology and Venereology for the year 1967," by K. Kirai, et al. VESTN DERM VENER. 43:60-62, February, 1969.

BIBLIOGRAPHY

"Studies of patients with penicillin allergy with a review of literature," by H. Strassmann. HAUTARZT. 20:323-329, July, 1969.

"Tasks of the journal 'Vestnik dermatologii i venereologii' in 1969," by B. M. Pashkov. VESTN DERM VENER. 43:3-5, January, 1969.

"Therapy of early syphilis--review of the literature," by M. Pacenovska, et al. CESK DERM. 45:171-180, August, 1970.

"Therapy of skin and venereal diseases. Review of the literature of 1967-1968," by H. Walther. DEUTSCH MED J. 20:480-485, August, 1969.

"Venereal disease books available in schools." SCI N L. 89:56, January 22, 1966.

BICILLINS

"Bicillin-6 in therapy of gonorrhea in women," by F. V. Potapnev, et al. VESTN DERM VENER. 43:52-55, January, 1969.

"Bicillin-6 in the treatment of gonorrhea in men," by M. U. Mirsagatov, et al. VESTN DERM VENER. 41:70-72, October, 1967.

"Bicillin-6 therapy in combination with pyrogenale and prodigiosane of patients with contagious forms of syphilis," by O. K. Loseva, et al. VESTN DERM VENER. 42:71-75, 1968.

"Clinico-laboratory studies of syphilis patients treated with bicillin-6," by A. A. Akovbian, et al. VESTN DERM VENER. 41:63-67, July, 1967.

"Comparative assessment of the treatment of syphilis patients with bicillin-3, -4, and -6," by A. A. Akovbian, et al. VESTN DERM VENER. 43:44-48, November, 1969.

"Experience of continuous treatment of early forms of syphilis with penicillin and bicillin," by L. A. Rozina. VESTN DERM VENER. 42:62-65, 1968.

"Histochemical studies of syphilids during treatment with bicillin-4 and bicillin-6," by A. A. Avokbian, et al. VESTN DERM VENER. 42:38-41, December, 1968.

BICILLINS

"The penetration of bicillin-6 into the cerebrospinal fluid," by O. K. Loseva. VESTN DERM VENER. 41:47-51, August, 1967.

"Penicillin-bicillin treatment of patients with infectious forms of syphilis," by G. I. Egorov. VESTN DERM VENER. 41:42-46, February, 1967.

"Remote results of bicillin-3 therapy of patients with active forms of syphilis," by V. A. Rakhmanov, et al. VESTN DERM VENER. 40:43-45, October, 1966.

"Remote results of the continuous treatment of fresh forms of syphilis with penicillin and bicillin," by S. T. Pavlov, et al. VESTN DERM VENER. 41:8-11, April, 1967.

"Remote results of treatment of syphilis patients with bicillin-1 and bicillin-3," by E. P. Nikol'skaia, et al. VESTN DERM VENER. 41:46-48, February, 1967.

"Some remote results of the treatment of syphilis with bicillin-1, bicillin-3, and bicillin-4," by KhN Khidyrov, et al. VESTN DERM VENER. 41:47-50, June, 1967.

"Study of the therapeutic effectiveness of bicillin-6 in patients with communicable forms of syphilis," by O. K. Loseva. VESTN DERM VENER. 41:59-62, May, 1967.

"Treatment of gonorrhea with bicillin," by I. I. Shkliar. VESTN DERM VENER. 40:84-85, January, 1966.

"Therapeutic effects of bicillin-6 in treatment of gonorrhea in men," by S. L. Kozin, et al. VESTN DERM VENER. 44:75-79, May, 1970.

BISMUTH

"Gummous syphilis of the penis refractory to penicillin and bismuth preparations," by A. I. Levykin. VESTN DERM VENER. 43:82-86, January, 1969.

"Immediate and remote results of the treatment of syphilis with antibiotics alone and in combination with bismuth," by G. B. Nesterenko, et al. VESTN DERM VENER. 43:37-40, May, 1969.

"Immediate results of treating patients with contagious forms of syphilis using simultaneously penicillin and

BISMUTH

bismuth preparations," by T. V. Vasil'ev, et al. VESTN DERM VENER. 44:50-55, April, 1970.

"Results of the treatment of recent syphilids with bismuth alone," by G. Falchi. G ITAL DERM. 107:683-689, September-December, 1966.

"Spinal fluid findings five years or more after infection in patients with early symptomatic syphilis treated with neo-arsphenamine bismuth," by F. M. Haagsma, et al. DERMATOLOGICA. 135:115-120, 1967.

BLASTOMYCOSIS
SEE: MINOR VENEREAL DISEASES & INFECTIONS

BLENNORRHAGIA
SEE: GONORRHEA

BLOOD DONORS AND TRANSFUSIONS

"Control of blood donors. 3. Syphilis transmitted by blood transfusion," by E. Skog. LAKARTIDNINGEN. 64: 1970-1972, May 10, 1967.

"Course in a number of cases of serologic syphilis in blood donors (1962-1968)," by R. Andre, et al. REV FRANC TRANSFUS. 13:93-95, March, 1970.

"Problem of syphilis in blood donors in the light of data of the Provinc Blood Service Center in Gdánsk," by J. Kozakiewicz, et al. WIAD LEK. 21:645-648, April 15, 1968.

"Serological and epidemiological evaluation of the present methods of examination of blood donors," by S. Jasser, et al. POL TYG LEK. 22:1237-1239, August 14, 1967.

"Serology of syphilis in blood transfusion service," by F. Kail. BIBL HAEMAT. 32:247-249, 1969.

"Simplified complex of serological syphilis reactions in mass donor examination," by A. M. Chistiakov. LAB DELO. 2:83-86, 1969.

"Study of the existence of treponemic antibodies in dry blood," by A. Utrilla. ACTAS DERMOSIF. 58:167-170, May-June, 1967.

"Transmission of syphilis by fresh blood components,"

BLOOD DONORS AND TRANSFUSIONS

    by R. W. Chambers, et al. TRANSFUSION. 9:32-34, January-February, 1969.

CANCER & PRE-CANCER

    "Adolescent coitus and cervical cancer: associations of related events with increased risk," by I. D. Rotkin. CANCER RES. 27:603-617, April, 1967.

    "Association of carcinoma of the uterine cervix and trichomonas vaginalis infestations. Frequency of trichomonas vaginalis in preinvasive and invasive cervical carcinoma," by O. Berggren. AMER J OBSTET GYNEC. 105:166-168, September, 1969.

    "The association of genital herpesvirus with cervical atypia and carcinoma in situ," by I. Royston, et al. AMER J EPIDEM. 91:531-538, June, 1970.

    "Canine venereal lymphoma as a model of experimental cancer," by H. Marquez-Monter. GAC MED MEX. 100:168-183, February, 1970.

    "Comparative cyto-histological studies on the precancerous and early stages of cervix carcinoma with simultaneous trichomonas vaginitis," by E. Boquoi. Z GEBRUTSH GYNAEK. 169:59-74, 1968.

    "Considerations on a case of primary syphiloma of the cervix uteri in pregnancy with special reference to the differential diagnosis from cervical carcinoma," by E. Rocco. MINERVA GINEC. 19:30-34, January 15, 1967.

    "Epidemiology of cervical cancer: Study of a prison population," by K. S. Moghissi, et al. AMER J OBSTET GYNEC. 100:607-614, March 1, 1968.

    "False-positive reaction to VDRL test with prozone phenomena. Association with lymphosarcoma," by K. D. Wuepper, et al. JAMA. 195:868-869, March 7, 1968.

    "Findings on trichomonas vaginitis--from the view of uterine cancer examination," by Y. Yokoyama, et al. SAISHIN IGAKU. 21:1585-1591, July, 1966.

    "High titer of Wassermann antibodies in a case of advanced myelomatosis," by A. B. Laurell, et al. ACTA DERMATOVENER. 46:406-411, 1966.

CANCER & PRE-CANCER

"Hutchinson's syndrome." OTOLARYNGOLOGY. 39:1299, December, 1967.

"Hutchinson's teeth." ORAL SURG. 24:635-636, November, 1967.

"The incidence of trichomonas vaginalis in cases of pre-invasive and invasive cervical cancer. Relationship between cervical cancer and trichomonas vaginalis," by O. Berggren. LAKARTIDNINGEN. 64:3335-3340, August 31, 1967.

"Influence of trichomonas vaginalis on preinvasive nonradical treatment of carcinoma of the cervix uteri," by M. Wawrzkiewicz, et al. WIAD PARAZYT. 16:195-197, 1970.

"On the etiologic relationship between leukoplakia, syphilis and cancer of the oral cavity," by K. Anastassov, et al. REV FRANC ODONTOSTOMAT. 14:1530-1536, November, 1967.

"Prevention of cancer of the cervix uteri in patients with chronic gonorrhea," by A. D. Tselishcheva. VESTN DERM VENER. 40:57-62, March, 1966.

"Prickle-cell carcinoma of the supre-and infra-clavicular fossa resembling the pancoasttobias syndrome in a patient with syphilis of the nervous system," by S. Zelazny, et al. PRZEGLAD LEK. 22:514-515, 1966.

"Relation of various epidemiologic factors to cervical cancer as determined by a screening program," by S. M. Naguib, et al. OBSTET GYNEC. 28:451-459, October, 1966.

"The role of colonic-rectal adenomas as a precarcinomatous condition," by M. Reifferscheid. ERGEBN CHIR ORTHOP. 50:83-105, 1967.

"The role of trichomoniasis in the development of precancerous state of the uterine cervix," by I. Szell, et al. ORV HETIL. 108:150-156, January 22, 1967.

"The role of urogenital trichomonas in the genesis of changes in the portio epithelium," by B. Toth, et al. ZBL GYNAEK. 91:547-551, April 26, 1969.

CANCER & PRE-CANCER

"The role of urogenital trichomonas infections in the incidence of changes in the cervix epithelium," by B. Toth, et al. ORV HETIL. 108:924-926, May 14, 1967.

"Sarcoid granuloma in secondary syphilis," by L. R. Lantis, et al. ARCH DERM. 99:748-752, June, 1969.

"A search for viruses in smegma, premalignant and early malignant cervical tissues. The isolation of herpesviruses with distinct antigenic properties," by W. E. Rawls, et al. AMER J EPIDEM. 87:647-655, May, 1968.

"Studies on carcinoma of the urinary bladder. I. Statistical and epidemiological studies on cancer of the bladder in Japanese," by O. Yoshida. ACTA UROL JAP. 12:1040-1064, October, 1966.

"Studies on granuloma inguinale. 8. Serological reactivity of sera from patients with carcinoma of penis when tested with Donovania antigens," by J. Goldberg. BRIT J VENER DIS. 42:205-209, September, 1966.

"Survey on information on health among citizens of a large city with special reference to cancer and venereal disease." J JAP MED ASS. 59:117-121, January 1, 1968.

"Swelling in the lower abdomen of the patients with cervix cancer is not necessarily an indication of metastasis," by M. Jin, et al. SANFUJIN JISSAI. 15:1102-1105, December, 1966.

"Treatment of venereal sarcoma in a bitch by vulvo-vagino-ovario-hysterectomy with perineal urethrostomy. A case report," by P. J. Philip. INDIAN VET J. 45:874-877, October, 1968.

"Trichomonas invasion and intraepithelial cancer of the cervix uteri," by R. M. Sokolovskii, et al. VOP ONKOL. 12:37-43, 1966.

CANDIDIASIS
SEE ALSO: TRICHOMONIASIS
          MINOR VENEREAL DISEASES & INFECTIONS

"Candida albicans and the contraceptive pill," by R. D. Catterall. LANCET. 2:830-831, October 15, 1966.

"Candidamycoses. Candidiasistinea (candidamycetica)

CANDIDIASIS

of the skin including genitalia," by H. Grimmer. Z HAUT GESCHLECHTSKR. 40:15-26, January 15, 1966.

"Candidiases of the skin and mucosae," by D. Grigoriou. REV MED SUISSE ROM. 86:619-631, September, 1966.

"Epidemiologic significance of the candida albicans infection of the vagina in pregnant women," by W. Mierzejewski, et al. GINEK POL. 37:501-506, May, 1966.

"Etiopathogenetic data concerning eczematous candidiasis of the genitals," by C. L. Meneghini, et al. DERM INT. 5:163-166, July-September, 1966.

"Experiences with pimafucin in candida and trichomonas vaginitis," by T. Ozbay, et al. MED WELT. 50:2741-2743, December 13, 1969.

"On the clinical use of a new antibiotic, pimaricin, in the therapy of vaginitis caused by candida albicans and by trichomonas," by B. Ferrari, et al. QUAD CLIN OSTET GINEC. 21:929-945, November, 1966.

"Preliminary observations on the use of pimaricin in vaginitis due to candida albicans, trichomonas vaginalis and in aspecific vaginitis," by B. I. De Luca. MINERVA GINEC. 18:840-846, August 15, 1967.

"The role of trichomonas and candida albicans as the principal cause of rupture of some perineorrhaphies after delivery," by D. Maroudi, et al. GYNEC OBSTET. 65:651-654, November-December, 1966.

"A study of 183 cases of leucorrhea: incidence of trichomonas vaginalis, candida spp., and hemophilus vaginalis," by Z. D. Desai, et al. J POSTGRAD MED. 12:91-98, April, 1966.

"Trichomonas and candida albicans as a cause of conjugal sterility. Proposal of a new fundic test," by S. Gaffuri, et al. MINERVA GINEC. 20:1260-1268, July 31, 1968.

CARBAMAZEPINE
"Carbamazepine for tabetic pain," by D. Alarcon-Segovia, et al. JAMA. 203:57, January 1, 1968.

CEFAZOLIN
"Cefazolin, a new semisynthetic cephalosporin anti-

CEFAZOLIN

biotic. II. In vitro and in vivo antimicrobial activity," by M. Nishida, et al. J ANTIBIOT. 23:137-148, March, 1970.

CELLINI, B.

"Cellini and his syphilis. Malevolent mercurial cure?," by G. W. Geelhoed. JAMA. 204:Suppl:245-246, May 13, 1968.

CEPHALEXIN

"Cephalexin and cephaloglycin activity in vitro and absorption and urinary excretion of single oral doses in normal young adults," by P. Braun, et al. APPL MICROBIOL. 16:1684-1694, November, 1968.

"Cephalexin--a new oral antibiotic," by A. Bailey, et al. POSTGRAD MED J, Minneapolis. 46:157-158, March, 1970; also in POUMON COEUR. 26:299-303, 1970.

"Intraocular penetration of cephalexin in man," by G. L. Boyle, et al. AMER J OPHTHAL. 69:868-872, January-June, 1970.

CEPHALORIDINE

"Cephaloridine in early syphilis," by L. Z. Oller. POSTGRAD MED J. 43:Suppl:43:128-129, August, 1967.

"Cephaloridine in gonorrhoea in females," by A. Jouhar, et al. BRIT J VENER DIS. 44:223-225, September, 1968.

"Cephaloridine in the treatment of non-gonococcal urethritis," by G. W. Csonka, et al. POSTGRAD MED J. 43:123-124, August, 1967.

"Cephaloridine treatment of experimental rabbit syphilis," by S. Kuwahara, et al. POSTGRAD MED J. 43:Suppl:43:130-133, August, 1967.

"Cephaloridine treatment of gonorrhoea in the female," by D. G. McLone, et al. BRIT J VENER DIS. 44:220-222, September, 1968.

"Effect of cephalothin and cephaloridine against rabbit syphilis," by T. Ikeda, et al. ACTA DERM. 61:310-313, November, 1966.

"First observations of the therapy of secondary syphilis with cephaloridine," by F. Flarer, et al. DIS

CEPHALORIDINE

NERV SYST. 27:271-277, September, 1966.

"Further experience with cephaloridine in gonorrhoea," by L. Z. Oller. POSTGRAD MED J. 43:Suppl:43:124-128, August, 1967.

"On the antitreponemic action of cephaloridine," by F. Flarer. POSTGRAD MED J. 43:Suppl:43-133-134, August, 1967.

"Parenteral cephaloridine treatment of patients with early syphilis," by J. M. Glicksman, et al. ARCH INTERN MED. 121:342-344, April, 1968.

"Single doses of cephaloridine in the treatment of gonococcal urethritis in males," by M. J. Marshall, et al. POSTGRAD MED J. 43:Suppl:43:121-122, August, 1967.

"Therapy of early syphilis with cephaloridine," by O. A. Gonzalez, et al. REV INVEST SALUD PUBLICA. 27:201-214, July-September, 1967, also in POSTGRAD MED J. 43:Suppl:43:134-135, August, 1967.

"Treatment of gonorrhea in males with cephaloridine," by J. B. Lucas, et al. JAMA. 195:919-921, March 14, 1966.

"The treatment of gonorrhea with cephaloridine intramuscularly," by H. Pariser, et al. SOUTHERN MED J. 63:384-386, April, 1970.

"Treatment of ophthalmic syphilis with special reference to cephaloridine therapy," by M. Mikuni, et al. OPHTHALMOLOGY. 12:724-731, September, 1970.

CEPHALOSPORINS
SEE ALSO: SPECIFIC ONES

"Further findings on the anti-treponemic action in vitro of cephalosporins," by F. Galla, et al. ANTIBIOTICA. 4:309-313, December, 1966.

"On the immunological reactivity of penicillin, cephalosporin and tetracycline antibiotics," by J. Lochmannova, et al. J HYG EPIDEM. 14:201-210, 1970.

CEPHALOTHIN
"Cephalothin in gonococcal urethritis," by E. B. Smith.

CEPHALOTHIN

CURR THER RES. 9:79-81, February, 1967.

"Effect of cephalothin and cephaloridine against rabbit syphilis," by T. Ikeda, et al. ACTA DERM. 61: 310-313, November, 1966.

CHAGAS' DISEASE
"Epidemiologic survey on Chagas' disease and syphilis in Ribeirao Preto," by N. Haddad. REV INST MED TROP. 9:333-342, September-October, 1967.

CHANCROID
"Disappearance of chancroid in Algeria," by F. G. Marill, et al. BULL SOC FRANC DERM SYPH. 77:236-237, 1970.

"Extra- and peri-genital chancre (2 cases)," by P. P. de Oliveira. AN BRASIL DERM. 43:273-276, December, 1968.

"Simplified laboratory technique for diagnosis of chanchroid," by K. A. Borchardt, et al. ARCH DERM. 102: 188-192, August, 1970.

"Treatment of chancroid. A comparison of tetracycline and sulfisoxazole," by R. E. Kerber, et al. ARCH DERM. 100:604-607, November, 1969.

CHARCOT'S JOINTS
SEE S: ARTHROPATHY

CHILDREN
"The problems of urogenital trichomonasis in pre-puberal girls," by B. Beric, et al. GYNEC PRAT. 21:217-222, 1970.

"A survey of trichomonal and Neisserian infection in antenatal patients," by R. Gaal, et al. MED J AUST. 1:634-635, April 13, 1968.

"A survey of trichomonal and Neisserian infection in antenatal patients," by R. A. Osborn, et al. MED J AUST. 2:92, July 13, 1968.

"Tonsillectomy--a bloody mess," by H. Faigel. CLIN PEDIAT. 5:562-563, November, 1966.

"Vulvovaginitis in the premenarcheal child," by R. H. Heller, et al. J PEDIAT. 74:370-377, March, 1969.

CHLORAMPHENICOL

CHLORAMPHENICOL
"Intramuscular injection of procaine penicillin combined with oral administration of chloramphenicol in the treatment of gonorrhoea," by H. C. Gjessing, et al. BRIT J VENER DIS. 42:107-109, June, 1966.

"Oral chloramphenicol alone and with intramuscular procaine penicillin in the treatment of gonorrhoea," by H. C. Gjessing, et al. BRIT J VENER DIS. 43:133-136, June, 1967.

"A study of the trichomonicidal activity of the association of chloramphenicol and 1-hydroxy-ethyl-2methyl-5nitro-imidazole," by F. Filadoro. ANTIBIOTICA. 5:105-113, June, 1967.

CHLOROCIDE
"Treatment of dermato-venereal diseases with chlorocide injections," by G. Maramarosi. THER HUNG. 14:11-15, 1966.

CHLOROQUINE
"The influence of chloroquine and related drugs on psoriasis and keratoderma blenorrhagicum," by H. Baker. BRIT J DERM. 78:161-166, March, 1966.

CHLOROSULFONAMIDES
"Effect of new chlorosulfonamides on the female vagina. Considering trichomoniasis complicated by mycosis. Experimental part," by A. Kurnatowska. WIAD PARAZYT. 15:19-33, 1969.

CIRRHOSIS, HEPATIC
"The association of syphilis with hepatic cirrhosis: a report of six cases and a review of the literature," by G. Karmi, et al. POSTGRAD MED J. 45:675-679, October, 1969.

CITRAL
"Treatment of trichomoniasis with citral," by V. I. Danilin. SOVET MED. 31:139-140, May, 1968.

CLINDAMYCIN
"In-vitro comparison of erythromycin, lincomycin and clindamycin," by L. Phillips, et al. BRIT MED J. 2:89-90, April 11, 1970.

CLINICS, INSTITUTES & SOCIETIES
"Activities of the board of All-Russian Scientific

CLINICS, INSTITUTES & SOCIETIES

Society of Dermatologists-Venereologists," by B. M. Pashkov. VESTN DERM VENER. 43:75-79, June, 1969.

"Activities of the Board of the All-Union Scientific Medical Society of Dermatologists-Venereologists for 1966-1968," by A. A. Studnitsin, et al. VESTN DERM VENER. 43:69-74, June, 1969.

"The activities of the Moscow Scientific Society of Dermatologists and Venereologists (1917-1967)," by V. A. Rakhmanov, et al. VESTN DERM VENER. 41:73-77, October, 1967.

"Activity of the V.M. Tarnovskii Leningrad Dermatological and Venereal Society during World War II," by G. V. Shiman. VESTN DERM VENER. 45:52-54, December, 1969.

"Case records of the Massachusetts General Hospital. Weekly clinicopathological exercises. Case 52-1969." NEW ENG J MED. 281:1414-1419, December 18, 1969.

"Clinic for dermatologic and venereal diseases." GOD ZBORN MED FAK SKOPJE. 14:51-53, 1968.

"Fundamental achievements of the Central Dermato-Venereal Institute in the scientific study of venereal diseases," by A. A. Studnitsin, et al. VESTN DERM VENER. 45:3-8, December, 1969.

"The main achievements of the Central Scientific-Research Dermatovenereological Institute (CDVI) in the field of scientific investigations in dermatology," by A. A. Studnitsin, et al. VESTN DERM VENER. 43:3-14, April, 1969.

"Manual use of punched cards in dermato-venereological dispensaries," by M. I. Arans. VESTN DERM VENER. 40:68-70, November, 1966.

"Social board of the dermato-venereologic institution," by I. A. L. Iudin. VESTN DERM VENER. 40:59-61, January, 1966.

"The special clinic," by J. F. Foulkes. NM. 131:22+, July 3, 1970.

"Some basic trends, results and prospectives of scientific-research at the Chair of Dermatologic and

CLINICS, INSTITUTES & SOCIETIES

Venereal Diseases of the Patrice Lumumba University of Friendship of Peoples," by R. S. Babaiants. VESTN DERM VENER. 43:3-7, November, 1969.

"Some results and perspectives of scientific investigations at the Faculty of Skin and Venereal Diseases of the N. I. Pirogov II Moscow Medical Institute," by IuK Shripkin, et al. VESTN DERM VENER. 43:3-6, September, 1969.

"Some results and prospects of research work of the Chair of Skin and Venereal Diseases of the Donetsk Medical Institute," by N. A. Torsuev, et al. VESTN DERM VENER. 43:11-16, January, 1969.

"Some results and prospects of scientific work of the Chair of Skin and Venereal diseases of the Leningrad Institute of Physician Training for 1962-1967," by P. V. Kozhevnikov. VESTN DERM VENER. 43:5-11, January, 1969.

"Theoretic and practical aspects of the scientific activity of the Gor'kii Institute of Dermatology and Venereology," by O. D. Kochura, et al. VESTN DERM VENER. 44:9-14, January, 1970.

"Use of the venereal disease clinic of San Mateo County, California," by D. L. White, et al. PUBLIC HEALTH REP. 83:954-956, November, 1968.

"VD Clinic," by D. Bashforth. DIST NURS. 8:285-286, February, 1966.

"VD Clinic, James Pringle house, the Middlesex Hospital," by H. Elliott, et al. NURS TIMES. 64:827-828, June 21, 1968.

"Visit to a clinic: Northwest Washington, D.C. venereal disease clinic," by D. Sanford. NEW REPUB. 159:12-13, December 7, 1968.

CLOMOCYCLINE
"Clinical trial of clomocycline (megaclor) in gonococcal and non-gonococcal urethritis," by G. S. Andrew, et al. BRIT J VENER DIS. 45:154-156, June, 1969.

COLPITIS
SEE: MINOR VD

CONFERENCES

CONFERENCES
SEE ALSO: HISTORY
SYMPOSIA

"APHA Conference Report, 1968. Laboratory." PUBLIC HEALTH REP. 84:272-279, March, 1969.

"Clinical neuropathological conference," by S. M. Aronson, et al. DIS NERV SYST. 28:688-694, October, 1967.

"Clinicopathologic conference," by E. H. Eigenbrodt, et al. TEXAS MED. 65:84-90, July, 1969.

"Clinicopathologic conference," by D. Jones, et al. TEXAS MED. 62:92-96, October, 1966.

"Clinicopathologic conference. Case presentation. (JHH 631077)," by V. A. McKusick, et al. BULL HOPKINS HOSP. 119:150-160, August, 1966.

"Conclusions of the venerological conference held during the period of May 24-30, 1969 at Destný, Orlické Hory," by J. Obrtel. CESK DERM. 45:145-153, August, 1970.

"Hamburg dermatologic society. 3. Practice forum on 17-9-1966 on board the motor boat 'Tom Kyle'," by A. Wiskemann. DERM WSCHR. 153:1097-1101, September 30, 1967.

CONTRACEPTION
SEE ALSO: OCCURRENCE
AND SOCIOLOGY

"Candida albicans and the contraceptive pill," by R. D. Catterall. LANCET. 2:830-831, October 15, 1966.

"Oral contraception among special clinic patients. With particular reference to the diagnosis of gonorrhoea," by A. B. Hewitt. BRIT J VENER DIS. 46:106-107, April, 1970.

"Prescribing contraception for teenagers--a moral compromise," by R. J. Pion. OBSTET GYNEC. 30:752-755, November, 1967.

"Promiscuity and contraception in a sample of patients attending a clinic for venereal diseases," by A. Linken, et al. BRIT J VENER DIS. 46:243-246, June, 1970.

COPPER OXIDASE

COPPER OXIDASE
"Effect of copper oxidase in the blood and cerebrospinal fluid of patients with syphilitic lesions of the central nervous system," by N. I. Tumasheva, et al. ZH NEVROPAT PSIKHIAT KORSAKOV. 66:391-393, 1966.

CREDE'S PROPHYLAXIS
"Crede's prophylaxis after 85 years," by K. Znamenacek, et al. CESK PEDIAT. 22:46-54, January, 1967.

--Discussion." CESK OFTAL. 22:335-338, September, 1966.

"The hazards of Crede's prophylaxis of neonatal blennorrhea," by V. J. Mathesius. GYNAECOLOGIA. 164: 274-278, 1967.

DEBECILLIN
"Herxheimer-Lukasiewicz reaction after injection of debecillin in early acquired syphilis," by E. Peisert, et al. POL TYG LEK. 22:344-347, March 6, 1967.

"Effect of debecycline on treponema pallidum," by J. Suchanek, et al. POL TYG LEK. 22:14-16, January 2, 1967.

DEFLAMON
"The use of a new drug (deflamon) in the treatment of vaginal trichomoniasis," by A. Segre. MINERVA GINEC. 20:52-59, January 15, 1968.

DEMETHYLCHLORTETRACYCLINE
SEE: LEDERMYCIN

DENTISTRY
SEE: ORAL

DE SANTA CRUZ Y ESPEJO, FRANCISCO XAVIER EUGENI
"Doctor Francisco Xavier Eugenio de Santa Cruz y Espejo," by N. H. de Huerta. REV ECUAT HIG. 26:55-58, January-April, 1969.

DETREOMYCIN
"TPI and FTA tests in the evaluation of effectiveness of the oral treatment of early symptomatic syphilis with detreomycin, erythromycin and oxytetracycline with consideration of the clinical picture," by J. Lebioda, et al. PRZEGL DERM. Suppl:39-51, 1969.

DIABETES

DIABETES
"Positive fluorescent treponemal antibody reactions in diabetes," by M. K. Hughes, et al. APPL MICROBIOL. 19:425-428, March, 1970.

DIAGNOSIS
"Clinical and laboratory diagnosis of venereal diseases," by M. B. Moore, Jr. BOL OFIC SANIT PANAMER. 60:316-327, April, 1966.

"Clinical peculiarities of skin and venereal diseases detected among persons arriving from tropical countries," by R. S. Babaiants. VESTN DERM VENER. 43:18-23, July, 1969.

"Clinical picture of sepsis in a two-month-old infant. What could be the cause of edema, ascites, iceterus and anemia?." CLIN PEDIAT. 9:214-225, April, 1970.

"Consequences of a diagnostic error--ulcus durum diagnosed as erosion of cervix uteri," by P. Botsov, et al. AKUSH GINEK. 9:58-60, 1970.

"Differential diagnostic problem: impetiginized eczematic scabies--lues II--psoriasis vulgaris," by V. Misgeld. MED KLIN. 64:2189-2192, November 21, 1969.

"Drugs and the Coombs antiglobulin test." NEW ENG J MED. 277:157-158, July 20, 1967.

"Laboratory diagnosis of venereal disease," by G. W. Schepers. MED ANN DC. 35:357-366 passim, July, 1966.

"On the venereal ulcer of the vulva," by G. Adinolfi, et al. ARCH OSTET GINEC. 72:173-181, March-April, 1967.

"The role of public health laboratories in the diagnosis of venereal diseases," by A. M. Vilches. BOL OFIC SANIT PANAMER. 60:328-334, April, 1966.

"Sexually transmitted disease in antenatal patients," by R. N. Thin, et al. BRIT J VENER DIS. 46:126-128, April, 1970.

"Usability of Boroviczeny's rapid hematological staining method for routine protozoological diagnosis," by W. Granz, et al. Z TROPENMED PARASITOL. 21:261-

DIAGNOSIS

266, September, 1970.

"Use of immunofluorescent antibody technic in the diagnosis of bacterial and viral diseases," by B. Babudieri. G MAL INFETT. 20:35-49, January, 1968.

"Value of positive serologic reactions in systematic examinations of Africans," by H. Van Wymeersch, et al. PRESSE MED. 76:1774, October 5, 1968.

"Which diagnosis would you make?" MED KLIN. 64:2311 passim, December 5, 1969.

DIMETHYL SULFOXIDE
"Effect of dimethyl sulfoxide on skin. A macroscopic and microscopic investigation on human skin" by E. Skog, et al. ACTA DERMATOVENER. 47:426-434, 1967.

DIRIBIOTINE
"Clinical experiments with diribiotine tablets," by J. Govers. THER UNSCH. 23:149-150, April, 1966.

DONOVANOSIS
SEE: GRANULOMA INGUINALE

DOXICILLIN
"Dermatologic iconography. Donovanosis (granuloma venerum tropical). Treatment using doxicillin," by L. H. Paschoal, et al. AN BRASIL DERM. 43:Suppl:1-3, January-March, 1968.

DOXYCYCLINE
SEE ALSO: OXYTETRACYCLINE
TETRACYCLINE

"Controls gonorrhea." AM DRUGGIST. 160:50, October 6, 1969.

"Doxycycline treatment of gonorrhoea in cases with decreased penicillin susceptibility of gonococci," by A. Lassus. CHEMOTHERAPY. 15:125-128, 1970.

"'Instant treatment' of gonorrhea with a new oxytetracycline derivate--doxycycline (preliminary report)," by L. Sylvestre, et al. INT Z KLIN PHARMAKOL THER TOXIK. 1:401-403, July, 1968.

"Study on doxycycline in the treatment of acute infections of the respiratory system and lymphogranuloma

DOXYCYCLINE

venereum," by J. Neves, et al. REV ASS MED BRASIL. 14:65-70, June, 1968.

"The treatment of gonorrhoea with doxycycline as a single dose," by A. Lassus. CHEMOTHERAPY. 13:366-368, 1968.

"Use of doxycycline in the treatment of syphilis," by L. H. Paschoal, et al. HOSPITAL. 75:1965-1967, June, 1969.

"Use of a single dose of doxycycline monohydrate for treating gonorrheal urethritis in men," by G. Domescik, et al. PUBLIC HEALTH REP. 84:182-183, February, 1969.

DRUG ADDICTION

"Drug dependence among patients attending a Department of Venereology," by L. I. Ponting, et al. BRIT J VENER DIS. 46:111-113, April, 1970.

"Drug-taking by patients with venereal disease," by D. C. Rawlins. BRIT J VENER DIS. 45:238-240, September, 1969.

"Narcotic addiction with false-positive reaction for syphilis. Immunologic studies," by D. L. Tuffanelli. ACTA DERMATOVENER. 48:542-546, 1968.

"Psychiatric drugs and trends. The alarming comeback of gonorrhea," by E. L. Dembicki. J PSYCHIAT NURS. 6:176-177, May-June, 1968.

"Serologic investigations in narcotic addicts. I. Syphilis, lymphogranuloma, venereum, herpes simplex, and Q fever," by C. E. Cherubin, et al. ANN INTERN MED. 69:739-742, October, 1968.

"Serologic tests for syphilis among narcotic addicts," by W. D. Harris, et al. NEW YORK J MED. 67:2967-2974, November 15, 1967.

"A study of drug-taking among young patients attending a clinic for venereal diseases," by A. Linken. BRIT J VENER DIS. 44:337-341, December, 1968.

ECMONOVOCILLIN

"Protein fractions of blood serum in patients with syphilis during ecmonovocillin therapy," by T. A. Maly-

ECMONOVOCILLIN

gina, et al. VRACH DELO. 11:132-133, November, 1968.

"Remote results of the treatment of syphilitic patients with ecmonovocillin and heavy metal salts," by T. V. Vasil'ev. VESTN DERM VENER. 40:52-57, March, 1966.

EDUCATION
SEE ALSO: PREVENTION & CONTROL
SOCIOLOGY
YOUTH

"Attitudes of prospective school teachers on teaching venereal disease information," by W. B. Neser, et al. PUBLIC HEALTH REP. 82:917-920, October, 1967.

"The bases of a suitable marital and premarital education in Turin. Activities of the AIEMP," by I. Terzi, et al. G BATT VIROL IMMUN. 62:703-709, September-October, 1969.

"Beginning of dermatological and venerological instruction at the University of Halle," by W. Kaiser, et al. MED MSCHR. 23:352-358, August, 1969.

"Breakthrough in VD education in Los Angeles county," by E. Reinig, et al. PUBLIC HEALTH REP. 82:505-512, June, 1967.

"Classroom sex education," by A. E. Gravatt. J AMER COLL HEALTH ASS. 15:61-65, May, 1967.

"Considerations on some helpful measures in the propaganda against venereal diseases. (On experiences in the high schools of the Province of Venezia)," by A. Serena. ARCH ITAL DERM VENER. 34:395-398, 1966.

"Controlling venereal disease through education," by P. E. Lenz. PUBLIC HEALTH REP. 81:996-998, November, 1966.

"A diploma in venereology," by C. D. Alergant. BRIT J VENER DIS. 46:162-163, April, 1970.

"Educating teen-agers about venereal disease," by D. Rosenblatt, et al. J SCH HLTH. 37:432+, November, 1967.

"Education can help cure VD," by L. M. Garner. SCH & COM. 52:16-17, May, 1966.

EDUCATION

"Education has vital role in correcting misconceptions about venereal diseases," by W. L. Porter, et al. DELAWARE MED J. 39:232-234, September, 1967.

"Education of the public about venereal diseases. Some views of venereologists," by R. S. Morton. BRIT J VENER DIS. 42:238-243, December, 1966.

"Education on venereal diseases in the school curriculum," by J. H. Milor, et al. J SEC ED. 42:135-139, March, 1967.

"Education vs. venereal disease," by S. Tolchin. FORECAST HOME ECON. 14:F30-31+, April, 1969.

"Experience in application of the elements of programmed instruction of students," by L. D. Butovetskii, et al. VESTN DERM VENER. 43:54-56, February, 1969.

"Factors influencing the spread of gonorrhea. I. Educational and social behavior," by L. Juhlin. ACTA DERMATOVENER. 48:75-81, 1968.

"Forward planning in the United Kingdom for anti-V.D. education," by A. J. Dalzell-Ward. BRIT J VENER DIS. 46:159-161, April, 1970.

"Health education and spreading of venereal diseases among youth," by L. Dyskin, et al. PRZEGL DERM. 55: 273-280, May-June, 1968.

"Health education and venereal disease." BRIT MED J. 1:493-494, February 25, 1967.

"Health education and venereal diseases," by R. S. Morton. NT. 63:957+, July 21, 1967.

"Health education by public health nurses as a preventive measure against venereal diseases," by K. Imazu, et al. JAP J NURS ART. 8:21-25, August, 1969.

"How to plan a program for VD education," by F. B. Benell. NATIONS SCH. 77:72-73+, February, 1966.

"The importance of health education in the prevention of venereal diseases," by E. Sulutiu. MUNCA SANIT. 17:745-747, December, 1969.

"The instruction of dermatovenereology in medical

EDUCATION

schools," by RKh Abudsametov, et al. VESTN DERM VENER. 43:71-72, April, 1969.

"Is education the answer to the venereal disease problem?," by H. Manser. J AMER OSTEOPATH ASS. 67:1031-1037, May, 1968.

"The method of antivenereal propaganda at the present time," by E. K. Reznikov. VESTN DERM VENER. 43:52-59, November, 1969.

"The new specialist education: Dermato-venereology," by K. Thomsen. YNG LAEG. 10:839-840, 1968.

"Organization of continuing education for dermato-venereologists," by A. I. Kartamyshev, et al. VESTN DERM VENER. 42:58-62, 1968.

"Overcoming teacher reluctancy toward VD education," by F. B. Benell. J SCH HEALTH. 40:483-486, November, 1970.

"Patients with venereal disease or a health education problem," by T. Z. Capinski, et al. PRZEGL DERM. 53:87-94, January-February, 1966.

"Pedagogic considerations on a lecture on syphilis," by J. Danda. CESK DERM. 41:189-190, July, 1966.

"Programmed instruction and prospects of its application in teaching of dermato-venereology," by V. A. Rakhmanov, et al. VESTN DERM VENER. 42:52-57, 1968.

"Programmed text gives students facts about VD," OHIO SCH. 44:15+, March, 1966.

"Public education in venereal disease," by F. S. Rowntree. BRIT J VENER DIS. 42:246-250, December, 1966.

"Resource guide on venereal disease control," by New York Board of Education. N Y C BD ED CURRIC BUL. no.9:18p. 1967-1968.

"The school nurse and VD education," by E. W. Collum. S CAROLINA NURS. 20:7, 30-33, Spring, 1968.

"The school nurse-teacher's role in controlling venereal disease," by D. E. Barlow. J NY SCH NURSE-TEACH ASS. 1:16-19, June, 1970.

EDUCATION

"Sex and V.D. education in Central Newfoundland schools."
CANAD J PUBL HLTH. 58:265+, June, 1967.

"Shall our schools teach about venereal disease?," by
S. Podair. SAT R. 49:72-73+, March 19, 1966.

"Some problems of organizing programmed instruction at
the Department of Dermatology and Venereal Diseases,"
by N. A. Torsuev, et al. VESTN DERM VENER. 42:49-52, February, 1968.

"Studies of the education of young people concerning
venereal diseases," by P. Many, et al. BULL SOC FRANC
DERM SYPH. 74:772-780, 1967.

"'Target' sites for anti-V.D. propaganda," by B. P.
Wells, et al. HEALTH BULL. 28:75-77, January, 1970.

"Teaching about venereal disease and its control," by
B. Webster. ARCH ENVIRON HEALTH, Chicago. 13:367-371, September, 1966.

"Teaching of the clinical, epidemiological, public
health, and social aspects of the venereal diseases
in the medical schools throughout the world. Interim
report of the continuing cooperative study between
WHO and the IUVDT," by B. Webster. BRIT J VENER DIS.
46:156-158, April, 1970.

"Teaching of dermatovenerology in the school of medicine. Goals and methods," by J. Obrtel, et al. CESK
DERM. 44:37-40, February, 1969.

"Teaching of venereal disease in medical schools throughout the world, Preliminary report," by B. Webster.
BRIT J VENER DIS. 42:132-133, June, 1966.

"Unique course focuses on the VD interview," by L.
Alexander. RN. 29:47-52, April, 1966.

"Use of testing and teaching devices at the Department
of Dermatology and Venereal Diseases," by I. I. Il'in.
VESTN DERM VENER. 43:49-53, February, 1969.

"VD: wages of ignorance; excerpt from address," by W. F.
Schwartz. PTA MAG. 61:14-17, September, 1966.

"Venereal disease books available in schools." SCI N
L. 89:56, January 22, 1966.

EDUCATION

"Venereal disease education in schools of the state of New Jersey," by W. E. Ferinden, Jr. J SCH HEALTH. 38:611-614, November, 1968.

"Venereal diseases educational project--Hutt Health District September, 1967," by E. M. Andrews. OCCUP HEALTH NURSE. 1:11, December, 1967.

"What you should know about VD and why," by B. Webster. SR SCHOL. 91:Suppl:27, November 30, 1967.

EHRLICH PAUL

"Ehrlich, his life and his work," by J. Montes, et al. ALERGIA. 15:29-42, November, 1967.

"Paul Ehrlich (1854-1915)," by D. Kirchheim. INVEST UROL. 7:257-259, November, 1969.

ENDURACIDIN

"Enduracidin, a new antibiotic. 3. In vitro and in vivo antimicrobial activity," by K. Tsuchiya, et al. J ANTIBIOT. 21:147-153, February, 1968.

ENZYMOLOGY

"Enzymatic activity of ceruloplasmin in patients with syphilis and gonorrhea," by A. M. Borisenko, et al. VESTN DERM VENER. 41:66-69, September, 1967.

"Lytic effect of trypsin, lysozyme, and complement on treponema pallidum," by R. H. Jones, et al. BRIT J VENER DIS. 44:193-200, September, 1968.

EPILEPSY

"Epilepsy and neurosyphilis," by E. Negulici-Baliff, et al. ACTA NEUROL BELG. 67:1138-1152, 1967.

ERYTHROMYCIN

"Erythromycin," by R. S. Griffith, et al. MED CLIN NORTH AM. 54:1199-1215, September, 1970.

"Erythromycin and oleandomycin in therapy of fresh gonorrhea in women," by L. D. Kuntsevich. VESTN DERM VENER. 42:84-86, July, 1968.

"Erythromycin controls gonorrhea." AM DRUGGIST. 159:44, February 24, 1969.

"Erythromycin in the acqueous humour," by N. Shorr, et al. BRIT J OPHTHAL. 53:331-334, May, 1969.

ERYTHROMYCIN

"Erythromycin in early syphilis," by W. L. Fernando. BRIT J VENER DIS. 45:200-201, September, 1969.

"Erythromycin in the therapy of gonorrhea in women," by E. N. Turanova, et al. SOVET MED. 29:123-125, September, 1966.

"Erythromycin in the therapy of inquinal lymphogranuloma," by I. I. Il'in. VESTN DERM VENER. 40:69-70, August, 1966.

"Erythromycin in the treatment of acute gonococcal urethritis in males," by D. O. Smith, Jr., et al. CURR THER RES. 11:1-4, January, 1969.

"Erythromycin in the treatment of gonorrhea in women," by B. A. Afanas'ev. VESTN DERM VENER. 41:83-86, April, 1967.

"Erythromycin in the treatment of non-gonococcal urethritis," by R. R. Willcox. BRIT J VENER DIS. 44:157-159, June, 1968.

"Erythromycin stearate in 'single dose' in the treatment of acute masculine gonococcal urethritis," by R. Bialski. REV BRASIL MED. 26:256-258, April, 1969.

"In-vitro comparison of erythromycin, lincomycin, and clindamycin," by L. Phillips, et al. BRIT MED J. 2:89-90, April 11, 1970.

"Orally administered erythromycin level in body fluids," by J. Bowszyc, et al. POL TYG LEK. 25:241-243, February 16, 1970.

"Possible mycoplasma hominis urethritis revealed by differing responses of abacterial urethritis to treatment with tetracycline and erythromycin," by A. S. Grimble. BRIT J VENER DIS. 44:230-231, September, 1968.

"Relationships between the sensitivities in vitro of Neisseria gonorrhoeae to spiramycin, penicillin, streptomycin, tetracycline, and erythromycin," by A. Reyn, et al. BRIT J VENER DIS. 45:223-227, September, 1969.

"Studies of the value of erythromycin and oxytetracycline in treatment of early syphilis," by J. Bowszyc, et al. POL TYG LEK. 25:1394-1396, September, 1970.

ERYTHROMYCIN

"T-strain mycoplasma. Selective inhibition by erythromycin in vitro," by M. C. Shepard, et al. BRIT J VENER DIS. 42:21-24, March, 1966.

"TPI and FTA tests in the evaluation of effectiveness of the oral treatment of early symptomatic syphilis with detreomycin, erythromycin and oxytetracycline with consideration of the clinical picture," by J. Lebioda, et al. PRZEGL DERM. Suppl:39-51, 1969.

"Treatment of acute male gonococcal urethritis with a single dose of erythromycin-stearate," by J. Martini, et al. REV MED. 96:525-527, August, 1968.

FLAGYL
SEE: METRONIDAZOLE

FRAMBESIA
SEE: YAWS
SEE ALSO: MINOR VENEREAL DISEASES & INFECTIONS

FURACIN
"Ophthalmia neonatorum. Prevention with 5-nitro-2-furaldehyde semicarbazone (furacin)," by O. R. Baptista. HOSPITAL. 71:187-193, January, 1967.

FURADONIN
"Experience with the use of furadonin in trichomoniasis," by B. I. Il'In. UROL NEFROL. 32:40-43, March-April, 1967.

FURAZOLIDONE
"Furazolidone in the therapy of trichomonas urethritis in men," by A. I. Poliakov, et al. VESTN DERM VENER. 40:70, July, 1966.

"Furazolidone in the therapy of trichomoniasis in men," by S. A. Artem'ev, et al. SOVIET MED. 29:128-130, October, 1966.

FUSIDIC ACID
"A study of the relationships between the sensitivities of Neisseria gonorrhoeae to sodium penicillin G, four semi-synthetic penicillins, spiramycin, and fusidic acid," by A. Reyn, et al. BRIT J VENER DIS. 44:140-150, June, 1968.

GERIATRICS
"Granuloma venereum in an 81-year-old man," by U. Brauer,

GERIATRICS

et al. DERM WSCHR. 152:780-784, July 23, 1966.

"Non-specific reactions to the quantitative fluorescent antibody test (FTA) in the elderly," by E. I. Grin, et al. BRIT J VENER DIS. 44:216-217, September, 1968.

"Proper interpretation of serologic tests for syphilis in the aged," by L. Nicholas. J AMER GERIAT SOC. 15:224-229, March, 1967.

"Serological tests for syphilis in the elderly," by E. A. Johansson, et al. ANN CLIN RES. 2:47-50, March, 1970.

"Syphilitic aortic insufficiency. Its increased incidence in the elderly," by T. A. Prewitt. JAMA. 211:637-639, January 26, 1970.

"Venereal infection in the elderly," by M. U. Krishnan, et al. GERONT CLIN. 12:76-79, 1970.

"Venereal infection in elderly people," by A. M. Mechie, et al. GERONT CLIN. 8:207-214, 1966.

"Venereal infection in old age: an autopsy study," by A. M. Mechie, et al. GERIATRICS. 22:176-179, September, 1967.

GIARDIASIS

"Evaluation of the nitrimidazine activity in giardiasis and genital trichomoniasis," by J. M. Salles, et al. HOSPITAL. 77:1689-1697, May, 1970.

GLITISOL

"Glitisol in syphilis," by M. Spiezia. ANN MED NAV. 71:247-252, March-April, 1966.

GONORRHEA

"Benign gonococcaemia," by J. Verbov, et al. BRIT MED J. 3:407, August 15, 1970.

"Boswell's gonorrhea," by W. B. Ober. BULL NY ACAD MED. 45:587-636, June, 1969.

"Clinical aspects of ascending gonorrhea in women during the past 18 years (1947-1964)," by A. V. Chastikova. VESTN DERM VENER. 41:54-57, June, 1967.

GONORRHEA

"Clinical course of gonorrhea combined with trichomoniasis in males," by Ial Khasin, et al. VESTN DERM VENER. 41:69-70, December, 1967.

"The current clinical picture of gonorrhea in males and females," by V. Sedlácek. CESK DERM. 42:100-107, April, 1967.

"Enlightened views on gonorrhoea," by D. Hill. NURSING TIMES. 62:566+, April 29, 1966.

"The fate of gonococci in polymorphonuclear leucocytes," by P. J. Watt. J MED MICROBIOL. 3:501-509, August, 1970.

"Gonococcal diseases from the clinical and bacteriological viewpoint," by H. Modde, et al. SCHWEIZ MED WSCHR. 99:1242-1245, August 30, 1969.

"Gonococcal infections." MED LETT DRUGS THER. 8:79-80, September 23, 1966.

"Gonorrhoea." LANCET. 1:280-281, February 7, 1970.

"Gonorrhoea." LANCET. 1:675-676, March 30, 1968.

"Gonorrhoea," by R. S. Morton. LANCET. 1:824, April 13, 1968.

"Gonorrhea," by A. L. Schroeter, et al. ANN INTERN MED. 72:553-559, April, 1970.

"Gonorrhea in adult women," by V. Sebek. CESK GYNEK. 31:609-615, October, 1966.

"Gonorrhea--a new look at an old problem," by C. Lindman. J MAINE MED ASS. 61:162-163, August, 1970.

"Latent gonorrhea in women," by L. Clark. JAMA. 209:563, July 28, 1969.

"Little Miss Muffet sure is a tough-it," by N. B. Rawls. NORTHWEST MED. 69:352, May, 1970.

"Psychiatric drugs and trends. The alarming comeback of gonorrhea," by E. L. Dembicki. J PSYCHIAT NURS. 6:176-177, May-June, 1968.

"Resistance of human Neisseria species against desicca-

GONORRHEA

tion," by U. Berger, et al. ARCH HYG BAKT. 153:556-559, December, 1969.

"The sexually transmitted diseases. Infectious urethritis. Part 3. NM. 128:24+, February 14, 1969.

"The sins of the fathers," by A. D. G. Gunn. NM. 122:221, June 10, 1966.

"Trichomoniasis and gonorrhea," by D. F. Hawkins. BRIT MED J. 2:116, April 12, 1969.

"Trichomoniasis and gonorrhoea," by W. Tsao. BRIT MED J. 1:642-643, March 8, 1969.

"Virulence of gonococci," by D. S. Kellogg, Jr., et al. ANN REV MED. 20:323-328, 1969.

GONORRHEA: ANO-RECTAL

"Ano-rectal gonococcia," by J. Soullard, et al. ARCH FRANC MAL APPAR DIG. 59:Suppl:7-8:31+, July-August, 1970.

"Culture of gonococci from the rectum on Thayer and Martin's selective medium," by A. L. Heimans. DERMATOLOGICA. 133:319-324, 1966.

"Experience with a selective medium in the routine diagnosis of gonorrhoeae, with special regard to rectal gonorrhoae, with special regard to rectal gonorrhoae in women," by S. O. Roepstorff, et al. ACTA PATH MICROBIOL SCAND. 67:563-568, 1966.

"Some observations on the diagnosis of rectal gonorrhoea in both sexes using a selective culture medium," by J. Scott, et al. BRIT J VENER DIS. 42:103-106, June, 1966.

GONORRHEA: ARTHRITIC

"Arthritis and gonococcal infection." NEW ENG J MED. 279:268, August 1, 1968.

"Arthritis associated with gonorrhoea," by J. O. Partain, et al. ANN RHEUM DIS. 27:156-162, March, 1968.

"Arthritis gonorrhoea. Report of a case in pregnancy with negative GR in serum and positive GR in the synovial fluid," by A. Nielsen. UGESKR LAEG. 130:1867-1868, October 31, 1968.

GONORRHEA: ARTHRITIC

"Clinical forms of gonococcal arthritis," by H. Keiser, et al. NEW ENG J MED. 279:234-240, August 1, 1968.

"Clinical studies on gonococcal arthritis and Reiter's syndrome and measurement of gonococcal and Bedsonia antibodies," by J. T. Sharp, et al. ARTHRITIS RHEUM. 11:569-578, August, 1968.

"Gonococcal arthritis," by A. H. Johnson. J S CAROLINA MED ASS. 66:74-76, March, 1970.

"Gonococcal arthritis," by A. B. Kirsner, et al. MOD TREATM. 6:1130-1139, September, 1969.

"Gonococcal arthritis," by I. Kushner. J INFECT DIS. 120:387-388, September, 1969; also in MED TIMES. 98:111-116, June, 1970.

"Gonococcal arthritis," by R. M. Poske, et al. GP. 39:91-95, June, 1969.

"Gonococcal arthritis after treatment of gonorrhoea," by D. F. Marcus, et al. LANCET. 1:43-44, January 3, 1970.

"Gonococcal arthritis: a cause of monarticular disease," by J. H. Warner. J AMER COLL HEALTH ASS. 14:209-212, February, 1966.

"Gonococcal arthritis complicating gonorrheal pharyngitis," by A. L. Metzger. ANN INTERN MED. 73:267-269, August, 1970.

"Gonococcal arthritis in the newborn. Report of a case and review of the literature," by S. Glaser, et al. AMER J DIS CHILD. 112:185-188, September, 1966.

"Gonococcal arthritis in pregnancy," by J. H. Niles, et al. MED ANN DC. 35:69-70 passim, February, 1966.

"Gonococcal arthritis in pregnancy," by H. A. Taylor, et al. OBSTET GYNEC. 27:776-782, June, 1966.

"Gonococcal arthritis in pregnancy. Report of a case," by E. W. Parker, et al. N CAROLINA MED J. 28:433-436, October, 1967.

"Gonococcal arthritis in the young," by J. J. Calabro. NEW ENG J MED. 279:1002, October 31, 1968.

GONORRHEA: ARTHRITIC

"Gonococcal arthritis with pericarditis," by W. M. Vietzke. ARCH INTERN MED. 117:270-272, February, 1966.

"Gonorrhea: arthritis, septicemia and cutaneous manifestations, a case report," by B. C. Frichot 3rd, et al. J OKLA MED ASS. 60:597-600, November, 1967.

"Gonorrheal arthritis," by J. Grossman. NEW ENG J MED. 279:721, September 26, 1968.

"Gonorrheal arthritis. Report of a case in pregnancy with negative GR in serum and positive GR in the synovial fluid," by A. Nielsen. UGESKR LAEG. 130:1867-1868, October 31, 1968.

"Recent clinical experience in the management of gonococcal arthritis," by R. D. Altman. J FLORIDA MED ASS. 56:318-322, May, 1969.

GONORRHEA: BARTHOLINITIS

"Gonococcal bartholinitis," by E. Rees. BRIT J VENER DIS. 43:150-156, September, 1967.

"The treatment of bartholin abscesses and bartholin cysts," by H. G. Mayer. MED KLIN. 65:200-203, January 30, 1970.

GONORRHEA: CARDIOVASCULAR

"Gonococcal endocarditis with severe aortic regurgitation: Early valve replacement," by G. C. Voigt, et al. JOHNS HOPKINS MED J. 126:305-311, June, 1970.

GONORRHEA: CHILDREN

"The current prevalence of gonococcal infections in children," by L. F. Nazarian. PEDIATRICS. 39:372-377, March, 1967.

"Gonococcal peritonitis in a prepubertal child," by G. L. Fuld. AMER J DIS CHILD. 115:621-622, May, 1968.

"Gonorrhea in childhood," by R. Peter. CESK GYNEK. 31:606-609, October, 1966.

"Laboratory diagnosis of gonorrhea in premenarchal females and in adults," by T. C. Gallanis, et al. OBSTET GYNEC. 29:401-404, March, 1967.

"Sexually acquired gonorrhoeal urethritis in a 6-year-

GONORRHEA: CHILDREN

old boy," by N. J. Fiumara, et al. BRIT J VENER DIS. 45:254, September, 1969.

GONORRHEA: COMPLICATIONS

"Benign gonococcal sepsis with skin lesions," by A. Bjornberg, et al. BRIT J VENER DIS. 42:100-102, June, 1966.

"A case of chronic gonococcal folliculitis," by M. Skencić, et al. SRPSKI ARTH CELOK LEK. 94:403-407, April, 1966.

"The clinical picture of adnexitis as a complication of female gonorrhea," by J. Divis, et al. CESK GYNEK. 35:1-4, February, 1970.

"Complications of gonorrhea," by V. Starck. NORD MED. 76:811-812, July 14, 1966.

"Fulminating meningitis with Waterhouse-Friderichsen syndrome due to Neisseria gonorrhoeae," by J. A. Swierczewski, et al. AMER J CLIN PATH. 54:202-204, August, 1970.

"Gonococcal hemorrhagic bullae," by C. L. Roeth. NEW ENG J MED. 282:1105, May 7, 1970.

"Gonococcal salpingitis," by E. Rees, et al. BRIT J VENER DIS. 45:205-215, September, 1969.

"Gonococcus sepsis," by M. Svanbom, et al. NORD MED. 84:988, July 30, 1970.

"Gonococcal skin lesions. Report of a case of gonococcal ecthyma," by J. M. Glicksman, et al. ARCH DERM. 96:74-76, July, 1967.

"Gonococcus sepsis," by M. Svanbom, et al. NORD MED. 84:988, July 30, 1970.

"Gonorrhoea and non-specific urethritis," by B. H. Hill. NEW ZEAL MED J. 69:198-204, April, 1969.

"Gonorrhea: arthritis, septicemia and cutaneous manifestations, a case report," by B. C. Frichot, 3rd, et al. J OKLA MED ASS. 60:597-600, November, 1967.

"Gonorrhoea with skin and joint manifestations," by C. B. Wolff, et al. BRIT MED J. 1:271-273, May, 1970.

GONORRHEA: COMPLICATIONS

"Guide to adequate treatment of gonorrhoea complicated by staphylococcus albus," by R. L. Tawes, Jr. BRIT J VENER DIS. 42:155-161, September, 1966.

"Hemorrhagic bullae in gonococcemia," by A. B. Ackerman. NEW ENG J MED. 282:793-794, April 2, 1970.

"Herpesvirus cervicitis with gonorrhoea," by D. C. Hutfield. LANCET. 1:1311-1312, June 15, 1968.

"Herpesvirus hominis infection of the cervix associated with gonorrhoea," by J. O. Beilby, et al. LANCET. 1:1065-1066, May 18, 1968.

"Non-gonococcal urethritis acquired concomitantly with gonorrhoea in males," by J. D. Mahony. ULSTER MED J. 38:148-149, Summer, 1969.

"On postgonorrheo-posttrichomonas urethritis in men," by A. I. Lopatin. SOVET MED. 30:113-117, September, 1967.

"On the problem of gonorrheal and postgonorrheal urethritis," by J. Soltz-Szots, et al. WIEN MED WSCHR. 117:1030-1033, November 18, 1967.

"On the problem of isolated involvement of the paraurethal passages in gonorrheal infection," by A. V. Klimenko, et al. VESTN DERM VENER. 42:56-57, May, 1968.

"Post-gonorrhoea urethral stricture and hypertension in Nigeria," by E. A. Elebute. TRANS ROY SOC TROP MED HYG. 60:678-680, 1966.

"Problems of postgonorrhea urethritides," by V. Semrádová. CESK DERM. 45:181-183, August, 1970.

"Studies of venereal disease. II. Observations on the incidence, etiology, and treatment of the postgonococcal urethritis syndrome," by K. K. Holmes, et al. JAMA. 202:467-473, November 6, 1967.

"Two interesting case reports," by K. D. Lahiri. INDIAN J DERM. 15:31-32, October, 1969.

GONORRHEA: CONTRACEPTION
"Gonorrhoea and the intrauterine contraceptive device," by R. Statham, et al. BRIT MED J. 4:623-625, December 7, 1968.

GONORRHEA: CONTRACEPTION

"Influence of contraceptive gestogen pills on sexual behaviour and the spread of gonorrhoea," by L. Juhlin, et al. BRIT J VENER DIS. 45:321-324, December, 1969.

"The 'pill', promiscuity, and venereal disease," by L. Cohen. BRIT J VENER DIS. 46:108-110, April, 1970.

GONORRHEA: DIAGNOSIS

"Advances in bacteriologic diagnosis of gonorrhea," by U. Berger. DEUTSCH MED WSCHR. 92:847-850, May 5, 1967.

"Asymptomatic gonorrhea," by R. W. Thatcher, et al. JAMA. 210:315-317, October 13, 1969.

"Asymptomatic gonorrhea, the gonococcal carrier state, and gonococcemia in men," by A. B. Ackerman, et al. JAMA. 196:101-103, April 4, 1966.

"Bacteriological diagnosis, and treatment of gonococcal urethritis in the male," by O. J. Bravo, et al. MED TROP. 43:143-151, March-April, 1967.

"Benign gonococcal sepsis. A report of 36 cases," by A. Bjornberg. ACTA DERMATOVENER. 50:313-316, 1970.

"Chacko-Nair egg-enriched selected medium in the diagnosis of pathogenic Neisserieae," by C. W. Chacko, et al. BRIT J VENER DIS. 44:67-71, March, 1968.

"Combined use of fluorescent antibody technique and culture on selective medium for the identification of Neisseria gonorrhoeae," by I. Lind. ACTA PATH MICROBIOL SCAND. 76:279-287, 1969.

"Comments on the paper of Z. Truksa, P. Belák, P. Havlík: 'Contribution to the problem of supplementing the conventional diagnosis of gonorrhea by the fluorescent antibody technic'," by A. Kabátova. CESK EPIDEM. 17:63-64, January, 1968.

"Comparison of four culture media for the isolation of Neisseria gonorrhoeae: Correlation with the direct smear method," by S. A. Grady. CANAD J MED TECHN. 32:119-126, June, 1970.

"A complex diagnostic problem: the differentiation among gonococcal arthritis, Reiter's syndrome, and rheumatoid arthritis," by J. C. Brooks, Jr. J MED ASS. 56:291-296, July, 1967.

"Complications of gonorrhea." BRIT MED J. 3:420, August 22, 1970.

"Contribution to the bacterial diagnosis of gonorrhea," by M. Miljković, et al. VOJNOSANIT PREGL. 24:328-330, June, 1967.

"Contribution to laboratory problems in the diagnosis of gonorrhea," by E. Geizer, et al. CESK DERM. 43: 249-254, August, 1968.

"Contribution to the problems of supplementing the conventional diagnosis of gonorrhea by the fluorescent antibody technic," by Z. Truksa, et al. CESK EPIDEM. 16:81-90, March, 1967.

"Contribution to the problem of supplementing the conventional diagnosis of gonorrhea by the fluorescent antibody technic. Reply to comments of graduate biologist A. Kabátová," by Z. Truksa. CESK EPIDEM. 17: 64, January, 1968.

"Cultivation of gonococci on selective media," by A. Wierer, et al. CESK DERM. 43:27-30, February, 1968.

"A culture method suitable in general practice for the diagnosis of gonorrhea," by H. A. Hirsch, et al. ARCH HYG BAKT. 153:473-477, October, 1969.

"Culture of gonococci. Advantages of culture in the diagnosis and treatment of gonorrhea," by K. Odegaard. T NORSK LAEGEFOREN. 86:791-793, May 15, 1966.

"Culture of gonococci from the rectum on Thayer and Martin's selective medium," by A. L. Heimans. DERMATOLOGICA. 133:319-324, 1966.

"Current problems of the diagnosis and therapy of gonorrhea," by I. M. Porudominskii, et al. VESTN DERM VENER. 41:40-46, May, 1967.

"Cytomorphologic analyses of smears from the male urethra in urethritis of gonococcal and non-gonococcal origin," by B. Lagerholm, et al. ACTA DERMATOVENER. 46:457-459, 1966.

GONORRHEA: DIAGNOSIS

"Demonstration of gonorrhea using the immunofluorescent technic. I. Methodical remarks," by V. Potuznik, et al. CESK EPIDEM. 16:163-167, May, 1967.

"Detection of Neisseria gonorrhoeae by means of fluorescent antibody technique. II. Clinical appraisal," by I. Saito. JAP J UROL. 58:1079-1091, October, 1967.

"Detection of Neisseria gonorrhoeae in clinical material by fluorescent antibodies," by L. Zelenkova, et al. CESK EPIDEM. 16:345-349, November, 1967.

"The diagnosis and management of gonorrhea," by A. B. Greaves. MED ANN DC. 35:369-371, July, 1966.

"Diagnosis and therapy of chronic female gonorrhea," by J. Kvicera, et al. CESK DERM. 45:241-242, September, 1970.

"Diagnosis and treatment of gonorrhea in the female," by J. B. Lucas, et al. NEW ENG J MED. 276:1454-1459, June 29, 1967.

"Diagnosis of gonorrhea by a fluorescent antibody technique," by R. P. Mouton. DERMATOLOGICA. 132:343-352. 1966.

"Diagnosis of gonorrhea by the immunofluorescente technic. 3. Delayed immunofluorescence test and its comparison with cultivation on a selective medium," by V. Potuznik, et al. CESK DERM. 43:273-276, August, 1968.

"Diagnosis of gonorrhea in the asymptomatic female: comparison of slide and culture technics," by H. Pariser, et al. SOUTHERN MED J. 61:505-506, May, 1968.

"The diagnosis of gonorrhea in females," by O. I. Haavelsrud. T NORSK LAEGEFOREN. 90:1220-1222, June 1, 1970.

"Diagnosis of gonorrhea in women," by V. N. Aristova. FELDSH AKUSH. 33:19-21, February, 1968.

"Diagnosis of gonorrhea with fluorescent antibodies," by D. Danielsson. NORD MED. 76:805-806, July 14, 1966.

"Diagnosis of vaginal discharge," by R. D. Catterall.

GONORRHEA: DIAGNOSIS

BRIT J VENER DIS. 46:122-124, April, 1970.

"Diagnosis of vaginal discharges. Another approach to an old problem," by G. J. Dennerstein. MED J AUST. 1:992-994, May 16, 1970.

"Diagnostic and therapeutic problems in gonorrhea," by K. Holzegel. DEUTSCH GESUNDH. 23:1172-1176, June 20, 1968.

"Diagnostic problems in gonorrhea," by L. O. Kallings, et al. NORD MED. 76:800-803, July 14, 1966.

"Do results of culture for gonococci vary with sampling phase of menstrual cycle?," by V. Falk, et al. ACTA DERMATOVENER. 47:190-193, 1967.

"An easily prepared selective medium for the cultivation of Neisseria gonorrhoeae," by C. R. Amies, et al. BRIT J VENER DIS. 43:137-139, June, 1967.

"Epidemic pediculosis and gonorrhea," by A. Altchek. OBSTET GYNEC. 35:638-641, April, 1970.

"An evaluation of gonorrhea case findings in the chronically infected female," by D. W. Johnson, et al. AMER J EPIDEM. 90:438-448, November, 1969.

"Experience with a rapid direct immunofluorescent test for the gonococcus as a 'bench'procedure in venereal disease clinics," by R. A. Henderson, et al. BRIT J VENER DIS. 46:205-208, June, 1970.

"Experience with a selective medium in the routine diagnosis of gonorrhoeae, with special regard to rectal gonorrhoae in women," by S. O. Roepstorff, et al. ACTA PATH MICROBIOL SCAND. 67:563-568, 1966.

"Gonococcal complement fixation reaction in patients with lung diseases in Greenland," by P. K. Lange, et al. UGESKR LAEG. 128:409-415, April 7, 1966.

"The gonococcal dermatitis syndrome. Demonstration of gonococci in skin lesions by immunofluorescence," by D. Danielsson, et al. ACTA DERMATOVENER. 46:256-261, 1966.

"Gonorrhoea," by E. Rees. LANCET. 1:572-573, March 14, 1970.

GONORRHEA: DIAGNOSIS

"Gonorrhea in the obstetric clinic," by D. S. Friendly. JAMA. 211:124, January 5, 1970.

"Gonorrheal arthritis. Report of a case in pregnancy with negative GR in serum and positive GR in the synovial fluid," by A. Nielsen. UGESKR LAEG. 130: 1867-1868, October 31, 1968.

"Identification of Neisseria gonorrhoeae by means of fluorescent antibody technique," by I. Lind. ACTA PATH MICROBIOL SCAND. 70:613-629, 1967.

"The immunofluorescence technic of gonococcus determination," by C. Simon, et al. MUNCHEN MED WSCHR. 109: 856-859, April 14, 1967.

"Immunofluorescent antibody technique in the diagnosis of gonorrhoea by direct smears from the female," by J. M. Gallwey, et al. BRIT J VENER DIS. 43:168-169, September, 1967.

"Immunofluorescent method for diagnosis of gonorrhoea in women," by R. N. Thin. BRIT J VENER DIS. 46:27-30, February, 1970.

"Improved medium selective for cultivation of N. gonorrhoeae and N. meningitidis," by J. D. Thayer, et al. PUBLIC HEALTH REP. 81:559-562, June, 1966.

"Improved methods for gonococcal sampling and examination on a large scale," by B. Gastrin, et al. ACTA PATH MICROBIOL SCAND. 74:362-370, 1968.

"Isolation of Neisseria gonorrhoeae in asymptomatic women," by R. V. Victoria, et al. REV INVEST SALUD PUBLICA. 28:119-126, April-June, 1968.

"Laboratory diagnosis of chronic forms of female gonorrhea," by K. L. Keburlia. VESTN DERM VENER. 41:50-53, March, 1967.

"The laboratory diagnosis of gonorrhoea in the female," by J. T. O'Brien, et al. NEW ZEAL MED J. 69:204-206, April, 1969.

"Laboratory diagnosis of gonorrhea in premenarchal females and in adults," by T. C. Gallanis, et al. OBSTET GYNEC. 29:401-404, March, 1967.

GONORRHEA: DIAGNOSIS

"Long-term cultivation of N. gonorrhoeae in tissue culture," by M. Gavrilescu, et al. BRIT J VENER DIS. 42:171-174, September, 1966.

"Method for preparing Neisseria gonorrhoeae fluorescent antibody conjugate," by W. L. Peacock, Jr. PUBLIC HEALTH REP. 85:733-738, August, 1970.

"Modified gram staining of smears in the diagnosis of gonorrhea," by M. K. Kuznetsova. LAB DELO. 9:554-555, 1966.

"Necessity for and technic of cultural diagnosis of gonococcus," by F. Fegeler. ARCH KLIN EXP DERM. 227:630-633, 1966.

"Neisseria gonorrhoeae. II. Colonial variation and pathogenicity during 35 months in vitro," by D. S. Kellogg, Jr., et al. J BACT. 96:596-605, September, 1968.

"A new fluid medium for cultivating gonococci," by M. Lazar, et al. RUM MED REV. 13:47-48, July-September, 1969.

"Observations on the culture diagnosis of gonorrhea in women," by J. D. Schmale, et al. JAMA. 210:312-314, October 13, 1969.

"The occurrence of Neisseria gonorrhoeae in 'routine' genital cultures," by P. D. Ellner. AMER J CLIN PATH. 52:174-175, August, 1969.

"The occurrence of oxidase-positive nongonococcal strains on Thayer-Martin selective media used in the laboratory diagnosis of N. gonorrhoeae," by E. Geizer. ZBL BAKT. 214:75-78, 1970.

"On my initial experiences with the immunofluorescence method for detection of gonococci," by H. Medebach. MED WELT. 39:2100-2105, September 28, 1968.

"On the value of routinely conducted swab examinations of the urethra and cervix of all clinical admissions in gynecology to discover all formerly unknown cases of gonorrhea," by C. Zwahr. ZBL GYNAEK. 90:1192-1196, August 31, 1968.

"Oral contraception among special clinic patients. With

particular reference to the diagnosis of gonorrhoea," by A. B. Hewitt. BRIT J VENER DIS. 46:106-107, April, 1970.

"Preliminary report on a mass program for detection of gonorrhea," by J. Zackler, et al. PUBLIC HEALTH REP. 85:681-684, August, 1970.

"Present problems of the epidemiology and diagnosis of gonorrhea," by J. Bartunek, et al. CESK DERM. 43: 31-38, February, 1968.

"Primary isolation of N. gonorrhoeae with a new commercial medium," by J. E. Martin, Jr., et al. PUBLIC HEALTH REP. 82:361-363, April, 1967.

"Primary isolation of Neisseria gonorrhoeae on hemoglobin-free Thayer-Martin medium," by D. M. Pariser, et al. PUBLIC HEALTH REP. 85:532-534, June, 1970.

"Proof of gonorrhea by the immunofluorescent technic. II. Comparison of the cultivation and immunofluorescent technics," by V. Potuznik, et al. CESK DERM. 42:86-90, April, 1967.

"Quick cytochrome oxidase test for the detection of gonococcal urethritis," by G. C. Fuga, et al. MINERVA DERM. 42:647-648, December, 1967.

"Rapid biochemical presumptive test for gonorrheal urethritis in the male," by A. H. Pedersen, et al. PUBLIC HEALTH REP. 81:318-322, April, 1966.

"Reappearance of gonorrhea and its diagnosis using the gonorrhea reaction," by E. Russo. HOSPITAL. 76:1693-1713, November, 1969.

"Recent developments in the laboratory diagnosis of gonococcal infections," by A. Reyn. BULL WHO. 40: 245-255, 1969.

"Recovery of the gonococcus from exudates dried on filter paper," by C. F. Pait, et al. HEALTH LAB SCI. 7:30-33, January, 1970.

"Reliable and practical procedure for the diagnosis of gonorrhea," by H. A. Hirsch, et al. MED KLIN. 64: 2193-2196, November 21, 1969.

GONORRHEA: DIAGNOSIS

"Screening test for gonorrhea in male suspects," by D. S. Kwalick, JAMA. 213:626, July 27, 1970.

"Selective culture media in the microbiologic diagnosis of gonorrhea," by V. Potuznik. CESK DERM. 42:173-174, June, 1967.

"Septic gonococcal dermatitis. Demonstration of gonococci and gonococcal antigens in skin lesions by immunofluorescence," by G. Kahn, et al. ARCH DERM. 99:421-425, April, 1969.

"Sero-diagnosis of gonorrhoea with a microprecipitin test using a lipopolysaccharide antigen from N. gonorrhoeae," by C. W. Chacko, et al. BRIT J VENER DIS. 45:33-39, March, 1969.

"Serologic detection of gonorrhea," by E. V. Hess, et al. ANN INTERN MED. 73:340-341, August, 1970.

"Serologic detection of gonorrhea," by J. D. Schmale. ANN INTERN MED. 72:593-595, April, 1970.

"Serological cross-reactions of aqueous ether extracted endotoxin from Neisseria gonorrhoeae strains," by J. A. Maeland. ACTA PATH MICROBIOL SCAND. 77:505-517, 1969.

"Serological properties of aqueous ether extracted endotoxin from Neisseria gonorrhoeae," by J. A. Maeland. ACTA PATH MICROBIOL SCAND. 77:495-504, 1969.

"Simplified method for the preparation of selective culture media used in microbiological diagnosis of gonorrhea," by V. Potuznik. CESK DERM. 43:321-322, October, 1968.

"A study of the causes of diagnostic discrepancies in the examination of women who are sources of gonorrhea infection," by E. N. Turanova, et al. VESTN DERM VENER. 41:69-71, September, 1967.

"Typing the gonococcus (letter to editor)," by R. I. Hutchinson. BRIT MED J. 3:107, July 11, 1970.

"Urethritis in infection with germs of the Miamae group as a contribution to the differential diagnosis of gonorrhea," by U. Heyl, et al. HAUTARZT. 19:463-465, October, 1968.

GONORRHEA: DIAGNOSIS

"'Urinary tract infection' in women caused by gonococci," by V. Starck. LAKARTIDNINGEN. 67:3206-3210, July 8, 1970.

"Use of vancomyin, colistimethate, nystatin medium to transport gonococcal specimens," by M. H. Robinson, et al. PUBLIC HEALTH REP. 85:390-392, May, 1970.

"Usefulness of the fluorescent antibody method for the demonstration of gonococci in routine work," by K. L. Wendland, et al. ARCH HYG BAKT. 151:118-123, May, 1967.

GONORRHEA: EDUCATION
SEE ALSO: YOUTH

"Factors influencing the spread of gonorrhea. I. Educational and social behavior," by L. Juhlin. ACTA DERMATOVENER. 48:75-81, 1968.

"Gonorrhea: growing menace to your students." SCH MGT. 12:36-42, August, 1968; also in PA SCH J. 117:414-419, March, 1969.

"Participation of health education in prevention of gonorrhea in the age catagories 15-24 years," by M. Beniak. CESK ZDRAV. 15:249-254, May, 1967.

GONORRHEA: ENDOCARDITIS
"Bacterial endocarditis due to Neisseria perflava in a patient hypersensitive to penicillin," by A. B. Breslin, et al. AUST ANN MED. 16:245-249, August, 1967.

GONORRHEA: EXPERIMENTAL
"Serum antibody response in experimental human gonorrhoea. Immunoglobulins G, A, and M," by I. R. Cohen, et al. BRIT J VENER DIS. 45:325-327, December, 1969.

GONORRHEA: HEPATIC
"Gonococcal perihepatitis in a male. The Fitz-Hugh-Curtis syndrome," by M. W. Kimball, et al. NEW ENG J MED. 282:1082-1084, May 7, 1970.

GONORRHEA: HISTORY
SEE ALSO: OCCURRENCE
SOCIOLOGY
STATISTICS

"Albert Neisser (1855-1916, the discoverer of the diplo-

GONORRHEA: HISTORY

coccus of gonorrhea," by E. Stocki. WIAD LEK. 20: 397-398, February 15, 1967.

"Boswell's clap," by W. B. Ober. JAMA. 212:91-95, April 6, 1970.

"The gonorrhea problem. 2-years data," by H. B. Svindland. T NORSK LAEGEFOREN. 24:2252-2255, December 15, 1968.

"Occurrence of gonorrhea in the last 10 years," by J. Obrtel, et al. CESK DERM. 43:22-26, February, 1968.

"Occurrence of gonorrhea in our material during the past 10 years," by V. Plintovic, et al. CESK GYNEK. 35:269-271, 1970.

GONORRHEA: IMMUNOLOGY

"Antibodies in human sera against antigens in gonococci, demonstrated by a passive haemolysis test," by J. A. Maeland. ACTA PATH MICROBIOL SCAND. 67:102-110, 1966.

"Development of gonococcal sensitivity," by P. Durel, et al. PATH BIOL. 15:1197-1203, December, 1967.

"Development of resistance of gonococci to penicillin: an eight-year study," by C. R. Amies. CANAD MED ASS J. 96:33-35, January 7, 1967.

"Immunochemical characterization of aqueous ether extracted endotoxin from Neisseria gonorrhoeae," by J. A. Maeland. ACTA PATH MICROBIOL SCAND. 76:484-492, 1969.

"Is gonococcal sensitivity to antibiotics increasing in Norway," by K. Odegaard, et al. BRIT J VENER DIS. 43:284-286, December, 1967.

"Isolation of an antigen of Neisseria gonorrhoeae involved in the human immune response to gonococcal infection," by J. D. Schmale, et al. J BACT. 99:469-471, August, 1969.

"Natural and immune human antibodies reactive with antigens of virulent Neisseria gonorrhoeae: immunoglobulins G, M, and A," by I. R. Cohen. J BACT. 94:141-148, July, 1967.

"The relationship between complete and incomplete anti-

GONORRHEA: IMMUNOLOGY

bodies in various manifestations of gonorrhea," by N. I. Tumasheva, et al. VESTN DERM VENER. 42:69-73. November, 1968.

"Serum antibody response in experimental human gonorrhea. Immunoglobulins G, A, and M," by I. R. Cohen, et al. BRIT J VENER DIS. 45:325-327, December, 1969.

GONORRHEA: MICROBIOLOGY

"Gonococci in urethral exudates possess a virulence factor lost on subculture," by M. E. Ward, et al. NATURE. 227:382-384, July 25, 1970.

"Microbiology of the Neisseria group," by H. Storck, et al. ARCH KLIN EXP DERM. 227:623-630, 1966.

GONORRHEA: MORPHOLOGY

"Colonial morphology of Neisseria gonorrhoeae isolated from males and females," by P. F. Sparling, et al. J BACT. 93:513, January, 1967.

GONORRHEA: NEONATAL

"The clinical picture of gonorrhea with special reference to infections of eye in newborn infants," by V. Resl. CESK OFTAL. 22:333-334, September, 1966.

"Crede's method for the prevention of gonorrheal blennorrhea in newborn infants," by J. van Doesschate. NEDERL T GENEESK. 112:1088-1090, June 8, 1968.

"Gonoblenorrhea neonatorum in spite of Crede's preventive method," by P. Kober. MED KLIN. 62:424-426, March 17, 1967.

"Gonococcal arthritis in the newborn. Report of a case and review of the literature," by S. Glaser, et al. AMER J DIS CHILD. 112:185-188, September, 1966.

"Gonococcal conjunctivitis of the newborn," by D. S. Friendly. CLIN PROC CHILD HOSP DC. 25:1-9, January, 1969.

"Gonococcal ophthalmia among newborn infants at Los Angeles County General Hospital, 1957-1963," by W. M. Brown, Jr., et al. PUBLIC HEALTH REP. 81:926-928, October, 1966.

"The hazards of Crede's prophylaxis of neonatal blennorrhea," by V. J. Mathesius. GYNAECOLOGIA. 164:

GONORRHEA: NEONATAL

274-278, 1967.

"Mediosocial background to gonococcal ophthalmia neonatorum," by C. B. Schofield. LANCET. 2:1182-1185, November 29, 1969.

"The occurrence of gonorrhoeal ophthalmia neonatorum and the efficiency of prophylaxis," by K. Osterlund, et al. ANN PAEDIAT FENN. 14:23-25, 1968.

GONORRHEA: OCCURRENCE
SEE ALSO: EDUCATION
HISTORY
PREVENTION & CONTROL
SOCIOLOGY

"Analysis of the causes for the increase of gonorrhea in Slovakia," by E. Hegyi, et al. BRATISL LEK LISTY. 47:341-354, March 31, 1967.

"Comparative study of the composition of groups of patients with gonorrhea who came for treatment in 1954-1956 and 1964-1966," by C. H. Beek. NEDERL T GENEESK. 112:989-991, May 25, 1968.

"Effect of the development of social hygiene on the occurrence of gonorrhea," by A. Perdrup. ARCH KLIN EXP DERM. 227:640-644, 1966.

"Epidemiologic problems of venereal diseases," by K. Kalbarczyk. PRZEGL DERM. 54:655-658, November-December, 1967.

"Epidemiology of lues and gonorrhea in Northrhine Westphalia from 1948 to 1968," by K. Gedicke. OEFF GESUNDHEITSWESEN. 32:218-226, May, 1970.

"An estimate of the risk of men acquiring gonorrhea by sexual contact with infected females," by K. K. Holmes, et al. AMER J EPIDEM. 91:170-174, February, 1970.

"Factors influencing the incidence of gonorrhoea and non-gonococcal urethritis in men in an industrial city," by L. Z. Oller, et al. BRIT J VENER DIS. 46:96-102, April, 1970.

"Factors influencing the spread of gonorrhea. I. Educational and social behavior," by L. Juhlin. ACTA

GONORRHEA: OCCURRENCE

DERMATOVENER. 48:75-81, 1968.

"Factors influencing the spread of gonorrhea. II. Sexual behavior at different ages," by L. Juhlin. ACTA DERMATOVENER. 48:82-89, 1968.

"Gonorrhea--an alarming comeback." AM DRUGGIST. 157: 37+, March 25, 1968.

"Gonorrhoea and the iceberg phenomenon," by W. J Brown. BRIT J VENER DIS. 46:118-121, April, 1970.

"Gonorrhea--frequently unrecognized reservoirs," by H. Pariser, et al. SOUTHERN MED J. 63:198-201, February, 1970.

"Gonorrhoea in a country town," by M. J. Loughlin. NEW ZEAL MED J. 69:195-198, April, 1969.

"Gonorrhea in Czechoslovakia during the years 1960-1966," by K. Kopecký, et al. CESK EPIDEM. 17:356-363, October, 1968.

"Gonorrhoea in 1964. Cases treated at the Department of Dermatology, Karoliska Sjukhuset," by A. Lodin, et al. ACTA DERMATOVENER. 46:245-249, 1966.

"Gonorrhoea in 1966. Cases treated at the Department of Dermatology, Karolinska Sjukhuset," by L. Gip, et al. ACTA DERMATOVENER. 48:272-276, 1968.

"Gonorrhoea in 1968," by L. Molin. ACTA DERMATOVENER. 50:157-160, 1970.

"Gonorrhea in the obstetric and gynecologic clinic. Incidence in a voluntary hospital in an urban community," by V. G. Cave, et al. JAMA. 210:309-311, October 13, 1969.

"Gonorrhea in recent years," by H. Okuma. JAP J UROL. 58:937, September, 1967.

"The gonorrhea situation in Greenland and the epidemiological control of this disease," by G. Lomholt. ARCH KLIN EXP DERM. 227:644-645, 1966.

"Gonorrhoea situation in South Greenland in the summer of 1964," by G. Lomholt, et al. BRIT J VENER DIS. 42:1-7, March, 1966.

GONORRHEA: OCCURRENCE

"Gonorrhoea study, 1966." BRIT J VENER DIS. 44:55-62, March, 1968.

"Gonorrhoea study, 1967," by British Cooperative Clinical Group. BRIT J VENER DIS. 44:299-306, December, 1968.

"Gonorrhoea study, 1968," by British Cooperative Clinical Group. BRIT J VENER DIS. 46:62-68, February, 197.

"Gonorrhoeal frequency continues to increase. The importance of medical factors," by S. Lidén. LAKARTIDNINGEN. 66:907-911, February 26, 1969.

"Gonorrheal reinfections among men treated at the dispensary of the Department of Dermatology in Cracow in 1962-1967," by I. Prorok. PRZEGL DERM. 56:735-739, 1969.

"Incidence of gonococci relatively resistant to penicillin occurring in the Southampton area of England during 1958 to 1965," by R. M. Warren. BRIT J VENER DIS. 44:80-81, March, 1968.

"Increase in gonorrhea in the Eastern Bohemian region and some problems of the antivenereal fight," by Z. Kraus. CESK DERM. 43:56-61, February, 1968.

"Influence of contraceptive gestogen pills on sexual behaviour and the spread of gonorrhoea," by L. Juhlin, et al. BRIT J VENER DIS. 45:321-324, December, 1969.

"Medico-epidemiologic problems posed by masculine gonococcal urethritis (apropos of 10,000 cases)," by A. Siboulet, et al. BULL INST NAT SANTE. 21:737-780, July-August, 1966.

"On the epidemiologic situation in the sector of venereal disease in the Western Slovakia region," by E. Hegyi, et al. CESK DERM. 43:65-71, February, 1968.

"On gonorrhea and moniliasis in Finnish battalion 8 on Cyprus in winter 1967-1968," by E. E. Vuori, et al. SOTILASIAAK AIKAK. 43:126-129, 1968.

"On the morbidity of gonorrhea in railway workers," by M. M. Vilenskii, et al. VESTN DERM VENER. 43:61-

GONORRHEA: OCCURRENCE

62, January, 1969.

"On the status of gonorrhea in women," by B. Holzegel, et al. Z AERZTI FORTBILD. 60:82-88, January 15, 1966.

"One hundred teenagers in Copenhagen infected with gonorrhoea. A socio-psychiatric study," by K. Ekstrom. BRIT J VENER DIS. 42:162-166, September, 1966.

"Relative incidence of Corynebacterium vaginale (Haemophilus vaginalis), Neisseria gonorrhoeae, and trichomonas spp. among women attending a venereal disease clinic," by W. E. Dunkelberg, Jr., et al. BRIT J VENER DIS. 46:187-190, June, 1970.

"Remarks on the reports of regional dermatovenerologists," by J. Obrtel. CESK DERM. 43:39-42, February, 1968.

"Report on a phantom epidemic of gonorrhea," by J. S. Mausner, et al. AMER J EPIDEM. 85:320-331, March, 1967.

"Sociomedical study of young gonorrhea patients," by B. H. Hatt. NORD MED. 76:816, July 14, 1966.

"A survey of trichomonal and Neisserian infection in antenatal patients," by R. Gaal, et al. MED J AUST. 1:634-635, April 13, 1968.

"A survey of trichomonal and Neisserian infection in antenatal patients," by R. A. Osborn, et al. MED J AUST. 2:92, July 13, 1968.

"Town and country in the spreading of venereal diseases," by J. Kolankowski. PRZEGL DERM. 54:651-653, November-December, 1967.

GONORRHEA: OPHTHALMOLOGY

"The clinical picture of gonorrhea with special reference to infections of eye in newborn infants," by V. Resl. CESK OFTAL. 22:333-334, September, 1966.

"Gonococcal conjunctivitis of the newborn," by D. S. Friendly. CLIN PROC CHILD HOSP DC. 25:1-9, January, 1969.

"Gonococcal ophthalmia among newborn infants at Los

GONORRHEA: OPHTHALMOLOGY

Angeles County General Hospital, 1957-1963," by W. M. Brown, Jr., et al. PUBLIC HEALTH REP. 81:926-928, October, 1966.

"Gonorrheal conjunctivitis an old disease returned," by T. Hansen, et al. JAMA. 195:1156, March 28, 1966.

"Medicosocial background to gonococcal ophthalmia neonatorum," by C. B. Schofield. LANCET. 2:1182-1185, November 29, 1969.

"The occurrence of gonorrhoeal ophthalmia neonatorum and the efficiency of prophylaxis," by K. Osterlund, et al. ANN PAEDIAT FENN. 14:23-25, 1968.

"Prophylaxis against gonorrhoeal ophthalmia," by V. G. Cave. JAMA. 212:630, April 27, 1970.

"Pseudogonococcal ophthalmia infection with Herellea vaginicola," by J. P. Canby. MED J AUST. 2:1104-1105, December 14, 1968.

"Specific prophylaxis of gonorrheal ophthalmia neonatorum. A review," by P. C. Barsam. NEW ENG J MED. 274:731-734, March 31, 1966.

"Treatment of penicillin-resistant gonococcal conjunctivitis with ampicillin," by G. L. Spaeth. AMER J OPHTHAL. 66:427-429, September, 1968.

GONORRHEA: PENILE

"Gonococcal penile ulcer," by S. Haim, et al. BRIT J VENER DIS. 46:336-337, August, 1970.

"Gonorrhoea of a congenital duct in the raphe penis," by H. Diabalová, et al. ACTA DERMATOVENER. 49:202-205, 1969.

"Gonorrheal abscess of preputium as a late complication of gonorrheal urethritis," by M. Skencič. SRPSKI ARH CELOK LEK. 97:805-809, July-August, 1969.

GONORRHEA: PERITONITIS

"Gonococcal peritonitis in a prepubertal child," by G. L. Fuld. AMER J DIS CHILD. 115:621-622, May, 1968.

GONORRHEA: PHARYNGEAL

"Gonococcal arthritis complicting gonorrheal pharyn-

GONORRHEA: PHARYNGEAL

gitis," by A. L. Metzger. ANN INTERN MED. 73:267-269, August, 1970.

"Gonorrheal pharyngitis," by N. J. Fiumara, et al. NEW ENG J MED. 276:1248-1250, June 1, 1967.

GONORRHEA: PREGNANCY

"Arthritis gonorrhoea. Report of a case in pregnancy with negative GR in serum and positive GR in the synovial fluid," by A. Nielsen. UGESKR LAEG. 130: 1867-1868, October 31, 1968.

"Gonococcal arthritis in pregnancy," by J. H. Niles, et al. MED ANN DC. 35:69-70 passim, February, 1966.

"Gonococcal arthritis in pregnancy," by H. A. Taylor, et al. OBSTET GYNEC. 27:776-782, June, 1966.

"Gonococcal arthritis in pregnancy. Report of a case," by E. W. Parker, et al. N CAROLINA MED J. 28:433-436, October, 1967.

"Gonococcal infection in a prenatal clinic," by J. R. Waters, et al. AMER J OBSTET GYNEC. 103:532-536, February 15, 1969.

"Gonorrhea during pregnancy," by G. W. Kraus, et al. OBSTET GYNEC. 31:258-260, February, 1968.

"Gonorrhea in the obstetric and gynecologic clinic. Incidence in a voluntary hospital in an urban community," by V. G. Cave, et al. JAMA. 210:309-311, October 13, 1969.

"Gonorrhea in the obstetric clinic," by D. S. Friendly. JAMA. 211:124, January 5, 1970.

"Gonorrhoea, trichomoniasis and yeast infection in late pregnancy in an unselected series of gravidae," by E. Purola, et al. ANN CHIR GYNAEC FENN. 56:95-98, 1967.

"Gonorrheal arthritis. Report of a case in pregnancy with negative GR in serum and positive GR in the synovial fluid," by A. Nielsen. UGESKR LAEG. 130: 1867-1868, October 31, 1968.

"Perinatal mastocytosis. Gonococcal infection in the mother," by C. Grupper, et al. BULL SOC FRANC DERM

GONORRHEA: PREGNANCY

SYPH. 73:847-849, December, 1966.

"Symptomatic gonorrhea during pregnancy," by P. M. Sarrel, et al. OBSTET GYNEC. 32:670-673, November, 1968.

GONORRHEA: PREVENTION & CONTROL

"Achievements in the field of gonorrhea control," by I. M. Porudominskii, et al. VESTN DERM VENER. 41: 27-36, October, 1967.

"Alabama Department of Public Health: state activates gonorrhoea control project," by C. G. Lamar. J MED ASS ALABAMA. 38:631-632, January, 1969.

"Contact investigation of male West Indian patients with gonorrhoea," by R. R. Willcox, et al. BRIT J VENER DIS. 42:167-170, September, 1966.

"Control examinations in gonorrhea," by G. Brundin, et al. LAKARTIDNINGEN. 66:912-917, February 26, 1969.

"Cooperation of the gynecologist, dermato-venerologist and bacteriologist in the fight against gonorrhea in the woman," by J. Obrtel. CESK DERM. 42:351-356, October, 1967.

"The essence of gonorrhoea control. 3. The delineation of the male: female source ratio," by R. R. Willcox. ACTA DERMATOVENER. 46:250-256, 1966.

--IV. The promiscuous female pool." ACTA DERMATOVENER. 46:460-465, 1966.

--V. The influence of promiscuity." ACTA DERMATOVENER. 47:65-69, 1967.

"Gonorrhea getting out of control." AM DRUGGIST. 161: 49-50, April 6, 1970.

"Gonorrhea: not yet controllable," by W. J. Brown. ANN INTERN MED. 72:280-281, February, 1970.

"Gonorrhea--a public-health problem." J IOWA MED SOC. 57:376-377, April, 1967.

"Identification of the asymptomatic female carrier of N. gonorrhoeae. Treatment with ampicillin," by E. S.

GONORRHEA: PREVENTION & CONTROL

Allen. BRIT J VENER DIS. 46:334-335, August, 1970.

"Neisseria control," by S. E. Acres. MED SERV J CANADA. 22:288-289, April, 1966.

"New data in the area of dermatology-venereology obtained at the chair of the Lvov Medical Institute," by A. A. Shtein. VESTN DERM VENER. 43:3-6, June, 1969.

"New developments in venereal disease research," by J. B. Lucas. MED ANN DC. 35:375-378 passim, July, 1966.

"On methods of control of cure of female gonorrhea," by IuN. Dobrovol'skii. VESTN DERM VENER. 40:73-75, January, 1966.

"On some organizational measures necessary for further reduction of gonorrhea incidence," by Z. P. Poliakova. VESTN DERM VENER. 40:84-87, September, 1966.

GONORRHEA: PROSTITUTES
"Gonorrhoea among prostitutes," by B. G. Wren. MED J AUST. 1:847-849, April 29, 1967.

"Sensitivity of gonococci to antibiotics in strains isolated from 'prosititutes' in Copenhagen," by A. Nielsen. BRIT J VENER DIS. 46:153-155, April, 1970.

GONORRHEA: PSEUDOGONORRHEA
"Casuistic contribution on the practical significance of so-called pseudogonorrhea," by H. J. Conraths. ARCH KLIN EXP DERM. 227:645-650, 1966.

GONORRHEA: SERODIAGNOSIS
SEE: DIAGNOSIS

GONORRHEA: SEROLOGY
"Antigenic determinants of aqueous ether extracted endotoxin from Neisseria gonorrhoeae," by J. A. Maeland. ACTA PATH MICROBIAL SCAND. 76:475-483, 1969.

"Antigenic properties of various preparations of Neisseria gonorrhoeae endotoxin," by J. A. Maeland. ACTA PATH MICROBIOL SCAND. 73:413-422, 1968.

"Antigens of Neisseria gonorrhoeae: Characterization by gel filtration, complement fixation, and agar-gel diffusion of antigens of gonococcal protoplasm," by

GONORRHEA: SEROLOGY

    D. G. Danielsson, et al. J BACT. 97:1012-1017, March, 1969.

GONORRHEA: SERVICEMEN
"Gonococcal urethritis in males in Vietnam: three penicillin regimens and one tetracycline regimen," by L. H. Maurer, et al. JAMA. 207:946-948, February 3, 1969.

"Gonococcal urethritis in Vietnam," by R. W. Dang. JAMA. 208:867, May 5, 1969.

GONORRHEA: SOCIOLOGY
SEE ALSO: HISTORY
          OCCURRENCE
          STATISTICS

"An analysis of some characteristics of males with gonorrhoea," by L. H. Glass. BRIT J VENER DIS. 43:128-132, June, 1967.

"The changes in age structure of patients with gonorrhea during the past years," by V. Sedlácek. CESK DERM. 42:108-114, April, 1967.

"Comparative study of the composition of groups of patients with gonorrhea who came for treatment in 1954-1956 and 1964-1966," by C. H. Beek. NEDERL T GENEESK. 112:989-991, May 25, 1968.

"Effect of the development of social hygiene on the occurrence of gonorrhea," by A. Perdrup. ARCH KLIN EXP DERM. 227:640-644, 1966.

"Emotional problems of gonorrhoea," by S. E. Mbanefo. J ROY COLL GEN PRACT. 15:272-279, April, 1968.

"Factors influencing the spread of gonorrhea. I. Educational and social behavior," by L. Juhlin. ACTA DERMATOVENER. 48:75-81, 1968.

--II. Sexual behavior at different ages." ACTA DERMATOVENER. 48:82-89, 1968.

"One hundred teenagers in Copenhagen infected with gonorrhoea. A socio-psychiatric study," by K. Ekstrom. BRIT J VENER DIS. 42:162-166, September, 1966.

GONORRHEA: SOCIOLOGY

"Sociomedical study of young gonorrhea patients," by B. H. Hatt. NORD MED. 76:816, July 14, 1966.

"Sociopsychiatric investigation of teenage girls with gonorrhea," by L. Palmgren. ACTA PSYCHIAT SCAND. 42:295-314, 1966.

GONORRHEA: TONGUE

"Gonococcal ulceration of the tongue in the gonococcal dermatitis syndrome," by L. Cowan. BRIT J VENER DIS. 45:228-231, September, 1969.

GONORRHEA: TREATMENT

"Acute gonococcal urethritis: Failure of response to phosphonomycin therapy," by P. M. Southern, Jr., et al. ANTIMICROB AGENTS CHEMOTHER. 9:343-345, 1969.

"Ampicillin in the treatment of gonorrhoea," by A. Finger. MED J AUST. 2:250-251, August 1, 1970.

"Ampicillin in the treatment of 'penicillin-resistant' gonorrhea," by E. B. Smith. MILIT MED. 131:345-347, April, 1966.

"Antibiotic sensitivity of gonococcal strains isolated in the South-east Asia and western Pacific regions in 1961-1968," by A. Reyn. BULL WHO. 40:257-262, 1969.

"Antibiotic sensitivity of gonococci and treatment of gonorrhoea in Uganda," by O. P. Arya, et al. BRIT J VENER DIS. 46:149-152, April, 1970.

"Antibiotic sensitivity of gonococci in Kampala," by I. Phillips, et al. E AFR MED J. 46:38-45, January, 1969.

"Antibiotic sensitivity of gonococci in women with various forms of gonorrhea," by Z. A. Pesina, et al. ANTIBIOTIKI. 10:852-855, September, 1965.

"Antibiotic sensitivity of Neisseria gonorrhoeae strains in the Essen area with special reference to penicillin sensitivity," by D. Hantschke. Z HAUT GESCHLECHTSKR. 45:49-62, January 1, 1970.

"Antibiotic susceptibilities of Neisseria gonorrhoeae isolates," by A. Ronald, et al. NORTHWEST MED. 66: 352-356, April, 1967.

GONORRHEA: TREATMENT

"Are there any scientific and practical reasons for objections against the current instructions and schedules for the treatment of gonorrhea?," by I. M. Porudominskii. VESTN DERM VENER. 39:48-53, October, 1965.

"Attempt to induce in vitro penicillin resistance in Neisseria gonorrhoeae," by F. Vymola, et al. J HYG EPIDEM. 12:426-430, 1968.

"Bicillin in the treatment of acute gonorrhea," by V. F. Maksimov. VESTN DERM VENER. 41:86-87, April, 1967.

"Bicillin-6 in therapy of gonorrhea in women," by F. V. Potapnev, et al. VESTN DERM VENER. 43:52-55, January, 1969.

"Bicillin-6 in the treatment of gonorrhea in men," by M. U. Mirsagatov, et al. VESTN DERM VENER. 41:70-72, October, 1967.

"Case contribution to the problem of penicillin resistance in gonorrhea," by E. Friedrich, et al. Z HAUT GESCHLECHTSKR. 40:194-200, March 15, 1966.

"Catamnestic remarks on the therapy of gonorrhea in 572 cases," by D. Kiesewalter. DEUTSCH GESUNDH. 23:1408-1412, July 25, 1968.

"Cephaloridine in gonorrhoea in females," by A. Jouhar, et al. BRIT J VENER DIS. 44:223-225, September, 1969.

"Cephaloridine treatment of gonorrhoea in the female," by D. G. McLone, et al. BRIT J VENER DIS. 44:220-222, September, 1968.

"Cephalothin in gonococcal urethritis," by E. B. Smith. CURR THER RES. 9:79-81, February, 1967.

"Clinical bacterial study of drug resistance of gonococci. Preliminary note," by M. Fazio, et al. G ITAL DERM. 45:163-164, March, 1970.

"Clinical course and treatment of female gonorrhea," by J. Obrtel. CESK GYNEK. 33:463-467, July, 1968.

"Clinical evaluation of treatment of gonorrhea in the female," by L. H. Shapiro, et al. AMER J OBSTET

GONORRHEA: TREATMENT

GYNEC. 97:968-973, April 1, 1967.

"Clinical experience with a new antibiotic in blennorrhagic infections," by N. M. Prandini. HOSPITAL. 74:1327-1331, October, 1968.

"Clinical experience with spiramycin in the 'minute therapy' of gonorrhea," by E. Heinke, et al. DEUTSCH MED WSCHR. 94:1182-1185, May 30, 1969.

"Clinical findings using demethylchlortetracycline in acute gonococcal urethritis," by J. Berger. REV BRASIL MED. 26:249-250, April, 1969.

"Clinical significance of lincomycin-resistant Neisseria gonorrhoeae," by E. Kutscher, et al. ANTIMIMICROB AGENTS CHEMOTHER. 8:331-334, 1968.

"Clinical trial of clomocycline (Megaclor) in gonococcal and non-gonococcal urethritis," by G. S. Andrew, et al. BRIT J VENER DIS. 45:154-156, June, 1969.

"The combination of hetacillin and kanamycin in the treatment of gonococcal urethritis," by D. C. Rodriguez, et al. REV VENEZ UROL. 21:136-141, January-June, 1969.

"Comparative study of the sensitivity of gonococci to various antibiotics," by S. S. Lur'e, et al. VESTN DERM VENER. 43:46-49, February, 1969.

"Comparative study of the therapeutic effect of a single dose of hetacillin and ampicillin in gonococcal urethritis," by D. C. Rodriguez, et al. REV VENEZ UROL. 21:143-151, January-June, 1969.

"Comparative study of two therapies for gonorrhea," by M. Nelson. PUBLIC HEALTH REP. 84:980-984, November, 1969.

"Complications after modern gonorrhea therapy," by J. Soltz-Szots. ARCH KLIN EXP DERM. 227:652-656, 1966.

"Contribution to the views on current therapy of gonorrhea by antibiotics," by M. Skencić. SRPSKI ARH CELOK LEK. 94:363-367, April, 1966.

"Controls gonorrhea (doxycycline)." AM DRUGGIST. 160: 50, October 6, 1969.

GONORRHEA: TREATMENT

"Cross-allergy caused by cephaloridine, cephalothin and penicillin," by H. Vogt. HAUTARZT. 20:407-408, September, 1969.

"Culture of gonococci. Advantages of culture in the diagnosis and treatment of gonorrhea," by K. Odegaard. T NORSK LAEGEFOREN. 86:791-793, May 15, 1966.

"Current problems in the treatment of gonorrhea," by H. Storck, et al. SCHWEIZ MED WSCHR. 96:1635-1641, December 10, 1966.

"Current problems of the diagnosis and therapy of gonorrhea," by I. M. Porudominskii, et al. VESTN DERM VENER. 41:40-46, May, 1967.

"Current status of the in vitro sensitivity of gonococci to penicillin in Finland," by O. V. Renkonen, et al. ACTA DERMATOVENER. 50:151-153, 1970.

"Current treatment of gonorrhea," by H. Szarmach. POL TYG LEK. 24:1250-1253, August 11, 1969.

"Decreased gonococcus sensitivity to penicillin and penicillin dosage, development and present situation," by E. Friedrich, et al. Z AERZTL FORTBILD. 63:861-868, August 15, 1969.

"Demethylchlortetracycline compared with penicillin in the treatment of gonorrhoea in women," by W. Enfors, et al. BRIT J VENER DIS. 46:209-211, June, 1970.

"Demethylchlortetracycline in the treatment of gonorrhoea," by R. R. Willcox. BRIT J VENER DIS. 43:157-160, September, 1967.

"The diagnosis and management of gonorrhea," by A. B. Greaves. MED ANN DC. 35:369-371, July, 1966.

"Diagnosis and therapy of chronic female gonorrhea," by J. Kvicera, et al. CESK DERM. 45:241-242, September, 1970.

"Diagnosis and treatment of gonorrhea in the female," by J. B. Lucas, et al. NEW ENG J MED. 276:1454-1459, June 29, 1967.

"Diagnostic and therapeutic problems in gonorrhea," by K. Holzegel. DEUTSCH GESUNDH. 23:1172-1176, June 20, 1968.

GONORRHEA: TREATMENT

"Doxycycline treatment of gonorrhoea in cases with decreased penicillin susceptibility of gonococci," by A. Lassus. CHEMOTHERAPY. 15:125-128, 1970.

"Erythromycin and oleandomycin in therapy of fresh gonorrhea in women," by L. D. Kuntsevich. VESTN DERM VENER. 42:84-86, July, 1968.

"Erythromycin controls gonorrhea." AM DRUGGIST. 159:44, February 24, 1969.

"Erythromycin in the therapy of gonorrhea in women," by E. N. Turanova, et al. SOVET MED. 29:123-125, September, 1966.

"Erythromycin in the treatment of acute gonococcal urethritis in males," by D. O. Smith, Jr., et al. CURR THER RES. 11:1-4, January, 1969.

"Erythromycin in the treatment of gonorrhea in women," by B. A. Afanas'ev. VESTN DERM VENER. 41:83-86, April, 1967.

"Erythromycin stearate in 'single dose' in the treatment of acute masculine gonococcal urethritis," by R. Bialski. REV BRASIL MED. 26:256-258, April, 1969.

"Experience in gonorrhea treatment in an outpatient department," by L. Gip, et al. LAKARTIDNINGEN. 65:1226-1230, March 20, 1968.

"Experience in the treatment of gonorrhea in males with oletetrin," by I. I. Mavrov. VESTN DERM VENER. 43:80-82, November, 1969.

"Experiences with the use of sodium ampicillin in acute gonococcal infections in Vietnam," by R. G. Kercull. MILIT MED. 133:985-986, December, 1968.

"Experimental under-treatment of early syphilis with probenecid and penicillin in anti-gonorrhoea dosages. A study to assess the best follow-up examination time for syphilis after gonorrhoea treatment in Greenland," by L. Hallinger. ACTA DERMATOVENER. 48:260-267, 1968.

"Fever therapy technique in syphilis and a gonococcic infections," by H. W. Kendell, et al. ARCH PHYS MED. 50:603-608, October, 1969.

GONORRHEA: TREATMENT

"Final report on the effectiveness of oxytetracycline in the treatment of gonorrhea in females," by L. H. Shapiro, et al. AMER J OBSTET GYNEC. 94:536-538, February 15, 1966.

"Further experience with cephaloridine in gonorrhoea," by L. Z. Oller. POSTGRAD MED J. 43:Suppl:43:124-128, August, 1967.

"Further studies of the sensitivity of gonococci to penicillin," by N. M. Ovcinnikov, et al. UROL NEFROL. 31:40-43, September-October, 1966.

"Gonococcal perihepatitis in a male. The Fitz-Hugh-Curtis syndrome," by M. W. Kimball, et al. NEW ENG J MED. 282:1082-1084, May 7, 1970.

"Gonococcal resistance to penicillin," by H. Storck, et al. DERMATOLOGICA. 139:254-259, 1969.

"Gonococcal urethritis in males in Vietnam: three penicillin regimens and one tetracycline regimen," by L. H. Maurer, et al. JAMA. 207:946-948, February 3, 1969.

"Gonorrhoea in females treated with one oral dose of tetracycline," by D. G. McLone, et al. BRIT J VENER DIS. 44:218-219, September, 1968.

"Gonorrhea: the minimum effective dose," by R. H. Meade, 3d. NEW ENG J MED. 283:42-43, July 2, 1970.

"Gonorrhea: the office management of acute infections," by L. Davis. CALIF MED. 107:4-7, July, 1967.

"Gonorrhea therapy with a combination of probenecid and benzylsodiumpenicillin. A report from Greenland," by G. A. Olsen, et al. UGESKR LAEG. 130:1465-1468, September 5, 1968.

"Gonorrhoea treated by a combination of probenecid and sodium penicillin G," by G. A. Olsen, et al. BRIT J VENER DIS. 45:144-148, June, 1969.

"Gonorrhea. A treatment problem," by N. H. Dyer, et al. W VIRGINIA MED J. 64:182-183, May, 1968.

"Gonorrheal and non-gonorrheal urethritis," by J. Bonelli, et al. HOSPITAL. 70:921-935, October, 1966.

GONORRHEA: TREATMENT

"Gonorrheal urethritis in males treated with one oral dose of ampicillin," by D. G. McLone, et al. SOUTHERN MED J. 61:278-280, March, 1968.

"Gonorrhoeal urethritis in males treated with one oral dose of oxytetracycline," by D. G. McLone, et al. BRIT J VENER DIS. 43:166-167, September, 1967.

"Gonorrheal urethritis in males treated with a single oral dose of minocycline," by R. W. Thatcher, et al. PUBLIC HEALTH REP. 85:160-162, February, 1970.

"Guide to adequate treatment of gonorrhoea complicated by staphylococcus albus," by R. L. Tawes, Jr. BRIT J VENER DIS. 42:155-161, September, 1966.

"Gynecologists and cases of gonorrhea," by L. Nilsson. LAKARTIDNINGEN. 65:1090-1091, March 13, 1968.

"High dosage procaine penicillin combined with ampicillin in the treatment of gonorrhoea after failure with standard procaine penicillin dosage," by J. L. Fluker, et al. BRIT J VENER DIS. 45:317-320, December, 1969.

"In-vitro activity of twelve antibacterial agents against Neisseria gonorrhoeae," by I. Phillips, et al. LANCET. 1:263-265, February 7, 1970.

"In vitro susceptibility of Neisseria gonorrhoeae to different antibiotics," by C. W. Halverson, et al. MILIT MED. 134:1427-1429, November, 1969.

"In vitro susceptibility of Neisseria gonorrhoeae to nine antimicrobial agents," by J. E. Martin, et al. APPL MICROBIOL. 18:21-23, July, 1969.

"The influence of chloroquine and related frugs on psoriasis and keratoderma blenorrhagicum," by H. Baker. BRIT J DERM. 78:161-166, March, 1966.

"Inhibition by acetazolamide of the growth of Neisseriae at increasing environmental concentration of CO_2," by A. Forkman. ACTA PATH MICROBIOL SCAND. 73:298-302, 1968.

"Inhibition of Neisseria gonorrhoeae by nifuratel," by G. M. Churcher, et al. BRIT J VENER DIS. 45:149-150, June, 1969.

GONORRHEA: TREATMENT

"'Instant treatment' ('traitement minute') of gonorrhea with a new oxytetracycline derivate--doxycycline (preliminary report)," by L. Sylvestre, et al. INT Z KLIN PHARMAKOL THER TOXIK. 1:401-403, July, 1968.

"Intramuscular injection of procaine penicillin combined with oral administration of chloramphenicol in the treatment of gonorrhoea," by H. C. Gjessing, et al. BRIT J VENER DIS. 42:107-109, June, 1966.

"Is there a penicillin resistance in gonorrhea?," by P. Wodniansky. ARCH KLIN EXP DERM. 227:650-652, 1966.

"Large doses of penicillin for treatment of gonorrhea in women," by L. H. Shapiro, et al. OBSTET GYNEC. 30:89-92, July, 1967.

"Management of blennorrhagia using a dose of rimactan," by L. Migliano. HOSPITAL. 75:297-300, January, 1969.

"Methacycline (rondomycin) in gonorrhoea," by R. S. Morton, et al. BRIT J VENER DIS. 42:175-177, September, 1966.

"Minute treatment of gonorrhea. Supplementary observations on the article by H. Biehler and E. Heinke: Single treatment of gonorrhea of the man with high doses of penicillins, Munchen Med Wschr 109 (1967) 296-300," by E. G. Jung, et al. MUNCHEN MED WSCHR. 110:152-153, January 19, 1968.

"Minute treatment of male gonococcal urethritis (600 cases)," by A. Siboulet. SEM THER. 41:307-309, May, 1965.

"Neisseria gonorrhoeae. A comparative study of the sensitivity of freshly isolated strains to antibiotics," by M. Hejzlar, et al. CESK DERM. 43:179-186, June, 1968.

"Neisseria gonorrhoea strain showing an exceptional resistance to streptomycin and a considerably decreased susceptibility to some other antibiotics," by M. Pekowski, et al. PRZEGL DERM. 57:49-54, January-February, 1970.

"New methods in therapy of gonorrhea," by J. Danda, et al. CESK DERM. 45:49-57, April, 1970.

GONORRHEA: TREATMENT

"New prospects in therapy of blennorrhagic urethritis," by R. Santini, et al. G ITAL DERMATOL. 45:590-594, October, 1970.

"New ways in the management of acute gonorrhea?," by W. Belda. HOSPITAL. 73:2001-2011, June, 1968.

"Note on the treatment of male gonococcic urethritis with vulcacycline," by F. Labouche, et al. BULL SOC FRANC DERM SYPH. 74:665-667, 1967.

"Notes on the treatment of gonorrhea with injectable thiophenicol," by H. Thiers, et al. LYON MED. 217:589-591, February 19, 1967.

"Observations on the bacteriology of penicillin-resistant gonococcal infections," by K. Kinda. REV MEDICOCHIR IASI. 73:967-970, October-December, 1969.

"Oletetrin in the therapy of gonorrhea," by A. I. Poliakov, et al. VESTN DERM VENER. 41:71-73, June, 1967.

"Oletetrine in the therapy of patients with gonorrhea," by Z. V. Ermol'eva, et al. VESTN DERM VENER. 42:81-86, April, 1968.

"Oletetrin in treatment of fresh gonorrhea in men," by T. A. Kislova, et al. ANTIBIOTIKI. 14:467-469, May, 1969.

"On the effectiveness of low doses of thiamphenicol in the treatment of urethritis," by A. Riboldi. MINERVA DERM. 41:35-37, January, 1966.

"On the question of penicillin resistance in gonorrhea," by P. Wodniansky. Z HAUT GESCHLECHTSKR. 41:16-21, July 1, 1966.

"On the sensitivity to penicillin of the gonococcus and the clinical dosage effect of penicillin," by G. Ludwig. DERM WSCHR. 152:1-4, January 8, 1966.

"On the therapy of gonorrhea in males," by V. I. Zhukov. VOENNOMED ZH. 3:70-72, March, 1966.

"'One minute treatment' of gonococcal urethritis by spiramycin," by L. Sylvestre, et al. UN MED CANADA. 96:199-201, February, 1967.

GONORRHEA: TREATMENT

"One-session treatment of gonorrhoea in males with procaine penicillin plus probenecid," by R. J. Cobbold, et al. POSTGRAD MED J. 46:142-145, March, 1970.

"Oral administration of a single dosage of ampicillin K in the treatment of gonorrhea," by J. M. De Barros, et al. REV SAUDE PUBLICA. 4:31-34, June, 1970.

"Oral ampicillin in gonorrhoea. Clinical evaluation," by O. Groth, et al. BRIT J VENER DIS. 46:21-26, February, 1970.

"Oral chloramphenicol alone and with intramuscular procaine penicillin in the treatment of gonorrhoea," by H. C. Gjessing, et al. BRIT J VENER DIS. 43:133-136, June, 1967.

"Pasomycin treatment of women with gonorrhea," by B. S. Kaliner. VESTN DERM VENER. 42:57-58, May, 1968.

"Penicillin dosage in fresh gonorrhea in men," by T. Putkonen, et al. DUODECIM. 84:512-516, 1968.

"Penicillin dosage in treatment of gonorrhea," by I. Juhlin. NORD MED. 76:806-808, July 14, 1966.

"Penicillin is losing effect on gonorrheal infections." AM DRUGGIST. 159:57, May 5, 1969.

"Penicillin-resistant gonorrhea," by N. Blumberg. J UROL. 101:106, January, 1969.

"Penicillin-resistant gonorrhoea and post-gonococcal urethritis." MED J AUST. 1:275-276, February 17, 1968.

"Penicillin sensitivity of gonococci and its significance in the clinic and treatment of gonorrhea in women," by A. V. Chastikova, et al. ANTIBIOTIKI. 15:561-564, June, 1970.

"Penicillinase-producing staphylococci in the male urethra and their effect on penicillin treatment of gonorrhoea," by B. Lagerholm, et al. ACTA DERMATOVENER. 46:345-347, 1966.

"The possible scope of trimethoprim-sulphonamide treatment," by L. P. Garrod. POSTGRAD MED J SUPPL. 45: 52-55, November, 1969.

GONORRHEA: TREATMENT

"Practical aspects of gonorrhea treatment," by G. Krook. NORD MED. 76:809-810, July 14, 1966.

"Present sensitivity to antibiotics of 65 strains of Neisseria gonorrhoeae isolated in Marseille region," by P. Le Noc, et al. MARSEILLE MED. 107:43-46, 1970.

"Present status of gonorrhea therapy with special reference to penicillin-sensitivity loss of specific gonococci strains," by J. Meyer-Rohn. Z HAUT GESCHLECHTSKR. 45:533-534, July 15, 1970.

"Prevention of cancer of the cervix uteri in patients with chronic gonorrhea," by A.D. Tselishcheva. VESTN DERM VENER. 40:57-62, March, 1966.

"Principles for treating gonorrhea," by L. Molin. LAKARTIDNINGEN. 66:1008-1010, March 5, 1969.

"Principles for treatment of gonorrhea. Comments and alternatives," by I. Juhlin. LAKARTIDNINGEN. 66:2078-2081, May 14, 1969.

"The problem of failures in the treatment of gonorrhea," by F. Miedziński, et al. POL MED J. 5:206-211, 1966.

"The problem of penicillin resistant gonococci," by C. S. Nicol, et al. BRIT J VENER DIS. 44:315-318, December, 1968.

"Problems in the management of patients with gonorrhea," by W. L. Porter. DELAWARE MED J. 41:157-158, May, 1969.

"Purple permanganate." JAMA. 195:214-215, January 17, 1966.

"Reactivity of two selected antigens of Neisseria gonorrhoeae," by G. Reising, et al. APPL MICROBIOL. 18:337-339, September, 1969.

"Recent clinicolaboratory observations in the treatment of acute gonococcal urethritis in men," by G. Ashamalla, et al. JAMA. 195:1115-1116, March 28, 1966.

"Recent developments in the treatment of gonorrhoea," by R. R. Willcox. BRIT J VENER DIS. 46:141-144, April, 1970.

GONORRHEA: TREATMENT

"Relapse of gonorrhoea after treatment with penicillin or streptomycin," by A. J. Evans. BRIT J VENER DIS. 42:251-262, December, 1966.

"Relationships between the sensitivities in vitro of Neisseria gonorrhoeae to spiramycin, penicillin, streptomycin, tetracycline, and erythromycin," by A. Reyn. BRIT J VENER DIS. 45:223-227, September, 1969.

"Results of studies of the sensitivity of Neisseria gonorrhoeae to penicillin in soldiers ill with gonorrhea," by J. Rodovsky, et al. CESK DERM. 43:9-14, February, 1968.

"The results of treatment of gonorrhea," by J. Forssell, et al. LAKARTIDNINGEN. 66:4198+, October 8, 1969.

"Results of treatment with tetraverin," by E. Chodyn, et al. PRZEGL DERM. Suppl:69-73, 1969.

"Rifampicin (rimactane) in the treatment of gonorrhoea," by R. R. Willcox, et al. BRIT J VENER DIS. 46:145-148, April, 1970.

"Rolitetracycline by injection and tetracycline phosphate complex by mouth given in a single session in the treatment of gonorrhoea in males," by R. R. Willcox. ACTA DERMATOVENER. 50:154-156, 1970.

"Rovamycin in the treatment of gonorrhea," by B. Raszeja-Koteiba. PRZEGL DERM. Suppl:75-78, 1969.

"Self-medication by patients attending a venereal diseases clinic," by K. Anderson. BRIT J VENER DIS. 42:44-45, March, 1966.

"Sensitivity of gonococcus to penicillin in patients with gonorrhea," by L.D. Kuntsevich, et al. VESTN DERM VENER. 43:44-45, February, 1969.

"Sensitivity of Neisseria gonorrhoeae to penicillin and other antibiotics. Studies carried out in Toronto during the period 1961 to 1968," by C. R. Amies. BRIT J VENER DIS. 45:216-222, September, 1969.

"Sensitivity of Neisseria gonorrhoeae to penicillin and other drugs," by V. G. Cave, et al. NEW YORK J MED. 70:844-847, April 1, 1970.

GONORRHEA: TREATMENT

"Sensitivity of strains of N. gonorrhoeae to some antibiotics," by S. Hausnerova, et al. CESK DERM. 44: 91-94, May, 1969.

"Sensitivity to penicillin of Neisseria gonorrhoeae. Relationship to the results of treatment," by D. A. Leigh, et al. BRIT J VENER DIS. 45:151-153, June, 1969.

"Should cases of gonorrhea in men be treated by urologists?," by L. Andersson, et al. LAKARTIDNINGEN. 65:1381, April 3, 1968.

"Significance of the 'defaulter' in the assessment of efficiency of treatment in gonorrhoea," by A. B. Hewitt. BRIT J VENER DIS. 45:40-41, March, 1969.

"Single-dose antibiotic treatment of asymptomatic gonorrhea in hospitalized women," by D. W. Johnson, et al. NEW ENG J MED. 283:1-6, July 2, 1970.

"Single dose therapy of gonorrhea with rovamycin," by P. Schmid. DERMATOLOGICA. 134:279-282, 1967.

"Single dose treatment of gonorrhea with selected antibiotic agents," by T. F. Keys, et al. JAMA. 210: 857-861, November 3, 1969.

"Single doses of cephaloridine in the treatment of gonococcal urethritis in males," by M. J. Marshall, et al. POSTGRAD MED J. 43:Suppl:43:121-122, August, 1967.

"Single treatment of gonorrhea in males with high doses of penicillin," by H. Biehler, et al. MUNCHEN MED WSCHR. 109:296-300, February 10, 1967.

"Six-city study of treatment of gonorrhoea in men using single oral doses of 1.5 or 3 G tetracycline hydrochloride," by C. E. Cornelius, 3d. BRIT J VENER DIS. 46:330-333, August, 1970.

"Some observations of the effectiveness of monomycin in the treatment of gonorrhea in men," by V. E. Grigor'ev, et al. VESTN DERM VENER. 44:59-62, April, 1970.

"Spectinomycin hydrochloride in the treatment of uncomplicated gonorrhoea," by C. E. Cornelius, 3d, et al. BRIT J VENER DIS. 46:212-213, June, 1970.

GONORRHEA: TREATMENT

"Spiramycin in the minute treatment of gonorrhoea," by E. Heinke, et al. GERMAN MED MONTHLY. 14:479-482, October, 1969.

"Spiramycin in the therapy of gonococcal infection," by V. Terminello. MINERVA MED. 61:1423-1425, April 11, 1970.

"Spiramycin in the treatment of gonorrhoea." BRIT MED J. 2:129, April 18, 1970.

"Streptomycin in the treatment of gonorrhoea in London in 1966," by R. J. Spitzer, et al. ACTA DERMATO-VENER. 48:537-541, 1968.

"Studies of venereal disease. I. Probenecid-procaine penicillin G combination and tetracycline hydrochloride in the treatment of 'penicillin-resistant' gonorrhea in men," by K. K. Holmes, et al. JAMA. 202: 461-473, November 6, 1967.

"Study of the concentration of oletetrine in the blood serum from patients with gonorrhea," by Z. V. Ermol'eva, et al. VESTN DERM VENER. 40:77-79, September, 1966.

"A study of the relationships between the sensitivities of Neisserian gonorrhoeae to sodium penicillin G, four semisynthetic penicillins, spiramycin, and fusidic acid," by A. Reyn, et al. BRIT J VENER DIS. 44:140-150, June, 1968.

"Sulphamethoxazole combined with 2-4-diamino-pyrimidines in the treatment of gonorrhoea," by D. J. Wright, et al. BRIT J VENER DIS. 46:34-36, February, 1970.

"A survey of problems in the antibiotic treatment of gonorrhoea. With special reference to South-East Asia," by R. R. Willcox. BRIT J VENER DIS. 46:217-242, June, 1970.

"A survey of the range of sensitivity in vitro of N. gonorrhoea to penicillin," by C. W. Chacko, et al. INDIAN J MED RES. 54:823-838, September, 1966.

"Susceptibility to N. gonorrhoeae to penicillin and tetracycline," by A. R. Ronald, et al. ANTIMICROB AGENTS CHEMOTHER. 8:431-434, 1968.

"Ten-year study of Neisseria gonorrhoeae sensitivity

to antibiotics in Czechoslovakia," by M. Hejzlar, et al. J HYG EPIDEM. 12:296-305, 1968.

"Therapeutic effects of bicillin-6 in treatment of gonorrhea in men," by S. L. Kozin, et al. VESTN DERM VENER. 44:75-79, May, 1970.

"Therapeutic failures in gonorrhea. Discussion on symposium II," by H. Biehler. ARCH KLIN EXP DERM. 227:656-662, 1966.

"Therapeutic trial of trimethoprim as a potentiator of sulphonamides in gonorrhoea," by G. W. Csonka, et al. BRIT J VENER DIS. 43:161-165, September, 1967.

"Therapy of gonococcal infection with rifamycin in a single dose," by A. Califano, et al. MINERVA DERM. 43:516-519, October, 1968.

"Treatment of acute gonococcal urethritis," by L. A. Blanco Gutierrez. REV VENEZ UROL. 21:93-100, January-June, 1969.

"Treatment of acute male gonococcal urethritis with a single dosis of erythromycin-stearate," by J. Martini, et al. REV MED CHILE. 96:525-527, August, 1968.

"Treatment of gonococcal urethritis with single injections of 2-4 mega units of aqueous procaine penicillin," by G. D. Morrison, et al. BRIT J VENER DIS. 44:319-323, December, 1968.

"Treatment of gonococcia with tetroid lactic," by H. Thiers, et al. LYON MED. 222:1172-1173, December 14, 1969.

"Treatment of gonorrhoea." BRIT MED J. 1:398-399, February 17, 1968.

"Treatment of gonorrhea," by V. Kaupas. JAMA. 213:2272, September 28, 1970.

"Treatment of gonorrhea," by W. Minkin. JAMA. 208:535, April 21, 1969.

"Treatment of gonorrhea," by P. Muller, et al. THER UMSCH. 26:75-80, February, 1969.

GONORRHEA: TREATMENT

"The treatment of gonorrhea and nongonorrheal urethral diseases," by H. Kresbach, et al. Z HAUT GESCHLECHTSKR. 43:865-873, November 1, 1968.

"Treatment of gonorrhoea by one oral dose of ampicillin and probenecid combined," by T. Gundersen, et al. BRIT J VENER DIS. 45:235-237, September, 1969.

"Treatment of gonorrhoea by penicillin and a renal blocking agent (probenecid), by G. Hatos. MED J AUST. 1:1096-1099, May 30, 1970.

"Treatment of gonorrhea by penicillin in a single large dose," by W. Minkin. MILIT MED. 133:382-386, May, 1968.

"Treatment of gonorrhea in males with cephaloridine," by J. B. Lucas, et al. JAMA. 195:919-921, March 14, 1966.

"The treatment of gonorrhoea in women with sulphamethoxazole-trimethoprim," by C. B. Schofield, et al. POSTGRAD MED J. 45:Suppl:81-86, November, 1969.

"Treatment of gonorrhoea patients with intolerance to penicillin," by G. Rajka. ACTA DERMATOVENER. 48:532-536, 1968.

"Treatment of gonorrhoea today." BRIT MED J. 2:391-392, August 17, 1968.

"Treatment of gonorrhea with bicilein," by I. I. Shkliar. VESTN DERM VENER. 40:84-85, January, 1966.

"The treatment of gonorrhea with cephaloridine intramuscularly," by H. Pariser, et al. SOUTHERN MED J. 63:384-386, April, 1970.

"Treatment of gonorrhoea with double doses of demethylchlortetracycline," by R. R. Willcox. ACTA DERMATOVENER. 49:103-105, 1969.

"The treatment of gonorrhoea with doxycycline as a single dose," by A. Lassus. CHEMOTHERAPY. 13:366-368, 1968.

"Treatment of gonorrhea with semisynthetic penicillin," by J. Kozerski. PRZEGL DERM. 55:551-555, July-September, 1968.

GONORRHEA: TREATMENT

"The treatment of gonorrhea with a single high-dosed penicillin injection (so-called 'one-shot' treatment)," by F. Nemec. Z HAUT GESCHLECHTSKR. 44:507-512, 1969.

"Treatment of gonorrhoea with single oral doses of rifampicin," by R. J. Cobbold, et al. BRIT MED J. 4:681-682, December 14, 1968.

"Treatment of gonorrhoea with trimethoprim-sulphamethoxazole in Uganda," by O. P. Arya, et al. BRIT J VENER DIS. 46:214-216, June, 1970.

"Treatment of gonorrheal urethritis evaluated in 230 men," by E. B. Berry. JAMA. 202:657-659, November 13, 1970.

"Treatment of 'penicillin-resistant' gonorrhea in military personnel in S.E. Asia: a cooperative evaluation of tetracycline and of penicillin plus probenecid in 1263 men," by K. K. Holmes, et al. MILIT MED. 133:642-646, August, 1968.

"Trimethoprim-sulphamethoxazole in the treatment of non-gonococcal urethritis and gonorrhoea," by B. R. Carroll, et al. BRIT J VENER DIS. 46:31-33, February, 1970.

"Use of methacycline in blennorrhagic infection," by E. Ferrea, et al. MINERVA DERM. 43:285-287, June, 1968.

"Use of a single dose of doxycycline monohydrate for treating gonorrheal urethritis in men," by G. Domescik, et al. PUBLIC HEALTH REP. 84:182-183, February, 1969.

"Usefulness of long-acting penicillin in combination with short-acting preparations for treatment of gonorrhea," by E. Fowinkle, et al. J TENN MED ASS. 59:1115-1118, November, 1966.

"Who ought to take care of the gonorrhea cases?," by H. Moller. LAKARTIDNINGEN. 65:2628-2629, June 5, 1968.

"Why sulphonamides, when combined with 2-4-diaminopyrimidines, are effective in sulphonamide-resistant gonorrhoea," by D. J. Wright. GUY HOSP REP. 118:287-291, 1969.

GONORRHEA: YOUTH

GONORRHEA: YOUTH
"Gonococcal arthritis in the young," by J. J. Calabro. NEW ENG J MED. 279:1002, October 31, 1968

"Gonorrhea: growing menace to your students." SCH MGT. 12:36-42, August, 1968; also in PA SCH J. 117:414-419, March, 1969.

GRANULOMA INGUINALE
"Ampicillin in the treatment of granuloma inguinale," by M. A. Thew, et al. JAMA. 210:866-867, November 3, 1969.

"Case reports from the Institute of Venereology (India). Uncommon features of Donovanosis," by P. N. Rangiah, et al. MEDISCOPE. 8:658-662, February, 1966.

"Dermatologic iconography. Donovanosis (Granuloma Venerum Tropical). Treatment using doxicillin," by L. H. Paschoal, et al. AN BRASIL DERM. 43:Suppl:1-3, January-March, 1968.

"Donovanosis," by I. Sluis. DERMATOLOGICA. 133:325-326, 1966.

"Donovanosis and other venereal diseases in southern India. 3rd part of a travel report," by H. J. Weise. Z HAUT GESCHLECHTSKR. 43:425-428, May 15, 1968.

"Donovanosis (granuloma inguinale): a rare cause of osteolytic bone lesions," by D. J. Kirkpatrick. CLIN RADIOL. 21:101-105, January, 1970.

"Granuloma inguinale," by W. P. Hogarth, et al. CANAD MED ASS J. 94:916-917, April 22, 1966.

"Granuloma inguinale," by S. Peck. ARCH DERM. 98:555-557, November, 1968.

"Granuloma inguinale. A clinical, histological and ultrastructural study," by C. M. Davis. JAMA. 211: 632-636, January 26, 1970.

"Granuloma inguinale. Report of a case in California with notes on pathogenesis," by W. M. Gould, et al. CALIF MED. 104:392-395, May, 1966.

"Granuloma inguinale: an ultrastructural study of Calymmatobacterium granulomatis," by C. M. Davis, et al.

GRANULOMA INGUINALE

J INVEST DERM. 53:315-321, November, 1969.

"Granuloma venereum," by O. I. Haavelsrud. T NORSK LAEGERFOREN. 88:2121-2122, November 15, 1968.

"Granuloma venereum in an 81-year-old man," by U. Brauer, et al. DERM WSCHR. 152:780-784, July 23, 1966.

"Methacycline in the management of Donovanosis (granuloma inguinale)," by J. M. Santos, et al. HOSPITAL. 74:1661-1668, November, 1968.

"Peculiarities in dermatology. A case of granuloma inguinale (Donovanosis)," by H. J. Kingsley. CENT AFR J MED. 13:145-146, June, 1967.

"Skin granuloma in the Nile Valley," by A. M. Mofty, et al. INT J DERM. 9:33-40, January-March, 1970.

"Studies on granuloma inguinale 8. Serological reactivity of sera from patient with carcinoma of penis when tested with Donovania antigens," by J. Goldberg, et al. BRIT J VENER DIS. 42:205-209, September, 1966.

"Tropical gynaecology. Ulcerative and hypertrophic lesions of the vulva," by D. B. Stewart. PROC ROY SOC MED. 61:363-365, April, 1968.

GRANULOMA VENERUM TROPICAL
SEE: GRANULOMA INGUINALE

HAMYCIN
"Leucorrhoea due to trichomonas vaginalis--clinical trial with hamycin," by D. Ganju, et al. HINDUSTAN ANTIBIOT BULL. 9:69-75, November, 1966.

HERPES
"The association of herpesvirus type 2 and carcinoma of the uterine cervix," by W. F. Rawls, et al. AMER J EPIDEM. 89:547-554, May, 1969.

"The association of genital herpesvirus with cervical atypia and carcinoma in situ," by I. Royston, et al. AMER J EPIDEM. 91:531-538, June, 1970.

"Diagnosis of skin changes caused by herpes simplex virus by means of fluorescence antibody technic," by

HERPES

O. P. Salo, et al. HAUTARZT. 20:112-113, March, 1969.

"Genital herpesvirus hominis infection: a venereal disease?," by S. Jeansson, et al. LANCET. 1:1064-1065, May 16, 1970.

"Genital infection with type 2 herpes virus hominis. A commonly occurring venereal disease," by A. J. Nahmias, et al. BRIT J VENER DIS. 45:294-298, December, 1969.

"Herpes genitalis," by D. C. Hutfield. BRIT J VENER DIS. 44:241-250, September, 1968.

"Herpes genitalis in Ibadan," by A. O. Osoba, et al. WEST AFR MED J. 19:117-119, August, 1970.

"Herpes progenitalis," by W. Minkin, et al. JAMA. 203:526, February 12, 1968.

"Herpesvirus cervicitis with gonorrhoea," by D. C. Hutfield. LANCET. 1:1311-1312, June 15, 1968.

"Herpesvirus hominis infection of the cervix associated with gonorrhoea," by J. O. Beilby, et al. LANCET. 1065-1066, May 18, 1968.

"History of herpes genitalis," by D. C. Hutfield. BRIT J VENER DIS. 42:263-268, December, 1966.

"Newborn infection with herpesvirus hominis types 1 and 2," by A. J. Nahmias, et al. J PEDIAT. 75:1194-1203, December, 1969.

"Serologic investigations in narcotic addicts. I. Syphilis, lymphogranuloma venereum, herpes simplex, and Q fever," by C. E. Cherubin, et al. ANN INTERN MED. 69:739-742, October, 1968.

"Virus diseases of the external female genitalia. 1. Herpes (simplex) genitalis (herpes progenitalis, herpes venereus, vulvitis or vulvovaginitis herpetica)," by H. Grimmer. Z HAUT GESCHLECHTSKR. 45:23-28, March 1, 1970.

HETACILLIN

"The combination of hetacillin and kanamycin in the treatment of gonococcal urethritis," by D. C. Rodri-

HETACILLIN

guez, et al. REV VENEZ UROL. 21:136-141, January-June, 1969.

"Comparative study of the therapeutic effect of a single dose of hetacillin and ampicillin in gonococcal urethritis," by D. C. Rodriguez, et al. REV VENEZ UROL. 21:143-151, January-June, 1969.

"Use of hetacillin in urogenital infections," by L. H. Rodriguez Diaz, et al. REV VENEZ UROL. 19:163-180, January-June, 1967.

HISTORY
"Achievements of famous Polish surgeons in venerology in the 19th century," by K. Lejman. PRZEGL DERM. 55:621-629, September-October, 1968.

"Beginning of dermatological and venerological instruction at the University of Halle," by W. Kaiser, et al. MED MSCHR. 23:352-358, August, 1969.

"Dermato-venerologic education as reflected by records of the University of Halle at the end of the 18th century," by W. Kaiser. DERM MSCHR. 155:569-579, 1969.

"Fifty years of V.D. service." BRIT MED J. 2:1344, December 3, 1966.

"The first venereologists," by R. S. Roberts. BRIT J VENER DIS. 45:58-60, March, 1969.

"40 years of dermato-venereological service in the Arkhangelsk region," by I. A. Lipskii, et al. VESTN DERM VENER. 40:63-66, November, 1966.

"From the diary of a regional ambulatory clinic for venereal diseases with special reference to the years 1956-1965," by W. DeWald. DEUTSCH GESUNDH. 21:1178-1181, June 23, 1966.

"From Ehrlich to Abraham," by P. Ehrlich, et al. HIPPOKRATES. 38:736-739, September 30, 1967.

"History--venereal diseases." NEW ZEALAND NURS J. 61: 18+, April, 1968.

"Infection of the sex organs in the years 1964-1966 and 1967-1969," by E. Zuber, et al. POL TYG LEK. 25:

HISTORY

1457-1458, September, 1970.

"Observations on the development in dermatovenereology in the period from 1912 to 1956," by J. Gate-Lyon. HAUTARZT. 17:81-83, February, 1966.

"The oldest department for skin- and venereal diseases in Russia," by V. A. Rakhmanov, et al. VESTN DERM VENER. 44:51-58, May, 1970.

"On the history of the All-Union Scientific-Medici Dermatovenerologic Society," by A. A. Studnitsin, et al. VESTN DERM VENER. 41:3-13, August, 1967.

"On the ideological history of the early period of chemotherapy," by P. Klein. DEUTSCH MED WSCHR. 91:2281-2284, December 23, 1966.

"On the investigation of uncertainties in the effect and treatment of venereal diseases and other ailments in the 19th century," by R. Brachwitz. Z HAUT GESCHLECHTSKR. 44:513-516, 1969.

"The 100th anniversary of the Department of Skin and Venereal Diseases of the Military Medical Academy," by O. K. Shaposhnikov. VESTN DERM VENER. 43:54-60, July, 1969.

"Polish dermatology and venerology for 25 years in the Polish People's Republic," by B. Michalowski, et al. PRZEGL DERM. 56:437-440, July-August, 1969.

"Pre- or post-Columbian? 1st appearance of syphilis in Europe," by T. Mildner. MED KLIN. 63:1392-1395, August 30, 1968.

"Progressive paralysis--Past and present," by S. Stojiljkovic, et al. SRPSKI ARH CELOK LEK. 94:211-218, March, 1966.

"Results of scientific research work of the Uzbek Dermatologic-Venereologic Institute for the period 1962-1968," by N. T. Tursunov, et al. VESTN DERM VENER. 43:6-7, June, 1969.

"Results of scientific studies at the Faculty of Skin and Venereal Diseases of the I. M. Sechenov I Moscow Medical Institute," by V. A. Rakhmanov, et al. VESTN DERM VENER. 44:8-13, April, 1970.

HISTORY

"Results of 3 years of activity (1964-1966) at the Centro di Medicina Preventiva del Comune di Novara," by C. Meloni, et al. ANN SANIT PUBBLICA. 29:43-59, January-February, 1968.

"A review of the activities of the Kuibyshev branch of the All-Russia Society of Dermatologists and Venereologists," by A. S. Zenin. VESTN DERM VENER. 41: 77-79, October, 1967.

"Scientific activity of the Department of Dermatology and Venereal Diseases of the Leningrad Sanitary-Hygiene Medical Institute for the period 1963-1968," by S. E. Gorbovitskii, et al. VESTN DERM VENER. 43:3-8, March, 1969.

"Scientific research of the Department of Dermatology and Venereology at the Kiev Medical Institute in 1961-1969," by I. I. Pototskii. VESTN DERM VENER. 44:3-8, May, 1970.

"Sergei Timofeevich Pavlow." VESTN DERM VENER. 41:89, June, 1967.

"Serological and experimental studies in the field of syphilis and gonorrhea in the USSR," by N. M. Ovchinnikov. VESTN DERM VENER. 41:23-37, September, 1967.

"The sexually transmitted diseases. Part 1. History and epidemiology," by J. K. Oates. NURS MIRROR. 128:17-19, January 31, 1969.

--Part 2. Syphilis." NURS MIRROR. 128:24+, February 7, 1969.

--Part 3. Infectious urethritis." NURS MIRROR. 128: 24+, February 14, 1969.

"Skin diseases and venereal diseases in Cracow during the 2d World War," by K. Capińska. PRZEGL LEK. 26: 34-39, 1970.

"Twenty-five years of dermatovenereology in India. A review," by S. C. Desai. J ASSOC PHYSICIANS INDIA. 18:135-153, January, 1970.

"Vladimir Nikolaevich Dobronravov." VESTN DERM VENER. 41:90, June, 1967.

HISTORY

"Who discovered the causative agent of syphilis? (Fritz Schaudinn)," by J. Kenéz. ORV HETIL. 107:1477-1480, July 31, 1966.

HOMOSEXUALITY

"The effects of hypnotherapy on homosexuality," by P. Roper. CANAD MED ASS J. 96:319-327, February 11, 1967.

"Homosexual practice and venereal disease." BRIT MED J. 2:5-6, April 1, 1967.

"Homosexuality and its relation to venereal disease," by I. Rácz. ORV HETIL. 110:2146-2149, September 14, 1969.

"Homosexuality as seen in a New Zealand city practice," by E. Philipp. NEW ZEAL MED J. 67:397-401, March, 1968.

"Homosexuality--a current venereological problem?," by F. Schiller, et al. DERM WSCHR. 153:1161-1165, October 21, 1967.

"Homosexually-acquired venereal disease," by F. J. Jefferiss. BRIT J VENER DIS. 42:46-47, March, 1966.

"Homosexuals and venereal diseases," by D. F. Contreras. ACTAS DERMOSIF. 59:467-470, July-August, 1968.

"Recent trends in homosexuality in West London," by J. L. Fluker. BRIT J VENER DIS. 42:48-49, March, 1966.

"Treatment of male homosexuals in groups," by S. B. Hadden. INT J GROUP PSYCHOTHER. 16:13-22, January, 1966.

"Venereal diseases and homosexuality (considerations apropos of 2 cases recorded in minors," by A. Serena. ARCH ITAL DERM VENER. 34:159-168, 1966.

HUTCHINSON, JONATHAN

"Jonathan Hutchinson on vaccination syphilis," by C. T. Nelson. ARCH DERM. 99:529-535, May, 1969.

IMIDAZOLE

"Therapeutic and diagnostic problems of vaginal trichomoniasis treated with imidazole (Klion)," by B. Toth,

IMIDAZOLE

et al. ORV HETIL. 108:452-455, March 5, 1967.

"The treatment of trichomonas infestations with klion," by P. Salacz, et al. Z AERZTLFORTBILD. 60:805-808, July 1, 1966.

IMMUNOLOGY

"Immunologic studies in a patient sensitive to tetracycline and penicillin," by M. J. Fellner, et al. ARCH KLIN EXP DERM. 224:157-167, February 3, 1966.

"Immunological and immunochemical investigations of patients suffering from general paralysis," by H. Schmidt, et al. BRIT J VENER DIS. 46:135-137, April, 1970.

"Immunology, clinical features and therapy of penicillin allergy," by G. Filipp. MED WELT. 50:2763-2773, December 14, 1968.

"Natural human antibodies to gram-negative bacteria: immunoglobulins G, A, and M," by I. R. Cohen, et al. SCIENCE. 152:1257-1259, May 27, 1966.

"On the immunological reactivity of penicillin, cephalosporin and tetracycline antibiotics," by J. Lochmannova, et al. J HYG EPIDEM. 14:201-210, 1970.

"Treatment of penicillin anaphylaxis with injection of the same antigen (penicillin) in high doses," by L. Katsilabors. REV MED MOYEN ORIENT. 24:346-348, July-August, 1967.

INFANTS

"Action of primaricin on postpartum mycoses," by M. E. Rochet, et al. LYON MED. 216:1179-1183, November 20, 1966.

"Clinical picture of sepsis in a two-month-old infant. What could be the cause of edema, ascites, iceterus and anemia?." CLIN PEDIAT. 9:214-225, April, 1970.

INFERTILITY
SEE ALSO: STERILITY

"Contribution of observations on the cases of male infertility," by L. Semmola. MINERVA DERM. 42:393-397, August, 1967.

INFERTILITY

"Mycoplasmas and human reproductive failure," by R. B. Kundsin, et al. SURG GYNEC OBSTET. 131:89-92, July, 1970.

"On the question of sterility and infertility," by H. Muth. HIPPOKRATES. 37:501-509, July 15, 1966.

"Phagocytic capability of the vaginal trichomonas and its role in female infertility," by A. P. Kolesov. UKRANIAN PEDIAT AKUSH GINEK. 2:63, March-April, 1966.

"Relations between trichomoniasis and male infertility. Preliminary note," by G. Argenziano, et al. MINERVA DERM. 42:388-391, August, 1967.

"Studies on the pathogenic significance of female urogenital trichomoniasis with special reference to its effects of fertility," by D. Hofmann, et al. ARCH GYNAEK. 203:1-19, 1966.

INSTITUTES
SEE: CLINICS
SOCIETIES
SEE ALSO: HISTORY

INTERSTITIAL KERATITIS
SEE SYPHILIS: OPHTHALMOLOGY

IODINOL
"Comparative assessment of the treatment of trichomonad urethritis in males with iodinol and ACD preparations," by L. M. Korik, et al. VESTN DERM VENER. 40:62-65, March, 1966.

IODOPOVIDONE
"Clinical tests using iodopovidone in patients with vaginal trichomoniasis," by A. A. Rustrian, et al. GINEC OBSTET MEX. 27:467-470, April, 1970.

JACKSONS SYNDROME
SEE: NEUROSYPHILIS

JARISCH-HERXHEIMER REACTION
SEE: REACTIONS

JASOMYCIN
"Treatment of latent syphilis with jasomycin," by R. Osako, et al. J JAP ASS INFECT DIS. 43:44-48, May, 1969.

KANAMYCIN

KANAMYCIN

"The combination of hetacillin and kanamycin in the treatment of gonococcal urethritis," by D. C. Rodriguez, et al. REV VENEZ UROL. 21:136-141, January-June, 1969.

KLION
SEE: IMIDAZOLE

LAW

"Anaphylactic reactions after penicillin as a clinical and medicolegal problem," by Z. Starzycki. PRZEGL DERM. 55:559-563, July-September, 1968.

"Are venereal diseases increasing? A change of legislation on the control of venereal diseases," by W. Becker. MED KLIN. 64:609-611, March 28, 1969.

"Law, medicine and minors. I.," by D. H. Russell. NEW ENG J MED. 278:35-36, January 4, 1968.

--II." NEW ENG J MED. 278:265-266, February 1, 1968.

"Legal aspects of reporting and treating venereal disease," by G. E. Hall. JAMA. 195:309-310, March 28, 1966; also in ARCH ENVIRON HEALTH, Chicago. 13:388-392, September, 1966.

"Liability for penicillin reactions," by A. R. Holder. JAMA. 212:2015-2016, June 15, 1970.

"Medical and legal problems in the treatment of delinquent girls in Scotland. I. Girls in custodial institutions," by D. H. Robertson. BRIT J VENER DIS. 45:129-139, June, 1969.

--II. Sexually transmitted disease in girls in custodial institutions," by D. H. Robertson, et al. BRIT J VENER DIS. 46:46-53, February, 1970.

"The serologic syphilis test required for marriage in other states," by R. L. Cavenaugh. MARYLAND MED J. 18:33, May, 1969.

"Some legal problems in venereal disease control," by Golebiowska-Podgorczyk. PRZEGL DERM. Suppl:101-105, 1969.

LEDERMYCIN

LEDERMYCIN

"Clinical findings using demethylchlortetracycline in acute gonococcal urethritis," by J. Berger. REV BRASIL MED. 26:249-250, April, 1969.

"Demethylchlortetracycline compared with penicillin in the treatment of gonorrhoea in women," by W. Enfors, et al. BRIT J VENER DIS. 46:209-211, June, 1970.

"Demethylchlortetracycline in the treatment of gonorrhea," by R. R. Willcox. BRIT J VENER DIS. 43:157-160, September, 1967.

"Treatment of syphilis with demethyltetracycline (ledermycin)," by S. Nolting. MED KLIN. 61:2043-2044, December 23, 1966.

LEPROSY

"A case report of gangrenous balanitis in progressive reaction in leprosy," by D. S. Chaudhury, et al. LEPROSY REV. 37:225-226, October, 1966.

"Clinical and serological profiles in leprosy," by L. J. Matthews, et al. LANCET. 2:915-917, November 6, 1965.

"Influence of treatment of biologic false positive syphilis tests in leprosy," by H. G. Ruge. INT J LEPROSY. 36:328-332, July-September, 1968.

"Occurrence of biologic false positive reactions with RPR (circle) card test on leprosy patients," by A. Achimastos, et al. PUBLIC HEALTH REP. 85:66-68, January, 1970.

"Serologic tests with sera from patients with lepromatous leprosy during the periods of exacerbation," by G. V. Mertslin, et al. VESTN DERM VENER. 40:41-43, October, 1966.

"Serological tests for treponemal infection in leprosy patients. An evaluation of the fluorescent treponemal antibody absorption (FTA-ABS) test," by M. F. Garner, et al. BRIT J VENER DIS. 45:19-22, March, 1969.

"Serology in leprosy," by H. Schmidt. DERM INT. 7:43-45, January-March, 1968.

LEPROSY

"Syphilis and biologic false positive reactors among leprosy patients," by A. T. Scotti, et al. ARCH DERM. 101:328-330, March, 1970.

"Syphilis reactions in leprosy sera. Mass screening tests," by H. Ruge. MED WELT. 48:2620-2627, November 26, 1966.

"Treponemal immobilization tests in leprosy," by H. G. Ruge. BRIT J VENER DIS. 43:191-196, September, 1967.

LEUKOPLAKIA

"On the etiologic relationship between leukoplakia syphilis and cancer of the ora cavity," by K. Anastassov, et al. REV FRANC ODONTOSTOMAT. 14:1530-1536, November, 1967.

LEUTIC GLOSSITIS
SEE: SYPHILIS

LEVORIN

"A clinical study of the efficacy of Levorin in urogenital trichomoniasis," by I.I. Il'in. VESTN DERM VENER. 41:87-88, September, 1967.

"Levorin in the therapy of trichomoniasis in men, and in post-trichomonas secondary infections," by L. M. Korik, et al. UROL NEFROL. 34:48-49, July-August, 1969.

"Levorin in the treatment of women with trichomoniasis and candidiasis of the sexual organs," by V. A. Lenartovich, et al. VESTN DERM VENER. 43:39-43, February, 1969.

LINCOMYCIN

"In-vitro comparison of erythromycin, lincomycin, and clindamycin," by L. Phillips, et al. BRIT MED J. 2:89-90, April 11, 1970.

"Lincomycin: activity in vitro and absorption and excretion in normal young men," by C. E. McCall, et al. AMER J MED SCI. 254:144-155, August, 1967.

"Lincomycin, non-gonococcal urethritis, and mycoplasmata," by G. W. Csonka, et al. BRIT J VENER DIS. 45:52-54, March, 1969.

"Selective inhibition in vitro of mycoplasma hominis

LINCOMYCIN

  by lincomycin," by G. Csonka, et al. BRIT J VENER DIS. 46:203-204, June, 1970.

LUPUS ERYTHEMATOSUS
SEE: MINOR VENEREAL DISEASE

LYMPHOGRANULOMA VENEREUM
  "Abdominoperineal resection of the rectum," by R. K. Gilchrist. SURG CLIN N AMER. 46:1191-1199, October, 1966.

  "Anogenital sinuses and polypi. Crohn's disease," by B. A. Thomas. BRIT J DERM. 80:414-415, June, 1968.

  "Auto-immune serum factors and IgA elevation in lymphogranuloma venereum," by A. Lassus, et al. ANN CLIN RES. 2:51-56, March, 1970.

  "A Bedsonia isolated from a patient with clinical-lymphogranuloma venereum," by J. Schachter. OPHTHAL. 63:1049-1053, May, 1967.

  "Canine venereal lymphoma as a model of experimental cancer," by H. Márquez-Monter. GAC MED MEX. 100:168-183, February, 1970.

  "Erythromycin in the therapy of inguinal lymphogranuloma," by I. I. Il'in. VESTN DERM VENER. 40:69-70, August, 1966.

  "Isolation of the agent of lymphogranuloma venereum in Australia," by I. Cook, et al. MED J AUST. 1:771-772, April 12, 1969.

  "Isolation of lymphogranuloma venereum agent in the Sudan," by A. R. Salim. J TROP MED HYG. 72:134-136, June, 1969.

  "Lymphogranuloma inguinale," by W. F. Schoning, et al. MED WELT. 31:1713-1714, August 2, 1969.

  "Lymphogranuloma venereum," by A. J. Abrams. JAMA. 205:199-202, July 22, 1968.

  "Lymphogranuloma venereum," by E. G. Weinstein, et al. J AMER GERIAT SOC. 14:80-84, January, 1966.

  "Lymphogranuloma venereum. I. Comparison of the Frei test, complement fixation test, and isolation of the agent," by J. Schachter, et al. J INFECT DIS. 120: 372-375, September, 1969.

--II. Characterization of some recently isolated strains." J BACT. 99:636-638, September, 1969.

"Lymphographic findings in venereal diseases," by L. Kerk, et al. FORTSCHR ROENTGENSTR. 111:22-29, July, 1969.

"Lymphographic studies in lymphopathia venerea," by J. J. Herzberg. DERM WSCHR. 153:854-857, July 29, 1967.

"Lymphography and lymphoscintigraphy of the pelvis in venereal lymphopathy in the buboes condition," by K. Vessal, et al. HAUTARZT. 18:256-259, June, 1967.

"Nicolas-Favre disease," by J. Duhamel, et al. ARCH FRANC MAL APPAR DIG. 59:Suppl:7-8:55+, July-August, 1970.

"Nicolas-Favre disease in Bordeaux," by P. Le Coulant, et al. BULL SOC FRANC DERM SYPH. 75:365-367, 1968.

"On the clinical early diagnosis of venereal lymphopathy," by H. Roder, et al. Z HAUT GESCHLECHTSKR. 40:158-164, March 1, 1966.

"On the present status of our knowledge of lymphogranuloma venereum," by W. Schmidt. THER UMSCH. 26:81-88, February, 1969.

"Recurrent lymphogranuloma venereum. Report of a case," by L. Z. Oller. BRIT J VENER DIS. 44:154-156, June, 1968.

"Serologic investigations in narcotic addicts. I. Syphilis, lymphogranuloma venereum, herpes simplex, and Q fever," by C. E. Cherubin, et al. ANN INTERN MED. 69:739-742, October, 1968.

"Serologic reactions to specific complement-fixing antigens from micro-organisms of the psittacosis-lymphogranuloma venereum-trachoma (PLT) group," by R. N. Philip, et al. AMER J OPTHAL. 63:1499-1504, May, 1967.

"Spontaneous fecal contamination of cerebrospinal fluid: An unusual complication of lymphogranuloma venereum,"

LYMPHOGRANULOMA VENEREUM

by E. Lozada, et al. AMER J DIG DIS. 14:30-34, January, 1969.

"Studies with an intradermal test of infections caused by viruses of the psittacosis-ornithosis-venereal lymphogranulomatosis type," by S. D'Agostino, et al. G MAL INFETT. 18:777-779, November, 1966.

"Study on doxycycline in the treatment of acute infection of the respiratory system and lymphogranuloma venereum," by J. Neves, et al. REV ASS MED BRASIL. 14:65-70, June, 1968.

"Study with an intradermal test of infections caused by viruses of the psittacosis-ornithosis- lymphogranuloma venereum group," by S. D'Agostino, et al. G MAL INFETT. 18:777-779, November, 1966.

"Uridine nucleotide synthesis in cells infected by the agent of benign inguinal lymphogranulomatosis," by G. A. Galegov, et al. VOP MED KHIM. 15:201-203, March-April, 1969.

MACMIROR
"Macmiror in the therapy of vaginal trichomoniasis," by A. Baron. MINERVA GINEC. 22:269-271, February 28, 1970.

"Treatment of trichomoniasis in women with Macmiror," by A. Baron. WIAD PARAZYT. 15:379-380, 1969.

MAGMILOR
SEE: NIFURATEL

MARCUS GUNN PHENOMENON
SEE: OPHTHALMOLOGY

MEDICAL DOCTORS & VENEREAL DISEASE
SEE ALSO: EDUCATION
PREVENTION & CONTROL

"Experience in raising the qualifications of dermatologists-venereologists in Leningrad," by I. G. Tsiura, et al. VESTN DERM VENER. 43:59-61, January, 1969.

"Family physicians' role in the control of VD," by M. P. Vora. J INDIAN MED ASS. 46:370-373, April 1, 1966.

"How can we get doctors genuinely concerned about the

VD problem," by W. L. Porter. MED TIMES. 94:1218-1219, October, 1966.

"Iatrogenic errors in the management of dermatovenereal diseases," by H. Rockl, et al. MUNCHEN MED WSCHR. 110:2010-2015, September 6, 1968.

"Iatrogenic infections and hazards in venerology," by Z. Somogyi. ORV HETIL. 107:2371-2373, December 11, 1966.

"Iatrogenic venereological complaints," by W. K. Bernfeld. BRIT J VENER DIS. 44:82, March, 1968.

"The new specialist education: Dermato-venereology," by K. Thomsen. YNG LAEG. 10:839-840, 1968.

"Organization of continuing education for dermato-venereologists," by A. I. Kartamyshev, et al. VESTN DERM VENER. 42:58-62, 1968.

"Physician reporting of venereal disease in the USA," by J. S. McKenzie-Pollock. BRIT J VENER DIS. 46:114-116, April, 1970.

"Physicians' attitudes toward venereal disease reporting. A survey by the national opinion research center," by R. L. Cleere, et al. JAMA. 202:941-946, December 4, 1967.

"A pilot survey of venereal disease in general practice," by B. W. Christmas. NEW ZEAL MED J. 67:188-191, February, 1968.

"The private physician and venereal disease control in the Western Pacific Region," by R. R. Willcox. BRIT J CLIN PRACT. 24:97-99, March, 1970.

"Programmed instruction and prospects of its application in teaching of dermato-venereology," by V. A. Rakhmanov, et al. VESTN DERM VENER. 42:52-57, 1968.

"The role of the general practitioner in the prevention and treatment of venereal diseases," by E. Pertl. MED GLAS. 22:121-125, May, 1968.

"Scientific organization of the work of physicians of dermatovenerological institutions," by A. I. Sul'zhenko, et al. SOVET ZDRAVOOKHR. 27:31-35, 1968.

MEDICAL DOCTORS & VENEREAL DISEASE

"Sex and the medical student," by W. M. Sheppe, Jr., et al. J MED EDUC. 41:457-464, May, 1966.

"Sex and the practicing physician," by W. F. Sheeley, et al. JAMA. 195:195-196, January 17, 1966.

"Some comments on the cooperation of microbiologists and dermatovenerologists in the prevention of gonorrhea," by V. Potuznik. CESK DERM. 42:217-223, August, 1967.

"Some problems of organizing programmed instruction at the Department of Dermatology and Venereal Diseases," by N. A. Torsuev, et al. VESTN DERM VENER. 42:49-52, February, 1968.

"Stresses role of MD in VD control," by J. A. Cowan. MICH MED. 65:552, July, 1966.

"Syphilophobia in the practice of the dermatovenereologist," by V. D. Kochetkov, et al. VESTN DERM VENER. 42:62-67, November, 1968.

"Teaching of the clinical, epidemiological, public health, and social aspects of the venereal diseases in the medical schools throughout the world. Interim report of the continuing cooperative study between WHO and the IUVDT," by B. Webster. BRIT J VENER DIS. 46:156-158, April, 1970.

"Teaching of dermatovenerology in the school of medicine. Goals and methods," by J. Obrtel, et al. CESK DERM. 44:37-40, February, 1969.

"Teaching of venereal disease in medical schools throughout the world. Preliminary report," by B. Webster. BRIT J VENER DIS. 42:132-133, June, 1966.

"Use of testing and teaching devices at the Department of Dermatology and Venereal Diseases," by I. I. Il'in. VESTN DERM VENER. 43:49-53, February, 1969.

"VD detectives; doctors and nurses in Boston." TIME. 90:32, September 1, 1967.

"The venereal disease problem facing the private physician and his patient," by A.N. Johnson. ARCH ENVIRON HEALTH, Chicago. 13:393-396, September, 1966.

MEDICAL DOCTORS & VENEREAL DISEASE

"We who treat but don't report are responsible for the rising venereal disease incidence. Editorial," by A. C. Curtis. UNIV MICH MED CENT J. 32:215-216, September-October, 1966.

MEGACLOR
SEE: CLOMOCYCLINE

METHACYCLINE

"Methacycline in the management of Donovanosis (granuloma inguinale)," by J. M. Santos, et al. HOSPITAL. 74:1661-1668, November, 1968.

"Methacycline (rondomycin) in gonorrhoea," by R. S. Morton, et al. BRIT J VENER DIS. 42:175-177, September, 1966.

"Methylenecycline in urology (rondomycin)," by R. Schilliro. J UROL NEPHROL. 74:498-501, June, 1968.

"Use of methacycline in blennorrhagic infection," by E. Ferrea, et al. MINERVA DERM. 43:285-287, June, 1968.

METRONIDAZOLE

"Action and secondary action of metronidazol in the therapy of trichomoniasis," by K. Wiesner, et al. FORTSCHR ARZNEIMITTELFORSCH. 9:361-391, 1966.

"Changes in the nuclear ultrastructure observed in trichomonas vaginalis after treatment with metronidazole," by D. Panaitescu, et al. MICROBIOLOGIA. 15:43-48, January-February, 1970.

"Clinical evaluation of metronidazole 'Polfa' in the treatment of trichomoniasis in women," by C. Zwierz, et al. WIAD PARAZYT. 15:387-388, 1969.

"Comparative efficacy of the use of metronidazole of diverse manufacture in the treatment of patients with trichomoniasis," by M. M. Dadashzade. UROL NEFROL. 32:39-41, July-August, 1967.

"Contribution to the resistance of trichomonas vaginalis to metronidazole," by M. Valent, et al. BRATISL LEK LISTY. 52:58-61, July, 1969.

"Control of concomitant vaginal moniliasis during metronidazole therapy for trichomonas vaginalis," by J. F.

METRONIDAZOLE

Clark, et al. J NAT MED ASS. 58:464-465 passim, November, 1966.

"The effect of metronidazole on the inflammatory changes in trichomonas vaginitis," by J. Mleziva, et al. ZBL GYNAEK. 90:425-431, March 23, 1968.

"The effect of metronidazole therapy on cervical histology in trichomoniasis," by B. Gray, et al. J OBSTET GYNAEC BRIT COMM. 74:98-103, February, 1967.

"Experience in the treatment of trichomonas urogenital infections in males with flagyl," by M. M. Dadashzade. VESTN DERM VENER. 41:87-89, August, 1967.

"Experience in the treatment of trichomoniasis in women with flagyl," by A. M. Mezhebovskii, et al. AKUSH GINEK. 42:45-46, February, 1966.

"Flagyl in the therapy of trichomoniasis (results of a complex work)." VESTN DERM VENER. 40:88-92, November, 1966.

"Further observations on strain sensitivity of trichomonas vaginalis to metronidazole," by J. A. McFadzean, et al. BRIT J VENER DIS. 45:161-162, June, 1969.

"Immediate and remote results of the treatment of urogenital trichomoniasis with flagyl (metronidazole)," by B. A. Teokharov, et al. VESTN DERM VENER. 41:52-58, April, 1967.

"The isolation and identification of the urinary oxidative metabolites of metronidazole in man," by J. E. Stambaugh, et al. J PHARMACOL EXP THER. 161:373-381, June, 1968.

"Metronidazole and syphilis." BRIT MED J. 4:4-5, October 7, 1967.

"Metronidazole and treponema pallidum." BRIT J VENER DIS. 43:149, September, 1967.

"Metronidazole in human infections with syphilis," by A. H. Davies. BRIT J VENER DIS. 43:197-200, September, 1967.

"Metronidazole in pregnancy," by W. F. Peterson, et al. AMER J OBSTET GYNEC. 94:242-249, February 1, 1966.

METRONIDAZOLE

"Metronidazole in the treatment of trichomoniasis in men," by A. I. Poliakov, et al. VESTN DERM VENER. 42:86-87, November, 1968.

"Metronidazole treatment of trichomonal vaginitis. A comparison of cure rates in 1961 and 1967," by J. C. Aure, et al. ACTA OBSTET GYNEC SCAND. 48:440-445, 1969.

"Metronidazole treatment of vaginal trichomoniasis. II. Oral vs vaginal therapy," by S. Porapakkham. OBSTET GYNEC. 29:213-216, February, 1967.

"Nifuratel compared with metronidazole in the treatment of trichomonal vaginitis," by B. A. Evans, et al. BRIT MED J. 1:335-336, May 9, 1970.

"A note on the effect of metronidazole on the Nichols strain of treponema pallidum in vitro and in vivo," by A. E. Wilkinson, et al. BRIT J VENER DIS. 43: 201-203, September, 1967.

"On the sensitivity of trichomonas vaginalis strains to metronidazole," by E. Kovacs, et al. ORV HETIL. 110:66-68, January 12, 1969.

"On the therapeutic value of flagyl in trichomoniasis in the male," by L. M. Rozhinskii. VESTN DERM VENER. 40:59-60, April, 1966.

"Pregnancy, trichomoniasis, and metronidazole. A novel dose schedule," by R. X. Sands. AMER J OBSTET GYNEC. 94:350-353, February 1, 1966.

"Prevention of post-metronidazole candidosis with amphotericin B pessaries," by L. Z. Oller. BRIT J VENER DIS. 45:163-166, June, 1969.

"The rapid detection of metronidazole in urine," by P. Durel, et al. BRIT J VENER DIS. 43:111-113, June, 1967.

"625 cases of trichomoniasis treated with metronidazole (statistical discussion)," by M. Gaudefroy, et al. GYNEC PRAT. 19:339-362, 1968.

"Treatment of female and male trichomoniasis with metronidazole," by W. Lapuszek. POL TYG LEK. 24:533-534, April, 1969.

METRONIDAZOLE

"Treatment of trichomonas infection in males with metronidazole," by M. E. Babichenko. VESTN DERM VENER. 41:86, August, 1967.

"Treatment of trichomonas vaginitis in the pregnant woman with metronidazole (8 823 RP). Absence of teratogenic effects," by P. Magnin, et al. REV FRANC GYNEC OBSTET. 61:861-867, December, 1966.

"Treatment of trichomoniasis in women with flagyl," by J. Zawadzki, et al. PRZEGL LEK. 22:367-369, 1966.

"Treatment of urogenital trichomoniasis with flagyl," by L. Slucki. WIAD LEK. 19:855-858, June 1, 1966.

"Treatment of vaginal trichomoniasis with metronidazole flagyl in gel form. Preliminary results," by C. G. de Netto. HOSPITAL. 70:447-449, August, 1966.

"The trichomonacidal action of flagyl," by G. A. Voskresenskaia. VESTN DERM VENER. 39:54-58, October, 1965.

"Trichomonas vaginalis: resistance to metronidazole," by A. W. Diddle. AMER J OBSTET GYNEC. 98:583-585, June 15, 1967.

"Trichomoniasis urogenitalis and metronidazole therapy in dermato-venerologic practice," by G. Elste. DERM WSCHR. 152:263-266, March 12, 1966.

"Use of metronidazole in trichomonas vaginitis," by R. J. Moreno. REV OBSTET GINEC VENEZ. 28:275-290, 1968.

"Use of metronidazole in vaginal trichomoniasis," by R. J. Moreno. REV OBSTET GINEC VENEZ. 29:275-290, 1968.

MINOCYCLINE

"Gonorrheal urethritis in males treated with a single dose of minocycline," by R. W. Thatcher, et al. PUBLIC HEALTH REP. 85:160-162, February, 1970.

MINOR VENEREAL INFECTIONS & DISEASES
SEE ALSO: URETHRITIS, NON-GONOCOCCAL

"Action of pimaricin on postpartum mycoses," by M. E. Rochet, et al. LYON MED. 216:1179-1183, November 20, 1966

MINOR VENEREAL INFECTIONS & DISEASES

"Activity of nifuratel against infective vulvovaginitis due to yeasts, trichomonas and bacteria," by J. E. Murphy. BRIT J CLIN PRACT. 22:431-432, October, 1968.

"Acute vaginitis and its treatment by a gynecologic terramycin foam. Clinical study and therapeutic results," by P. Magnier. GYNEC PRAT. 17:315-335, 1966.

"Apropos of a case of balantis," by A. Siboulet. BULL SOC FRANC DERM SYPH. 74:339-342, 1967.

"Apropos of uveitis in childhood," by S. Braun-Vallon, et al. ANN OCULIST. 200:764-777, July, 1967.

"Atypical FTA-ABS test fluorescence in lupus erythematosus patients," by S. J. Kraus, et al. JAMA. 211: 2140-2141, March 30, 1970.

"Bacteriologic studies on the etiology of colpitis," by M. Pinter. GEBURTSH FRAUENHEILK. 26:27-31, January, 1966.

"Balanoposthitis of bifid urethra," by L. Linguiti. NUNT RADIOL. 34:1839-1845, December, 1968.

"Bejel in Sheffield," by P. M. Wray. BRIT J VENER DIS. 42:25-27, March, 1966.

"A case report of gangrenous balanitis in progressive reaction in leprosy," by D. S. Chaudhury, et al. LEPROSY REV. 37:225-226, October, 1966.

"Cervical and peritoneal bacterial flora associated with salpingitis," by J. Lip, et al. OBSTET GYNEC. 28:561-563, October, 1966.

"Chemotherapy of chlamydial infections," by E. Jawetz. ADVANCES PHARMACOL. 7:253-282, 1969.

"Clinical and laboratory study of vaginitis. Evaluation of diagnostic methods and results of treatment," by S. G. Burgess, et al. NEW YORK J MED. 70:2086-2091, August 15, 1970.

"Clinical and virologic study of patients seen in the Yale-New Haven hospital women's clinic (1963-1964)," by M. E. Wade, et al. AMER J OBSTET GYNEC. 99:595-597, October 15, 1967.

MINOR VENEREAL INFECTIONS & DISEASES

"Clinical experience with nifuratel," by J. Wainstock, et al. REV BRAS MED. 26:675-681, November, 1969.

"Clinical use of pimaricin in parasitic vaginitis," by D. Colavita, et al. MINERVA GINEC. 18:473-476, May 15, 1966.

"A clinico-serologic study of pinta in the Alto Beni Region, Bolivia," by W. F. Edmundson, et al. DERM INT. 6:64-76, April-June, 1967.

"Complement fixing antibodies against miyagawanella ornithosis in a group of subjects in Accra (Ghana)," by V. Russo, et al. ANN MED NAV. 73:437-443, September-October, 1968.

"Conditions of genital organs in women working in foundries," by R. Wawryk, et al. POL TYG LEK. 22:1208-1211, August 7, 1967.

"Condylomata acuminata," by B. A. Teokharov. AKUSH GINEK. 42:41-44, February, 1966.

"Condylomata acuminata--past and present," by B. Bafverstedt. ACTA DERMATOVENER. 47:376-381, 1967.

"Conjugal blastomycosis," by M. W. Craig, et al. AMER REV RESP DIS. 102:86-90, July, 1970.

"Contractures of the fingers associated with tramboesial palmar hyperkeratosis," by S. G. Browne. DERM INT. 7:104-108, April-June, 1968.

"Control of concomitant vaginal moniliasis during metronidazole therapy for trichomonas vaginalis," by J. F. Clark, et al. J NAT MED ASS. 58:464-465 passim, November, 1966.

"Current etiological diversity of infectious urethritis," by A. Siboulet, et al. J UROL NEPHROL. 72:425-430, December, 1966.

"Development of pinta in Mexico," by O. G. Gosset. SALUD PUBLICA MEX. 9:751-753, September-October, 1967.

"Diagnosis and therapy of trichomonal monilial vaginitis," by F. Branger. PRAXIS. 57:1196-1198, September 3, 1968.

MINOR VENEREAL INFECTIONS & DISEASES

"Diagnosis and treatment of vaginitis," by J. C. Hartgill. PRACTITIONER. 202:363-371, March, 1969.

"The diagnosis of borreliosis by immunofluorescence," by M. Allinne, et al. ANN INST PASTEUR. 111:Suppl: 28-35, November, 1966.

"Diagnosis of vaginal discharges," by E. A. Shipton. MED J AUST. 1:1175-1176, June 6, 1970.

"Effect of new chlorosulfonamides on the female vagina. Considering trichomoniasis complicated by mycosis. Experimental part," by A. Kurnatowska. WIAD PARAZYT. 15:19-33, 1969.

"Emphysematous vaginitis," by E. F. Christensen, et al. JAMA. 200:1001-1002, June 12, 1967.

"Emphysematous vaginitis," by J. P. Whalen, et al. OBSTET GYNEC. 29:9-11, January, 1967.

"Endemic pinta. Present situation in Mexico," by O. G. Gosset. SALUD PUBLICA MEX. 11:211-215, March-April, 1969.

"Endometrial blastomycosis acquired by sexual contact," by E. R. Farber, et al. OBSTET GYNEC. 32:195-199, August, 1968.

"Experimental pinta in the chimpanzee," by G. Varela. SALUD PUBLICA MEX. 11:37-38, January-February, 1969.

"Experimental pinta in the chimpanzee," by U. S. Kuhn, 3d, et al. JAMA. 206:829, October 21, 1968.

"Immunologic aspects of pinta," by A. P. Goncalves. DERMATOLOGICA. 135:199-204, 1967.

"Infections of the uterus and accessory organs," by H. Hirai. JAP J NURS ART. 7:39-50, July, 1970.

"Isolation of mima polymorpha var, oxydans from 2 cases of urethritis and 1 of vaginitis," by L. Vergara. REV LAT AMER MICROBIOL. 11:141-144, July-September, 1969.

"Isolation of TRIC agents from the human genital tract," by D. K. Ford, et al. BRIT J VENER DIS. 45:44-46, March, 1969.

MINOR VENEREAL INFECTIONS & DISEASES

"Method for isolation and identification of corynebacterium vaginale (haemophilus vaginalis)," by W. E. Dunkelberg, Jr., et al. APPL MICROBIOL. 19:47-52, January, 1970.

"Molluscum contagiosum," by P. H. Jacobs. AEROSPACE MED. 41:1196-1197, October, 1970.

"Molluscum contagiosum as a sexually transmitted disease," by R. J. Cobbold, et al. PRACTITIONER. 204: 416-419, March, 1970.

"Molluscum contagiosum of the adult. Probably venereal transmission," by P. J. Lynch, et al. ARCH DERM. 98:141-143, August, 1968.

"Mycotic diseases of the male genital organs with specific reference to non-gonorrheal or mycotic urethritis," by J. Rossberg. CESK DERM. 43:168-170, June, 1968.

"Necrotic cervicitis due to primary infection with the virus of herpes simplex," by R. R. Willcox. BRIT MED J. 1:610-612, March 9, 1968.

"New therapeutic and diagnostic points of view in gynecology," by A. Stockli. THER UMSCH. 24:18-23, January, 1967.

"Non-gonococcal infections of the female genitalia," by B. A. Teokharov. BRIT J VENER DIS. 45:334-340, December, 1969.

"Objectivized diagnosis of acute pelvic inflammatory disease. Diagnostic and prognostic value of routine laparoscopy," by L. Jacobson, et al. AMER J OBSTET GYNEC. 105:1088-1098, December 1, 1969.

"Occurrence of vaginal trichomoniasis and mycosis in our material," by M. Valent, et al. BRATISL LEK LISTY. 53:573-577, May, 1970.

"On the etiology of the urethrooculosynovial syndrome," by I. A. Zhodzishskii. UROL NEFROL. 31:36-40, January-February, 1966.

"On the treatment of fluor vaginalis," by A. Bradenburg. MED KLIN. 61:307-308, February 25, 1966.

MINOR VENEREAL INFECTIONS & DISEASES

"Palmar lesions in lupus erythematosus," by L. C. Parish, et al. ARCH DERM. 96:273-276, September, 1967.

"Pinta in Puerto Rico," by A. L. Carrion. BOL ASOC MED P RICO. 60:456-461, October, 1968.

"Relation of TRIC agent to 'non-specific genital infection'," by E. M. Dunlop, et al. BRIT J VENER DIS. 42:77-87, June, 1966.

"Resistant monilial vaginitis. The male aspect," by C. A. Gilpin. J FLORIDA MED ASS. 54:337-338, April, 1967.

"The role of colonic-rectal adenomas as a precarcinomatous condition," by M. Reifferscheid. ERGEBN CHIR ORTHOP. 50:83-105, 1967.

"Serological activity of mycobacterial cardiolipin in comparison with cardiolipin from the cardiac muscle," by M. Sasaki, et al. SCI REP RES INST TOHOKU UNIV. 16:68-71, October, 1969.

"Sexually transmitted disease in gynaecological outpatients with vaginal discharge," by A. M. Driscoll, et al. BRIT J VENER DIS. 46:125, April, 1970.

"The sexually transmitted disease, Part IV. Minor infections," by J. K. Oates. NURS MIRROR. 128:38-39, February 21, 1969.

"Specific and aspecific cervico-vaginitis. Diagnostic aspects and new therapeutic trends," by A. Aluigi. MINERVA GINEC. 18:913-918, August 31, 1966.

"A study and new description of corynebacterium vaginale (haemophilus vaginalis)," by W. E. Dunkelberg, Jr., et al. AMER J CLIN PATH. 53:370-377, March, 1970.

"A study of 183 cases of leucorrhea: incidence of trichomonas vaginalis, candida spp., and hemophilus vaginalis," by Z. D. Desai, et al. J POSTGRAD MED. 12:91-98, April, 1966.

"Therapy of fluor vaginalis," by S. Iversen. T NORSK LAEGEFOREN. 88:769-773, May 1, 1968.

"Treatment of urethritis in males," by R. L. Dougherty, Jr. MED TIMES. 98:171-173, July, 1970.

MINOR VENEREAL INFECTIONS & DISEASES

"Tropical gynaecology. Pelvic inflammatory disease," by R. R. Trussell. PROC ROY SOC MED. 61:365-368, April, 1968.

"Tropical treponematoses," by K. F. Schaller. ARCH KLIN EXP DERM. 237:332-340, 1970.

"Vaginal corynebacteria with distinctive properties," by B. Brzin. ZBL BAKT. 210:202-206, June, 1969.

"Vaginal diseases," by W. R. Lang. J AMER COLL HEALTH ASS. 15:Suppl:22-25, May, 1967.

"Vaginitis diagnosis and treatment," by R. E. Burmeister, et al. POSTGRAD MED, Minneapolis. 48:159-163, August, 1970.

"Vaginitis in general practice," by J. H. Kelley. J MED ASS GEORGIA. 57:339-341, July, 1968.

"Vaginostic diagnostic kit." MED LETT DRUGS THER. 10:19-20, March 8, 1968.

"Various therapeutic aspects of bacterial, mycotic and protozoan cervico-vaginitis," by G. Candela, et al. MINERVA GINEC. 20:1626-1629, October 31, 1968.

"Viral and virus-like infections of the female genital tract," by W. E. Josey, et al. CLIN OBSTET GYNEC. 12:161-178, March, 1969.

"Viral urethritis of a venereal origin," by I. I. Il'In. UROL NEFROL. 35:41-44, May-June, 1970.

"Vulvitis and vaginitis," by E. Landes. MED WELT. 27:1450-1453, July 2, 1966.

"Vulvovaginitis in the premenarcheal child," by R. H. Heller, et al. J PEDIAT. 74:370-377, March, 1969.

MONOMYCIN

"Some observations of the effectiveness of monomycin in the treatment of gonorrhea in men," by V. E. Grigor'ev, et al. VESTN DERM VENER. 44:59-62, April, 1970.

MONONUCLEOSIS

"Biologic false-positive reactions and infectious mononucleosis," by H. A. Cabrera, et al. TECHN BULL

MONONUCLEOSIS

    REGIST MED TECHN. 38:261-263, October, 1968.

MYCOPLASMAS

"Clinical syndromes with mycoplasma infections," by D. A. Tyrrell. POSTGRAD MED J, London. 43:104-106, March, 1967.

"Colonization of newborn infants by mycoplasmas," by J. O. Klein, et al. NEW ENG J MED. 280:1025-1030, May 8, 1969.

"Detection of mycoplasma infection in routine laboratory testing," by R. Wik, et al. MUNCHEN MED WSCHR. 112:888-889, May 8, 1970.

"Detection of mycoplasmas in upper parts of the urinary tract," by W. Witzleb, et al. ZBL BAKT. 208:427-430, 1968.

"Genital mycoplasma in pathology of the woman, fetus, and neonate (literature review)," by M. A. Bashakova. VOP OKHR MATERIN DETS. 15:71-74, June, 1970.

"Genital mycoplasmosis in cattle and man," by R. S. Hirth, et al. J AMER VET MED ASS. 148:277-282, February 1, 1966.

"Incidence and role of mycoplasma in urogenital diseases," by A. Stangalini, et al. MINERVA GINEC. 21:1701-1706, December 31, 1969.

"Infections and first trimester losses: Possible role of mycoplasmas," by S. G. Driscoll, et al. FERTIL STERIL. 20:1017-1019, November-December, 1969.

"Intrauterine infection of the fetus with genital mycoplasma," by M. A. Bashmakova, et al. VOP OKHR MATERIN DETS. 14:69-73, November, 1969.

"Isolation and propagation of mycoplasma," by A. C. Ruys, et al. ANN NY ACAD SCI. 143:390-393, July 28, 1967.

"Isolation of mycoplasmas and their significance in male urethritis," by G. Catalano, et al. G MAL INFETT. 20:1009-1013, December, 1968.

"Isolation of TRIC agents and mycoplasma from the genitourinary tracts of patients of a venereal disease clinic," by S. Holt, et al. AMER J OPHTHAL. 63:Suppl: 1057-1064, May, 1967.

"Lincomycin, non-gonococcal urethritis, and mycoplasmata," by G. W. Csonka, et al. BRIT J VENER DIS. 45:52-54, March, 1969.

"Methodologic investigations and prevalence of genital mycoplasmas in pregnancy," by P. Braun, et al. J INFECT DIS. 121:391-400, April, 1970.

"Mycoplasma hominis and abortion," by H. J. Harwick, et al. J INFECT DIS. 121:260-268, March, 1970.

"Mycoplasma hominis in abortion," by D. M. Jones. BRIT MED J. 1:338-340, February 11, 1967.

"Mycoplasma in clinical and experimental gynecology," by C. Trinka. CAS LEK CESK. 109:463-466, May, 1970.

"Mycoplasma in human urogenital pathology," by P. Altucci, et al. G MAL INFETT. 19:487-497, August, 1967.

"Mycoplasma in urogenital tract," by M. E. Thomas, et al. LANCET. 2:366-367, August 15, 1970.

"Mycoplasma recovery from the male genitourinary tract: Voided urine versus the urethral swab," by J. E. Gregory, et al. APPL MICROBIOL. 19:268-270, February, 1970.

"Mycoplasmas and arthritis," by J. T. Sharp. ARTHRITIS RHEUM. 13:263-271, May-June, 1970.

"Mycoplasmas and diseases of the urogenital tract," by I. Farber, et al. DEUTSCH GESUNDH. 24:2054-2057, October 23, 1969.

"Mycoplasmas and human reproductive failure," by R. B. Kundsin, et al. SURG GYNEC OBSTET. 131:89-92, July, 1970.

"Mycoplasmas and 'non-specific' genital infection. I. Previous studies and laboratory aspects," by D. Taylor-Robinson, et al. BRIT J VENER DIS. 45:265-273, December, 1969.

--II. Clinical aspects," by E. M. Dunlop, et al. BRIT

J VENER DIS. 45:274-281, December, 1969.

--III. Post-gonococcal urethritis. A prospective study," by M. J. Hare, et al. BRIT J VENER DIS. 45:282-286, December, 1969.

"Mycoplasmas in the female urogenital tract," by C. Del Bianco, et al. G MAL INFETT. 20:1006-1009, December, 1968.

"Mycoplasmas in human pathology," by P. L. Altucci. G MAL INFETT. 20:557-571, June, 1968.

"Mycoplasmas of the human urogenital tract and oropharynx and their possible role in disease: A review with some recent observations," by D. Taylor-Robinson, et al. PROC ROY SOC MED. 59:1112-1116, November, 1966.

"Nongonococcal urethritis associated with human strains of 'T' mycoplasmas," by M. C. Shepard. JAMA. 211: 1335-1340, February 23, 1970; also in US NAVAL MED FIELD RES LAB. 18:1-17, September, 1968.

"Occurrence of T-strains and other mycoplasmata in non-gonococcal urethritis," by F. T. Black, et al. BRIT J VENER DIS. 44:324-330, December, 1968.

"On the pathogenicity of L-form bacteria and mycoplasmataceae and their role in infectious pathology. II. The significance of mycoplasmataceae (PPLO) in infectious pathology," by V. D. Timakov, et al. ZH MIKROBIOL. 43:1-7, January, 1966.

"Possible mycoplasma hominis urethritis revealed by differing responses of 'abacterial urethritis' to treatment with tetracycline and erythromycin," by A. S. Grimble. BRIT J VENER DIS. 44:230-231, September, 1968.

"Relationships between mycoplasma and the etiology of nongonococcal urethritis and Reiter's syndrome," by D. K. Ford. ANN NY ACAD SCI. 143:501-504, July 28, 1967.

"Role of mycoplasma in nongonococcal urethritis," by J. Thivolet, et al. PRESSE MED. 76:1755-1776, October 5, 1968.

"Role of mycoplasma in urethritis. I. Mycoplasma

MYCOPLASMAS

hominis type I," by M. Sepetjian, et al. PATH BIOL. 17:953-959, November, 1969.

"Selective inhibition in vitro of mycoplasma hominis by lincomycin," by G. Csonka, et al. BRIT J VENER DIS. 46:203-204, June, 1970.

"Significance of mycoplasma (PPLO) in diseases of men," by G. Schabinski, et al. Z AERZTL FORTBILD. 63: 1076-1081, October 15, 1969.

"T-strain mycoplasma. Selective inhibition by erythromycin in vitro," by M. C. Shepard, et al. BRIT J VENER DIS. 42:21-24, March, 1966.

"T-strain mycoplasma in non-gonococcal urethritis," by G. W. Csonka, et al. ANN NY ACAD SCI. 143:794-798, July 28, 1967.

"T-strain mycoplasma in non-gonococcal urethritis, Pathogen or commensal?," by W. Fowler, et al. BRIT J VENER DIS. 45:287-293, December, 1969.

"T-strain mycoplasmas in non-specific urethritis," by A. Shipley, et al. MED J AUST. 1:794-796, May 11, 1968.

"Tubal and cervical cultures in acute salpingitis with special reference to mycoplasma hominis and T-strain mycoplasmas," by P. A. Mardh, et al. BRIT J VENER DIS. 46:179-186, June, 1970.

"Work on mycoplasma at the Rackham Arthritis Research Unit," by L. E. Bartholomew. UNIV MICH MED CENT J. 229:30, 1968.

MYCOSIS
  SEE: MINOR VENEREAL DISEASES & INFECTIONS
  SEE ALSO: CANDIDIASIS
          MYCOPLASMAS
          TRICHOMONIASIS
          URETHRA, NON-GONORRHEAL

NAXOGIN
"Treatment of vaginal trichomoniasis using a new drug. Results using naxogin. (K-1900)," by F. V. Rodrigues, et al. HOSPITAL. 77:417-424, February, 1970.

NEISSER, ALBERT

NEISSER, ALBERT
"Albert Neisser (1855-1916) the discoverer of the diplococcus of gonorrhea," by E. Stocki. WIAD LEK. 20: 397-398, February 15, 1967.

NEONATAL
SEE ALSO: OPHTHALMIA NEONATORUM UNDER OPHTHALMOLOGY

"Bedsoniae inclusions in two newborn infants in Lebanon," by N. A. Haddad. AMER J OPHTHAL. 64:124-128, July, 1967.

"A correlative immunologic, microbiologic and clinical approach to the diagnosis of acute and chronic infections in newborn infants," by C. A. Alford, et al. NEW ENG J MED. 277:437-449, August 31, 1967.

"Drug toxicity in the human fetus and newborn child," by J. T. Litchfield, Jr. APPL THER. 9:922-926, November, 1967.

"On the problem of credeization in newborn infants," by V. Dvorak. CESK OFTAL. 22:329-330, September, 1966.

NIFURATEL
"Activity of nifuratel against infective vulvovaginitis due to yeasts, trichomonas and bacteria," by J. E. Murphy. BRIT J CLIN PRACT. 22:431-432, October, 1968.

"Clinical experience with nifuratel," by J. Wainstock, et al. REV BRAS MED. 26:675-681, November, 1969.

"Inhibition of Neisseria gonorrhoeae by nifuratel," by G. M. Churcher, et al. BRIT J VENER DIS. 45:149-150, June, 1969.

"Nifuratel compared with metronidazole in the treatment of trichomonal vaginitis," by B. A. Evans, et al. BRIT MED J. 1:335-336, May 9, 1970.

"Nifuratel for trichomonal vaginitis," by M. Arnold. BRIT MED J. 2:792, June 27, 1970.

"Nifuratel for trichomonal vaginitis," by A. Grimble, et al. BRIT MED J. 2:542, May 30, 1970.

"Nifuratel for trichomonal vaginitis," by S. M. Laird. BRIT MED J. 2:731, June 20, 1970.

NIFURATEL

"Nifuratel for trichomonal vaginitis," by I. Sagone. BRIT MED J. 2:792, June 27, 1970.

"Nifuratel (magmilor) in trichomonal vaginitis," by W. Fowler, et al. BRIT J VENER DIS. 44:331-333, December, 1968.

"Preliminary clinical findings using nifuratel in vaginal trichomoniasis," by C. G. De Netto, et al. REV BRASIL MED. 26:190-192, March, 1969.

"Therapy of trichomonas and thrush colpitis using nifuratel," by A. Weidenbach, et al. MUNCHEN MED WSCHR. 110:343-345, February 9, 1968.

"Treatment of trichomonas vaginitis with nifuratel," by H. Gjonnaess, et al. ACTA OBSTET GYNEC SCAND. 48:85-94, 1969.

"Treatment of vaginal trichomonadosis with nifuratel," by H. Schmidt, et al. WIAD PARAZYT. 15:373-376, 1969.

NIRIDAZOLE

"The amoebicidal, trichomonicidal, and antibacterial effects of niridazole in laboratory animals," by F. Kradolfer, et al. ANN NY ACAD SCI. 160:740-748, October 6, 1969.

NITRIMIDAZINE

"Evaluation of the nitrimidazine activity in giardiasis and genital trichomoniasis," by J. M. Salles, et al. HOSPITAL. 77:1689-1697, May, 1970.

"Nitrimadazone, a new systemic trichomonacide," by A. Cantone, et al. G MAL INFETT PARASSIT. 21:954-958, December, 1969.

"Observations on the problem of trichomoniasis and its systemic treatment with nitrimidazine," by I. Signorelli, et al. MINERVA GINEC. 21:1649-1654, December 15, 1969.

"Treatment of genital trichomonas using a new drug: nitrimidazine," by M. A. Fonngera, et al. REV COLUMBIA OBSTET. 21:141-146, March-April, 1970.

NITROFURAN

"Studies on the trichomonacidal effects of various ni-

NITROFURAN

trofuran preparations," by H. Birnbaum. ZBL GYNAEK. 89:1303-1313, September 9, 1967.

"Treatment of vaginal trichomoniasis with nitrofurazone," by Z. Malachowski, et al. POL TYG LEK. 24:1823-1824, October 24, 1969.

NITROMIDAZOLE

"Antiprotozoan activity of nitroimidazoles," by I. De Carneri. ARZNEIMITTELFORSCHUNG. 19:382-386, March, 1969.

"Clinical test of a drug; nitroimidazine (1-N-Beta-Ethylmorpholin-5-Nitroimidazole) in genital trichomoniasis," by J. E. Zuniga, et al. REV COLUMBIA OBSTET GINEC. 21:193-196, March-April, 1970.

"Effect of a nitro-imidazole on primary experimental syphilis in rabbits," by A. R. Yobs, et al. BRIT J VENER DIS. 42:122-124, June, 1966.

NON-GONORRHEAL INFECTIONS & DISEASES (+NON-VENEREAL GENITAL DISEASES)
SEE ALSO: MINOR VENEREAL DISEASES & INFECTIONS
MYCOPLASMAS
TRICHOMONIASIS
URETHRITIS, NON-GONOCOCCAL

"The nonvenereal genital diseases as an historical problem," by E. Seidler. HAUTARZT. 17:123-125, March, 1966.

"The status of the sexual organs of women whose husbands have nongonorrheal inflammatory diseases of the urogenital system," by S. N. Kheifets, et al. VESTN DERM VENER. 43:51-55, May, 1969.

NON-GONORRHEAL URETHRITIS
SEE: URETHRITIS, NON-GONOCOCCAL

NURSES

"Health education by public health nurses as a preventive measure against venereal diseases," by K. Imazu, et al. JAP J NURS ART. 8:21-25, August, 1969.

"The nurse and venereal disease control," by F. A. Walsh. S CAROLINA NURS. 18:11-13, Winter 1965-1966.

"The nurse's role in the control of venereal disease,"

NURSES

by J. Towpik. PIELEG POLOZ. 11:6-7, 1966; also in PIELEG POLOZ. 2:13-15, 1967.

"The school nurse and VD education," by E. W. Collum. S CAROLINA NURS. 20:7, 30-33, Spring, 1968.

"The school nurse-teacher's role in controlling venereal disease," by D. E. Barlow. J NY SCH NURSE-TEACH ASS. 1:16-19, June, 1970.

"Unique course focuses on the VD interview," by L. Alexander. RN. 29:47-52, April, 1966.

"The work of a screening nurse in venerology," by F. Novotny. CESK DERM. 41:84-91, April, 1966.

OBSTETRICS
SEE: PREGNANCY

OCCURRENCE

"Attempt at the evaluation of the influence of environment on the incidence of syphilis in soldiers of obligatory service," by J. Lańcucki, et al. PRZEGL DERM. Suppl:93-99, 1969.

"Brucellosis, treponematosis, rickettsiosis and psittacosis in Surinam. A serological survey," by P. Kooy. TROP GEOGR MED. 22:172-178, June, 1970.

"Centers of rickettsiosis and treponematosis in the east of the Central African Republic (Bangassou, 1966)," by A. Retel-Laurentin. BULL SOC PATH EXOT. 61:321-339, 1968.

"Data concerning venereal diseases in metropolitan France for the year 1966," by G. Martin-Bouyer. BULL INST NAT SANTE. 22:1021-1055, September-October, 1967.

"Developmental trends in the occurrence of syphilis and gonorrhea in Czechoslovakia in the years 1948-1964," by J. Beniakovà. CESK DERM. 42:263-270, August, 1967.

"Epidemiological situation of venereal diseases," by H. C. Sturde, et al. OEFF GESUNDHEITSWESEN. 31:348-353, July-August, 1969.

"Epidemiology of venereal diseases in France from 1963 to 1967." BULL INST NATE SANTE RECH MED. 23:1477-1498, November-December, 1968.

OCCURRENCE

"Health of immigrants," by F. J. Kinsella. PROC ROY SOC MED. 61:23, January, 1968.

"Highest venereal disease rates for United States and Georgia in younger age groups," J MED ASS GEORGIA. 56:302, July, 1967.

"Immigrants and venereal disease." BRIT MED J. 3:129-130, July 19, 1969.

"Immigration and venereal disease in Great Britain," by R. R. Willcox. BRIT J VENER DIS. 42:225-237, December, 1966.

"Importance and epidemiological characteristics of venereal disease," by W. J. Brown. BOL OFIC SANIT PANAMER. 60:93-106, February, 1966.

"Incidence of venereal and skin diseases among the population of the town of Stupino, Moscow region," by E. I. A. Filina. VESTN DERM VENER. 40:62-65, January, 1966.

"The incidence of venereal diseases in India and their control," by V.K. Tatochenko. VESTN DERM VENER. 41:72-77, September, 1967.

"Incidence of venereal diseases in the Netherlands," by H. Bijkerk. BRIT J VENER DIS. 46:247-261, June, 1970.

"Male-female ratios in the V.D. clinics of England and Wales," by R. S. Morton. BRIT J VENER DIS. 46:103-105, April, 1970.

"Observations in the Haight-Ashbury Medical Clinic of San Francisco. Health problems in a 'hippie' subculture," by D. Smith, et al. CLIN PEDIAT. 7:313-316, June, 1968.

"Observations on the occurrence of venereal diseases in Berlin 1933-1939," by M. Sturzbecher. MED MSCHR. 23:259-264, June, 1969.

"Occurrence of venereal diseases in the Central Bohemian Region," by J. Obrtel. CESK DERM. 43:48-50, February, 1968.

"On the epidemiology of syphilis and gonorrhea in Nordrhein-Westfalia," by K. Gedicke. OEFF GESUNDHEITS-WESEN. 29:28-33, January, 1967.

"Patterns of venereal disease morbidity in recent years." STATIST BULL METROP LIFE INSUR CO. 50:5-7, April, 1969.

"Peculiarities of skin and venereal morbidity of the population of some countries of Asia, Africa and Latin America," by R. S. Babaiants. VESTN DERM VENER. 41:49-54, February, 1967.

"Preliminary study on the epidemiology of venereal diseases in Turin from 1958 to 1968," by B. Erber, et al. G BATT VIROL IMMUN. 62:3-15, January-February, 1969.

"Present-day situation regarding venereal diseases in Mexico," by S. A. Campos, et al. SALUD PUBLICA MEX. 8:553-560, July-August, 1966.

"Problem of venereal diseases in the area of Stalowa Wola," by K. Wojas. ZDROW PUBLICZNE. 4:493-499, April, 1967.

"The problem of venereal diseases in the capital Prague," by J. Konopik. CESK DERM. 43:46-47, February, 1968.

"Problems of public health resulting from migration of workers," by A. Roussel. BULL INST NAT SANTE. 21: 1121-1138, November-December, 1966.

"Problems with gonorrhea in the Southern Moravian region," by J. Horacek. CESK DERM. 43:62-64, February, 1968.

"Problems with venereal diseases in the Eastern Slovakian region in 1966 according to districts," by E. Maly. CESK DERM. 43:72-76, February, 1968.

"Psychiatric differences in Ashkenazim and Sephardim," by F. Grewel. PSYCHIAT NEUROL NEUROCHIR. 70:339-347, September-October, 1967.

"Recapitulation of data received during the year 1965, concerning statistics for venereal disease in metropolitan France," by P. Chassagne. BULL INST NAT SANTE. 21:709-736, July-August, 1966.

OCCURRENCE

"Research on Mimeae-Herellae in venereal diseases," by F. Caprilli, et al. MINERVA DERM. 42:663-664, December, 1967.

"Rural health in northern Nigeria: some recent developments and problems," by K. D. Thomson. TRANS ROY SOC TROP MED HYG. 61:277-302, 1967.

"A tale of two cities," by G. S. Hayes. QUEENSLAND NURSES J. 8:29+, June, 1966.

"Venereal disease among seafarers on board of Polish ships," by S. Tomaszunas. BULL INST MAR MED GDANSK. 18:67-72, 1967.

"Venereal disease and treponematosis in African countries," by A. P. Shchepin. VESTN DERM VENER. 42:71-75, June, 1968.

"Venereal disease in an Australian metropolis," by A. Adams. MED J AUST. 1:145-151, January 28, 1967.

"Venereal disease in New Zealand," by W. M. Platts. BRIT J VENER DIS. 45:61-66, March, 1969.

"Venereal diseases." NEW ZEALAND MED J. 69:234-235, April, 1969.

"Venereal diseases-environmental changes," by T. Guthe, et al. T NORSK LAEGEFOREN. 89:1784-1789 passim, December 1, 1969.

"Venereal diseases in Dresden 1946 to 1965," by H. Roder. DEUTSCH GESUNDH. 22:313-317, February 16, 1967.

"Venereal diseases in England and Wales. Extract from the Annual Report of the Chief Medical Officer for the year 1964," BRIT J VENER DIS. 42:50-57, March, 1966.

--Extract from the annual report of the Chief Medical Officer for the year 1966." BRIT J VENER DIS. 44:83-91, March, 1968.

--Extract from the annual report of the Chief Medical Officer for the year 1967." BRIT J VENER DIS. 45:67-75, March, 1969.

"Venereal diseases in Finland," by A. Lassus. SAIRAAN-

OCCURRENCE

HOITAJA. 45:520-521, August 11, 1969.

"Venereal diseases in N.Z." NEW ZEALAND NURS J. 61: 120+, November, 1968.

"Venereal diseases in Vojvodina," by S. Cvejić, et al. MED PREGL. 22:229-241, 1969.

"Venereal diseases in women," by K. S. Krishna. INDIAN PRACT. 19:173-176, February, 1966.

"Venereology and the sexually transmitted diseases in Denmark, Sweden and Holland. Part 1," by N. O. J. Hallis. NT. 66:105, July 23, 1970.

--Part 2." NT. 66:109+, July 30, 1970.

"Why South Carolina's high VD rate," by R. W. Ball. J S CAROLINA MED ASS. 62:175-176, April, 1966.

"Work disability due to dermatologic and venereal diseases in Czechoslovakia during 1955-1964," by J. Stach. CESK DERM. 41:343-349, October, 1966.

"Work experience of a dermatologist--venereologist in a screening room," by G. I. Filatov. VESTN DERM VENER. 43:57-59, January, 1969.

OLEANDOMYCIN
"Erythromycin and oleandomycin in therapy of fresh gonorrhea in women," by L. D. Kuntsevich. VESTN DERM VENER. 42:84-86, July, 1968.

OLETETRIN
"Experience in the treatment of gonorrhea in males with oletetrin," by I. I. Mavrov. VESTN DERM VENER. 43: 80-82, November, 1969.

"Oletetrin in the therapy of gonorrhea," by A. I. Poliakov, et al. VESTN DERM VENER. 41:71-73, June, 1967.

"Oletetrin in the therapy of patients with gonorrhea," by Z. V. Ermol'eva, et al. VESTN DERM VENER. 42:81-86, April, 1968.

"Oletetrin in treatment of fresh gonorrhea in men," by T. A. Kislova, et al. ANTIBIOTIKI. 14:467-469, May, 1969.

OLETETRIN

"Study of the concentration of oletetrin in the blood serum from patients with gonorrhea," by Z. V. Ermol'ev, et al. VESTN DERM VENER. 40:77-79, September, 1966.

OPHTHALMIA NEONATORUM
SEE: OPHTHALMOLOGY

OPHTHALMOLOGY

"Acute and subacute demyelination of the optic nerves," by W. H. Melanowski. KLIN OCZNA. 37:517-525, 1967.

"Acute bilateral perivasculitis retinae probably of a gonococcal origin," by S. Kamel. BULL OPHTHAL SOC EGYPT. 59:Suppl:63:107+, 1966.

"Acute conjunctivitis among Cairo adult inhabitants increase in bacteriologically negative cases," by A. Mortada. BULL OPHTHAL SOC EGYPT. 58:37-45, 1965.

"Acute conjunctivitis among Cairo children. Decrease in K.W. and gonococcal infections and increase in bacteriologically negative cases," by A. Mortada, et al. BULL OPHTHAL SOC EGYPT. 58:25-35, 1965.

"Argyll Robertson pupil," by D. Leak. NM. 123:lv, February 17, 1967.

"The Argyll Robertson pupil, 1869-1969. A critical survey of the literature," by I. E. Loewenfeld. SURVEY OPHTHAL. 14:199-200, November, 1969.

"A case of Marcus Gunn phenomenon with oculomotor paralysis," by J. Kaouzny. KLIN OCZNA. 37:389-393, 1967.

"Comparison of procedures for laboratory diagnosis of oculogenital infections with inclusion conjunctivitis agents," by J. Schachter, et al. AMER J EPIDEM. 85: 453-458, May, 1967.

"Dislocation of the lens. A study of 166 hospitalized cases," by W. H. Jarrett, II. ARCH OPHTHAL. 78:289-296, September, 1967.

"Endogenous uveitis. V. Laboratory tests (W.R.,G.R., E.S.R.,S.A.T.,HB Per cent)," by M. S. Norn. ACTA OPHTHAL. 47:848-864, 1969.

"Implications of spiral forms in the eye," by B. Golden, et al. SURVEY OPHTHAL. 14:179-183, November, 1969.

OPHTHALMOLOGY

"Incidence of bacterial causes of ophthalmia neonatorum," by J. A. Kagwa-Nyanzi. E AFR MED J. 47:159-162, March, 1970.

"Infection by bedsoniae and the possibility of spurious isolation. 2. Genital infection, disease of the eye, Reiter's disease," by E. M. Dunlop, et al. AMER J OPHTHAL. 63:Suppl:1073-1081, May, 1967.

"Infection by TRIC agent and other members of the bedsonia group, with a note on Reiter's disease. 1. Ocular disease in the adult," by B. R. Jones, et al. TRANS OPHTHAL SOC UK. 86:291-312, 1966.

--2. Ophthalmia neonatorum due to TRIC agent," by A. Freedman, et al. TRANS OPHTHAL SOC UK. 86:313-320, 1966.

--3. Genital infection and disease of the eye," by E. M. Dunlop, et al. TRANS OPHTHAL SOC UK. 86:321-334, 1966.

--4. Laboratory aspects," by I. A. Harper, et al. TRANS OPHTHAL SOC UK. 86:335-348, 1966.

"Intraocular penetration of cephalexin in man," by G. L. Boyle, et al. AMER J OPHTHAL. 69:868-872, January-June, 1970.

"Neonatal ophthalmia." LANCET. 2:630, September 20, 1969.

"Ophthalmia neonatorum. Prevention with 5-nitro-2-furaldehyde semicarbazone (furacin)," by O. R. Baptista. HOSPITAL. 71:187-193, January, 1967.

"Ophthalmia neonatorum in Glasgow," by J. A. Smith. SCOT MED J. 14:272-276, August, 1969.

"Proliferation of pigmented cells in the corneal endothelium," by M. L. Restivo-Manfridi, et al. ANN OTTAL. 92:1007-1011, November, 1966.

"Retino-choroidal pigmented paravenous degeneration," by M. Ardouin, et al. BULL SOC OPHTAL FRANC. 67:742-744, September, 1967.

"Use of Nelson's test in the diagnosis of specific diseases of the cornea," by F. Beauchamp, et al.

OPHTHALMOLOGY

MED TROP. 27:679-681, November-December, 1967.

"VD and vision." J MED SOC NEW JERSEY. 66:266, June, 1969.

"The venereal nature of inclusion conjunctivitis," by J. Schachter, et al. AMER J EPIDEM. 85:445-452, May, 1967.

"Why prophylaxis for ophthalmia neonatorum?," by R. H. Dennis. J MAINE MED ASS. 57:27-28, February, 1966.

ORAL
"Be alert to the dental patient with venereal disease," by D. R. Wallace. DENT ASSIST. 35:23, November, 1966.

"Value of medical diagnostic screening tests for dental patients," by W. R. Sabes, et al. J AMER DENT ASS. 80:133-136, January, 1970.

OXYGEN THERAPY
"Anaerobic pelvic infections and developments in hyperbaric oxygen therapy," by R. T. Parker, et al. AMER J OBSTET GYNEC. 96:645-659, November 1, 1966.

OXYGUINOLINE
"Long-term treatment of trichomonas infection with a diiodine derivative of oxyguinoline," by M. Arnold. PRAXIS. 57:1663-1666, November 26, 1968.

OXYTERRACINE
"Studies on the disappearance of treponema pallidum from the eruption of early syphilis under the effect of various antibiotics. Effect of oxyterracine on treponema pallidum," by J. Suchanek, et al. POL TYG LEK. 22:1103-1106, July 17, 1967.

OXYTETRACYCLINE
SEE ALSO: DOXYCYCLINE
TETRACYCLINE

"Final report on the effectiveness of oxytetracycline in the treatment of gonorrhea in females," by L. H. Shapiro, et al. AMER J OBSTET GYNEC. 94:536-538, February 15, 1966.

"Gonorrhoeal urethritis in males treated with one oral dose of oxytetracycline," by D. G. McLone, et al.

OXYTETRACYCLINE

BRIT J VENER DIS. 43:166-167, September, 1967.

"'Instant treatment' of gonorrhea with a new oxytetracycline derivate--doxycycline (preliminary report)," by L. Sylvestre, et al. INT Z KLIN PHARMAKOL THER TOXIK. 1:401-403, July, 1968.

"Studies of the value of erythromycin and oxytetracycline in treatment of early syphilis," by J. Bowszyc, et al. POL TYG LEK. 25:1394-1396, September, 1970.

"TPI and FTA tests in the evaluation of effectiveness of the oral treatment of early symptomatic syphilis with detreomycin, erythromycin and oxytetracycline with consideration of the clinical picture," by J. Lebioda, et al. PRZEGL DERM. Suppl:39-51, 1969.

"The treatment of early lues with oxytetracycline," by K. Bosse. HAUTARZT. 17:306-309, July, 1966.

PARESIS
SEE ALSO: NEUROSYPHILIS

"A case of congenital paresis in 1966," by M. M. Carruthers, et al. ANN INTERN MED. 66:1204-1206, June, 1967.

"General paralysis and cerebral angiomatosis in a child. Apropos of a case," by H. Collomb, et al. BULL SOC MED AFR NOIRE LANG FRANC. 12:506-511, 1967.

"General paralysis in Victoria, Australia: historical study," by A. Stoller, et al. MED J AUST. 2:607-611, September 20, 1969.

"General paralysis of the insane with gumma of the skull," by S. B. Mahapatra. BRIT J VENER DIS. 43:178-180, September, 1967.

"Immunological and immunochemical investigations of patients suffering from general paralysis," by H. Schmidt, et al. BRIT J VENER DIS. 46:135-137, April, 1970.

"Paresis of the recurrent nerve as the first symptom of luetic aortic aneurysm," by Z. Jina. CESK OTOLARYNG. 16:247-251, August, 1967.

"Presence of spirochaetes in paresis despite penicillin therapy," by W. E. Gager, et al. BRIT J VENER DIS.

PARESIS

    44:277-282, December, 1968.

"Progressive paralysis--past and present," by S. Stojiljkovic, et al. SRPSKI ARH CELOK LEK. 94:211-218, March, 1966.

"Report on a study of cerebral biopsy in general paretics," by R. A. Venkoba, et al. NEUROL INDIA. 17: 26-27, January-March, 1969.

"Study of the non-inflammatory lesions of neurosyphilis. 3. Case of progressive paralysis association with Huntington's chorea," by T. Matsuoka, et al. BRAIN NERVE. 20:925-930, 1968.

PARETICS
SEE: PARESIS

PAROMOMYCIN
"Is paromomycin appropriate for the treatment of trichomona infection in women. II. Clinical experiences," by H. Spitzbart, et al. ZBL GYNAEK. 88:563-566, April 30, 1966.

PASOMYSIN
"Pasomycin treatment of women with gonorrhoea," by B. S. Kaliner. VESTN DERM VENER. 42:57-58, May, 1968.

PAVLOV, SERGEI T.
"Sergei Timofeevich Pavlov." VESTN DERM VENER. 41:89, June, 1967.

PEDICULOSIS
"Epidemic pediculosis and gonorrhea," by A. Altchek. OBSTET GYNEC. 35:638-641, April, 1970.

PENICILLIN
SEE ALSO: REACTIONS: PENICILLIN

"Attempt to induce in vitro penicillin resistance in Neisseria gonorrhoeae," by F. Vymola, et al. J HYG EPIDEM. 12:427-430, 1968.

"Case contribution to the problem of penicillin resistance in gonorrhea," by E. Friedrich, et al. Z HAUT GESCHLECHTSKR. 40:194-200, March 15, 1966.

"Catamnestic studies of syphilis patients treated with arsenobenzene-penicillin-bismuth," by J. Rossberg.

PENICILLIN

DERM WSCHR. 153:161-164, February 18, 1967.

"Cerebrospinal fluid findings after treatment of early syphilis with penicillin. A further series of 80 cases," by W. L. Fernando. BRIT J VENER DIS. 42: 134-135, June, 1968.

"Clinical and epidemiologic impact of penicillins old and new," by G. T. Stewart. PEDIAT CLIN N AMER. 15: 13-29, February, 1968.

"Clinical and experimental studies on the thrombosis formation influenced by penicillin," by B. Nagay. ROCZN POM AKAD MED SWIERCZEWSKI. 13:289-306, 1967.

"Clinical application of methyldichlorphenylisonxizolyl penicillin (dicloxacillin, staphcillin A) for urinary tract infections, especially for non-gonorrheal urethritis," by J. Ishigami, et al. J ANTIBIOT. 19:354-357, October, 1966.

"Current status of the in vitro sensitivity of gonococci to penicillin in Finland," by O. V. Renkonen, et al. ACTA DERMATOVENER. 50:151-153, 1970.

"Decreased gonococcus sensitivity to penicillin and penicillin dosage, development and present situation," by E. Friedrich, et al. Z AERZTL FORTBILD. 63:861-868, August 15, 1969.

"Demethylchlortetracycline compared with penicillin in the treatment of gonorrhoea in women," by W. Enfors, et al. BRIT J VENER DIS. 46:209-211, June, 1970.

"Development of resistance of gonococci to penicillin: An eight-year study," by C. R. Amies. CANAD MED ASS J. 96:33-35, January 7, 1967.

"Experience of continuous treatment of early forms of syphilis with penicillin and bicillin," by L. A. Rozina. VESTN DERM VENER. 42:62-65, 1968.

"Experimental under-treatment of early syphilis with probenecid and penicillin in anti-gonorrhoea dosages. A study to assess the best follow-up examination time for syphilis after gonorrhoea treatment in Greenland," by L. Hallinger. ACTA DERMATOVENER. 48:260-267, 1968.

PENICILLIN

"Failure of penicillin in a newborn with congenital syphilis," by J. B. Hardy, et al. JAMA. 212:1345-1349, May 25, 1970.

"The formation of penicillin antigens," by A. L. De Weck. PROC ROY SOC MED. 61:894-897, September, 1968.

"Further studies of the sensitivity of gonococci to penicillin," by N. M. Ovchinnikov, et al. UROL NEFROL. 31:40-43, September-October, 1966.

"Gonococcal resistance to penicillin," by H. Storck, et al. DERMATOLOGICA. 139:254-259, 1969.

"Gonococcal urethritis in males in Vietnam: three penicillin regimens and one tetracycline regimen," by L. H. Maurer, et al. JAMA. 207:946-948, February 3, 1969.

"Gonorrhea therapy with a combination of probenecid and benzylsodiumpenicillin. A report from Greenland," by G. A. Olsen, et al. UGESKR LAEG. 130:1465-1468, September 5, 1968.

"Gonorrhoea treated by a combination of probenecid and sodium penicillin G," by G. A. Olsen, et al. BRIT J VENER DIS. 45:144-148, June, 1969.

"Gummous syphilis of the penis regractory to penicillin and bismuth preparations," by A. I. Levykin. VESTN DERM VENER. 43:82-86, January, 1969.

"Hemagglutinating antipenicillin antibodies (HAPA). Incidence and significance in four groups of patients," by W. Q. Ascari, et al. TRANSFUSION. 9:35-39, January-February, 1969.

"High dosage procaine penicillin combined with ampicillin in the treatment of gonorrhoea after failure with standard procaine penicillin dosage," by J. L. Fluker, et al. BRIT J VENER DIS. 45:317-320, December, 1969.

"Immediate results of treating patients with contagious forms of syphilis using simultaneously penicillin and bismuth preparations," by T. V. Vasil'ev, et al. VESTN DERM VENER. 44:50-55, April, 1970.

"The immunofluorescence reaction of the blood serum of

syphilitic patients following therapy with various durable penicillin preparations," by T. V. Vasil'ev, et al. VESTN DERM VENER. 40:40-45, August, 1966.

"Inactivation of penicillins by carbohydrate solutions at alkaline pH," by M. S. Simberkoff, et al. NEW ENG J MED. 283:116-119, July 16, 1970.

"Intramuscular injection of procaine penicillin combined with oral administration of chloramphenicol in the treatment of gonorrhoea," by H. C. Gjessing, et al. BRIT J VENER DIS. 42:107-109, June, 1966.

"Is there a penicillin resistance in gonorrhea?," by P. Wodniansky. ARCH KLIN EXP DERM. 227:650-652, 1966.

"Large doses of penicillin for treatment of gonorrhea in women," by L. H. Shapiro, et al. OBSTET GYNEC. 30:89-92, July, 1967.

"Minute treatment of gonorrhea. Supplementary observations on the article by H. Biehler and E. Heinke: singe treatment of gonorrhea of the man with high doses of penicillins," by E. G. Jung, et al. MUNCHEN MED WSCHR. 109:296-300, 1967; also in MUNCHEN MED WSCHR. 110:152-152, January 19, 1968.

"Neurosyphilis, the search for adequate treatment. A review and report of a study using benzathine penicillin," by G. D. Short, et al. ARCH DERM. 93:87-91, January, 1966.

"On the immunological reactivity of penicillin, cephalosporin and tetracycline antibiotics," by J. Lochmannova, et al. J HYG EPIDEM. 14:201-210, 1970.

"On the question of penicillin resistance in gonorrhea," by P. Wodniansky. Z HAUT GESCHLECHTSKR. 41:16-21, July, 1966.

"On sensitivity to penicillin of the gonococcus and the clinical dosage effect of penicillin," by G. Ludwig. DERM WSCHR. 152:1-4, January 8, 1966.

"On the timing of penicillin treatment of syphilis during pregnancy," by H. Walther. ARCH KLIN EXP DERM. 227:307-308, 1966.

PENICILLIN

"On the use of benzathine penicillin 'penduran' for the long term therapy of syphilis," by A. Kern. DEUTSCH GESUNDH. 21:1739-1750, September 15, 1966.

"One-session treatment of gonorrhoea in males with procaine penicillin plus probenecid," by R. J. Cobbold, et al. POSTGRAD MED J. 46:142-145, March, 1970.

"Oral chloramphenicol alone and with intramuscular procaine penicillin in the treatment of gonorrhoea," by H. C. Gjessing, et al. BRIT J VENER DIS. 43:133-136, June, 1967.

"Penicillin and urethritis," by H. N. de Carvalho. HOSPITAL. 76:763-768, August, 1969.

"Penicillin-bicillin treatment of patients with infectious forms of syphilis," by G. I. Egorov. VESTN DERM VENER. 41:42-46, February, 1967.

"Penicillin dosage in fresh gonorrhea in men," by T. Putkonen, et al. DUODECIM. 84:512-516, 1968.

"Penicillin dosage in treatment of gonorrhea," by I. Juhlin. NORD MED. 76:806-808, July 14, 1966.

"Penicillin is losing effect on gonorrheal infections." AM DRUGGIST. 159:57, May 5, 1969.

"Penicillin-resistant gonorrhea," by N. Blumberg. J UROL. 101:106, January, 1969.

"Penicillin-resistant gonorrhoea and post-gonococcal urethritis." MED J AUST. 1:275-276, February 17, 1968.

"Penicillin-resistant syphilis," by M. A. Rozentul, et al. VESTN DERM VENER. 40:55-58, April, 1966.

"Penicillin sensitivity of gonococci and its significance in the clinic and treatment of gonorrhea in women," by A. V. Chastikova, et al. ANTIBIOTIKI. 15:561-564, June, 1970.

"Penicillin treatment in neurosyphilis," by W. Schubert. MED KLIN. 63:806-810, May 17, 1968.

"Preliminary results of penicillin treatment in symptomatic early syphilis in 1959-1963," by J. Towpik.

PENICILLIN

PRZEGL DERM. 53:29-32, January-February, 1966.

"Presence of spirochaetes in paresis despite penicillin therapy," by W. E. Gager, et al. BRIT J VENER DIS. 44:277-282, December, 1968.

"Present status of gonorrhea therapy with special reference to penicillin-sensitivity loss of specific gonococci strains," by J. Meyer-Rohn. Z HAUT GESCHLECHTSKR. 45;533-534, July 15, 1970.

"The problem of penicillin resistant gonococci," by C. S. Nicol, et al. BRIT J VENER DIS. 44:315-318, December, 1968.

"Relapse of gonorrhoea after treatment with penicillin or streptomycin," by A. J. Evans. BRIT J VENER DIS. 42:251-262, December, 1966.

"Relationships between the sensitivities in vitro of Neisseria gonorrhoeae to spiramycin, penicillin, streptomycin, tetracycline, and erythromycin," by A. Reyn, et al. BRIT J VENER DIS. 45:223-227, September, 1969.

"Remission possibilities in early seropositive syphilis using high doses of penicillin," by E. Malý, et al. CESK DERM. 45:63-69, April, 1970.

"Remote results of the continuous treatment of fresh forms of syphilis with penicillin and bicillin," by S. T. Pavlov, et al. VESTN DERM VENER. 41:8-11, April, 1967.

"Remote results of pyro-penicillin therapy of syphilis," by I. I. Pototski. VESTN DERM VENER. 42:60-62, April, 1968.

"Resistance of the manifestations of syphilis to the action of penicillin," by M. N. Bukharovich. SOVET MED. 31:137-138, March, 1968.

"Results of studies of the sensitivity of Neisseria gonorrheae to penicillin in soldiers ill with gonorrhea," by J. Rodovský, et al. CESK DERM. 43:9-14, February, 1968.

"Secondary syphilis after 1 injection of 2,4000,000 units of penicillin for primary preserologic syphilis,"

PENICILLIN

by R. Degos, et al. BULL SOC FRANC DERM SYPH. 75: 289-290, 1968.

"Sensitivity of gonococcus to penicillin in patients with gonorrhea," by L. D. Kuntsevich, et al. VESTN DERM VENER. 43:44-45, February, 1969.

"Sensitivity of Neisseria gonorrhoeae to penicillin and other antibiotics. Studies carried out in Toronto during the period 1961 to 1968," by C. R. Amies. BRIT J VENER DIS. 45:216-222, September, 1969.

"Sensitivity of Neisseria gonorrhoeae to penicillin and other drugs," by V. G. Cave, et al. NEW YORK J MED. 70:844-847, April 1, 1970.

"Sensitivity to penicillin of Neisseria gonorrhoeae. Relationship to the results of treatment," by D. A. Leigh, et al. BRIT J VENER DIS. 45:151-153, June, 1969.

"The significance of serum penicillin levels in syphilis therapy," by K. Mach, et al. Z HAUT GESCHLECHTSKR. 44:81-86, February 1, 1969.

"Single treatment of gonorrhea in males with high doses of penicillin," by H. Biehler, et al. MUNCHEN MED WSCHR. 109:296-300, February 10, 1967.

"Spirochetes in the aqueous humor in seronegative ocular syphilis. Persistence after penicillin therapy," by J. L. Smith, et al. ARCH OPHTHAL. 77:474-477, April, 1967.

"Spirochetes in late seronegative syphilis, despite penicillin therapy," by J. L. Smith. MED TIMES. 96:611-623, June, 1968.

"Studies of venereal disease. I. Probenecid-procaine penicillin G combination and tetracycline hydrochloride in the treatment of penicillin-resistant gonorrhea in men," by K. K. Holmes, et al. JAMA. 202:461-473, November 6, 1967.

" A study of the relationships between the sensitivities of Neisseria gonorrhoeae to sodium penicillin G, four semisynthetic penicillins, spiramycin, and fusidic acid," by A. Reyn, et al. BRIT J VENER DIS. 44:140-150, June, 1968.

PENICILLIN

"A survey of the range of sensitivity in vitro of N. gonorrhoea to penicillin," by C. W. Chacko, et al. INDIAN J MED RES. 54:823-838, September, 1966.

"Susceptibility of N. gonorrhoeae to penicillin and tetracycline," by A. R. Ronald, et al. ANTIMICROB AGENTS CHEMOTHER. 8:431-434, 1968.

"Syphilitic aortitis. 56 cases followed-up for 10 years after treatment with penicillin," by S. E. Vivas. ARCH CARIOL MEX. 36:316-321, May-June, 1966.

"Therapy of syphilis with penicillin with special consideration of the time factor," by A. Kern, et al. Z AERZTL FORTBILD. 60:1201-1206, November 15, 1966.

"Treatment of gonococcal urethritis with single injections of 2-4 mega units of aqueous procaine penicillin," by G. D. Morrison, et al. BRIT J VENER DIS. 44:319-323, December, 1968.

"Treatment of gonorrhoea by penicillin and a renal blocking agent (probenecid)," by G. Hatos. MED J AUST. 1:1096-1099, May 30, 1970.

"Treatment of gonorrhea by penicillin in a single large dose," by W. Minkin. MILIT MED. 133:382-386, May, 1968.

"Treatment of gonorrhea with semisynthetic penicillin," by J. Kozerski. PRZEGL DERM. 55:551-555, July-September, 1968.

"The treatment of gonorrhea with a single high-dosed penicillin injection (so-called 'one-shot' treatment," by F. Nemec. Z HAUT GESCHLECHTSKR. 44:507-512, 1969.

"Treatment of penicillin anaphylaxis with injection of the same antigen (penicillin) in high doses," by L. Katsilabors. REV MED MOYEN ORIENT. 24:346-348, July-August, 1967.

"Treatment of penicillin-resistant gonococcal conjunctivitis with ampicillin," by G. L. Spaeth. AMER J OPHTHAL. 66:427-429, September, 1968.

"Treatment of 'penicillin-resistant' gonorrhea in military personnel in SE Asia: a cooperative evaluation of tetracycline and of penicillin plus probenecid in

PENICILLIN

1263 men," by K. K. Holmes, et al. MILIT MED. 133: 642-646, August, 1968.

"Treatment of syphilitic patients with a single course of penicillin," by G. I. Egorov. VESTN DERM VENER. 40:68-71, May, 1966.

"The treponema pallidum immobilization test of cerebrospinal fluid in syphilis patients treated with various delayed-action penicillin preparations," by T. V. Vasil'ev, et al. VESTN DERM VENER. 41:40-45, March, 1967.

"Trial treatment of primo-secondary syphilis with intravenous perfusion of penicillin. Long persistence of seropositivity in favor of actual clinical penicillin resistance of treponema," by M. Bolgert, et al. BULL SOC FRANC DERM SYPH. 74:325-328, 1967.

"Twenty-five years of penicillin in the service of venereology," by R. R. Willcox. BRIT J CLIN PRACT. 21:165-170, April, 1967.

"Usefulness of long-acting penicillin in combination with short-acting preparations for treatment of gonorrhea," by E. Fowinkle, et al. J TENN MED ASS. 59: 1115-1118, November, 1966.

"Value and possibility of long-lasting penicillin therapy in early syphilis," by A. Kern. PRZEGL DERM. 54:95-101, January-February, 1967.

"Value and security of a weekly injection interval in dispensing doses of 1.8 mega units of benzathine penicillin (Penduran-AWD) during long-term therapy of early syphilis," by A. Kern. DERM WSCHR. 154: 608-616, June 29, 1968.

PHOSPHONOMYCIN
"Acute gonococcal urethritis: Failure of response to phosphonomycin therapy," by P. M. Southern, Jr., et al. ANTIMICROB AGENTS CHEMOTHER. 9:343-345, 1969.

PIMAFUCIN
"Experiences with pimafucin in candida and trichomonas vaginitis," by T. Ozbay, et al. MED WELT. 50:2741-2743, December 13, 1969.

PIMARICIN

PIMARICIN
"Action of pimaricin on postpartum mycoses," by M. E. Rochet, et al. LYON MED. 216:1179-1183, November 20, 1966.

"Clinical use of pimaricin in parasitic vaginitis," by D. Colavita, et al. MINERVA GINEC. 18:473-476, May 15, 1966.

"Effect of an antifungal agent, pimaricin, on trichomonas vaginalis in vitro," by K. Asami, et al. J ANTIBIOT. 20:344-346, October, 1967.

"Effect of pimaricin on vaginal trichomoniasis," by H. Wada, et al. J ANTIBIOT. 20:281-284, August, 1967.

"Management of trichomonas vaginitis with pimaricin," by A. Papaloukas, et al. Z HAUT GESCHLECHTSKR. 43: 343-348, April 15, 1968.

"On the clinical use of a new antibiotic, pimaricin, in the therapy of vaginitis caused by candida albicans and by trichomonas," by B. Ferrari, et al. QUAD CLIN OSTET GINEC. 21:929-945, November, 1966.

"Pimaricin," by J. Bret. SEM THER. 41:427-428, October, 1965.

"Pimaricin, an antibiotic towards fungi and trichomonads," by W. Raab. ARZNEIMITTELFORSCHUNG. 17:538-543, May, 1967.

"Pimaricin in the treatment of trichomoniasis and vaginal moniliasis," by H. Zorn. Z ALLGEMEINMED. 45: 1640-1643, December 10, 1969.

"Preliminary observations on the use of pimaricin in vaginitis due to candida albicans, trichomonas vaginalis and in aspecific vaginitis," by B. I. De Luca. MINERVA GINEC. 18:840-846, August 15, 1967.

PINTA: SEE MINOR
       VENEREAL DISEASES & INFECTIONS
       YAWS

POLYRADICULNEURITIS
"Clinical investigation of inflammatory polyradiculoneuritis in France," by P. Castaigne, et al. REV NEUROL. 115:849-872, October, 1966.

PREDNISONE

PREDNISONE

"Congenital luetic hearing impairment. Treatment with prednisone," by M. E. Patterson. ARCH OTOLARYNG. 87:378-382, April, 1968; also in TRANS PACIF COAST OTOOPHTHAL SOC. 51:235-246, 1967.

"The effect of prednisone on the Jarisch-Herxheimer reaction," by H. Gudjonsson, et al. ACTA DERMATO-VENER. 48:15-18, 1968.

PREGNANCY

"Advantage of a routine Reiter protein complement-fixation test in the serodiagnosis of syphilis in pregnancy," by C. A. Morris. J CLIN PATH. 21:731-734, November, 1968.

"Apropos of false specific serology in a woman presenting habitual abortions," by G. Zographos, et al. BULL FED GYNEC OBSTET FRANC. 18:299-301, June-August, 1966.

"A case of anaphylactic shock in a pregnant women with a nephropathia after the administration of penicillin," by T. A. Avksent'Eva. AKUSH GINEK. 42:43, December, 1966.

"Diagnostic problems in a patient with habitual intrauterine fetal death," by A. M. Schellen, et al. BULL SOC ROY BELG GYNEC OBSTET. 36:187-194, 1966.

"Drug toxicity in the human fetus and newborn child," by J. T. Litchfield, Jr. APPL THER. 9:922-926, November, 1967.

"Fetal infections with bacteria and protozoa," by H. Kraubig. MSCHR KINDERHEILK. 116:211-214, June, 1968.

"Genital mycoplasma in pathology of the woman, fetus and neonate. (Literature review)," by M. A. Bashakova. VOP OKHR MATERIN DETS. 15:71-74, June, 1970.

"Importance of mass colpocytological examination in the diagnosis of uterine tumors in preclinical phases, of vaginal trichomoniasis and of prolonged pregnancy," by S. DeLeo, et al. MINERVA MED. 58:2821-2822, August 11, 1967.

"Intrauterine infection of the fetus with genital mycoplasma," by M. A. Bashmakova, et al. VOP OKHR MATERIN DETS. 14:69-73, November, 1969.

PREGNANCY

"Methodologic investigations and prevalence of genital mycoplasmas in pregnancy," by P. Braun, et al. J INFECT DIS. 121:391-400, April, 1970.

"Metronidazole in pregnancy," by W. F. Peterson, et al. AMER J OBSTET GYNEC. 94:243-249, February 1, 1966.

"Mycoplasma hominis and abortion," by H. J. Harwick, et al. J INFECT DIS. 121:260-268, March, 1970.

"Mycoplasma hominis in abortion," by D. M. Jones. BRIT MED J. 1:338-340, February 11, 1967.

"Pregnancy, trichomoniasis, and metronidazole. A novel dose schedule," by R. X. Sands. AMER J OBSTET GYNEC. 94:350-353, February 1, 1966.

"Premarital pregnancy and status before and after marriage," by L. C. Coombs, et al. AM J SOCIOL. 75:800-820, March, 1970.

"Problems of obstetrics and gynecology in an African developing country (Ethiopia)," by A. Huber, et al. BIBL GYNAEC. 47:1-128, 1968.

"Recognition of infectious pregnancy disorders," by O. Fenner. LANDARZT. 42:1430-1432, November 20, 1966.

"The role of trichomonas and candida albicans as the prinicpal cause of rupture of some perineorrhaphies after delivery," by D. Maroudi, et al. GYNEC OBSTET. 65:651-654, November-December, 1966.

"Significance of the treatment of trichomoniasis in gynecology and obstetrics," by J. Zawadski, et al. WIAD PARAZYT. 15:473-475, 1969.

"Treatment of trichomonas vaginitis in the pregnant woman with metronidazole (8 823 RP). Absence of teratogenic effects," by P. Magnin, et al. REV FRANC GYNEC OBSTET. 61:861-867, December, 1966.

"Treatment of trichomoniasis during puerperium," by R. Wawryk, et al. WIAD PARAZYT. 15:467-468, 1969.

"Trichomoniasis in pregnant women and its treatment with RP 8823," by M. Glowinski, et al. GYNEC PRAT. 15:239-246, 1964.

PREGNANCY

"Trichomoniasis, sterility and aborton," by G. Carvalho, et al. VIRGINIA MED MONTHLY. 96:444-448, August, 1969.

"Venereal diseases and their significance in obstetrics," by K. Grabner. OEST HEBAMMENZEITUNG. 15:13-14 passim, February, 1968.

"Venereology in midwifery. Part 1," by E. Gourlay. NT. 62:242+, February 25, 1966.

--Part 2." NT. 62:298+, March 4, 1966.

PREVENTION & CONTROL
SEE ALSO: EDUCATION

"Antivenereal fight in the Western Bohemian Region," by V. Resl. CESK DERM. 43:43-45, February, 1968.

"Are venereal diseases increasing? A change of legislation on the control of venereal diseases," by W. Becker. MED KLIN. 64:609-611, March 28, 1969.

"Can we really stamp out VD?," by H. S. Gorlick. RN. 29:39-45, April, 1966.

"Case-finding in venereal disease control with special reference to the District of Columbia Department of Public Health," by C. W. Freeman. MED ANN DC. 38: 183-186 passim, April, 1969.

"Certain problems of deontology," by A. A. Studnitsin. VESTN DERM VENER. 43:7-12, November, 1969.

"The chain of venereal disease control," by C. W. Freeman. MED ANN DC. 35:355-356, 374, July, 1966.

"The control of venereal disease." LANCET. 2:1289-1290, December 10, 1966.

"The control of venereal diseases in British Columbia," by H. K. Kennedy. CANAD J PUBLIC HEALTH. 60:482-485, December, 1969.

"Cooperation in venereal disease control," by S. L. Andelman. BULL MATERN CHILD HLTH. 4:17+, Summer, 1968.

"Cooperation of the Military Health Service in the control of venereal diseases during 25-years of the Polish People's Republic," by K. Płoński, et al. PRZEGL DERM. 56:713-714, 1969.

"Current problems of control of venereal diseases and spirochaeta infections in the light of world health organization data," by J. Towpik. POL TYG LEK. 21: 1513-1515, October 3, 1966.

"Effective drugs fail to stem VD rise." AM DRUGGIST. 154:35+, September 26, 1966.

"Enforced legal regulations in venerology," by F. Novotny. CESK DERM. 42:58-68, February, 1967.

"Failure to control venereal disease." BRIT MED J. 1:447-448, February 21, 1970.

"Failure to control venereal disease," by A. King. BRIT MED J. 1:451-457, February 21, 1970.

"Few notes on the prevention of venereal diseases," by F. Novotný. CESK DERM. 45:160-163, August, 1970.

"Fluorescent antibody methods in the detection and control of venereal diseases. A bibliographical review of the literature," by Z. P. Mora. BRIT J VENER DIS. 45:23-32, March, 1969.

"Intercountry exchange of reports on sources of infection for prevention and control of venereal diseases in 1967," by G. Elste. DEUTSCH GESUNDH. 23:2489-2491, December 27, 1968.

"The main problems of public health organizations and institutions in the field of controlling venereal and fungous diseases from 1967 to 1970," by N. V. Nikitina. VESTN DERM VENER. 41:3-7, March, 1967.

"The modern management of venereal diseases," by A. Luger. WIEN KLIN WSCHR. 79:529-535, June 30, 1967.

"New forms of work of dermatovenereological institutions on the control of venereal diseases of the urogenital organs," by S. L. Kozin, et al. VESTN DERM VENER. 44:79-82, January, 1970.

"New methods of contact tracing in infectious venereal diseases," by A. M. Lamb. BRIT J VENER DIS. 42:276-

PREVENTION & CONTROL

279, December, 1966.

"The nurse and venereal disease control," by F. A. Walsh. S CAROLINA NURS. 18:11-13, Winter, 1965-1966.

"The nurse's role in the control of venereal diseases," by J. Towpik. PIELEG POLOZ. 11:6-7, 1966.

"On epidemiology and control of venereal disease in the German Democratic Republic," by H. D. Jung. DERM WSCHR. 152:793-800, July 30, 1966.

"On the prevention of venereal diseases in a city," by J. Kvicera. CESK DERM. 42:404-410, December, 1967.

"On the results, principles, methods and problems of the venereal diseases control in the USSR," by V. A. Rakhmanov, et al. VESTN AKAD MED NAUK SSSR. 22:64-71, 1967.

"Physician reporting of venereal disease in the USA," by J. S. McKenzie-Pollock. BRIT J VENER DIS. 46:114-116, April, 1970.

"Physicians' attitudes toward venereal disease reporting. A survey by the national opinion research center," by R. L. Cleere, et al. JAMA. 202:941-946, December 4, 1967.

"The pox," by S. E. Acres. CANAD J PUBLIC HEALTH. 60:457-458, December, 1969.

"Present status of the control of venereal diseases in Mexico," by S. A. Campos. SALUD PUBLICA MEX. 7:371-380, May-June, 1965.

"The problems of the antivenereal fight in the Northern Bohemian Region," by V. Seycek. CESK DERM. 43:51-55, February, 1968.

"Progress in the diagnosis and management of venereal disease," by B. A. Smithurst. MED J AUST. 1:308-310, February 8, 1969.

"Public health and the Vietnam returnee," by D. L. Nathan. JAMA. 208:154, April 7, 1969.

"Public health aspects of syphilis," by W. J. Brown. SOUTHERN MED J. 59:639-642, June, 1966.

PREVENTION & CONTROL

"Public health problems relating to the Vietnam returnee," by J. H. Greenberg. JAMA. 207:697-702, January 27, 1969.

"Public health report," by L. Breslow. CALIF MED. 106:429-430, May, 1967.

"The public health service venereal disease program," by W. J. Brown. ARCH ENVIRON HEALTH, Chicago. 13: 372-375, September, 1966.

"Publicity material on VD," HEALTH BULL. 28:6, January, 1970.

"Referrals from VD to family planning. An obvious oversight," by O. J. Sikes, 3d. AMER J PUBLIC HEALTH. 58:1586-1587, September, 1968.

"Reporting venereal disease," by W. J. Brown. JAMA. 202:981-982, December 4, 1967.

"The role of the general practitioner in the prevention and treatment of venereal diseases," by E. Perti. MED GLAS. 22:121-125, May, 1968+.

"The role of the nurse in venereal disease control," by J. Towpik. PIELEG POLOZ. 2:13-15, 1967.

"Serology in control of venereal diseases," by N. C. Bhattacharyya. INDIAN J DERM. 14:129-132, April, 1969.

"Some aspects of the field work of the ancillary staff in the dermato-venereologic department in the family," by E. Sulutiu, et al. MUNCA SANIT. 16:357-360, June, 1968.

"Some aspects of the management of venereal disease," by S. Olansky. ARCH ENVIRON HEALTH, Chicago. 13: 376-380, September, 1966.

"Some comments on the cooperation of microbiologists and dermatovenerologists in the prevention of gonorrhea," by V. Potuznik. CESK DERM. 42:217-223, August, 1967.

"Some epidemiological and administrative aspects of venereal disease control," by C. L. Gonzalez. BOL SANIT PANAMER. 60:107-114, February, 1966.

PREVENTION & CONTROL

"Some legal problems in venereal disease control," by Golebiowska-Podgórczyk. PRZEGL DERM. Suppl:101-105, 1969.

"Some of the problems in the control of syphilis in the United States," by W. J. Brown. SALUD PUBLICA MEX. 10:615-618, September-October, 1968.

"Stresses role of MD in VD control," by J. A. Cowan. MICH MED. 65:552, July, 1966.

"Truth can stop VD," by P. Deutsch, et al. READ DIGEST. 90:55-59, January, 1967.

"Use of behavioral research in venereal disease control," by W. J. Brown, et al. PUBLIC HEALTH REP. 83:583-586, July, 1968.

"VD Clinic," by D. Bashforth. DIST NURS. 8:285-286, February, 1966.

"VD clinic, James Pringle house, the Middlesex hospital," by H. Elliott, et al. NURS TIMES. 64:827-828, June 21, 1968.

"VD; consent for care," by D. A. Dukelow. TODAYS HEALTH. 47:88, February, 1969.

"VD detectives; doctors and nurses in Boston." TIME. 90:32, September 1, 1967.

"VD in D.C. health department notes," by M. Grant. MED ANN DC. 35:388-389, July, 1966.

"VD must be reported," by M. I. Shanholtz. VIRGINIA MED MONTHLY. 94:188-190, March, 1967.

"Value of re-interviewing in contact tracing," by T. Z. Capiński, et al. BRIT J VENER DIS. 46:138-140, April, 1970.

"Venereal disease," by N. J. Fiumara. PEDIAT CLIN N AMER. 16:333-345, May, 1969.

"Venereal disease control," by W. J. Brown. BOL OFIC SANIT PANAMER. 68:288-296, April, 1970.

"Venereal disease control in Australia," by G. S. Hayes. MED J AUST. 1:1151-1152, May 31, 1969.

PREVENTION & CONTROL

"Venereal disease in public health practice today," by O. Ravenholt. ARCH ENVIRON HEALTH, Chicago. 13:397-398, September, 1966.

"Venereal disease program." J ARKANSAS MED SOC. 67:75-76, July, 1970.

"Venereal diseases campaign," by W. J. Brown. BOL OFIC SANIT PANAMER. 68:288-296, April, 1970.

"WHO meeting on Neisseria research." MED SERV J CANADA. 22:298-302, April, 1966.

"What would be the cost to a country of an inadequate syphilis control program?," by A. E. Callin. SALUD PUBLICA MEX. 10:611-614, September-October, 1968.

PROBENECID

"Clinical experience with ampicillin and probenecid in the management of treponeme-associated uveitis," by J. N. Goldman. TRANS AMER ACAD OPHTHAL OTOLARYNG. 74:509-514, May-June, 1970.

"Experimental under-treatment of early syphilis with probenecid and penicillin in anti-gonorrhoea dosages. A study to assess the best follow-up examination time for syphilis after gonorrhoea treatment in Greenland," by L. Hallinger. ACTA DERMATOVENER. 48:260-267, 1968.

"Gonorrhea therapy with a combination of probenecid and benzylsodiumpenicillin. A report from Greenland," by G. A. Olsen, et al. UGESKR LAEG. 130:1465-1468, September 5, 1968.

"Gonorrhoea treated by a combination of probenecid and sodium penicillin G," by G. A. Olsen, et al. BRIT J VENER DIS. 45:144-148, June, 1969.

"One-session treatment of gonorrhoea in males with procaine penicillin plus probenecid," by R. J. Cobbold, et al. POSTGRAD MED J. 46:142-145, March, 1970.

"Studies of venereal disease. I. Probenecid-procaine penicillin G combination and tetracycline hydrochloride in the treatment of penicillin-resistant gonorrhea in men," by K. K. Holmes, et al. JAMA. 202:461-473, November 6, 1967.

PROBENECID

"Treatment of gonorrhoea by one oral dose of ampicillin and probenecid combined," by T. Gundersen, et al. BRIT J VENER DIS. 45:235-237, September, 1969.

"Treatment of gonorrhoea by penicillin and a renal blocking agent (probenecid)," by G. Hatos. MED J AUST. 1:1096-1099, May 30, 1970.

"Treatment of 'penicillin-resistant' gonorrhea in military personnel in SE Asia: a cooperative evaluation of tetracycline and of penicillin plus probenecid in 1263 men," by K. K. Holmes, et al. MILIT MED. 133: 642-646, August, 1968.

PRODIGIOSANE

"Bicillin-6 therapy in combination with pyrogenale and prodigiosane of patients with contagious forms of syphilis," by O. K. Loseva, et al. VESTN DERM VENER. 42:71-75, 1968.

"Prodigiozane in the therapy of skin and venereal diseases," by M. A. Rozentul, et al. VESTN DERM VENER. 40:46-47, October, 1966.

PROSTITUTION

"Current aspects of prostitution. The moral aspects," by P. U. Rocco. MINERVA MED. 57:Varia:940+, July 21, 1966.

"Current legislation concerning prostitution," by C. Rotta. MINERVA MED. 57:Varia:954+, July 21, 1966.

"Health knowledge of prostitutes in Saigon, Vietnam. A study of health attitudes and habits relating to venereal diseases taken from a group of prostitutes," by R. S. Marcondes, et al. REV SAUDE PUBLICA. 1:18-23, June, 1967.

"Medical basis of the theory of abolition of the 'red light districts'," by T. Matsuda. JAP J NURS ART. 8:122-132, August, 1969.

PSORIASIS

"Differential diagnostic problem: impetiginized eczematic scabies--lues II-psoriasis vulgaris," by V. Misgeld. MED KLIN. 64:2189-2192, November 21, 1969.

"The influence of chloroquine and related drugs on psoriasis and keratoderma blenorrhagicum," by H. Baker.

PSORIASIS

BRIT J DERM. 78:161-166, March, 1966.

"A 20 years persisting tubero serpiginous syphilis treated as psoriasis," by W. G. Roth. DERM WSCHR. 154:459-463, May 18, 1968.

"Very grave pustular psoriasis probably caused by penicillin. Presentation of 6 fatal cases observed in black Africa," by Y. Privat, et al. BULL SOC FRANC DERM SYPH. 76:505-509, 1969.

PSYCHIATRY
SEE ALSO: NEUROSYPHILIS

"Psychiatric referral of patients in a venereal diseases clinic," by J. R. Pedder. BRIT J VENER DIS. 46:54-57, February, 1970.

"Psychosomatic aspects of female genital trichomoniasis," by G. Pinoli, et al. MINERVA GINEC. 21:508-511, April 30, 1969.

"A survey by questionnaire of psychiatric disturbance in patients attending a venereal diseases clinic," by J. R. Pedder, et al. BRIT J VENER DIS. 46:58-61, February, 1970.

PYROGENALE
"Bicillin-6 therapy in combination with pyrogenale and prodigiosane of patients with contagious forms of syphilis," by O. K. Loseva, et al. VESTN DERM VENER. 42:71-75, 1968.

"The use of pyrogenale in the treatment of late forms of syphilis," by A. K. Shcherbakova. VESTN DERM VENER. 41:43-47, June, 1967.

Q FEVER
"Serologic investigations in narcotic addicts. I. Syphilis, lymphogranuloma venereum, herpes simples, and Q fever," by C. E. Cherubin, et al. ANN INTERN MED. 69:739-742, October, 1968.

REACTIONS
"Anamnestic reactions in syphilis serology," by A. Lassus, et al. INT ARCH ALLERG. 36:394-398, 1969.

"Anaphylactic reactions after intradermal diagnostic tests with penicilloyl-polylysin. Preliminary report," by J. Bowszyc. PRZEGL DERM. 55:307-309, May-June, 1968.

"Anaphylactic shock and its treatment in field practice," by Z. Balcar. SBORN VED PRAC LEK FAK KARLOV UNIV. 11:665-675, 1968.

"Data on the study of the clinical aspects, diagnosis, therapy and prevention of allergic reactions in dermatology," by BIu. Sidaravichius, et al. VESTN DERM VENER. 43:3-7, July, 1969.

"Immunologic studies in a patient sensitive to tetracycline and penicillin," by M. J. Fellner, et al. ARCH KLIN EXP DERM. 224:157-167, February 3, 1966.

"Lymphocyte transformation test (LTT) for the diagnosis of drug allergy," by E. Schopf, et al. ARCH KLIN EXP DERM. 237:177-180, 1970.

"Multivalent antibiotic allergy with penicillin and tetracycline anaphylaxis," by J. Zelger, et al. DERMATOLOGICA. 139:365-373, 1969.

"Nicolau syndrome following retacillin compositum injection," by A. Niedner, et al. Z AERZTL FORTBILD. 64:39-42, January 1, 1970.

"Occurrence of agranulocytic reaction in connection with the use of biomycin and penicillin," by M. L. Aviosor, et al. KLIN MED. 46:139-140, May, 1968.

"On methods of lymphocyte culture as an allergy test," by H. J. Heitmann. HAUTARZT. 18:152-156, April, 1967.

"Penicillin allergy in the light of clinical investigations and results of skin tests with crystalline penicillin, novocaine and trichophytin," by Z. Starzycki. PRZEGL DERM. 57:203-209, March-April, 1970.

"Reactivity of two selected antigens of Neisseria gonorrhoeae," by G. Reising, et al. APPL MICROBIOL. 18:337-339, September, 1969.

"Renal failure and interstitial nephritis due to penicillin and methicillin," by D. S. Baldwin, et al. NEW ENG J MED. 279:1245-1252, December 5, 1968.

REACTIONS

"Side-effects of chemotherapeutic agents," by O. Mustala. DUODECIM. 86:192-202, 1970.

"Simultaneous occurrence of toxic hepatitis and Stevens-Johnson syndrome following therapy with sulfisoxazole and sulfamethoxazole," by D. J. Shaw, et al. JOHNS HOPKINS MED J. 126:130-133, March, 1970.

"Stevens-Johnson syndrome caused by allergy to sulfonamides and penicillin. Histological study with the electronic microscope," by T. J. Guillen, et al. ALLERGIA. 15:8-18, August, 1967.

"A study of sensitivity induced by certain drugs by intradermal skin tests," by B. Raj, et al. INDIAN J MED RES. 57:1769-1775, September, 1969.

"The value of the Shelley test in complications to intolerance of antibiotics," by G. Despierres, et al. J MED LYON. 48:1097-1104, July 5, 1967.

REACTIONS: AMPICILLIN

"Cross-reactivity between ampicillin and penicillin," by R. H. Stewart, et al. JAMA. 213:131, July 6, 1970.

"Renal damage associated with prolonged administration of ampicillin, cephaloridine, and cephalothin," by E. J. Benner. ANTIMICROB AGENTS CHEMOTHER. 9:417-420, 1969.

REACTIONS: ANTIBIOTICS

"Allergic reactions to antibiotics," by J. E. Kasik, et al. MED CLIN N AMER. 54:59-73, January, 1970.

"Anaphylactic shock during skin test with antibiotics," by I. U. A. Tereshchenko. SOVET MED. 32:137-139, August, 1969.

"Anaphylactic shock in antibiotic therapy," by V. V. Kuptsov. VRACH DELO. 7:127-128, July, 1968.

"Case of fatal anaphylactic shock caused by the administration of antibiotics," by E. M. Deliagina. KLIN MED. 48:129-131, March, 1970.

"Extremely severe hypersensitivity to antibiotics and its significance in the diagnosis of drug allergy," by E. Hegyi. BRATISL LEK LISTY. 53:216-218, Feb-

REACTIONS: ANTIBIOTICS

ruary, 1970.

"Hypersensitivity and toxicity of the beta-lactam antibiotics," by G. T. Stewart. POSTGRAD MED J, London. 43:31-36, August, 1967.

REACTIONS: ANTIMICROBIAL
"Clinically useful antimicrobial agents. Untoward reactions," POSTGRAD MED, Minneapolis. 42:396-419, November, 1967.

REACTIONS: BICILLINS
"Anaphylactic shock caused by the use of bicillin forte," by M. V. Ignat'ev. KLIN MED. 46:138, May, 1968.

"Characteristics of allergic reactions in bicillin therapy for the prevention of rheumatic exacerbations," by O. A. Kuvaldina. VOP REVM. 8:83-85, April-June, 1968.

"On the side effects of bicillin-1 and bicillin-3," by B. P. Skokh, et al. VOP OKHR MATERIN DETS. 11:53-56, June, 1966.

REACTIONS: CEPHALORIDINE
"Cross-allergy caused by cephaloridine, cephalothin and penicillin," by H. Vogt. HAUTARZT. 20:407-408, September, 1969.

"Renal damage associated with prolonged administration of ampicillin, cephaloridine, and cephalothin," by E. J. Benner. ANTIMICROB AGENTS CHEMOTHER. 9:417-420, 1969.

REACTIONS: CEPHALOTHIN
"Cross-allergy caused by cephaloridine, cephalothin and penicillin," by H. Vogt. HAUTARZT. 20:407-408, September, 1969.

"Renal damage associated with prolonged administration of ampicillin, cephaloridine, and cephalothin," by E. J. Benner. ANTIMICROB AGENTS CHEMOTHER. 9:417-420, 1969.

REACTIONS: CEPHALOSPORINS
"Allergenic factors in penicillins and cephalosporins," by G. T. Stewart. AMER HEART J. 75:429-431, March, 1968.

REACTIONS: CEPHALOSPORINS

"Allergy to antibiotics. I. Fact and conjecture on the sensitizing contaminants of penicillins and cephalsporins," by J. G. Feinberg. INT ARCH ALLERG. 33: 439-443, 1968.

REACTIONS: JARISCH-HERXHEIMER & HERXHEIMER-LUKASIEWICZ

"ACTH as a prophylactic against the Jarisch-Herxheimer reaction," by E. Sylvester. Z HAUT GESCHLECHTSKR. 44:125-126, February 15, 1969.

"Herxheimer-Lukasiewicz reaction after injection of debecillin in early acquired syphilis," by E. Peisert, et al. POL TYG LEK. 22:344-347, March 6, 1967.

"Jarisch-Herxheimer reaction." BRIT MED J. 1:384, February 18, 1967.

"Jarisch-Herxheimer reaction and syphilitic aortitis," by G. R. Hughes. BRIT MED J. 1:360, February 10, 1968.

"Jarisch-Herxheimer reaction with interesting blood count," by R. B. Davis. J INDIAN MED ASS. 53:83-85, July 16, 1969.

"Effect of encorton on the Lukasiewicz-Jarisch-Herxheimer reaction," by K. Bien, et al. PRZEGL DERM. 56:305-310, May-June, 1969.

"The effect of prednisolone on the Jarisch-Herxheimer reaction," by H. Gudjónsson, et al. ACTA DERMATOVENER. 48:15-18, 1968.

"Febrile Herxheimer reaction in different phases of primary and secondary syphilis," by T. Putkonen, et al. BRIT J VENER DIS. 42:181-184, September, 1966.

"Herxheimer-Lukasiewicz reaction after injection of debecillin in early acquired syphilis," by E. Peisert, et al. POL TYG LEK. 22:344-347, March 6, 1967.

"Herxheimer's reaction. Asymptomatic neurosyphilis treated with penicillin," by H. A. Podesta, et al. PRENSA MED ARGENT. 54:301-304, April 14, 1967.

"Herxheimer's reaction in maternal milk in early congenital syphilis," by R. Rollier, et al. BULL SOC FRANC DERM SYPH. 74:178-180, 1967.

REACTIONS: JARISCH-HERXHEIMER & HERXHEIMER-LUKASIEWICZ

"On the allergic origin of the Jarisch-Herxheimer reaction," by E. Skog, et al. ACTA DERMATOVENER. 46:136-143, 1966.

"The problem of Jarisch-Herxheimer-Lukasiewicz reaction in congenital syphilis in infants," by K. Lejman, et al. POL MED J. 6:1069-1073, 1967; also in PRZEGL DERM. 54:51-56, January-February, 1967.

"Serum proteinogram in the course of the febrile reaction of Jarisch-Herxheimer-Lukasiewicz," by W. Powrozny, et al. PRZEGL DERM. 55:677-680, September-October, 1968.

REACTIONS: NOVOCAIN

"A case of anaphylactic shock after penicillin and novocain injection," by A. G. Ostrovskii. ANTIBIOTIKI. 12:338-339, April, 1967.

"Penicillin allergy in the light of clinical investigations and results of skin tests with crystalline penicillin, novocaine and trichopytin," by Z. Starzycki. PRZEGL DERM. 57:203-209, March-April, 1970.

REACTIONS: PENICILLIN

"Acute embolic-toxic induced incident in treatment of stomach syphilis with penicillin," by W. Lindheimer. THER GEGENW. 106:755-759, June, 1967.

"Acute non-allergic reactions following I.M. administration of clemizole-penicillin G and streptomycin," by K. Bornemann, et al. MUNCHEN MED WSCHR. 108: 834-837, April 15, 1966.

"Acute psychotic reactions to aqueous procaine penicillin," by P. M. Utley, et al. SOUTHERN MED J. 59:1271-1274, November, 1966.

"Adverse reactions to penicillin," by J. Silverio. J AMER DENT ASS. 77:17, July, 1968.

"Allergenic factors in penicillins and cephalosporins," by G. T. Stewart. AMER HEART J. 75:429-431, March, 1968.

"Allergic cutaneous reactions to penicillin and their mechanisms," by M. J. Fellner, et al. DERMATOLOGICA. 135:362-368, 1967.

REACTIONS: PENICILLIN

"Allergic reaction during repeated administration of penicillin," by D. I. Khozeniuk. VRACH DELO. 11: 141-142, November, 1967.

"Allergic reactions in patients with syphilis treated with penicillin," by L. Ciecierski, et al. PRZEGL DERM. 53:189-192, March-April, 1966.

"Allergic reactions to penicillins. Advances in understanding and management," by A. L. De Weck, et al. MINN MED. 52:137-150, January, 1969.

"Allergy to antibiotics. I. Fact and conjecture on the sensitizing contaminants of penicillins and cephalosporins," by J. G. Feinberg. INT ARCH ALLERG. 33:439-443, 1968.

--II. Comparative immunogenicity of some penicillins." INT ARCH ALLERG. 33:444-453, 1968.

"Allergy to penicillin. Clinical study of 105 patients tested with penicilloylpolylysine," by E. B. Negreiros. REV BRASIL MED. 25:597-600, September, 1968.

"Allergy to penicillin in children," by J. Charles, et al. ARCH FRANC PEDIAT. 25:955-956, October, 1968.

"Anaphylactic reactions after penicillin as a clinical and medicolegal problem," by Z. Starzycki. PRZEGL DERM. 55:559-563, July-September, 1968.

"Anaphylactic shock after intramuscular administration of penicillin," by V. N. Groshev. TER ARKH. 39:122, February, 1967.

"Anaphylactic shock following administration of penicillin," by P. M. Liashuk, et al. VRACH DELO. 1:139, January, 1968.

"Anaphylactic shock in the administration of penicillin," by M. P. Golovinskii. VRACH DELO. 3:146-147, March, 1966.

"Anaphylactic shock in penicillin and streptomycin therapy," by B. V. Smirnov, et al. SOVET MED. 30:135-136, February, 1967.

"Antimicrobial therapy in patients allergic to penicillin," by P. A. Bunn. NEW YORK J MED. 69:1859-1865,

REACTIONS: PENICILLIN

July 1, 1969.

"Apropos of an unusual case of penicillin allergy," by M. Zivković. SRPSKI ARH CELOK LEK. 95:297-300, May, 1967.

"Bacterial endocarditis due to Neisseria perflava in a patient hypersensitive to penicillin," by A. B. Breslin, et al. AUST ANN MED. 16:245-249, August, 1967.

"Basophil degranulation test in penicillin sensitivity," by Z. Rumbolt, et al. LIJECNVJESN. 88:619-625, June, 1966.

"Cardiac asystole following intravenous administration of aqueous potassium penicillin." ANAESTH ANALG. 48:55-57, January-February, 1969.

"A case of anaphylactic shock after penicillin and novocain injection," by A. G. Ostrovskii. ANTIBIOTIKI. 12:338-339, April, 1967.

"A case of anaphylactic shock in a pregnant woman with nephropathia after the administration of penicillin," by T. A. Avksent'Eva. AKUSH GINEK. 42:43, December, 1966.

"A case of generalized thrombocytopenic diathesis after local application of crystalline penicillin solution," by T. Pytel-Dabrowska. PEDIAT POL. 43: 73-74, January, 1968.

"Central nervous system toxicity secondary to massive doses of penicillin 'G' in the treatment of overwhelming infections," by D. F. Cohill, et al. AMER J MED SCI. 254:692-694, November, 1967.

"Changes in the ECG during penicillin shock," by A. M. Korepanov. TER ARKH. 39:118-121, June, 1967.

"The clinical diagnosis of penicillin allergy," by J. Pedersen-Bjergaard. ACTA ALLERGOL. 25:89-130, June, 1970.

"Clinical manifestations and diagnosis of penicillin allergy and other penicillin side effects," by N. Sonnichsen, et al. DERM MSCHR. 155:739-750, 1969.

REACTIONS: PENICILLIN

"Clinical observations on the problem of penicillin allergy," by P. Sunder-Plassmann. MED KLIN. 61:892, June 3, 1966.

"Clinical treatment of patients with post-penicillin reactions after early syphilis therapy," by J. Bowszyc. PRZEGL DERM. 54:585-589, September-October, 1967.

"Clinical verification of the phenomenon of chemical saturation of antibodies during allergic shock caused by penicillin," by E. Seropian. MED INTERNA. 22:997-1000, August, 1970.

"Collapse after penicillin injection," by K. Naess. T NORSK LAEGEFOREN. 324:325, February 1, 1970.

"Comparative cutaneous sensitivity studies in man with benzylpenicillin and its purified counterpart," by O. P. Robinson. ANTIMICRO AGENTS CHEMOTHER. 7:550-552, 1967.

"Comparative studies of the value of methods used in the diagnosis of penicillin allergy," by E. Maciejowska. DERM MSCHR. 155:761-770, 1969.

"Coombs' positive hemolytic anemia due to penicillin," by L. J. Lyon. J MOUNT SINAI HOSP NY. 35:258-264, May-June, 1968.

"Cross-allergy caused by cephaloridine, cephalothin, and penicillin," by H. Vogt. HAUTARZT. 20:407-408. September, 1969.

"Cross reactivity between ampicillin and penicillin G," by R. H. Stewart, et al. JAMA. 213:131, July 6, 1970.

"Delayed hypersensitivity to penicillin. Clinical significance and hyposensitization after therapy," by M. J. Fellner, et al. JAMA. 210:2061,2062, December 15, 1969.

"Delayed skin reactions to benzylpenicillin in man," by A. P. Redmond, et al. INT ARCH ALLERG. 33:193-206, 1968.

"Diagnosis of intolerance to penicillin and other antibiotics," by G. Brehm. MED KLIN. 61:1180-1184,

REACTIONS: PENICILLIN

July 29, 1966.

"'Double reaction' to penicillin. Anaphylactic and serum sickness-like reactions due to a single dose," by M. J. Fellner, et al. ARCH DERM. 96:687-688, December, 1967.

"Drug reactions. 1. A protein contaminant causing penicillin hypersensitivity," by J. L. Turk, et al. BRIT J DERM. 80:199-201, March, 1968.

"Embolico-toxic reaction following depot penicillin administration," by R. Kaufer. DEUTSCH GESUNDH. 24: 1208-1211, June 26, 1969.

"Encephalopathy from penicillin (Editorial)," BRIT MED J. 3:198, July 27, 1968.

"Encephalopathy with transitory amaurosis, visual agnosia and oculomotor apraxia following high-dose intravenous penicillin therapy," by B. Cagianut, et al. SCHWEIZ MED WSCHR. 100:42-43, January 3, 1970.

"Exploration of the possible allergic consequences of utilization of clemizole-penicillin," by J. Jubelin, et al. MARSEILLE MED. 105:189-192, 1968.

"Fever following penicillin treatment as a symptom of syphilis," by K. Nordin, et al. LAKARTIDNINGEN. 63:490-491, February 9, 1966.

"Fixed eruption due to penicillin allergy," by W. L. Dennison, et al. ARCH DERM. 101:594-597, May, 1970.

"Hemiplegia following 1st injection of penicillin in a patient with secondary relapsing syphilis," by L. Ciecierski, et al. POL TYG LEK. 25:145-147, January 26, 1970.

"Hemolytic anemia caused by penicillin." JAMA. 204: 635, May 13, 1968.

"Hemolytic anemia caused by penicillin. Report of a case in which antipenicillin antibodies crossreacted with cephalothin sodium," by L. W. Nesmith, et al. JAMA. 203:27-30, January 1, 1968.

"Hoigne syndrome - nonallergic reaction to depot penicillin," by M. Ondrejicka, et al. BRATISL LEK LISTY.

REACTIONS: PENICILLIN

52:703-708, 1969.

"Hypokalaemia, metabolic alkalosis, and hypernatraemia due to 'massive' sodium penicillin therapy," by F. P. Brunner, et al. BRIT MED J. 4:550-552, November 30, 1968.

"Immediate reaction to penicillin. Association with penicilloyl-specific skin-sensitizing antibodies and low titers of blocking (IgG) antibodies," by M. J. Fellner, et al. JAMA. 202:909-911, November 27, 1967.

"Immunochemical mechanisms of penicillin induced Coombs positivity and hemolytic anemia in man," by B. Levine, et al. INT ARCH ALLERG. 31:594-606, 1967.

"Immunochemical mechanisms in penicillin allergies," by M. Ledvina, et al. CAS LEK CESK. 109:138-146, February, 1970.

"Immunohemolytic anemia following penicillin," by W. Straub. SCHWEIZ MED WSCHR. 97:1294, September 30, 1967.

"Immunologic examinations for the diagnosis of fatal shock caused by penicillin," by A. Franchini, et al. MED LEG DOMM CORPOR. 3:160-168, April-June, 1970.

"Immunologic studies in a patient sensitive to tetracycline and penicillin," by M. J. Fellner, et al. ARCH KLIN EXP DERM. 224:157-167, February 3, 1966.

"Immunology, clinical features and therapy of penicillin allergy," by G. Filipp. MED WELT. 50:2763-2773, December 14, 1968.

"Incidence of immediate systemic penicillin reactions," by W. Minkin, et al. MILIT MED. 133:557-560, July, 1968.

"The indirect basophil degranulation test for allergy to penicillin," by T. Feizi. TRANS ST JOHN HOSP DERM SOC. 53:162-164, 1967.

"An instance of fatal reaction to the penicillin scratch-test," by M. Dogliotti. DERMATOLOGICA. 136:489-496, 1968.

REACTIONS: PENICILLIN

"Laryngeal edema following intramuscular administration of penicillin," by P. A. Kravchuk. ZH USHN NOS GORL BOLEZ. 28:94-95, November-December, 1968.

"Liability for penicillin reactions," by A. R. Holder. JAMA. 212:2015-2016, June 15, 1970.

"Life-threatening infection. Choice of alternate drugs when penicillin cannot be given," by G. O. Westenfielder, et al. JAMA. 210:845-848, November 3, 1969.

"A localized Arthus-type hypersensitivity reaction to penicillin," by A. Lupovitch, et al. ANN ALLERG. 26:206-210, April, 1968.

"Loco-regional complication after benzathine penicillin," by G. Vasiliu, et al. PEDIATRIA. 17:75-78, January-February, 1968.

"Lupoid hepatitis following administration of penicillin. Case report and immunological studies," by J. P. Girard, et al. HELV MED ACTA. 34:23-35, December, 1967.

"The lymphocyte culture in penicillin allergy," by H. J. Heitmann, et al. HAUTARZT. 17:313-316, July, 1966.

"Management of syphilitic patients allergic to penicillin," by J. Lebioda, et al. PRZEGL DERM. 55:311-316, May-June, 1968.

"Mechanisms of clinical desensitization in urticarial hypersensitivity to penicillin," by M. J. Fellner, et al. J ALLERG. 45:55-61, January, 1970.

"The methodology of serologic tests in experimental penicillin allergy," by H. P. Werner, et al. Z IMMUNITAETSFORSCH. 139:14-24, December, 1969.

"Methods of detection of immediate hypersensitivity to penicillin," by E. Maciejowska. PRZEGL DERM. 56:757-764, 1969.

"Multivalent antibiotic allergy with penicillin and tetracycline anaphylaxis," by J. Zelger, et al. DE DERMATOLOGICA. 139:365-373, 1969.

"Myocarditis in penicillin sensitivity," by D. Banerjee.

REACTIONS: PENICILLIN

    INDIAN HEART J. 20:73-75, January, 1968.

    "Nature and extent of penicillin side effects with special reference to 151 fatal cases after anaphylactic shock," by O. Idsoe, et al. SCHWEIZ MED WSCHR. 99: 1190-1197, August 16, 1969; also in BULL WHO. 38:159-188, 1968.

    "Neurotoxic effects of large doses of penicillin administered intravenously (letter to editor)," by J. B. Borman, et al. ARCH SURG. 97:662-665, October, 1968.

    "Neurotoxicity of penicillin," by M. I. Marks, et al. NEW ENG J MED. 279:1002-1003, October 31, 1968.

    "New views on the problem of allergy to penicillin," by E. Maciejowska. PRZEGL DERM. 55:299-306, May-June, 1968.

    "Nonallergic fatal incidents following depot penicillin. Pathogenesis and prevention," by G. Ernst, et al. DEUTSCH MED WSCHR. 95:618 passim, March 20, 1970.

    "Occurrence of agranulocytic reaction in connection with the use of biomycin and penicillin," by M. L. Aviosor, et al. KLIN MED. 46:139-140, May, 1968.

    "On the problem of allergic reactions of the immediate type during treatment with penicillin and streptomycin," by I. I. Dantsig, et al. PROBL TUBERK. 44:70-71, 1966.

    "Oral penicillin and anaphylactoid reactions," by J. H. Dunn. JAMA. 202:552-553, November 6, 1967.

    "Passive cutaneous anaphylaxis with guinea-pig and rabbit antibodies to penicillin derivatives," by A. E. Cronin. AUST J DERM. 9:65-69, June, 1967.

    "The penetration of penicillin and other antimicrobials into joint fluid. Three case reports with a reappraisal of the literature," by D. J. Drutz, et al. J BONE JOINT SURG. 49:1415-1421, October, 1967.

    "Penicillin allergy." MED LETT DRUGS THER. 10:101-103, December 13, 1968.

    "Penicillin allergy," by J. Charpin, et al. MARSEILLE

REACTIONS: PENICILLIN

MED. 103:577-578, 1966.

"Penicillin allergy," by J. Jouglard, et al. MED LEG DOMM CORPOR. 2:252-273, July-September, 1969.

"Penicillin allergy (Commentary)," by G. T. Stewart. CLIN PHARMACOL THER. 11:307-311, May-June, 1970.

"Penicillin allergy. A report of thirteen cases of severe reactions," by A. H. Rosenblum. J ALLERG. 42:309-318, December, 1968.

"Penicillin allergy in the light of clinical investigations and results of skin tests with crystalline penicillin, novocaine, and trichophytin," by Z. Starzycki. PRZEGL DERM. 57:203-209, March-April, 1970.

"Penicillin encephalopathy in children," by S. R. Ullal. J INDIAN MED ASSOC. 54:513-515, July 1, 1970.

"Penicillin hypersensitivity," by M. G. Maheras. MINN MED. 52:1811-1817, November, 1969.

"Penicillin-induced granulopenia," by J. Forshaw. BRIT MED J. 3:184, July 20, 1968.

"Penicillin-induced haemolytic anaemia." BRIT MED J. 3:4, July 6, 1968.

"Penicillin-induced haemolytic anaemia," by H. E. Amos, et al. BRIT MED J. 2:436, August 17, 1968.

"Penicillin-induced haemolytic anaemia," by M. A. Rossiter, et al. BRIT MED J. 3:616-617, September 7, 1968.

"Penicillin-induced haemolytic anaemia," by J. M. White, et al. BRIT MED J. 3:26-29, July 6, 1968.

"Penicillin-induced seizures during cardiopulmonary bypass. A clinical and electroencephalographic study," by K. B. Seamans, et al. NEW ENG J MED. 278:861-868, April 18, 1968.

"Penicillin skin tests as predictive and diagnostic aids in penicillin allergy," by R. G. Van Dellen, et al. MED CLIN N AMER. 54:997-1007, July, 1970.

"Pencillinase-producing staphylococci in the male ure-

REACTIONS: PENICILLIN

thra and their effect on penicillin treatment of gonorrhoea," by B. Lagerholm, et al. ACTA DERMATOVENER. 46:345-347, 1966.

"Penicillins and aqueous humor," by E. E. Goldman, et al. AMER J OPHTHAL. 65:717-721, May, 1968.

"Possible advantages of highly purified penicillin in avoiding penicilloyl-specific sensitization and allergic reactions," by J. Pedersen-Bjergaard. ACTA ALLERG. 24:303-325, November, 1969.

"Prediction of penicillin allergy by immunological test," by B. B. Levine, et al. J ALLERG. 43:231-244, April, 1969.

"Problems caused by complications of penicillin therapy in antivenereal dispensaries," by F. X. Carton. BULL SOC FRANC DERM SYPH. 74:189-190, 1967.

"Pseudoanaphylactic reactions to procaine penicillin G," by R. Tompsett. ARCH INTERN MED. 120:565-567, November, 1967.

"Psychotic reaction to penicillin," by S. Jacobson. AMER J PSYCHIAT. 124:999, January, 1968.

"Reactions to penicillins." LANCET. 2:673, September 21, 1968.

"Renal failure and instertitial nephritis due to penicillin and methicillin," by D. S. Baldwin, et al. NEW ENG J MED. 279:1245-1252, December 5, 1968.

"Resuscitation in embolic and toxic complication caused by intravascular administration of a depot-penicillin," by G. Clauberg. ANAESTHESIST. 14:284-285, August, 1966.

"The risk of penicillin reactions (Editorial), by P. P. Van Arsdel, Jr. ANN INTERN MED. 69:1071-1073, November, 1968.

"Role of penicilloyl-polylysin in the detection of delayed hypersensitivity to penicillin," by E. Maciejowska. PRZEGL DERM. 57:55-59, January-February, 1970.

"The role of penicilloyl-polylysins for the diagnosis

REACTIONS: PENICILLIN

of penicillin allergy," by E. Maciejowska. DERM MSCHR. 155:751-760, 1969.

"The role of penicilloylated protein impurities, penicillin polymers and dimers in penicillin allergy," by A. I. DeWeck, et al. INT ARCH ALLERG. 33:535-567, 1968.

"Selected aspects of penicillin allergy," by R. L. Baer, et al. BRIT J DERM. 83:Suppl:37-47, 1970.

"Severe anaphylactic reaction to penicillin," by L. I. Geller, et al. KLIN MED. 44:138, January, 1966.

"Shock death after oral penicillin administration," by H. Bankl, et al. WIEN KLIN WSCHR. 80:43-44, January 19, 1968.

"Skin-sensitizing antibodies in serum from patients with penicillin allergy studied by passive transfer to monkey skin and compared with results obtained on human skin. (Prausnitz-Kustner technique)," by J. Pedersen-Bjergaard. ACTA ALLERG. 24:57-72, March, 1969.

"Skin testing in urticarial penicillin hypersensitivity," by T. Matner, et al. ARCH KLIN EXP DERM. 227:349-352, 1966.

"Some aspects of penicillin allergy," by F. R. Batchelor, et al. PROC ROY SOC MED. 61:897-899, September, 1968.

"Specific hyposensitization of patients with penicillin allergy," by J. Pedersen-Bjergaard. ACTA ALLERG. 24:333-361, November, 1969.

"Specificity for benzyl-penicillin, pencilloyl compounds, and benzyl-pencilloate in human allergy to pencillin," by J. Pedersen-Bjergaard. ACTA ALLERG. 24:87-106, May, 1969.

"Stevens-Johnson syndrome caused by allergy to sulfonamides and penicillin. Histological study with the electronic microscope," by T. J. Guillen, et al. ALLERGIA. 15:8-18, August, 1967.

"Studies of patients with penicillin allergy with a review of literature," by H. Strassmann. HAUTARZT.

REACTIONS: PENICILLIN

20:323-329, July, 1969.

"Sudden death occurring during 'massive dose' potassium penicillin G therapy. An argument implicating potassium intoxication," by G. L. Tullett. WISCONSIN MED J. 69:216-217, September, 1970.

"The tesa-film patch test for the demonstration of penicillin allergy in practice," by M. Reichenberger. Z HAUT GESCHLECHTSKR. 40:293-300, April 15, 1966.

"Three incidents after intracutaneous tests with penicilloyl-polylysine," by I. Luckerath, et al. HAUTARZT. 18:183-185, April, 1967.

"Toxic reactions from depot-penicillin," by R. Kiesewetter, et al. DEUTSCH GESUNDH. 23:631-634, April 4, 1968.

"Treatment of penicillin anaphylaxis with injection of the same antigen (penicillin) in high doses," by L. Katsilabors. REV MED MOYEN ORIENT. 24:346-348, July-August, 1967.

"Value of the intradermal test and scarification test in the determination of penicillin sensitivity," by A. R. Tuszkiewicz, et al. POL TYG LEK. 22:1197-1199, August 7, 1967.

"The value of penicilloyl-polylysine (PPL) in the detection of penicillin allergy in man," by H. Prochacki, et al. PRZEGL DERM. 57:325-329, May-June, 1970.

"Very grave pustular psoriasis probably caused by penicillin. Presentation of 6 fatal cases observed in black Africa," by Y. Privat, et al. BULL SOC FRANC DERM SYPH. 76:505-509, 1969.

REACTIONS: STREPTOMYCIN

"Acute, non-allergic reactions following I. M. administration of clemizole-penicillin G and streptomycin," by K. Bornemann, et al. MUNCHEN MED WSCHR. 108:834-837, April 15, 1966.

"Anaphylactic shock in penicillin and streptomycin therapy," by B. V. Smirnov, et al. SOVET MED. 30:135-136, February, 1967.

"On the problem of allergic reactions of the immediate

REACTIONS: STREPTOMYCIN

    type during treatment with penicillin and streptomycin," by I. I. Dantsig, et al. PROBL TUBERK. 44:70-71, 1966.

REITER'S DISEASE

"Clinical studies on gonococcal arthritis and Reiter's syndrome and measurement of gonococcal and Bedsonia antibodies," by J. T. Sharp, et al. ARTHRITIS RHEUM. 11:569-578, August, 1968.

"Complement-fixing antibodies to Bedsonia organisms in Reiter's syndrome and ankylosing spondylitis," by T. D. Kinsella, et al. ANN RHEUM DIS. 27:241-244, May, 1968.

"A complex diagnostic problem: the differentiation among gonococcal arthritis, Reiter's syndrome, and rheumatoid arthritis," by J. C. Brooks, Jr. J MED ASS GEORGIA. 56:291-296, July, 1967.

"Demonstration by cultures, of agents of the genus Bedsonia in joint fluid in cases of fiessinger-leroy-Reiter rheumatism," by B. Amor, et al. C R ACAD SCI. 264:1365-1367, March 6, 1967.

"Infection by Bedsoniae and the possibility of spurious isolation. 2. Genital infection, disease of the eye, Reiter's disease," by E. M. Dunlop, et al. AMER J OPHTHAL. 63:Suppl:1073-1081, May, 1967.

"Infection by TRIC agent and other members of the Bedsonia group, with a note on Reiter's disease. 1. Ocular disease in the adult," by B. R. Jones, et al. TRANS OPHTHAL SOC UK. 86:291-312, 1966.

--2. Ophthalmia neonatorum due to TRIC agent," by A. Freedman, et al. TRANS OPHTHAL SOC UK. 86:313-320, 1966.

--3. Genital infection and disease of the eye," by E. M. Dunlop, et al. TRANS OPHTHAL SOC UK. 86:321-324, 1966.

--4. "Laboratory aspects," by I. A. Harper, et al. TRANS OPHTHAL SOC UK. 86:335-348, 1966.

"Non-gonococcal urethritis and Reiter's syndrome: personal experience with etiological studies during 15 years," by D. K. Ford. CANAD MED ALL J. 99:900-910,

REITER'S DISEASE

November 9, 1968.

"Parallel studies on modifications of the behavior of Reiter's treponema (in vitro) and treponema pallidum (in vivo)," by P. Collart, et al. PATH BIOL. 15: 470-479, May, 1967.

"Reiter treponeme. A review of the literature," by A. L. Wallace, et al. BULL WHO. 36:Supplement No. 2, 1-103, 1967.

"Reiter's disease in two brothers," by A. G. Mowat, et al. BRIT J VENER DIS. 44:334-336, December, 1968.

"Reiter's syndrome," by E. P. Engleman, et al. CLIN ORTHOP. 57:19-29, March-April, 1968.

"Reiter's syndrome - an infection-induced defect in inflammation," by O. J. Stone. DERM INT. 7:137-140, July-September, 1968.

"Reiter's treponema," by M. Deluca. RASS INT CLIN TER. 48:643-644, May 31, 1968.

"Relationships between mycoplasma and the etiology of nongonococcal urethritis and Reiter's syndrome," by D. K. Ford. ANN NY ACAD SCI. 143:501-504, July 28. 1967.

"Sero-negative polyarthritis. The Bedsonia (chlamydia) group of agents and Reiter's disease. A progress report," by E. M. Dunlop, et al. ANN RHEUM. 27:234-239, May, 1968.

REVERIN
"Follow-up of reverin-treated patients in manifest, primary, secondary, tertiary and latent seropositive lues. IV," by V. Matanic. HAUTARZT. 17:121-123, March, 1966.

"Intravenous injection of reverin in syphilis," by Z. Matanic. MED GLAS. 20:193-198, May-June, 1966.

RICORD, PHILIPPE
"Philippe Ricord (1800-1889), syphilographer." JAMA. 211:115-116, January 5, 1970.

RIFAMPICIN
"Management of blennorrhagia using a dose of rimactan,"

RIFAMPICIN

by L. Migliano. HOSPITAL. 75:297-300, January, 1969.

"Observations on the use of rifampicin in dermatovenereology," by G. Bonu, et al. MINERVA MED. 60:4840-4844, December 1, 1969.

"Rifampicin in dermatology. Clinical trial," by E. Cappelli. ARCH MARAGLIANO PAT CLIN. 25:397-401, September-October, 1969.

"Rifampicin in dermatology and venereology," by L. Ayala. G ITAL DERM. 44:665-672, December, 1969.

"Rifampicin (rimactane) in the treatment of gonorrhoea," by R. R. Willcox, et al. BRIT J VENER DIS. 46:145-148, April, 1970.

"Treatment of gonorrhoea with single oral doses of rifampicin," by R. J. Cobbold, et al. BRIT MED J. 4:681-682, December 14, 1968.

RIFOMYCIN
"Clinical experimentation with rifomycin in dermatologic and venereal diseases," by L. Rasponi. G CLIN MED. 50:896-903, October, 1969.

"Therapy of gonococcal infection with rifamycin in a 'single dose'," by A. Califano, et al. MINERVA DERM. 43:516-519, October, 1968.

RIMACTAN
SEE: RIFAMPICIN

RONDOMYCIN
SEE: METHCYCLINE

ROVAMYCIN
"Rovamycin in the treatment of gonorrhea," by B. Raszeja-Kotelba. PRZEGL DERM. Suppl:75-78, 1969.

"Single dose therapy of gonorrhea with rovamycin," by P. Schmid. DERMATOLOGICA. 134:279-282, 1967.

SALPINGITIS
SEE: MINOR VENEREAL DISEASES & INFECTIONS

SCABIES
"A combined epidemic of scabies and syphilis. What therapeutic course to follow?," by R. Rollier. LYON

SCABIES

MED. 222:953-954, November 23, 1969.

"Differential diagnostic problem: impetiginized eczematic scabies--lues II--psoriasis vulgaris," by V. Misgeld. MED KLIN. 64:2189-2192, November 21, 1969.

SCIENTIFIC SOCIETY OF DERMATOLOGISTS-VENEROLOGISTS
SEE: CLINICS

SERODIAGNOSIS

"ABO and rhesus blood group distribution among patients attending venereal diseases clinics," by C. B. Schofield. J MED GENET. 3:101-103, June, 1966.

"Intracellular complement fixation by 'in vitro' stimulated lymphocytes (fluorescent serologic demonstration," by H.J. Heitmann. Z HAUT GESCHLECHTSKR. 44: 121-124, February 15, 1969.

"On the diagnostic value of serum phosphohexose isomerase in some liver diseases in childhood," by C. M. Berni, et al. BOLL SOX ITAL BIOL SPER. 42:1765-1768, December 15, 1966.

SEROLOGY
SEE ALSO: SERO-DIAGNOSIS

"Antibodies of the IgG, IgM, and IgA classes in newborn and adult sera reactive with gram-negative bacteria," by I. R. Cohen, et al. J CLIN INVEST. 47: 1053-1062, May, 1968.

"Brucellosis, treponematosis, rickettsiosis, and psittacosis in Surinam. A serological survey," by P. Kooy. TROP GEOGR MED. 22:172-178, June, 1970.

"Comparison of inconclusive smears from gynecological and obstetrical clinics of Johns Hopkins Hospital," by M. B. Skrocka. J MAINE MED ASS. 58:79-83, April, 1967.

"On the evaluation of results of serologic reactions. II. Qualitative demonstration of antibodies," by J. Morenz. Z IMMUNITAETSFORSCH. 131:376-389, October, 1966.

"Positive fluorescent treponemal antibody reactions in diabetes," by M. K. Hughes, et al. APPL MICROBIOL. 19:425-428, March, 1970.

SEROLOGY

"Report of a serological survey of Cape Verdeans living on the island of Sao Nicolau and in New England, U.S.A. treponematosis, yellow fever and tetanus antibodies," by C. V. Du Florey, et al. AN ESC NAC SAUDE PUBLICA MED TROP. 2:3-9, January-December, 1968.

"Serological activity of mycobacterial cardiolipin in comparison with cardiolipin from the cardiac muscle," by M. Sasaki, et al. SCI REP RES INST TOHOKU UNIV. 16:68-71, October, 1969.

"Serological techniques," by C. E. Taylor. J CLIN PATH. 3:Suppl:3:14-19, 1969.

"Serology in control of venereal diseases," by N. C. Bhattacharyya. INDIAN J DERM. 14:129-132, April, 1969.

"Serology in leprosy," by H. Schmidt, et al. DERM INT. 7:43-45, January-March, 1968.

"Serology of normal primates," by B. M. Levine, et al. BRIT J VENER DIS. 46:307-310, August, 1970.

"Skin-sensitizing antibodies in serum from patients with penicillin allergy studied by passive transfer to monkey skin and compared with results obtained on human skin (Prausnitz-Kustner technique)," by J. Pedersen-Bjergaard. ACTA ALLERG. 24:57-72, March, 1969.

"Survey of recent developments in some fields of serologic diagnosis of disease," by K. F. Petersen. HIPPOKRATES. 38:714-719, September 30, 1967.

SERVICEMEN

"Attempt at the evaluation of the influence of environment on the incidence of syphilis in soldiers of obligatory service," by J. Lancucki, et al. PRZEGL DERM. Suppl:93-99, 1969.

"Cooperation of the Military Health Service in the control of venereal diseases during 25 years of the Polish People's Republic," by K. Plonski, et al. PRZEGL DERM. 56:713-714, 1969.

"Experiences with the use of sodium ampicillin in acute gonococcal infections in Vietnam," by R. G. Kercull. MILIT MED. 133:985-986, December, 1968.

SERVICEMEN

"Findings on the management of syphilis in military personnel," by A. F. Giordano. REV SANIT MILIT ARGENT. 67:38-44, January-June, 1968.

"Health knowledge of prostitutes in Saigon, Vietnam. A study of health attitudes and habits relating to venereal diseases taken from a group of prostitutes," by R. S. Marcondes, et al. REV SAUDE PUBLICA. 1: 18-23, June, 1967.

"A nationwide serum survey of Colombian military recruits 1966. I. Description of sample and antibody patterns with arboviruses, polioviruses, respiratory viruses, tetanus, and treponematosis," by A. S. Evans, et al. AMER J EPIDEM. 90:292-303, October, 1969.

"On gonorrhea and moniliasis in Finnish battalion 8 on Cyprus in winter 1967-1968," by E. E. Vuori, et al. SOTILASLAAK AIKAK. 43:126-129, 1968.

"The prevention of venereal disease in the Royal Navy," by S. Dudley. J ROY NAV MED SERV. 53:36-42, Spring, 1967.

"Psychosocial background of servicemen contracting venereal diseases," by K. Singh, et al. J INDIAN MED ASS. 46:270-274, March 1, 1966.

"Public health and the Vietnam returnee," by D. L. Nathan. JAMA. 208:154, April 7, 1969.

"Public health problems relating to the Vietnam returnee," by J. H. Greenberg. JAMA. 207:697-702, January 27, 1969.

"Tests for syphilis in young males. An analysis of a seven-year series from a Central Military Hospital," by O. P. Salo, et al. MILIT MED. 132:258-261, April, 1967.

"Treatment of 'penicillin-resistant' gonorrhea in military personnel in SE Asia: a cooperative evaluation of tetracycline and of penicillin plus probenecid in 1263 men," by K. K. Holmes, et al. MILIT MED. 133: 642-646, August, 1968.

"Treatment of venereal diseases in the Royal Navy," by F. E. Willmott. J ROY NAV MED SERV. 54:254-257, Winter, 1968.

SERVICEMEN

"VD in Vietnam," by R. S. Cooperman. NEW ENG J MED. 283:546, September 3, 1970.

"V.D., a military-civilian problem," by W. J. Brown. MILIT MED. 132:316-317, April, 1967.

"Venereal disease control in the 2nd Marine Division, Camp Lejeune, North Carolina," by P. C. White, Jr., et al. MILIT MED. 132:252-257, April, 1967.

"Vietnam: Preventive medicine orientation," by D. N. Gilbert, et al. MILIT MED. 132:769-790, October, 1967.

SEX RESEARCH
"Before Kinsey: Continuity in American sex research," by A. Krich. PSYCHOANAL REV. 53:233-254, Summer, 1966.

SIGMAMYCIN
"Clinical experience with sigmamycin in skin and venereal diseases," by E. Heinke. MED WELT. 5:265-269, February 4, 1967.

SMALLPOX
"Studies of false positive serological tests for syphilis following smallpox vaccination," by O. P. Salo, et al. ANN MED EXP FENN. 44:304-306, 1966.

SOCIETIES, CLINICS & INSTITUTES
SEE: CLINICS
SEE ALSO: HISTORY

SOCIOLOGY & BEHAVIOR
SEE ALSO: OCCURRENCE

"Attitudes of college students in East Africa to sexual activity and venereal disease," by O. P. Arya, et al. BRIT J VENER DIS. 44:160-166, June, 1968.

"Attitudes of prospective school teachers on teaching venereal disease information," by W. B. Neser, et al. PUBLIC HEALTH REP. 82:917-920, October, 1967.

"Attitudes toward venereal disease," by W. L. Porter. DELAWARE MED J. 40:373-375, December, 1968.

"The bases of a suitable marital and premarital education in Turin. Activities of the AIEMP," by I. Terzi, et al. G BATT VIROL IMMUN. 62:703-709, September-October, 1969.

"The behavioural diseases. 2. The venereal diseases," by R. D. Catterall. NURS TIMES. 64:1041-1043, August 2, 1968.

"Factors influencing the spread of gonorrhea. I. Educational and social behavior," by L. Juhlin. ACTA DERMATOVENER. 48:75-81, 1969.

--II. Sexual behavior at different ages." ACTA DERMATOVENER. 48:82-89, 1968.

"Influence of contraceptive gestogen pills on sexual behaviour and the spread of gonorrhoea," by L. Juhlin, et al. BRIT J VENER DIS. 45:321-324, December, 1969.

"Investigation into the sexual behavior of young men," by P. Hertoft. DANISH MED BULL SUPPL. 1:1-96, March, 1969.

"Medicosocial background to gonococcal ophthalmia neonatorum," by C. B. Schofield. LANCET. 2:1182-1185, November, 1969.

"Patterns of sexual behaviour in relation to venereal disease," by K. Ekstrom. BRIT J VENER DIS. 46:93-95, April, 1970.

"Personality characteristics of V.D. patients," by B. W. Wells. BRIT J SOC CLIN PSYCHOL. 8:246-252, September, 1969.

"Premarital pregnancy and status before and after marriage," by L. C. Coombs, et al. AM J SOCIOL. 75:800-820, March, 1970.

"Promiscuity and contraception in a sample of patients attending a clinic for venereal diseases," by A. Linken, et al. BRIT J VENER DIS. 46:243-246, June, 1970.

"Psychosocial background of servicemen contracting venereal diseases," by K. Singh, et al. J INDIAN MED ASS. 46:270-274, March 1, 1966.

"Sex attitudes of young people: London, England," by

SOCIOLOGY & BEHAVIOR

M. Holmes, et al. ED RES. 11:38-42, November, 1968.

"Sexual assault on women and girls in the District of Columbia," by C. R. Hayman, et al. SOUTHERN MED J. 62:1227-1231, October, 1969.

"Sexually deviant behavior in expectant fathers," by A. A. Hartmen, et al. J ABNORM PSYCHOL. 71:232-234, June, 1966.

"Social behaviour and the use of medical services," by J. A. Savin. BRIT J PREV SOC MED. 23:53-55, February, 1969.

"Social diseases and the structure of society," by S. Gorbovitskii. VESTN DERM VENER. 44:5-8, January, 1970.

"Social problems of venereal diseases among New York youth," by W. Curth. ARCH KLIN EXP DERM. 227:637-640, 1966.

"Trends in the incidence and sociology of venereal diseases," by G. Wagner. THER UMSCH. 26:60-66, February, 1969.

"Use of behavioral research in venereal disease control," by W. J. Brown, et al. PUBLIC HEALTH REP. 83:583-586, July, 1968.

"VD is on the increase--social aspects," NEW ZEALAND NURS J. 61:12+, April, 1968.

"Venereal diseases. Social aspects," by M. Tottie. NORD MED. 76:817-818, July 14, 1966.

SPECTINOMYCIN
"Co-operative evaluation of treatment of early syphilis. Preliminary report with special reference to spectinomycin sulphate (actinospectacin)," by J. B. Lucas, et al. BRIT J VENER DIS. 43:244-248, December, 1967.

"Spectinomycin hydrochloride in the treatment of uncomplicated gonorrhoea," by C. E. Cornelius, 3rd, et al. BRIT J VENER DIS. 46:212-213, June, 1970.

SPIRAMYCIN
"Clinical experience with spiramycin in the 'minute

SPIRAMYCIN

therapy' of gonorrhea," by E. Heinke, et al. DEUTSCH MED WSCHR. 94:1182-1185, May 30, 1969.

"'One minute treatment' of gonococcal urethritis by spiramycin," by L. Sylvestre, et al. UN MED CANADA. 96:199-201, February, 1967.

"Relationships between the sensitivities in vitro of Neisseria gonorrhoeae to spiramycin, penicillin, streptomycin, tetracycline, and erythromycin," by A. Reyn, et al. BRIT J VENER DIS. 45:223-227, September, 1969.

"Spiramycin in the 'minute treatment' of gonorrhoea," by E. Heinke, et al. GERMAN MED MONTHLY. 14:479-482, October, 1969.

"Spiramycin in the therapy of gonococcal infection," by V. Terminello. MINERVA MED. 61:1423-1425, April 11, 1970.

"Spiramycin in the treatment of gonorrhoea." BRIT MED J. 2:129, April 18, 1970.

"A study of the relationships between the sensitivities of Neisseria gonorrhoeae to sodium penicillin G, four semisynthetic penicillins, spiramycin, and fusidic acid," by A. Reyn, et al. BRIT J VENER DIS. 44:140-150, June, 1968.

SPONDYLITIS

"Complement-fixing antibodies to Bedsonia organisms in Reiter's syndrome and ankylosing spondylitis," by T. D. Kinsella, et al. ANN RHEUM DIS. 27:241-244, May, 1968.

STATISTICS
  SEE ALSO: HISTORY
            OCCURRENCE

"Clinical statistics in the Department of Urology of Kanazawa University during the last 10 years (1955-1964)," by K. Kuroda, et al. JAP J UROL. 57:773-794, July, 1966.

"Congenital syphilis in the Istituto Provinciale Assistenza all' Infanzia of Rome. (Comparison between the decade 1943-1952 and that of 1957-1966). Statistical, clinical, therapeutic and prophylactic considerations,"

STATISTICS

by V. Menichella, et al. MINERVA NIPOL. 19:35-39, January-February, 1969.

"Current clinical aspects and statistics of early and late syphilis in Poland," by J. Towpik. POL TYG LEK. 22:1477-1480, September 25, 1967.

"Evolution of vaginal trichomoniasis from 1957 to 1964. Statistical discussion," by M. Gaudefroy, et al. J SCI MED LILLE. 84:409-422, September-October, 1966.

"Extent and development of late syphilis according to autopsy statistics (1945-1965)," by G. Fromm, et al. DEUTSCH MED WSCHR. 92:1181-1185, June 30, 1967.

"New statistical contribution on the relationships between the Nelson-Mayer test and classical serological reactions (13,000 cases)," by V. Resta, et al. MINERVA MED. 59:222-228, January 20, 1968.

"The prognosis of syphilitic infection. (Clinical, serological and statistical data)," by U. Boncinelli, et al. G ITAL DERM. 107:463-512, September-December, 1966.

"Recapitulation of data received during the year 1965, concerning statistics for venereal disease in metropolitan France," by P. Chassagne. BULL INST NAT SANTE. 21:709-736, July-August, 1966.

"Recent syphilis in pregnancy and early congenital syphilis in the province of Milan. Statistico-epidemiological findings for 1967 and 1968 (through November, 1968). Considerations and proposals," by C. Ducrey. G ITAL DERM. 45:156-163, March, 1970.

"625 cases of trichomoniasis treated with metronidazole (statistical discussion)," by M. Gaudefroy, et al. GYNEC PRAT. 19:339-362, 1968.

"Statistical considerations on the pathogenesis of epithelioma of the lip," by L. Tobia. MINERVA CHIR. 21:966-968, November 15, 1966.

"Statistical data on venereal diseases in Czechoslavakia in 1965," by J. Obrtel. CESK DERM. 42:72, February, 1967.

"Statistical evaluation of syphilis serodiagnosis," by

STATISTICS

S. Yamamoto, et al. JAP J CLIN PATH. 16:374, April, 1968.

"Statistical findings on the curability of syphilis," by G. Argenziano, et al. MINERVA DERM. 42:630-632, December, 1967.

"Studies on carcinoma of the urinary bladder. I. Statistical and epidemiological studies on cancer of the bladder in Japanese," by O. Yoshida. ACTA UROL JAP. 12:10-1040-1064, October, 1966.

"Study of the increase of primary-secondary and early congenital syphilis from 1938 to 1965 bases on the statistics of the Clinical Dermosifilopatica of the University of Genoa and of the Ospedale Pediatrico 'Giannina Gaslini' of Genoa," by E. Rampini, et al. MINERVA DERM. 41:442-444, December, 1966.

STERILITY
SEE ALSO: INFERTILITY

"Genital trichomoniasis and conjugal sterility," by G. Nicora, et al. GYNEC PRAT. 19:309-327, 1968.

"On the role of trichomonas infection of the sperm in sterility," by E. B. Bank. ZBL GYNAEK. 88:566-569, April 30, 1966.

"Role of trichomonas vaginalis in sterility," by P. Kostie. GYNEC PRAT. 15:467-469, 1964.

"Trichomonas and candida albicans as a cause of conjugal sterility. Proposal of a new fundic test," by S. Gaffuri, et al. MINERVA GINEC. 20:1260-1268, July 31, 1968.

"Trichomoniasis, sterility and abortion," by G. Carvalho, et al. VIRGINIA MED MONTHLY. 96:444-448, August, 1969.

STREPTOMYCIN

"Effect of streptomycin on treponema pallidum," by J. Suchanek, et al. POL TYG LEK. 22:89-91, January 16, 1967.

"Neisseria gonorrhoea strain showing an exceptional resistance to streptomycin and a considerable decreased susceptibility to some other antibiotics," by M. Pek-

STREPTOMYCIN

owski, et al. PRZEGL DERM. 57:49-54, January-February, 1970.

"Relapse of gonorrhoea after treatment with penicillin or streptomycin," by A. J. Evans. BRIT J VENER DIS. 42:251-262, December, 1966.

"Relationships between the sensitivities in vitro of Neisseria gonorrhoeae to spiramycin, penicillin, streptomycin, tetracycline, and erythromycin," by A. Reyn, et al. BRIT J VENER DIS. 45:223-227, September, 1969.

"Streptomycin in the treatment of gonorrhoea in London in 1966," by R. J. Spitzer, et al. ACTA DERMATOVENER. 48:537-541, 1968.

SULPHAMETHOXAZOLE

"Sulphamethoxazole combined with 2-4 diamino-pyrimidines in the treatment of gonorrhoea," by D. J. Wright, et al. BRIT J VENER DIS. 46:34-36, February, 1970.

"Therapeutic trial of some genital infections with trimethoprim-sulphamethoxazole," by G. W. Csonka. POSTGRAD MED J. 45:Suppl:77-80, November, 1969.

"The treatment of gonorrhoea in women with sulphamethoxazole-trimethoprim," by C. B. Schofield, et al. POSTGRAD MED J. 45:Suppl:81-86, November, 1969.

"Treatment of gonorrhoea with trimethoprim-sulphamethoxazole in Uganda," by O. P. Arya, et al. BRIT J VENER DIS. 46:214-216, June, 1970.

SULFANILAMIDE

"Remote results of the treatment of gonorrhea in girls with sulfanilamide preparations and antibiotics," by V. N. Matveev, et al. VESTN DERM VENER. 41:81-83, April, 1967.

SULFISOXAZOLE

"Treatment of chancroid. A comparison of tetracycline and sulfisoxazole," by R. E. Kerber, et al. ARCH DERM. 100:604-607, November, 1969.

SULPHONAMIDES

"Why sulphonamides, when combined with 2-4-diamino-pyrimidines, are effective in sulphonamide-resistant gonorrhoea," by D. J. Wright. GUY HOSP REP. 118:287-291, 1969.

SYMPOSIA

SYMPOSIA
"AMA National Symposium on Venereal Disease Control. Introductory speech," by J. H. Sterner. ARCH ENVIRON HEALTH, Chicago. 13:352, September, 1966.

--Opening address," by A. W. Christensen. ARCH ENVIRON HEALTH, Chicago. 13:354-356, September, 1966.

--Welcoming address," by C. C. Edwards. ARCH ENVIRON HEALTH, Chicago. 13:353, September, 1966.

--Venereal disease and environmental health," by J. G. Telfer. ARCH ENVIRON HEALTH, Chicago. 13:351-352, September, 1966.

"Round table on chemotherapy of venereal diseases." ANTIMICROB AGENTS CHEMOTHER. 5:1115-1119, 1965.

"Symposium on certain forms of infective kerato-uveitis or uveitis: I. An approach to the problem, and the technique of anterior chamber tap," by B. R. Jones, et al. TRANS OPHTHAL SOC UK. 88:235-242, 1969.

"Therapeutic failures in gonorrhea. Discussion on symposium II," by H. Biehler. ARCH KLIN EXP DERM. 227: 656-662, 1966.

SYPHILIS
"Apropos of a case of syphilitic reinfection," by P. Caubet. BULL SOC FRANC DERM SYPH. 73:110-111, January-February, 1966.

"Atypical sub-periosteal abscess simulating a syphilitic gumma," by J. M. Meshaka, et al. REV DENT LIBAN. 17: 26-30, April-September, 1967.

"Broad spectrum antibiotics. The editors view," by E. J. Best. DENT DIG. 74:268, June, 1968.

"A case of early malignant syphilis," by S. Boulle, et al. BULL SOC FRANC DERM SYPH. 74:32-34, 1967.

"A case of early malignant syphilis," by P. Laugier, et al. BULL SOC FRANC DERM SYPH. 77:15-16, July, 1970.

"Changing patterns of late syphilis," by J. Towpik, et al. BRIT J VENER DIS. 46:132-134, April, 1970.

SYPHILIS

"Considerations on a current problem. Syphilitic reinfections," by G. Tramier, et al. PRESSE MED. 74: 2085-2090, October 1, 1966.

"Contribution to the study of multiple pseudosclerosis of a syphilitic nature (7 cases)," by B. Pollingher, et al. NEUROLOGIA. 12:215-225, May-June, 1967.

"Current aspects in syphiligraphy," by M. J. Maleville. BORDEAUX MED. 3:1041-1042 passim, April, 1970.

"Current aspects of primo-secondary syphilis. I. Primary syphilis." PRESSE MED. 78:1848, October 10, 1970.

--II. Secondary syphilis." PRESSE MED. 78:1945, October 24, 1970.

"Current trends in venereology." UNIV NEWCASTLE TYNE MED GAS. 63:34-39, October, 1968.

"Early malignant syphilis with a fatal course (anatomic examination," by R. Degos, et al. BULL SOC FRANC DERM SYPH. 77:10-15, July, 1970.

"Electrocardiographic and serum enzyme study with special reference to glutamic-oxalacetic and glutamic-pyruvic transaminase, lactate dehydrogenase and creatine phosphokinase in syphilis. Preliminary results," by M. Aricò. MINERVA DERM. 42:48-49, February, 1967.

"How could this happen to our daughter?," by L. David. GOOD H. 169:86-87+, September, 1969.

"Immunogenic properties of the protein component of treponema pallidum," by M. Metzger, et al. BRIT J VENER DIS. 45:299-304, December, 1969.

"Late atrophying syphilids," by B. Duperrat, et al. BULL SOC FRANC DERM SYPH. 76:798, 1969.

"Latent syphilis," by J. A. Etcheverry, et al. PRENSA MED ARGENT. 54:777-785, June 23, 1967.

"Man, monkeys, and treponemal disease (Editorial)," LANCET. 1:562, March 15, 1969.

"Modern aspect of latent syphilis," by K. N. Suvorova.

SYPHILIS

VESTN DERM VENER. 43:70-73, March, 1969.

"New antibody in early syphilis," by D. J. Wright, et al. LANCET. 1:740-743, April 11, 1970.

"New trends in syphilogy," by V. G. Cave. J NAT MED ASS. 61:158-163 passim, March, 1969.

"Observations of the pathogenesis of syphilis in Aotus trivirgatus," by J. W. Clark, Jr., et al. BRIT J VENER DIS. 44:208-215, September, 1968.

"Present status and variation in syphilis patients," by H. Tsugami. JAP J NURS ART. 8:11-20, August, 1969.

"Secondary syphilis. Report of 2 cases," by P. H. Nexmand. UGESKR LAEG. 132:1157-1158, June 11, 1970.

"Serologic investigations in narcotic addicts. I. Syphilis, lymphogranuloma venereum, herpes simplex, and Q fever," by C. E. Cherubin, et al. ANN INTERN MED. 69:739-742, October, 1968.

"The sexually transmitted diseases. Part II. Syphilis. NURS MIRROR. 128:24, February 7, 1969.

"Some features of clinical picture and course of secondary syphilis nowadays," by V. A. Rakhmanov, et al. VESTN DERM VENER. 42:56-60, April, 1968.

"Study of the existence of treponemic antibodies in dry blood," by A. Utrilla. ACTAS DERMOSIF. 58:167-170, May-June, 1967.

"Syphilis." LYON MED. 215:69-117, January 9, 1966.

"Syphilis--an ancient enemy grows weaker. (Editorial)," by W. H. Kaufman. VIRGINIA MED MONTHLY. 96:499-500, August, 1969.

"Syphilis--the persistent problem." EYE EAR NOSE THROAT MONTHLY. 45:88 passim, November, 1966.

"Syphilis--rediscovered," by S. Olansky. DM. 3-30, May, 1967.

"Syphilis under our noses," by D. R. Richardson, et al. VIRGINIA MED MONTHLY. 95:607-609 passim, October, 1968.

SYPHILIS

"Syphilization," by J. R. Prakken. NEDERL T GENEESK. 114:1019-1023, June 13, 1970.

SYPHILIS: ANO-RECTAL
"Anal syphilis," by O. Delzant. ARCH FRANC MAL APPAR DIG. 59:Suppl:7-8:13+, July-August, 1970.

"Anogenital cutaneous lesions," by R. R. Kierland. JAMA. 203:213-218, January 15, 1968.

"Ano-rectal syphilis," by O. Delzant. ARCH FRANC MAL APPAR DIG. 59:Suppl:7-8, 13+, July-August, 1970.

"Anorectal syphilis," by B. Samenius, et al. NORD MED. 76:813, July 14, 1966.

"Manifestations of early syphilis in the anoperineal region," by E. B. Molina Leguizamon. PRENSA MED ARGENT. 55:898-900, July 5, 1968.

"Primary syphilis of the anorectal region," by B. Samenius. DIS COLON RECTUM. 11:462-466, November, 1968; also in PROC ROY SOC MED. 59:629-631, July, 1966.

"Swelling of the inguinal lymph nodes in syphilis of the anus," by A. H. Schmid. MED KLIN. 61:914-915, June 10, 1966.

SYPHILIS: ARTHRITIC
SEE ALSO: SYPHILIS: ARTHROPATHY
TABES

"Low frequency of chronic biological false positive reactors to serological tests for syphilis in rheumatoid arthritis and ankylosing spondylitis," by O. P. Salo, et al. ANN RHEUM DIS. 27:261-263, May, 1968.

"Syphilitic osteoarthritis of the hip joint," by A. Sobbe, et al. FORTSCHR ROENTGENSTR. 110:249-253, February, 1969.

"Treponemal infection and arthritis," by C. J. Goodwill, et al. PROC ROY SOC MED. 62:198-199, February, 1969.

SYPHILIS: ARTHROPATHY
SEE ALSO: SYPHILIS: ARTHRITIC
TABES

"Apropos of a case of tabetic arthropathy of both shoul-

SYPHILIS: ARTHROPATHY

ders," by S.D.E. Seze, et al. REV RHUM. 35:551-554, October, 1968.

"Arteriographic findings in an atrophic tabetic arthropathy," by H. J. Maurer, et al. Z ORTHOP. 107:139-144, November, 1969.

"Arthrodesis in tabetic arthropathy," by G. Friedebold, et al. ARCH ORTHOP UNFALLCHIR. 59:272-285, 1966.

"Case contribution to tabetic arthropathy of the spine and of both elbow joints," by K. Wallmann. BEITR ORTHOP TRAUMA. 14:441-448, August, 1967.

"A case of delayed diagnosis of tabetic arthropathy," by P. F. Triapichnikov. VESTN DERM VENER. 42:86-88, 1968.

"A case of polyarthropathy of cryptogenic tabetic type," by L. Canet, et al. REV RHUM. 36:613-615, November, 1969.

"Charcot joint of the lumbar spine," by D. P. McNeel, et al. J NEUROSURG. 30:55-61, January, 1969.

"Charcot joints," by G. O. Storey. RHEUMATOL PHYS MED. 10:312-320, August, 1970.

"Diagnostic difficulties in tabetic arthropathy," by W. Kozina, et al. REUMATOLOGIA. 7:369-373, 1969.

"Gumma of the shoulder joint," by J. Singh, et al. J INDIAN MED ASS. 48:592-593, June 16, 1967.

"Isolated lumbar tabetic arthropathy," by J. David-Chausse, et al. BULL SOC FRANC DERM SYPH. 77:105-107, July, 1970.

"Nerve compressions in tabetic arthropathy of the spine," by H. Serre, et al. BULL ACAD NAT MED. 154:212-216, March 17, 1970.

"Neurogenic arthropathies (Charcot's joints)," by P. C. Das, et al. J INDIAN MED ASSOC. 54:368-372, April 16, 1970.

"Neuropathic arthritis (Charcot's joint)," by R. Stien. T NORSK LAEGEFOREN. 88:1941-1943 passim, October 15, 1968.

SYPHILIS: ARTHROPATHY

"Osteoarthropathia tabetica of the ankle joint following a fracture," by T. Krezel. CHIR NARZAD RUCHU ORTOP POL. 31:757-761, 1966.

"Radicular and medullary complications of tabetic vertebral osteoarthropathies," by R. Thurel, et al. REV NEUROL. 114:62-65, January, 1966.

"Radicular compression due to tabetic arthropathies of the spine," by H. Serre, et al. REV RHUM MAL OSTEOARTIC. 37:525-533, August-September, 1970.

"A rare case of tabetic arthropathy of the hip," by G. Sgarbi, et al. OSPED ITAL CHIR. 16:615-625, June, 1967.

"Syphilitic arthropathy," by M. Makuch, et al. CHIR NARZAD RUCHU ORTOP POL. 33:673-677, 1968.

"Tabetic arthropathies," by E. Delvecchio. OSPED ITAL CHIR. 18:481-493, May, 1968.

"Tabetic arthropathy," by M. L. Livshits. VRACH DELO. 11:147-149, November, 1967.

"Tabetic arthropathy and secondary neurological manifestations," by M. Cardas, et al. NEUROLOGIA. 12: 341-353, July-August, 1967.

"An unusual case of tabetic polyarthropathy," by A. Osti. MINERVA ORTOP. 19:637-643, November, 1968.

SYPHILIS: AURAL

"Aural condylomata in secondary syphilis," by J. F. Jarvis, et al. J LARYNG. 82:157-159, February, 1968.

"Congenital luetic hearing impairment. Treatment with prednisone," by M. E. Patterson. ARCH OTOLARYNG. 87:378-382, April, 1968.

"Deafness and late congenital syphilis," by F. Baron, et al. REV LARYNG. 88:877-883, November-December, 1967.

"Deafness in congenital syphilis," by C. S. Karmody, et al. ARCH OTOLARGYN. 83:18-27, January, 1966.

"Rapidly progressive deafness caused by syphilitic neuro-labyrinthitis," by G. Pellegrini, et al. REV

SYPHILIS: AURAL

OTONEUROOPHTAL. 41:203-211, May-June, 1969.

"Steroid treatment in congenital syphilitic deafness," by R. S. Dawkins, et al. J LARYNG. 82:1095-1107, December, 1968.

BIBLIOGRAPHY
"Late syphilis: a review of some of the recent literature," by L. Nicholas, et al. AMER J MED SCI. 254: 549-569, October, 1967.

SYPHILIS: CARDIOVASCULAR
"An anatomo-clinical case of tabes and syphilitic aneurysm of the aorta. Its course under treatment," by M. Giroud, et al. LYON MED. 215:1603-1609, June 5, 1966.

"Aneurysm of the ascending aorta. Recession and direct anastomosis. Report of a case," by J. F. Saadi, et al. ARQ BRASIL CARDIOL. 21:215-220, June, 1968.

"Aneurysms of the descending thoracic aorta," by M. L. Dillon, et al. ANN THORAC SURG. 3:430-438, May, 1967.

"Aneurysms of the thoracic and abdominal aorta. I. Incidence of aortic aneurysm in 10,392 autopsies," by P. Tala, et al. ANN CHIR GYNAEC FENN. 56:270-277, 1967.

"Angiographic demonstration of aortic aneurysm," by E. Lohr, et al. FORTSCHR ROENTGENSTR. 110:71-78, January, 1969.

"Angiographic demonstration of coronary ostial stenosis. Report of a case probably due to syphilis," by C. A. Macleod, et al. AMER J CARDIOL. 22:122-125, July, 1968.

"Anti-anginal activity of a beta-adrenergic blocking agent, butydrine, alone and in association with pentaerythritol tetranitrate, in the aged," by A. Gatti, et al. CLIN TER. 41:363-374, May 31, 1967.

"Aortic aneurysm and block of the right branch in a 22-year-old man. Syphilis?," by G. Heuillet, et al. MARSEILLE MED. 106:437-444, 1969.

"Aortic arch replacement in leutic aneurysm," by G.

SYPHILIS: CARDIOVASCULAR

Heberer, et al. CHIRURG. 40:174-179, April, 1969.

"Aortic root aneurysm. Diagnosis and treatment," by H. Najafi. JAMA. 197:133-134, July 11, 1966.

"Aortic valve insufficiency in geriatrics. 3. Clinical observations on 206 cases over 60 years of age," by H. Ueda, et al. SAISHIN IGAKU. 22:2738-2744, December 10, 1967.

"Aortitis," by I. Ito. NAIKA. 19:1116-1118, June, 1967.

"Apropos of a case of specific arteritis," by A. Luise. CARDIOL PRAT. 17:215-220, April, 1966.

"Apropos of the treatment of late syphilis," by A. Meyer. PRESSE MED. 74:1306, May 21, 1966.

"The Austin Flint murmur in cardiac diagnosis," by D. N. Wysham, et al. INDIAN HEART J. 19:238-246, July, 1967.

"Brain tumor syndrome in syphilitic arteritis," by R. Suchenwirth. DEUTSCH Z NERVENHEILK. 190:338-348, 1967.

"Cardio-aortic syphilis." PENN MED. 72:75, February, 1969.

"Cardiovascular and neurological findings in Ethiopians with syphilitic heart disease," by D. Vukotich, et al. TROP GEOGR MED. 22:45-52, March, 1970.

"Cardiovascular syphilis in a 20-year-old man," by C. Hiltenbrand, et al. ARCH MAL COEUR. 60:1041-1048, July, 1967.

"A case of intravital diagnosis of dissecting aneurysm of the abdominal aorta," by E. B. Shnaider. KLIN MED. 44:124-125, January, 1966.

"A case of rupture of an aortic aneurysm into the trachea," by Z. S. Chichinadze. ZH USHN NOS GORL BOLEZ. 26:82-83, September-October, 1966.

"A case of thrombosis of the left median cerebral artery with active syphilis of the vessels," by Z. Konopka, et al. PRZEGL DERM. 54:343-346, May-June, 1967.

SYPHILIS: CARDIOVASCULAR

"A case of triple fusiform aneurysm of the aortic arch successfully operated with resection and grafting," by D. Guilmet, et al. MINERVA CARDIOANGIOL. 15:175-181, February, 1967.

"The change of the ground substance of the aorta in syphilitic aortitis," by L. Józsa, et al. VIRCHOW ARCH. 345:324-330, 1968.

"Chiasmal arachnoiditis as a manifestation of generalized arachnoiditis in systemic vascular disease. Clinico-pathological report of two cases," by M. Oliver, et al. BRIT J OPHTHAL. 52:227-235, March, 1968.

"Cholesterol embolism in the course of antiluetic therapy," by P. H. Berghuis, et al. NEDERL T GENEESK. 113:2046-2049, November 15, 1969.

"Cholesterol embolism in the course of antiluetic therapy," by D. J. Vermeer. NEDERL T GENEESK. 114:172, January 24, 1970.

"Clinical aspects of the dissecting aortic aneurysm," by M. I. Gorbunova. KLIN MED. 48:133-135, January, 1970.

"Clinicopathologic conference," by E. H. Eigenbrodt, et al. TEXAS MED. 65:84-90, July, 1969.

"Clinicopathologic conference. Case presentation (JHH 631077)," by V. A. McKusick, et al. BULL HOPKINS HOSP. 119:150-160, August, 1966.

"Complex shape and variability of the diastolic murmur of aortic regurgitation," by W. Dressler, et al. AMER J CARDIOL. 18:616-621, October, 1966.

"Considerations on the evolution of cardio-aortic and nervous syphilis in the city of Birlad in the past 15 years (1953-1967)," by I. Graur, et al. REV MEDICOCHIR IASI. 73:127-131, January-March, 1969.

"Contemporary principles and methods in treatment of syphilitic aortitis," by M. P. Frishman. VESTN DERM VENER. 44:47-51, May, 1970.

"Contribution on lues visceralis," by N. Kraus, et al. Z GES INN MED. 21:443-445, July 15, 1966.

SYPHILIS: CARDIOVASCULAR

"Jarisch-Herxheimer reaction and syphilitic aortitis," by G. R. Hughes. BRIT MED J. 1:360, February 10, 1968.

"Diagnosis and therapy of luetic aneurysm of the thoracic aorta," by G. Heberer, et al. DEUTSCH MED WSCHR. 95:1707-1713 passim, August 21, 1970.

"Diagnosis and treatment of cardiovascular syphilis," by J. Pautrat, et al. PRESSE MED. 74:269-270, January 29, 1966.

"Difficulty in swallowing due to a large luetic aneurysm of the thoracic aorta," by H. Wehling. MED WELT. 2:106-108, January 8, 1966.

"Diffuse arteritis of aorta with a large aortic aneurysm. Report of a case in an African," by M. Gelfand. CENT AFR J MED. 13:179-181, August, 1967.

"Diseases of the ascending aorta with aortic insufficiency," by Y. Marquis, et al. UN MED CANADA. 97:1776-1786, December, 1968.

"Dissecting aneurysm in a 29-year-old man with syphilis of main aorta," by H. Dzioba, et al. POL TYG LEK. 23:1148-1149, July 22, 1968.

"Dissecting aneurysm of the aorta in syphilitic mesaortitis," by S. G. Moisseev, et al. Z GES INN MED. 21:134-136, June 15, 1966.

"Electrocardiographic findings in syphilitic aortitis," by D. Knapikowá, et al. KARDIOL POL. 13:131-135, 1970.

"Etiological studies of atrio-ventricular blocks (clinical study of 573 cases)," by L. Prevosti, et al. FOLIA CARDIOL. 26:79-92, March-April, 1967.

"Hemodynamic study of aortic valvular cardiopathies by the isotope dilution curve," by J. Di Matteo, et al. ARCH MAL COEUR. 60:1061-1085, August, 1967.

"Intracerebral aneurysm of probably luetic origin," by S. Kopczynski, et al. POL TYG LEK. 25:1465-1466, September, 1970.

"Ischaemic heart disease due to syphilitic narrowing

SYPHILIS: CARDIOVASCULAR

of the coronary ostia," by K. K. Datey, et al. INDIAN HEART J. 21:253-258, July, 1969.

"Late complications of syphilis. A comparative epidemiological and serological study of cardiovascular syphilis and various forms of neurosyphilis," by K. Aho, et al. ACTA DERMATOVENER. 49:336-342, 1969.

"Linear calcification of the ascending aorta without syphilis," by J. A. Cohen. JAMA. 214:375, October 12, 1970.

"Luetic aneurysms of the aortic valve, sinus of Valsalva and aorta," by D. Sohn, et al. AMER J CLIN PATH. 46:99-102, July, 1966.

"Luetic stenosis of the abdominal aorta and of the renal arteries," by H. Rykowski, et al. POL TYG LEK. 25:694-695, May 11, 1970.

"Management of thoracic aneurysms," by J. Storer, et al. INT SURG. 47:344-355, April, 1967.

"Mesaortitis luica," by P. Ostendorf, et al. MED WELT. 11:419-422, March 14, 1970.

"Multiple aorto-cervical occlusions of syphilitic origin," by V. Maslenikov, et al. ACTA NEUROL LAT AMER. 12:48-55, 1966.

"Myocardial infarct in syphilitic aortitis," by J. M. Torre, et al. ARCH INST CARDIOL MEX. 36:300-307, May-June, 1966.

"Myocardial infarct on a background of syphilitic aortitis," by N. I. Ianushkevich, et al. KLIN MED. 45:119-120, February, 1967.

"Myocarditis in penicillin sensitivity," by D. Banerjee. INDIAN HEART J. 20:73-75, January, 1968.

"Nonsyphilitic aortitis," by C. Restrepo, et al. ARCH PATH. 87:1-12, January, 1969.

"Obliteration of the anterior cerebral artery by probable syphilitic arteritis," by G. Almard, et al. J MED LYON. 50:215-220, February 5, 1969.

"Ocular manifestations of polyarteritis nodosa," by

SYPHILIS: CARDIOVASCULAR

M. R. Nanjiani. BRIT J OPHTHAL. 51:696-697, October, 1967.

"On certain difficulties in the diagnosis of syphilitic aortitis," by S. V. Shestakov. KLIN MED. 45:117-122, June, 1967.

"Paresis of the recurrent nerve as the first symptom of luetic aortic aneurysm," by Z. Jina. CESK OTOLARYNG. 16:247-251, August, 1967.

"Personal experience in surgical treatment of thoracic aortic aneurysms. Observations on 16 cases," by R. Donatelli, et al. ANN ITAL CHIR. 43:987-1027, December, 1967.

"A rare case of aneurysm of the ascending aorta," by Z. Zaborowski, et al. WIAD LEK. 22:655-656, April 1, 1969.

"Remote results of the treatment of patients with various forms of syphilitic aortitis," by M. P. Frishman. VESTN DERM VENER. 41:76-80, January, 1967.

"Rupture of the aortic aneurysm into the superior vena cava," by A. Kropfl, et al. LIJECN VJESN. 89:233-239, 1967.

"Sero-positive syphilitic aorto-myocarditis in a woman treated during 20 years and after several years of negative serology," by R. Degos, et al. BULL SOC FRANC DERM SYPH. 77:32-33, July, 1970.

"Some changing aspects of aortic regurgitation," by J. A. Barondess, et al. ARCH INTERN MED. 124:600-605, November, 1969.

--An autopsy study." TRANS AMER CLIN CLIMAT ASS. 80:23-36, 1969.

"Spontaneous rupture of aortic aneurysm into the esophagus," by J. Komorowski, et al. BULL POL MED SCI HIST. 9:24-25, January, 1966.

"Swallowing disorders due to a large luetic aneurysm of the thoracic aorta," by H. Wehling. MED WELT. 2:106-108, January 8, 1966.

"Syphilitic aneurysm of the ascending aorta producing

SYPHILIS: CARDIOVASCULAR

pulmonic stenosis by compression," by T. Watanabe, et al. AMER J CARDIOL. 20:575-578, October, 1967.

"Syphilitic aortic insufficiency. Its increased incidence in the elderly," by T. A. Prewitt. JAMA. 211:637-639, January 26, 1970.

"Syphilitic aortic insufficiency. Some observations on a vanishing disorder," by B. Friedman. ALABAMA J MED SCI. 6:8-17, January, 1969.

"Syphilitic aortitis," by D. B. Reddy, et al. INDIAN HEART J. 19:86-95, April, 1967.

"Syphilitic aortitis, 56 cases followed-up for 10 years after treatment with penicillin," by S. E. Vivas. ARCH INST CARDIOL MEX. 36:316-321, May-June, 1966.

"Syphilitic coronary ostial occlusion," by V. Schrive, et al. S AFR MED J. 40:553-555, July 2, 1966.

"Syphilitic coronary ostial sclerosis," by R. W. Frater, et al. ANN THORAC SURG. 6:463-468, November, 1968.

"Syphilitic ostial coronaritis: 5 cases of surgical disobstruction, 2 of which including a valve replacement for aortic insufficiency," by P. Michaud, et al. ARCH MAL COEUR. 63:674-693, May, 1970; also in LYON CHIR. 66:3-9, January-February, 1970.

"Syphilitic temporal arteritis," by J. L. Smith, et al. ARCH OPHTHAL. 78:284-288, September, 1967.

"Takayasu's syndrome and disease," by A. Zuch. WIAD LEK. 20:1271-1273, July 1, 1967.

"The thyroid and phospho-calcic metabolism. IV. The behavior of the specific radioactivity of plasmatic calcium during infusion of swine thyrocalcitonin (TCT) in man," by C. Scandellari, et al. ACTA ISOTOP. 7: 153-161, December 15, 1967.

"2 cases of dissecting aneurysm of the aorta in syphilitic mesaortitis diagnosed during life," by S. G. Moiseev, et al. TER ARKH. 38:108-111, June, 1966.

"2 cases of syphilitic aortic aneurysm of a very prolonged development (15 and 30 years), 1 a juvenile

SYPHILIS: CARDIOVASCULAR

form," by G. Plauchu, et al. LYON MED. 215:1575-1601, June 5, 1966.

"Unusual complications of an aortic aneurysm of syphilitic origin," by E. Kodlová. VNITRNI LEK. 13:1015-1017, October, 1967.

"Vascular involvement in congenital syphilis--an autopsied case with aortic arch syndrome and coarctation of the aorta," by S. Kimata, et al. NAIKA. 22:1431-1436, December, 1968.

"Vertebro-basilar arterial insufficiency (subclavian steal syndrome) (6 cases)," by J. Caron, et al. J RADIOL ELECTR. 49:157-162, January-February, 1968.

SYPHILIS: CEREBROSPINAL FLUID

"Cerebrospinal fluid electrolyte disturbances in neurological disorders: with special reference to inorganic phosphate," by U. Breyer, et al. NEUROLOGY. 20:247-253, March, 1970.

"Cerebrospinal fluid findings after treatment of early syphilis with penicillin. A further series of 80 cases," by W. L. Fernando. BRIT J VENER DIS. 42:134-135, June, 1968.

"Cerebrospinal fluid findings in ophthalmology. In eye diseases," by S. Shimizu. ACTA SOC OPHTHAL JAP. 71:1825-1845, October, 1967.

"Comparative study of cerebrospinal fluid and blood in syphilis and cerebral cysticercosis," by E. Oberhauser, et al. NEUROCIRUGIA. 27:61-68, January-September, 1969.

"Contribution of cerebrospinal fluid electrophoresis to clinical diagnosis," by U. Consbruch, et al. DEUTSCH MED WSCHR. 93:2168-2172, November 8, 1968.

"The effect of antisyphilitic treatment on the frequency of detection of antibrain autoantibodies in the blood and cerebrospinal fluid of patients with syphilis," by N. I. Tumasheva, et al. VESTN DERM VENER. 42:43-47, 1968.

"Immobilizing antibodies to treponema pallidum in the cerebrospinal fluid in syphilis," by F. Muller. GERMAN MED MONTHLY. 12:120-124, March, 1967.

SYPHILIS: CEREBROSPINAL FLUID

"Immunoglobulins of cerebrospinal fluid in syphilis," by V. A. Oxelius, et al. BRIT J VENER DIS. 45:121-125, June, 1969.

"Spinal fluid findings five years or more after infection in patients with early symptomatic syphilis treated with neo-arsphenamine bismuth," by F. M. Haagsma, et al. DERMATOLOGICA. 135:115-120, 1967.

"Study of late ocular syphilis. Demonstration of treponemes in aqueous humour and cerebrospinal fluid. I. Methods of demonstration of treponemes," by A. E. Wilkinson. TRANS OPHTHAL SOC UK. 88:251-256, 1969.

--II. Ocular findings," by N. S. Rice, et al. TRANS OPHTHAL SOC UK. 88:257-273, 1969.

--III. General and serological findings," by E. M. Dunlop, et al. TRANS OPHTHAL SOC UK. 88:275-294, 1969.

SYPHILIS: CHILDREN

"Bilateral recurrent laryngeal nerve paralysis in early childhood following congenital syphilis," by B. Fioresi. MSCHR OHRENHEILK. 101:375-377, 1967.

"General paralysis and cerebral angiomatosis in a child, Apropos of a case," by H. Collomb, et al. BULL SOC MED. 12:506-511, 1967.

"Pediatric use of the rapid plasma reagin (circle) card test," by J. C. Herweg, et al. PEDIATRICS. 40:440-443, September, 1967.

"Remote results of prophylactic treatment of children born to mothers with syphilis or with a history of syphilis," by V. N. Ivanov. VESTN DERM VENER. 43:86-90, January, 1969.

"The rise and fall of the treponematoses. II. Endemic treponematoses of childhood," by T. Guthe, et al. BRIT J VENER DIS. 44:35-48, March, 1968.

"Tests for syphilis in children for adoption," by C. E. Cooper. LANCET. 2:261, August 1, 1970.

"Tests for syphilis in children for adoption," by O. P. Gray. LANCET. 2:673, September 26, 1970.

SYPHILIS: CHILDREN

"Tests for syphilis in children for adoption," by D. H. Robertson. LANCET. 2:568, September 12, 1970.

SYPHILIS: COMPLICATIONS

"Alcoholic lymphalgia in early syphilis," by D. J. Wright. POSTGRAD MED J. 45:191-192, March, 1969.

"A case of acquired syphilis revealed by unilateral keratitis," by P. Desbordes, et al. MED TROP. 28: 230-232, March-April, 1968.

"A case of pyloric stenosis due to syphilis," by W. Straczkowski, et al. WIAD LEK. 20:893-894, May 1, 1967.

"Coombs' positive hemolytic anemia due to penicillin," by L. J. Lyon. J MOUNT SINAI HOSP NY. 35:258-264, May-June, 1968.

"Cytomegaly, cirrhosis and cancer of the pancreas in a patient with gummatous visceral syphilis," by V. A. Samsonov. ARKH PAT. 28:59-62, 1966.

"Diffuse pseudo-angiomatous phlebectases," by J. Delacrétaz, et al. DERMATOLOGICA. 137:242-249, 1968.

"Disease dominant chronic inflammatory splenomegaly. Dysproteinanemic manifestations and lienal lues," by K. Bauch. MED KLIN. 62:47-50, January 13, 1967.

"Drug-induced hemolysis," by B. Dreyfus, et al. PRESSE MED. 76:1009-1012, April 27, 1968.

"Gardner's syndrome with concomitant tertiary lues: report of case," by J. F. Welborn, et al. J ORAL SURG. 28:131-133, February, 1970.

"General paralysis and cerebral angiomatosis in a child. Apropos of a case," by H. Collomb, et al. BULL SOC MED AFR NOIRE LANG FRANC. 12:506-511, 1967.

"Hair root status in secondary lues," by W. Kostanecki, et al. Z HAUT GESCHLECHTSKR. 41:380-382, November 15, 1966.

"Hematuria in congenital lues," by J. Szabo, et al. SCHWEIZ MED WSCHR. 96:1446-1450, October 29, 1966.

"Hepatitis as a complication of early syphilis," by P.

SYPHILIS: COMPLICATIONS

Davidoff. DAPIM REFUIIM. 24:530-533, December, 1965.

"Hyperparathyreosis of syphilitic etiology in a patient with tertiary syphilis," by B. S. Pankov. VESTN DERM VENER. 40:51-54, April, 1966.

"Incomplete pachydermoperiostosis," by J. A. Savin. PROC ROY SOC MED. 61:239, March, 1968.

"Involvement of the epididymis in secondary syphilis," by C. Korte, et al. HAUTARZT. 20:369-370, August, 1969.

"Labyrinthitis luetica," by R. Haye. J OSLO CITY HOSP. 19:68-72, April, 1969.

"Leukoplakia of the kidney pelvis; hydronephrosis and syphilis as a possible cause," by I. A. Rovinescu, et al. ACTA UROL BELG. 34:495-500, October, 1966.

"Multiple cranial ostolysis associated with secondary syphilis (apropos of 2 cases)," by B. Duperrat, et al. BULL SOC FRANC DERM SYPH. 74:484-486, 1967.

"On specific trochanteritis," by G. Rava, et al. MINERVA ORTOP. 18:143-147, March, 1967.

"Osteolytic lesions in early syphilis," by M. F. Bauer, et al. BRIT J VENER DIS. 43:175-177, September, 1967.

"Paroxysmal cold haemoglobinuria in Jamaica. A case report," by J. K. Wood. W INDIAN MED J. 17:175-179, September, 1968.

"Radiological case of the month. Congenital syphilis with Parrot's pseudoparalysis," by J. L. Gwinn, et al. AMER J DIS CHILD. 120:243-244, September, 1970.

"Rare case of Simmonds' disease possibly caused by syphilitic lesion. Clinical diagnosis: adrenal cortical insufficiency and autopsy study: severe atrophy of pituitary gland," by T. Oda, et al. CLIN ENDOCR. 14:479-486, June, 1966.

"Relations between hepatic cirrhosis and microcythemia," by A. Garagnani, et al. ARCH ITAL MAL APPAR DIG. 33:529-546, November-December, 1966.

SYPHILIS: COMPLICATIONS

"Research on syphilitic spondylitis," by F. G. Marill, et al. BULL SOC FRANC DERM SYPH. 75:311-314, 1968.

"Sarcoid granuloma in secondary syphilis," by L. R. Lantis, et al. ARCH DERM. 99:748-752, June, 1969.

"Sectorial pigmented retinopathy secondary to acquired syphilis," by R. Cristiani. ANN OTTAL. 93:1099-2108, October, 1967.

"Subacute inflammatory rheumatism due to secondary syphilis," by M. F. Kahn, et al. PRESSE MED. 78:750, March 28, 1970.

--4 cases". REV RHUM. 37:431-436, June-July, 1970.

"Symptomatic 'migrating' phlebitis," by R. Verjat. PHLEBOLOGIE. 19:159-160, April-June, 1966.

"Syphilitic amyotrophy," by A. Datta, et al. J INDIAN MED ASS. 47:287-290, September 16, 1966.

"Syphilitic amyotrophy. A case occurring after apparently successful treatment in primary syphilis," by A. B. Hewitt. BRIT J VENER DIS. 43:272-274, December, 1967.

"Syphilitic chancre complicated by fusospirochaetal infection from the same partner. Development of necrotizing ulcer perforating the prepuce," by K. Lejman, et al. BRIT J VENER DIS. 45:313-316, December, 1969.

"Tietze's syndrome and syphilis," by J. Vachtenheim. DEUTSCH GESUNDH. 21:1387-1388, July 21, 1966.

"Tuberous mucinosis in a syphilitic," by P. Franceschini, et al. BULL SOC FRANC DERM SYPH. 76:860-861, 1969.

"Tumoral form of syphilis of the cheek," by A. Tarel, et al. REV STOMATOODONT NORD FRANCE. 23:179-184, October-December, 1968.

"Unusual jaundice during primary syphilis," by J. Duverne, et al. BULL SOC FRANC DERM SYPH. 74:57-58, 1967.

SYPHILIS: CONGENITAL

SYPHILIS: CONGENITAL
SEE ALSO: FETAL
INFANTS
NEONATAL + SPECIFIC KINDS OF SYPHILIS

"Autopsy case of congenital syphilis with jaundice," by Y. Ishiwata, et al. JAP J CLIN MED. 24:784-790, April, 1966.

"Clinical observation of early congenital syphilis," by F. C. Yu, et al. ACTA PAEDIAT SINICA. 8:93-101, April-June, 1967.

"Congenital luetic macroglobulinemia and cryoglobulinemia. Literature review and personal contribution," by A. G. Marchi, et al. G MAL INFETT. 20:249-251, March, 1968.

"Congenital syphilis," by M. Hart. ARCH DERM. 100: 260, August, 1969.

"Congenital syphilis," by R. C. Robinson. ARCH DERM. 99:599-610, May, 1969.

"Congenital syphilis: a continuing problem," by A. J. Strauss, Jr., et al. VIRGINIA MED MONTHLY. 94:684-687, November, 1967.

"Congenital syphilis: a description of 18 cases and re-examination of an old but ever-present disease," by F. Saxoni, et al. CLIN PEDIAT. 6:687-691, December, 1967.

"Congenital syphilis has many faces," by R. McDonald. CLIN PEDIAT. 9:110-114, February, 1970.

"Congenital syphilis in an infant of a seronegative mother," by J. Hallock, et al. OBSTET GYNEC. 32: 336-338, September, 1968.

"Congenital syphilis in the Istituto Provinciale Assistenza all' Infanzia of Rome. (Comparison between the decade 1943-1952 and that of 1957-1966). Statistical, clinical, therapeutic and prophylactic considerations," by V. Menichella, et al. MINERVA NIPOL. 19:35-39, January-February, 1969.

"Congenital syphilis: observations on laboratory diagnosis of intrauterine infection," by B. D. Ackerman.

SYPHILIS: CONGENITAL

J PEDIAT. 74:459-462, March, 1969.

"Congenital syphilitic labryrinthitis," by A. G. Kerr, et al. ARCH OTOLARYNG. 91:474-478, May, 1970.

"Deafness and late congenital syphilis," by F. Baron, et al. REV LARYNG. 88:877-883, November-December, 1967.

"Deafness in congenital syphilis," by C. S. Karmody, et al. ARCH OTOLARYNG. 83:18-27, January, 1966.

"Early congenital syphilis," by C. Simao, et al. HOSPITAL. 75:1045-1057, March, 1969.

"Early congenital syphilis," by O. R. Turro, et al. ARCH ARGENT PEDIATR. 67:1-8, January-June, 1969.

"Early congenital syphilis and thrombocytopenia," by L. Juhlin. ACTA DERMATOVENER. 48:166-169, 1968.

"Early congenital syphilis in the newborn," by L. De Camillis, et al. QUAD CLIN OSTET GINEC. 21:1134-1152, December, 1966.

"Functional status of the liver in patients with congenital syphilis," by Kh L. Druian, et al. VRACH DELO. 1:145-146, January, 1966.

"Gamma-M-fluorescent treponemal antibody in the diagnosis of congenital syphilis," by C. A. Alford, Jr., et al. NEW ENG J MED. 280:1086-1091, May 15, 1969.

"Glossitis interstitialis luetica in the course of late congenital syphilis," by D. Niedzwiecka. PRZEGL DERM. 53:211-212, March-April, 1966.

"Hematuria in congenital lues," by J. Szabó, et al. SCHWEIZ MED WSCHR. 96:1446-1450, October 29, 1966.

"Herxheimer's reaction in maternal milk in early congenital syphilis," by R. Rollier, et al. BULL SOC FRANC DERM SYPH. 74:178-180, 1967.

"Higoumenakis' sign and its significance for the diagnosis of congenital syphilis," by K. G. Higoumenakis. DERM WSCHR. 154:697-705, July 27, 1968.

"Immunologic aspects of congenital syphilis," by F.

SYPHILIS: CONGENITAL

Aiuti, et al. HELV PAEDIAT ACTA. 21:66-71, April, 1966.

"In relation to the article by V. N. Ivanov: 'Remote results of preventive treatment of children born of mothers suffering from or having sustained syphilis' (Vestn Derm Vener No. 1, 1969)," by I. G. Bal'barer. VESTN DERM VENER. 43:63-64, November, 1969.

"Intraocular treponemes in treated congenital syphilis," by J. N. Goldman, et al. ARCH OPHTHAL. 78:47-50, July, 1967.

"Late congenital syphilis in the 2nd generation," by E. N. Oganesian. VESTN DERM VENER. 42:91-92, May, 1968.

"The lesions of congenital syphilis," by B. J. Cremin, et al. BRIT J RADIOL. 43:333-341, May, 1970.

"Multiple osteochondritis due to prenatal syphilis," by J. Mercadai-Peyri, et al. ACTAS DERMOSIF. 58: 101-104, March-April, 1967.

"Nephrotic syndrome associated with congenital syphilis," by P. Pollner. JAMA. 198:263-266, October 17, 1966.

"Occurrence of congenital syphilis in its dependence on the treatment of syphilitic mothers. I. Serologic evaluation of the prevention of congenital syphilis by means of the Nelson-Mayer test," by E. Malý, et al. CESK DERM. 44:108-117, May, 1969.

--II. Comparison of classical reagin seroreactions with the Nelsem-Mayer test in 612 children of syphilitic mothers," by E. Stammová, et al. CESK DERM. 45:164-170, August, 1970.

"On a case of congenital syphilis," by M. Passoni, et al. G MAL INFETT. 19:672-674, October, 1967.

"On a case of congenital syphilitic pemphigus," by G. Reynaud. MINERVA PEDIAT. 19:778-780, April 21, 1967.

"On the prevention of congenital syphilis," by C. Simon, et al. THER GEGENW. 105:1430-1435, November, 1966; also in MUNCHEN MED WSCHR. 107:1813-1815, September 17, 1965.

SYPHILIS: CONGENITAL

"On the recurrence of interstitial keratitis," by J. Sédan. BULL SOC OPHTHAL FRANC. 66:435-435, April, 1966.

"Oral disorders associated with ocular disease. II. Disorders affecting dentition," by B. Harcourt. BRIT J OPHTHAL. 51:284-285, April, 1967.

"The presence of spirochetes in late seronegative syphilis," by J. L. Smith, et al. JAMA. 199:126-130, March 27, 1967.

"Prophylaxis in congenital syphilis," by A. Chmielecki. WIAD LEK. 23:1487-1490, September 1, 1970.

"Reflections on 8 cases of early congenital syphilis recently observed," by M. Bethenod, et al. J MED LYON. 46:1743-1757, November 5, 1965.

"Remarks apropos of a case of early congenital syphilis," by P. Combe, et al. PEDIATRIC. 21:603-604, July-August, 1966.

"Role and functions in the prevention and control of congenital syphilis," by M. Oros, et al. MUNCA SANIT. 241-245, April, 1969.

"Somatopsychic aspect of hypopituitarism in a congenital syphilitic. Report of a case," by G. J. Taylor. NEW ZEAL MED J. 66:77-78, February, 1967.

"A special case of congenital lues," by P. M. Bakker. NEDERL T GENEESK. 110:1721-1722, September 24, 1966.

"Status of serological testing for congenital syphilis," by F. D. Hoffmann, et al. J PEDIAT. 71:686-690, November, 1967.

"Steroid treatment in congenital syphilitic deafness," by R. S. Dawkins, et al. J LARYNG. 82:1095-1107, December, 1968.

"Symmetrical synovitis of the knee in hereditary syphilis," by H. H. Clutton. CLIN ORTHOP. 57:5-8, March-April, 1968.

"Syphilis with macroglobulinemia," by R. Francois, et al. PEDIATRIE. 21:47-59, January-February, 1966.

SYPHILIS: CONGENITAL

"Thrombocytopenia and congenital syphilis in South African Bantu infants," by I. Freiman, et al. ARCH DIS CHILD. 41:87-90, February, 1966.

"Two darkfield-positive reinfections in treated congenital syphilis," by B. Schwimmer, et al. JAMA. 208:1705, June 2, 1969.

"An unusual case of congenital syphilis," by P. M. Bakker. DERMATOLOGICA. 133:430-432, 1966.

"An unusual picture of congenital syphilitic dysproteinemia: cryoglobulinemia. Report of a case," by A. G. Marchi, et al. MINERVA PEDIAT. 18:1155-1157, July 28, 1966.

SYPHILIS: CUTANEOUS

"Anatomoclinical case of secondary papulotuberculous syphilis," by P. Le Coulant, et al. BULL SOC FRANC DERM SYPH. 75:367-368, 1968.

"Chancriform gumma developing in 20 years at the site of former primary syphiloma," by B. S. Pankov. VESTN DERM VENER. 40:89-91, October, 1966.

"Current problems of syphilidology," by M. A. Rozentul, et al. VESTN DERM VENER. 41:3-7, April, 1967.

"Cutaneous gumma--a contemporary disease," by W. H. Eaglstein, et al. SOUTHERN MED J. 62:976-977, August, 1969.

"Cutaneous manifestations of recent luetic infection, their diagnosis and therapy," by V. Puccinelli. ATTI ACCAD MED LOMBARD. 22:Suppl:2779-2783, 1967.

"Electron microscopic observation of syphilid. I. The ultrastructure of treponema pallidum (Nicols strain)," by S. Abe. BULL PHARM RES INST. 60:1-6, January, 1966.

"Histopathology of serpiginous skin lesions in late syphilis (lues tubero-ulcero-serpiginosa)," by K. Lejman, et al. PRZEGL DERM. 53:419-423, July-August, 1966.

"Incidence of cutaneous manifestations of syphilis," by S. B. Mandal. INDIAN J DERM. 11:123-124, July, 1966.

SYPHILIS: CUTANEOUS

"Lues maligna. Presentation of a case and a review of the literature," by D. A. Fisher, et al. ARCH DERM. 90:70-73, January, 1969.

"Primo-secondary syphilis; digital chancre with unusual localization," by F. Labouche, et al. BULL SOC FRANC DERM SYPH. 74:154-155, 1967.

"Pseudo-gummatous scrotal pyodermitis associated with isolated pyodermitis of the right leg," by M. Bolgert, et al. BULL SOC FRANC DERM SYPH. 73:14-15, January-February, 1966.

"2 cases of tertiary cutaneous syphilis in a 63-year-old man and in a 22-year-old man," by M. Bolgert, et al. BULL SOC FRANC DERM SYPH. 76:794-796, 1969.

"An unusual solitary lesion of secondary syphilis," by W. Minkin, et al. ARCH DERM. 95:217, February, 1967.

"Zosteriform late cutaneous syphilide," by C. Kodandapani. BRIT MED J. 1:685, March 16, 1968.

SYPHILIS: DENTISTRY
SEE: ORAL

SYPHILIS: DIAGNOSIS

"Ancillary investigations in neurological diagnosis," by J. M. Sutherland, et al. MED J AUST. 2:452-546, September 16, 1967.

"Certain peculiarities of the clinical aspects and course of the initial period of syphilis at the present time," by V. A. Rakhmanov, et al. VESTN DERM VENER. 41:36-40, March, 1967.

"Clinical manifestations of visceral lues," by P. Kop. SRPSKI ARH CELOK LEK. 94:143-149, February, 1966.

"Colposcopic and cytological picture in 2 cases of primary luetic infection of uterine cervix," by J. Zadjelović. LIJECN VJESN. 90:433-437, May, 1968.

"Congenital syphilis," by M. Hart. ARCH DERM. 100:260, August, 1969.

"Considerations on a case of primary syphiloma of the cervix uteri in pregnancy, with special reference to the differential diagnosis from cervical carcinoma,"

SYPHILIS: DIAGNOSIS

by E. Rocco. MINERVA GINEC. 19:30-34, January 15, 1967.

"Cytological aspects of the adenogram in recent syphilis," by P. Morel, et al. LYON MED. 215:1363-1368, May 15, 1966.

"Darkfield examination and causes of the most frequent errors," by F. Vosmik. CESK DERM. 43:334-337, October, 1968.

"Demonstration of treponema pallidum in smear preparations (fluorescence serologic examination)," by H. J. Heitmann, et al. Z HAUT GESCHLECHTSKR. 44:529-532, August 1, 1969.

"Demonstration of treponeme-like forms in cases of treated and untreated late syphilis and of treated early syphilis," by N. S. Rice, et al. BRIT J VENER DIS. 46:1-9, February, 1970.

"Development of rheumatoid factor activity and cryoglobulins in primary and secondary syphilis," by A. Lassus. INT ARCH ALLERG. 36:515-522, 1969.

"Diagnosis and differential diagnosis of syphilitic diseases of the mouth mucosa," by K. W. Mach. OEST Z STOMAT. 65:350-357, September, 1968.

"Diagnosis, control of course, and therapy of syphilis," by R. Schroter. THER UMSCH. 26:70-75, February, 1969.

"The diagnosis of early syphilis," by S. Olansky. MED ANN DC. 35:367-368, July, 1966.

"Diagnosis of syphilis in the geriatric patient," by L. Nicholas, et al. GERIATRICS. 23:169-174, September, 1968.

"Diagnostic and therapeutic difficulties in late pulmonary syphilis in adults," by W. Kiesz, et al. WIAD LEK. 20:1181-1184, June 15, 1967.

"Differential diagnostic problem: impetiginized eczematic scabies--lues II--psoriasis vulgaris," by V. Misgeld. MED KLIN. 64:2189-2192, November 21, 1969.

"Difficulties in the diagnosis of syphilis," by L. M. Toporovskii, et al. TER ARKH. 41:76-79, August, 1969

SYPHILIS: DIAGNOSIS

"Early diagnosis and treatment of syphilis," by K. Higuchi. NAIKA. 23:1277-1284, June, 1969.

"Early diagnosis of neonatal syphilis. Evaluation of a gamma M-fluorescent treponemal antibody test," by P. Mamunes, et al. AMER J DIS CHILD. 120:17-21, July, 1970.

"Early primary syphilis--a fluorescent test to replace dark-ground examination of chancre exudate," by M. F. Garner. MED J AUST. 2:199-200, July 29, 1967.

"Errors in the diagnosis of syphilis in surgical practice," by L. M. Toporovskii, et al. SOVET MED. 29:132-135, May, 1966.

"Errors of dermatovenereologists in the diagnosis of syphilis," by N. A. Chaika, et al. VESTN DERM VENER. 42:86-89, January, 1968.

"Evaluation of a quantitative automated micro-hemagglutination assay for antibodies to treponema pallidum," by L. C. Logan, et al. AMER J CLIN PATH. 53:163-166, February, 1970.

"Experimental method of differentiation between various treponematoses: venereal syphilis, endemic syphilis and pain," by A. Paris-Hamelin, et al. BULL SOC FRANC DERM SYPH. 75:547-549, 1968.

"Experimental method for the differentiation of several treponemal infections: Venereal syphilis, endemic syphilis and yaws, by A. Paris-Hamelin, et al. BULL WHO. 38:808-809, 1968.

"Fever following penicillin treatment as a symptom of syphilis," by K. Nordin, et al. LAKARTIDNINGEN. 63:490-491, February 9, 1966.

"Flocculation Venereal Diseases Research Laboratory reaction for lues after vaccination against variola," by S. Smálik, et al. VNITRNI LEK. 12:152-155, February, 1966.

"Fluorescent examinations of pupils and pupillary reactions in the early stages of syphilis," by A. V. Braitsev, et al. VESTN DERM VENER. 42:47-51, June, 1968.

SYPHILIS: DIAGNOSIS

"A fluorescent technique for demonstrating treponemes in films made from suspected chacres," by M. F. Garner, et al. J CLIN PATH. 21:108-109, January, 1968.

"Gummata of tuberculous appearance in an 80-year-old syphilitic woman. Syphilo-tuberculous hybrid?," by E. Hadida, et al. BULL SOC FRAN DERM SYPH. 73:406-407, July-August, 1966.

"Higoumenakis's sign and its significance for the diagnosis of congenital syphilis," by K. G. Higoumenakis. DERM WSCHR. 154:697-705, July 27, 1968.

"Incidence of cutaneous manifestations of syphilis," by S. B. Mandal. INDIAN J DERM. 11:123-124, July, 1966.

"Infectivity tests in syphilis," by T. B. Turner, et al. BRIT J VENER DIS. 45:183-196, September, 1969.

"Laboratory diagnosis of syphilis," by L. Nicholas. INT J DERM. 9:64-68, January-March, 1970.

"Martorell-Fabre syndrome of syphilitic etiology," by A. Bohorquez, et al. ANGIOLOGIA. 20:255-260, September-October, 1968.

"Mouth mucosa findings in lues," by H. M. Hofmeier. HNO. 16:73-78, March, 1968.

"Ocular manifestations of polyarteritis nodosa," by M. R. Nanjiani. BRIT J OPHTHAL. 51:696-697, October, 1967.

"On the current picture of early syphilis," by H. Kresbach. Z HAUT GESCHLECHTSKR. 43:109-118, February 1, 1968.

"On the diagnosis of pulmonary syphilis," by F. Mersch. THORAXCHIRURGIE. 15:456-460, August, 1967.

"On a granuloma of the vulva by trichomonads. (Case history contribution to the differential diagnosis of primary syphilitic lesion)," by N. Sonnichsen, et al. Z HAUT GESCHLECHTSKR. 41:202-204, September 1, 1966.

"On the usefulness of a new agglutination test (S.p.A.) in the diagnosis of syphilis," by L. Caldera, et al.

SYPHILIS: DIAGNOSIS

FRACASTORO. 61:293-297, May-June, 1968.

"Present clinical and serological aspects of syphilis," by G. B. Cottini, et al. HAUTARZT. 17:74-79, February, 1966.

"Pseudo-neoplastic aspects of syphilis of the cervix," by D. Rossi, et al. RIV ITAL GINEC. 51:480-491, June-July, 1967.

"Quantitative automated reagin test for syphilis," by B. E. McGrew, et al. AMER J MED TECHN. 36:1-7, January, 1970.

"Recovery of spirochaetes in the monkey by passive transfer from human late sero-negative syphilis," by J. L. Smith, et al. BRIT J VENER DIS. 42:109-115, June, 1968.

"'Red eye' as the presenting sign of syphilis d'emblée," by K. D. Wuepper. CALIF MED. 107:518-520, December, 1967.

"Relationship between skin allergy tests and Boyden's test in syphilis," by N. I. Tumasheva, et al. VRACH DELO. 3:152, March, 1967.

"Results of serologic studies in endogenous ocular inflammations," by W. Paul, et al. KLIN MBL AUGENHEILK. 151:332-344, 1967.

"Secondary syphilis misdiagnosed as infectious mononucleosis," by M. A. Conant, et al. CALIF MED. 109: 462-464, December, 1968.

"Secondary syphilis misdiagnosed as lymphoma," by D. R. Goffinet, et al. NORTHWEST MED. 69:Suppl:22-23, May, 1970; also in ARIZONA MED. 27:22-23, May, 1970.

"Secondary syphilis with unusual clinical and laboratory findings," by L. Biro, et al. ARCH DERM. 99:240-243, February, 1969; also in JAMA. 206:889-891, October 21, 1968.

"A shortened and simplified treponema test in diagnostic practice," by J. Weberschinke, et al. J HYG EPIDEM. 10:483-487, 1966.

"Silent limb contracture as a diagnostic indicator of

tertiary syphilis," by K. Dawson-Butterworth. BRIT J CLIN PRACT. 22:471-473, November 11, 1968.

"Skull changes in early syphilis. A contribution to the differential diagnosis of localized clearings in the x-ray film of the skull," by E. Nagele, et al. RADIOLOGE. 6:242-245, June, 1966.

"Skull lacunae during secondary syphilis," by C. Bénichou, et al. REV RHUM. 37:330-333, April, 1970.

"Swelling of the inguinal lymph nodes in syphilis of the anus," by A. H. Schmid. MED KLIN. 61:914-915, June 10, 1966.

"Syphilis and biologic false positive reactors among leprosy patients," by A. T. Scotti, et al. ARCH DERM. 101:328-330, March, 1970.

"Syphilis as a differential diagnosis of neck masses," by C. T. Yarington, Jr., et al. ARCH OTOLARYNG. 86:219-221, August, 1967.

"Syphilis as an unusual cause of aches and pains," by A. Beardwell, et al. PROC ROY SOC MED. 62:197, February, 1969.

"Syphilis casefinding through the laboratory reporting system," by G. Pickett. MICH MED. 66:1416-1418, November, 1967.

"Syphilis: a difficult diagnosis?," by J. Smoler, et al. LARYNGOSCOPE. 78:404-410, March, 1968.

"Syphilis screening using the multi-channel blood-grouping machine," by J. W. Lockyer. BRIT J VENER DIS. 46:290-294, August, 1970.

"A 20 years persisting tubero serpiginous syphilis treated as psoriasis," by W. G. Roth. DERM WSCHR. 154:459-463, May 18, 1968.

"The unlabeled antibody enzyme method of immuno-histochemistry: Preparation and properties of soluble antigen-antibody complex (horseradish peroxidase-antihorseradish peroxidase) and its use in identification of spirochetes," by L. A. Sternberger, et al. J HISTOCHEM CYTOCHEM. 18:315-333, May, 1970.

SYPHILIS: DIAGNOSIS

"The usefulness of the isotope labelled lymphocyte-stimulation test in the diagnosis of syphilis," by N. Simon, et al. ARCH DLIN EXP DERM. 236:1-7, 1969.

"Various stages of syphilis and its diagnosis," by T. Tomizawa. JAP J NURS ART. 8:97-104, August, 1969.

"Vascular erythematous reaction by administration of vitamin PP (nicotinic acid). Demonstration of a pre- and post-clinical luetic roseola," by E. Ionescu. DERM WSCHR. 152:184-187, February 19, 1966.

SYPHILIS: DIAGNOSIS: CEREBROSPINAL FLUID
"The composition of the cerebrospinal fluid in the neuro-syphilitic psychoses," by K. Dewhurst. ACTA NEUROL SCAND. 45:119-123, 1969.

"On the demonstration of immobilizing antibodies against treponema pallidum in the cerebrospinal fluid in syphilis," by F. Muller. DEUTSCH MED WSCHR. 91:2292-2297, December 23, 1966.

"Quantitative determination of immunoglobulins in cerebrospinal fluid," by S. Takase, et al. TOHOKU J EXP MED. 98:189-198, June, 1969.

"Spinal puncture and cerebrospinal fluid diagnosis," by A. Bischoff. SCHWEIZ MED WSCHR. 99:1381-1388, September 27, 1969.

"Study of late ocular syphilis. Demonstration of treponemes in aqueous humour and cerebrospinal fluid. I. Methods of demonstration of treponemes," by A. E. Wilkinson. TRANS OPHTHAL UK. 88:251-256, 1969.

--3. General and serological findings," by E. M. Dunlop, et al. TRANS OPHTHAL SOC UK. 88:275-294, 1969.

"The treponema pallidum immobilization test of cerebrospinal fluid in syphilis patients treated with various delayed-action penicillin preparations," by T. V. Vasil'ev, et al. VESTN DERM VENER. 41:40-45, March, 1967.

SYPHILIS: EXPERIMENTAL
  SEE ALSO: TREATMENT
          SYPHILIS: IMMUNOLOGY
          FOR RESEARCH RESULTS, ETC: SEE: HISTORY

SYPHILIS: EXPERIMENTAL

"Accidental human infection in the laboratory with Nichols rabbit-adapted virulent strain of treponema pallidum," by C. W. Chacko. BULL WHO. 35:809-810, 1966.

"Anabolic hormones and gamma globulins in the course of experimental syphilis," by I. Orhel. RAD MED FAK ZAGREB. 15:203-211, 1967.

"Artificial immunization of rabbits against syphilis. I. Effect of increasing doses of treponemes given by the intramuscular route," by M. Metzger, et al. BRIT J VENER DIS. 45:308-312, December, 1969.

"Attempts for speeding up the development of experimentally maintained specific orchitis in rabbits, contaminated with 'Nichols' strain," by D. Naumova. NAUCH TR VISSH MED INST SOFIIA. 48:45-53, 1969.

"Cephaloridine treatment of experimental rabbit syphilis," by S. Kuwahara, et al. POSTGRAD MED J. 43: Suppl:43:130-133, August, 1967.

"Contribution to the study of strains of pathogenic treponema pallidum isolated in Rumania. II. Transmission of experimental syphilitic infection by intracorneal inoculation, in the rabbit, followed by symptoms of generalization," by D. I. Volosceanu, et al. ARCH ROUM PATH EXP MICROBIOL. 23:459-466, June, 1964.

"Effect of cephalothin and cephaloridine against rabbit syphilis," by T. Ikeda, et al. ACTA DERM. 61: 310-313, November, 1966.

"Effect of a nitro-imidazole on primary experimental syphilis in rabbits," by A. R. Yobs, et al. BRIT J VENER DIS. 42:122-124, June, 1966.

"The effect of x-irradiation on the development of orchitis in rabbits and on the quality of antigen for the treponema pallidum immobilization test," by L. D. Butovetskii. ZH MIKROBIOL. 43:131-134, March, 1966.

"Effects of griseofulvin in experimental rabbit syphilis," by T. Hasegawa. BRIT J VENER DIS. 42:178-180, September, 1966.

"Experimental ocular and neurosyphilis in the primate,"

SYPHILIS: EXPERIMENTAL

by J. A. Wells, et al. BRIT J VENER DIS. 43:10-17, March, 1967.

"Experimental studies in vivo on the effect upon treponema pallidum of some antibiotics other than penicillin," by A. Jakubowski, et al. PRZEGL DERM. 55: 1-6, January-February, 1968.

"Experimental studies on the masking effect of antibiotics on the course of treponemal infections," by R. Mielech, et al. PRZEGL DERM. Suppl:63-67, 1969.

"Experimental studies on the treatment of syphilis with various antibiotics," by A. Jakubowski, et al. PRZEGL DERM. Suppl:57-61, 1969.

"Experimental syphilis in the chimpanzee. Immunoglobulin class of early antibodies reactive with treponema pallidum," by W. J. Brown, et al. BRIT J VENER DIS. 46:198-200, June, 1970.

"Experimental under-treatment of early syphilis with probenecid and penicillin in anti-gonorrhoea dosages. A study to assess the best follow-up examination time for syphilis after gonorrhoea treatment in Greenland," by L. Hallinger. ACTA DERMATOVENER. 48:260-267, 1968.

"Experiments in accelerating the development of experimentally maintained specific orchitis in rabbits infected with the Nichols strain of treponema pallidum," by D. Naumova. VESTN DERM VENER. 43:40-44, May, 1969.

"Immunity in experimental syphilis. V. The immunogenicity of treponema pallidum attenuated by gamma-irradiation," by J. N. Miller. J IMMUN. 99:1012-1016, November, 1967.

"The immunologic response of goats to normal and syphilitic rabbit testicular tissue," by J. N. Miller, et al. J IMMUN. 97:184-188, August, 1966.

"Importance of the anti-complement immunofluorescence technic in serodiagnosis of experimental treponomatoses in various animal species," by A. Vaisman, et al. BULL SOC FRANC DERM SYPH. 74:803-806, 1967.

"Late ocular syphilis: transfer of infection from man

to experimental animals," by J. L. Smith. TRANS AMER OPHTHAL SOC. 67:658-697, 1969.

"Late syphilis in experiment and clinic," by P. Collart, et al. MUNCHEN MED WSCHR. 109:1555-1564, July 21, 1967.

"Lysozyme activity of serum in the course of experimental syphilis in rabbits. 1. Changing dynamics of lysozyme activity," by L. Pospi'sil, et al. Z IMMUNITAETSFORSCH. 131:444-448, December, 1966.

--2. Quantitative changes of lysozyme," by A. Jakubowski, et al. Z IMMUNITAETSFORSCH. 131:449-452, December, 1966.

"Multiple sensitization in experimental syphilis in rabbits. (An investigation on the mechanism of gumma formation)," by T. Yano. JAP J BACT. 24:345-353, 1969.

"Muramidase from tissue fluid of syphilitic rabbit testes. I. Purification and properties of the enzyme," by W. Kopeč. ARCH IMMUN THER EXP. 15:161-175, 1967.

--II. Comparative study of the enzyme and hen egg white muramidase," by W. Kopeč, et al. ARCH IMMUN THER EXP. 16:533-545, 1968.

"On the antigenic properties of a protein-polysaccharide complex of cultured treponema pallidum studies in experiments on rabbits. I.," by S. A. Ugrimov. LAB DELO. 3:173-175, 1968.

"Present state of experimental studies on the effect of antibiotics other than penicillin on treponema pallidum in vitro," by A. Jakubowski. PRZEGL DERM. Suppl:7-12, 1969.

"Recent studies on late experimental and human syphilis," by P. Collart, et al. MINERVA MED. 57:4478-4486, December 26, 1966.

"Recent studies on latent syphilis, experimental and human," by P. Collart, et al. REV CLIN ESP. 103:456-465, December 31, 1966.

"Results of inoculation of rabbits from biopsies of primo-secondary syphilitic lesions taken from untreated patients," by P. Collart, et al. ANN DERM SYPH. 95:285-292, 1968.

"Results of investigation of the nature of syphilitic reagins by means of thin layer Ion exchange and paper chromatography," by L. S. Reznikova, et al. VESTN DERM VENER. 41:46-51, May, 1967.

"Runting syndrome in neonatal rabbits infected with treponema pallidum," by H. Festenstein, et al. CLIN EXP IMMUN. 2:311-320, May, 1967.

"Serologic study after inoculation of treponema pallidum in normal mice and mice thymectomized at birth," by J. Thivolet, et al. EXPERIENTIA. 25:304-305, March 15, 1969.

"Serological fluorescence studies on syphilitic veinous changes in animals," by H. J Heitmann. DERMATOLOGICA. 137:129-132, 1968.

"Serological tests for syphilis in healthy rabbits," by J. W. Clark, Jr. BRIT J VENER DIS. 46:191-197, June, 1970.

"Studies on durable long term preservation of stained preparations of treponema pallidum. Experiment I. Detection of treponema pallidum in testes of syphilitic rabbits by fluorescent antibody reaction," by H. Furukawa. BULL PHARM RES INST. 61:1-12, March, 1966.

"Studies on immunity in experimental syphilis. 2. Transfer of antibodies to the fetus in rabbits," by T. Tomizawa, et al. JAP J BACT. 21:222-225, April, 1966.

"Transformation of antibody from IgM to IgG in experimental syphilitic rabbits. I. Syphilitic serum reaction," by M. Ogata, et al. ACTA MED OKAYAMA. 24:93-99, February, 1970.

"Ultrafine structure of te cell elements in hard chancres of the rabbit and their interrelationship with treponema pallidum," by N. M Ovcinnikov, et al. BULL WHO. 42:437-444, 1970.

"VDRL test in normal albino and pigmented rabbits," by B. M. Levine, et al. BRIT J VENER DIS. 45:197-199,

SYPHILIS: EXPERIMENTAL

September, 1969.

SYPHILIS: GASTROINTESTINAL

"Acute embolic-toxic induced incident in treatment of stomach syphilis with penicillin," by W. Lindheimer. THER GEGENW. 106:755-759, June, 1967.

"A case of undetected syphilis of the stomach," by L. A. Shifrin. KLIN KHIR. 8:61-63, August, 1966.

"Gastric syphilis: a case with pernicious anemia," by H. D. Frank, et al. CONN MED. 31:773-778, November, 1967.

"Syphilitic disease of the stomach," by W. Lindheimer. MUNCHEN MED WSCHR. 109:638-643, March 24, 1967.

SYPHILIS: GERIATRICS

"Diagnosis of syphilis in the geriatric patient," by L. Nicholas, et al. GERIATRICS. 23:169-174, September, 1968.

"Gummata of tuberculous appearance in an 80-year-old syphilitic woman. Syphilo-tuberculous hybrid?," by E. Hadida, et al. BULL SOC FRANC DERM SYPH. 73: 406-407, July-August, 1966.

"Proper interpretation of serologic tests for syphilis in the aged," by L. Nicholas. J AMER GERIAT SOC. 15:224-229, March, 1967.

"Serological tests for syphilis in the elderly," by E. A. Johansson, et al. ANN CLIN RES. 2:47-50, March, 1970.

"Silent limb contracture in syphilitic geriatric patients," by K. Dawson-Butterworth. PRACTITIONER. 199:68-70, July, 1967.

SYPHILIS: HISTORY

"Another look at the Morbus Gallicus," by R. S. Morton. BRIT J VENER DIS. 42:174-177, June, 1968.

"Cellini and his syphilis. Malevolent mercurial cure?," by G. W. Geelhoed. JAMA. 204:Suppl:245-246, May 13, 1968.

"Christopher Columbus and the history of syphilis," by E. H. Hudson. ACTA TROP. 25:1-16, 1968.

SYPHILIS: HISTORY

"Jean Astruc (March 19, 1684 to May 5, 1766) and his work 'De morbis venereis' on the 200th anniversary of his death," by L. Mendel. DERM WSCHR. 153:105-111, February 4, 1967.

"Early history of syphilis: a reappraisal. A," by W. Crosby, Jr. AM ANTHROP. 71:218-227, April, 1969.

"50 years of research work in the therapy of skin diseases and syphilis at the Faculty of Dermatology and Venereology of the I. M. Sechenov Moscow Medical Institute," by V. A. Rachmanov. CESK DERM. 42:361-367, December, 1967.

"The illness of Poliziano," by L. Szodoray. ORV HETIL. 109:771, April 7, 1968.

"In memory of Professor Paruir Gavrilovich Oganesian," by P. G. Oganesian. VESTN DERM VENER. 41:93, June, 1967.

"Incidence and pathomorphosis of congenital syphilis in the last 20 years," by D. Mazzacuva, et al. CLIN PEDIAT. 49:3-16, January, 1967.

"A new conception of the origin of syphilis in Europe," by A. Boneff. ANN DERM SYPH. 95:529-530, 1968.

"On the history of the development of serological help in the prevention of syphilis in Uzbekistan," by T. U. Usmanov. LAB DELO. 10:633-634, 1968.

"Outline of the history of syphilis," by K. Lejman. ARCH HIST MED. 32:125-145, 1969.

"Primary, secondary and congenital syphilis from 1938 to 1965 on the basis of statistics of the dermosyphilopathic clinic of Genoa and the 'Giannini Gaslini' Pediatric Hospital of Genoa," by E. Rampini, et al. MINERVA DERM. 41:442-444, December, 1966.

"Study of the increase of primary-secondary and early congenital syphilis from 1938 to 1965 based on the statistics of the Clinical Dermosifilopatica of the University of Genoa and of the Ospedale Pediatrico 'Giannini Gaslini' of Genoa," by E. Rampini, et al. MINERVA DERM. 41:442-444, December, 1966.

"Syphilis: current disease," by J. Grandbois. UN MED CANADA. 95:728-733, June, 1966.

SYPHILIS: HISTORY

"Syphilis maligna praecox. Syphilis of the great epidemic? An historical review," by D. J. Cripps, et al. ARCH INTERN MED. 119:411-418, April, 1967.

"The syphilis of Ulrich von Hutten. Sensational studies of a group of experts of the medical school of the University of Zurich," by H. Jung. HAUTARZT. 20:334-336, July, 1969.

"Syphilis past and present." LANCET. 2:503-504, September 2, 1967.

"Syphilis: was it endemic in pre-Columbian America or was it brought here from Europe?," by A. I. Weisman. BULL NY ACAD MED. 42:284-300, April, 1966.

"Syphilis yesterday and today," by M. G. Achten. J MED LYON. 49:685-702, April 20, 1968.

"Therapy of early syphilis during the last 21 years at the dermatologic clinic of Wiesbaden," by F. Nemec. Z HAUT GESCHLECHTSKR. 45:561-575, August 1, 1970.

"Treponematosis and man's social evolution," by E. H. Hudson. AM ANTHROP. 67:885-901, August, 1965.

--Reply," by J. B. Ford. AM ANTHROP. 68:1507-1508, December, 1966.

SYPHILIS: HOMOSEXUALITY

"Early syphilis and homosexuality in the Berlin district from 1961 till 1966," by G. Elste, et al. DEUTSCH GESUNDH. 23:1510-1513, August 8, 1968.

"Homosexuality among syphilitic patients," by I. Racz. BRIT J VENER DIS. 46:117, April, 1970.

"Importance of homosexuals and bisexuals in the epidemiology of syphilis," by W. B. Neser, et al. SOUTHERN MED J. 62:177-180, February, 1969.

"Reinfection with early syphilis in homosexuals," by G. Elste, et al. DERM WSCHR. 154:985-994, October 19, 1968.

"Syphilis and homosexuality," by I. Kirjakov, et al. CESK DERM. 41:25-27, February, 1966.

SYPHILIS: IMMUNOLOGY

SYPHILIS: IMMUNOLOGY
SEE ALSO: SYPHILIS: EXPERIMENTAL
SYPHILIS: SERODIAGNOSIS

"Autoimmune phenomena in syphilitic infection: rheumatoid factor and cryoglobulins in different stages of syphilis," by K. K. Mustakallio, et al. INT ARCH ALLERG. 31:417-426, 1967.

"Detection of antibodies against myocardial constituents by means of the complement fixation test," by A. Ieri, et al. FOLIA ALLERG. 14:579-585, November-December, 1967.

"Fetal production of immunoglobulins in the course of congenital infections," by G. B. Serra, et al. MINERVA PEDIAT. 19:591-592, March 31, 1967.

"Findings on changes in the complement activity of serums in dermatologic and syphilitic patients," by G. Cozza, et al. FOLIA ALLERG. 13:30-34, January-February, 1966.

"Fluorescence-serologic demonstration of an antibody against a heat-stable antigen of Reiter treponema present in the sera of subjects with syphilis," by W. Bredt, et al. ARCH KLIN EXP DERM. 229:117-125, 1967.

"Fluorescence serologic differentiation of various antibodies directed against treponema pallidum," by F. Muller. KLIN WSCHR. 46:209-210, February 15, 1968.

"Gamma globulin and the treponema immobilization test," by A. K. Shcherbakova, et al. VESTN DERM VENER. 40: 66-69, July, 1966.

"Immobilization of certain cultured treponemes in sera from syphilitic humans," by W. J. Guest, et al. J BACT. 93:1190-1191, March, 1967.

"Immobilizing antibodies to treponema pallidum in the cerebrospinal fluid in syphilis," by F. Muller. GERMAN MED MONTHLY. 12:120-124, March, 1967.

"Immunity in experimental syphilis. V. The immunogenicity of treponema pallidum attenuated by gamma-irradiation," by J. N. Miller. J IMMUN. 99:1012-

SYPHILIS: IMMUNOLOGY

1016, November, 1967.

"Immunobiological reactivity of chicks to treponema anserinum Sakharoff 1891," by I. Djankov, et al. ZBL VETERINAERMED. 14:677-681, November, 1967.

"Immunoelectrophoresis and simple radial immuno-diffusion tests of saliva of subjects with syphilis in the primary and secondary phases," by M. Pippione, et al. MINERVA DERM. 43:543, October, 1968.

"Immunoelectrophoretic pattern of Wassermann reagin and comparison of the appearance time between RPCF and FTA antibodies," by K. Kakusui. JAP J BACT. 24:28-36, January, 1969.

"Immunofluorescence in biological diagnosis. Its application to the serology of syphilis after absorption of nonspecific antibodies by ultrasonicated Reiter treponema," by A. Fribourg-Blanc, et al. BIOL MED. 55:235-252, May-June, 1966.

"Immunoglobulin class and light chain type of human antibodies. Studies with anti-gammaG, -gammaM, -gammaA-globulin, -beta 1CA, E-globulins and anti-kappa, -lambda chains reagents," by T. Matuhasi, et al. JAP J EXP MED. 36:407-421, August, 1966.

"Immunoglobulins in congenital syphilis: analysis with fluorescein-labeled antigammaglobulin fractions," by M. Lospalluti, et al. G ITAL DERM. 45:184-185, March, 1970.

"Immunoglobulins in syphilis," by J. J. Delhanty, et al. LANCET. 2:1099-1103, November 22, 1969.

"Immunologic aspects of congenital syphilis," by F. Aluti, et al. HELV PAEDIAT ACTA. 21:66-71, April, 1966.

"Immunologic response of the fetus in congenital syphilis," by B. J. Fogel, et al. J FLORIDA MED ASS. 56:777-779, October, 1969.

"The immunologic response of goats to normal and syphilitic rabbit testicular tissue," by J. N. Miller, et al. J IMMUN. 97:184-188, August, 1966.

"Immunologic responses and 'altered reactivity' in syphilis," by D. H. Short, et al. ANN ALLERG. 24:430-436, August, 1966.

"Immunological study on cardiolipin from Escherichia coli," by Y. Kanemasa. ACTA MED OKAYAMA. 22:241-249, October, 1968.

"Immunology of syphilis," by G. R. Cannefax, et al. ANN REV MED. 18:471-482, 1967.

"The importance of the fluorescent antibody technic (FAT) as a control of questionable Wassermann reactions in pregnancy," by I. Placentini. FRACASTORO. 59:615-618, September-October, 1966.

"Induction of anti-treponema pallidum antibodies in normal rabbits by RNA-immuno-carrier extraxcted from serum of syphilitic rabbits," by L. Michelazzi, et al. EXPERIENTIA. 23:207-208, March 15, 1967.

"The influencing of syphilitic orchitis by different animal material," by G. Naumann, et al. Z MED MIKROBIOL IMMUN. 153:169-174, 1967.

"Late syphilis in experiment and clinic," by P. Collart, et al. MUNCHEN MED WSCHR. 109:1555-1564, July 21, 1967.

"Localization of treponema pallidum immobilizing antibody in human immunoglobulins," by G. Tringali, et al. RIV IST SIEROTER ITAL. 43:161-168, July-August, 1968.

"Lymphocyte stimulation in vitro in syphilitic subjects," by G. C. Chieregato, et al. MINERVA DERM. 42:406-407, August, 1967.

"On certain properties and behavior of the so-called syphilitic reagins (the problem of seroresistance)," by M. Miklaszewska, et al. POL TYG LEK. 22:1867, November 27, 1967.

"Persistence of particular forms of treponema pallidum in syphilitic patients detected in the late stages of their infection and not treated in time," by S. G. Nicolau, et al. ANN DERM SYPH. 96:253-264, 1969.

"Persistence of treponemes and the infectivity test in syphilis." LANCET. 1:130-131, January 17, 1970.

SYPHILIS: IMMUNOLOGY

"Practical possibilities of the use of immunological phenomena in syphilis," by J. Towpik. POL TYG LEK. 22:360-363, March 6, 1967.

"Reduced lymphocyte transformation due to a plasma factor in patients with active syphilis," by G. M. Levene, et al. LANCET. 2:246-247, August 2, 1969.

"Relationship between in vitro treponema immobilizing action of antibiotics and rabbit immunity against treponema," by T. Ikeda, et al. ACTA DERM. 62:9-13, February, 1967.

"Rheumatoid factor in syphilitics," by Z. Hrncir, et al. CESK DERM. 43:190-198, June, 1968.

"Role of acquired immunity to T. pallidum in the control of syphilis," by J. F. Jekel. PUBLIC HEALTH REP. 83:627-632, August, 1968.

"The role of the bursa of fabricius in immunity against spirochetosis in fowls," by I. Soumrov, et al. ZBL VETERINAERMED. 14:672-676, November, 1967.

"Serum immunoelectrophoretic pattern in primary and secondary syphilis," by M. Pippione, et al. G ITAL DERM. 45:193-194, March, 1970.

"Serum immunoglobulin levels in syphilis," by A. B. Laurel, et al. ACTA DERMATOVENER. 48:268-271, 1968.

"Some current problems of syphilis immunology," by L. Pospisil. CESK DERM. 44:95-101, May, 1969.

"Studies of syphilitic antibodies. I. Anti-lipoidal antibodies in various stages of syphilis," by K. Aho. BRIT J VENER DIS. 43:259-263, December, 1967.

--II. Substances responsible for biological false positive sero-reactions." BRIT J VENER DIS. 44:49-54, March, 1968.

--III. Anamnestic reactions and 19S predominance of the anti-lipoidal antibodies in aged persons." BRIT J VENER.DIS. 44:283-286, December, 1968.

--IV. Evidence of reactant partner common for C-reactive protein and certain anti-lipoidal antibodies." BRIT J VENER DIS. 45:13-18, March, 1969.

SYPHILIS: IMMUNOLOGY

"Studies on reagin formation in rabbits immunized with pallidum and Reiter treponeme," by G. Tringali, et al. RIV IST SIEROTER ITAL. 43:144-149, May-June, 1968.

"Treponemal-like organisms in the aqueous of nonsyphilitic patients. An immunologic study," by B. Golden, et al. ARCH OPHTHAL. 80:727-731, December, 1968.

SYPHILIS: INFANTS

"Concerning congenital syphilis in infants," by J. P. Soares. BOL INST PUERICULT. 22:123-134, August-December, 1965.

"Morbidity and clinical symptoms of congenital syphilis in infancy," by K. Wechselberg, et al. DEUTSCH MED WSCHR. 95:1976-1981, September 25, 1970.

"The problem of Jarisch-Herxheimer-Lukasiewicz reaction in congenital syphilis in infants," by K. Lejman, et al. POL MED J. 6:1069-1073, 1967.

"Recent cases of congenital syphilis in infants," by M. Hori, et al. JAP J NURS ART. 8:60-69, August, 1969.

"3 cases of congenital syphilis in infants," by E. Majima. SAISHIN IGAKU. 22:1260-1265, June, 1967.

SYPHILIS: JAUNDICE

"Autopsy case of congenital syphilis with jaundice," by Y. Ishiwata, et al. JAP J CLIN MED. 24:784-790, April, 1966.

SYPHILIS: KIDNEY

"Nephrotic syndrome and acute hepatitis in secondary syphilis," by J. D. McCracken, et al. MILIT MED. 134:682-686, September, 1969.

"Nephrotic syndrome associated with congenital syphilis," by P. Pollner. JAMA. 198:263-266, October 17, 1966.

"The nephrotic syndrome associated with secondary syphilis. An immune deposit disease," by G. D. Braunstein, et al. AMER J MED. 48:643-648, May, 1970.

"Nephrotic syndrome in secondary syphilis," by D. F. de Andrade, et al. REV ASS MED BRASIL. 13:97-98, March, 1967.

SYPHILIS: KIDNEY

"Syphilitic lesions of the kidney," by K. S. Reddy. INDIAN J MED SCI. 20:424-426, June, 1968.

"Unusual case of nephrotic syndrome," by K. Fujita, et al. JAP J CLIN MED. 26:1220-1224, May, 1968.

SYPHILIS: LIVER

"The association of syphilis with hepatic cirrhosis: a report of six cases and a review of the literature," by G. Karmi, et al. POSTGRAD MED J. 45:675-679, October, 1969.

"Case of hepatic syphilis," by Y. Salembier. LILLE MED. 12:1215-1216, November, 1967.

"A case of renal lesion in secondary recurrent syphilis," by B. Batko, et al. WIAD LEK. 23:1043-1045, June 15, 1970.

"Early syphilitic hepatitis," by H. E. Zellmann, et al. LAHEY CLIN FOUND BULL. 16:255-259, 1967.

"Functional status of the liver in patients with congenital syphilis," by Kh L. Drulan, et al. VRACH DELO. 1:145-146, January, 1966.

"Nephrotic syndrome and acute hepatitis in secondary syphilis," by J. D. McCracken, et al. MILIT MED. 134:682-686, September, 1969.

"Syphilis and hepatic cirrhosis." LANCET. 1:28-29, January 3, 1970.

"Syphilis and hepatic cirrhosis," by I. A. Kellock, et al. LANCET. 1:369, February 14, 1970.

"Treatment of infectious granulomas of the liver and infectious mononucleosis. Treatment of hepatic schistosomiasis, tuberculosis, syphilis and echinococcus cyst," by M. A. Spellberg. AMER J GASTROENT. 52: 203-212, September, 1969.

"Two observations of gummatous disease of the liver, diagnosed during surgery," by M. P. Serdiuk. KHIRURGHA. 41:126-128, December, 1965.

SYPHILIS: LUNG
SEE: PULMONARY

SYPHILIS: LYMPH

SYPHILIS: LYMPH
"Luetic lymphadenitis: a clinical and histologic study of 20 cases," by R. J. Hartsock, et al. AMER J CLIN PATH. 53:304-314, March, 1970.

"The lymph node biopsy in infectious diseases," by D. J. Winslow, et al. MARYLAND MED J. 15:55-58, February, 1966.

"Lymph-node, cutaneous and splenic tertiary syphilis with the aspects of sarcoidosis," by R. Cazzola. FRIULI MED. 21:1129-1141, November-December, 1966.

SYPHILIS: MENINGITIS
"Chronic syphilitic multiple subdural meningitis," by G. Lemercier, et al. BULL SOC MED AFR NOIRE LANG FRANC. 11:62-65, 1966.

SYPHILIS: METABOLISM
"Iron metabolism in early symptomatic syphilis," by Z. Olszewska. POL MED J. 5:686, 1966; also in PRZEGL DERM. 53:15-20, January-February, 1966.

SYPHILIS: MICROBIOLOGY
"Electron microscopic observation of syphilid. I. The ultrastructure of treponema pallidum (Nicols strain)," by S. Abe. BULL PHARM RES INST. 60:1-6, January, 1966.

--II. The ultrastructure of rabbit syphilitic orchitis." BULL PHARM RES INST. 68:1-8, May, 1967.

--III. The ultrastructure of syphilitic chancre in man." BULL PHARM RES INST. 79:6-22, March, 1969.

"Electron microscopic observations on the lesions of condyloma latum," by T. Hasegawa. BRIT J DERM. 81:367-374, May, 1969.

"Electron microscopic studies on secondary retinitis pigmentosa," by S. Nishida, et al. ACTA SOC OPHTHAL JAP. 71:1410-1417, September, 1967.

"An electron microscopic study of a syphilitic chancre. Engulfment of treponema pallidum by plasma cells," by H. A. Azar, et al. ARCH PATH. 90:143-150, August, 1970.

"Electron microscopic study of treponema pallidum in

SYPHILIS: MICROBIOLOGY

rabbit chancre tissue," by N. M. Ovchinnikov, et al. VESTN DERM VENER. 43:14-19, March, 1969.

"Electron microscopic study of treponema pallidum isolated from human syphilids," by V. V. Delektorskii. VESTN DERM VENER. 40:63-66, July, 1966.

"Electron microscopy of treponema pallidum occurring in a human primary lesion," by L. M. Drusin, et al. J BACT. 97:951-955, February, 1969.

"A fluorescent technique for demonstrating treponemes in films made from suspected chancres," by M. F. Garner, et al. J CLIN PATH. 21:108-109, January, 1968.

"Further studies of the morphology of treponema pallidum under the electron microscope," by N. M. Ovcinnikov, et al. BRIT J VENER DIS. 45:87-116, June, 1969.

"Further study of ulrathin sections of treponema pallidum under the electron microscope," by N. M. Ovcinnikov, et al. BRIT J VENER DIS. 44:1-34, March, 1968.

"The observed incompatibility of viruses, bacteria and treponema pallidum in the syphilitic patient. Verified by a new in vitro technique for propagating the human pathogen, treponema pallidum," by G. Di Virgillio. GYNAECOLOGIA. 165:338-348, 1968.

"Temporal bone treponemes," by L. W. Mack, Jr., et al. ARCH OTOLARYNG. 90:11-14, July, 1969.

SYPHILIS: NASOPHARYNGEAL

"Nasopharyngeal syphilis with blindness," by W. E. Gager, et al. ARCH OTOLARYNG. 90:641-646, November, 1969.

"Syphilis of nose and paranasal sinus," by H. Y. Lee. OHIO MED J. 64:1264-1267, November, 1968.

SYPHILIS: NEONATAL
  SEE ALSO: OPHTHALMIA NEONATORUM UNDER SYPHILIS: OPHTHALMOLOGY

"Early congenital syphilis in the newborn. (Clinicoradiological study)," by L. De Camillis, et al. QUAD CLIN OSTET GINEC. 21:1134-1152, December, 1966.

SYPHILIS: NEONATAL

"Early diagnosis of neonatal syphilis. Evaluation of a gamma M-fluorescent treponemal antibody test," by P. Mamunes, et al. AMER J DIS CHILD. 120:17-21, July, 1970.

"Failure of penicillin in a newborn with congenital syphilis," by J. B. Hardy, et al. JAMA. 212:1345-1349, May 25, 1970.

"Fluorescent antibody test for neonatal congenital syphilis: a progress report," by A. Scotti, et al. J PEDIAT. 75:1129-1134, December, 1969.

"Investigation of neonatal conjunctivitis in the Gambia," by S. Sowa, et al. LANCET. 2:243-247, August 3, 1968.

"Investigation of a specific IgM antibody test in neonatal congenital syphilis," by M. Sepetjian, et al. BRIT J VENER DIS. 46:18-20, February, 1970.

"On a case of syphilitic pemphigus in a newborn infant with multiple osteochondritic lesions," by G. Sciafani. MINERVA PEDIAT. 22:902-903, April 28, 1970.

"Roentgenographic diagnosis of congenital syphilis in the newborn," by D. R. Coblentz, et al. JAMA. 212:1061-1064, May 11, 1970.

"Specific antiluetic antibody production in a newborn with congenital lues with hypergamma M globulinemia," by F. Aiuti, et al. G MAL INFETT. 19:332-333, May, 1967.

"A specific IgM antibody test in neonatal congenital syphilis," by A. T. Scotti, et al. J PEDIAT. 73:242-243, August, 1968.

"Syphilis in the new-born in La Paz, Bolivia," by G. G. de Murillo. J AMER MED WOM ASS. 24:420-422, May, 1969.

"Unusual bullous dermatitis of the fingers and face in a newborn with very important monocytosis," by F. Gianotti. ANN DERM SYPH. 96:395-398, 1969.

"Unusual electrophoretic aspects of the blood of newborn infants with cytomegalic disease and congenital syphilis," by G. Turbessi, et al. MINERVA PEDIAT.

SYPHILIS: NEONATAL

19:590-591, March 31, 1967.

SYPHILIS: NEPHROSIS
SEE: SYPHILIS: KIDNEY

SYPHILIS: NEUROSYPHILIS
"Accidents during the treatment of neurosyphilis," by J. Roland. MAROC MED. 45:221-222, March, 1966.

"Atypical serology in neurosyphilis," by K. Dewhurst. J NEUROL NEUROSURG PSYCHIAT. 31:496-500, October, 1968.

"Bilateral recurrent laryngeal nerve paralysis in early childhood following congenital syphilis," by B. Fioresi. MSCHR OHRENHEILK. 101:375-377, 1967.

"Changing clinical picture of neurosyphilis (Letter to Ed.)," by B. Levy. BRIT MED J. 2:491-492, May 25, 1968.

"Changing clinical picture of neurosyphilis: report of seven unusual cases," by R. Joffe, et al. BRIT MED J. 1:211-212, January 27, 1968.

"Clinical observations on symptomatic neurosyphilis," by D. Loesch. NEUROL NEUROCHIR PSYCHIAT POL. 16: 1047-1056, September, 1966.

"Clinico-pathological aspects of the neurosyphilitic psychoses," by K. Dewhurst. POSTGRAD MED J. 44: 898-902, December, 1968.

"The composition of the cerebrospinal fluid in the neurosyphilitic psychoses," by K. Dewhurst. ACTA NEUROL SCAND. 45:119-123, 1969.

"Does syphilis still erode the spine?," by M. Baledent, et al. SEM HOP PARIS. 46:2354-2357, September 10, 1970.

"Effect of copper oxidase in the blood and cerebrospinal fluid of patients with syphilitic lesions of the central nervous system," by N. I. Tumasheva, et al. ZH NEVROPAT PSIKHIAT KORSAKOV. 66:391-393, 1966.

"Epilepsy and neurosyphilis," by E. Negulici-Baliff, et al. ACTA NEUROL BELG. 67:1138-1152, 1967.

SYPHILIS: NEUROSYPHILIS

"Experimental ocular and neurosyphilis in the primate," by J. A. Wells, et al. BRIT J VENER DIS. 43:10-17, 1967.

"Four illustrious neuroluetics (Heinrich Heine, Jules De Goncourt, Alphonse Daudet, Guy de Maupassant," by H. Heine, et al. PROC ROY SOC MED. 62:669-673, July 7, 1969.

"General paralysis in Victoria, Australia: historical study," by A. Stoller, et al. MED J AUST. 2:607-611, September 20, 1969.

"General paralysis of the insane with gumma of skull," by S. B. Mahapatra. BRIT J VENER DIS. 43:178-180, September, 1967.

"Hanson's multineuritis in a syphilitic," by P. Warot, et al. LILLE MED. 14:558-562, 1969.

"Herxheimer's reaction. Asymptomatic neurosyphilis treated with penicillin," by H. A. Podesta, et al. PRENSA MED ARGENT. 54:301-304, April 14, 1967.

"The identification of sarcoid granulomas in the nervous system," by W. J. Williams. PROC ROY SOC MED. 60:1170-1172, November 1, 1967.

"Incidence of neurosyphilis and its clinical forms in Sao Paula," by E. Zukerman, et al. REV PAUL MED. 70:270-274, June, 1967.

"The intradermal treponemal color reaction in neurosyphilis," by C. Lazzaro, et al. ACTA NEUROL. 21:287-292, May-June, 1966.

"Late complications of syphilis. A comparative epidemiological and serological study of cardiovascular syphilis and various forms of neurosyphilis," by K. Aho, et al. ACTA DERMATOVENER. 49:336-342, 1969.

"Liquor diagnosis of neurosyphilis," by G. Ritter, et al. DEUTSCH MED WSCHR. 93:1595-1596 passim, August 23, 1968.

"Meningoradiculitis, a disease misnamed atypical polyradiculoneuritis," by F. Thiebaut, et al. REV NEUROL. 115:1070-1075, December, 1966.

SYPHILIS: NEUROSYPHILIS

"Neurologic disorders in the secondary stage of syphilis with the differential diagnosis of brain tumor," by G. Huffmann. MED WELT. 48:2614-2619, November 26, 1968.

"Neurosyphilis (Letter to Ed.)," by K. W. Heathfield. BRIT MED J. 1:765-766, March 23, 1968.

"Neurosyphilis. Its current frequency in our medical clinic," by J. Garrachon, et al. REV CLIN ESP. 101: 279-282, May 31, 1966.

"Neurosyphilis associated with haematemesis: report of a case," by J. L. Verbov, et al. BRIT J CLIN PRACT. 21:515-517, October, 1967.

"Neurosyphilis in cases from the Departments of Neurology and Psychiatry of Medical Schools in Poland in 1956-1965 (Clinical data)," by A. Dowzenko, et al. NEUROL NEUROCHIR POL. 3:559-566, September-October, 1969.

"Neurosyphilis in Uganda: a comparison of two five-year periods," by W. R. Billington. E AFR MED J. 43:469-473, November, 1966.

"Neurosyphilis lesions recorded in a group of 1,987 necropsies. (Statistical review and anatomical study)," by B. Rodriquez-Arias, et al. REV CLIN ESP. 108:153-156, January 31, 1968.

"Neurosyphilis, the search for adequate treatment. A review and report of a study using benzathine penicillin," by G. D. Short, et al. ARCH DERM. 93:87-91, January, 1966.

"The neurosyphilitic psychoses today. A survey of 91 cases," by K. Dewhurst. BRIT J PSYCHIAT. 115:31-38, January, 1969.

"A new technic to control malariotherapy in syphilogenic psychoses," by J. A. Garcia, et al. REV BRASIL MED. 24:902-906, November, 1967.

"On autoinhibition in classical syphilis reactions in neurologic-psychiatric patients," by J. Berndt, et al. ARCH PSYCHIAT NERVENKR. 210:198-210, 1967.

"On an incomplete luetic cerebrospinal fluid syndrome

SYPHILIS: NEUROSYPHILIS

in connection with a skull-brain trauma," by G. Ehrmann, et al. WIEN Z NERVENHEILK. 25:68-75, 1967.

"On the therapy of cerebrospinal positive late syphilis," by H. H. Wiek, et al. MED WELT. 35:1883, August 31, 1968.

"Parallelism of the pathologic changes in the spinal fluid, nonspecific, in patients with neurosyphilis and cerebral cysticercosis. Importance of the Weinberg test," by N. S. Filho. HOSPITAL. 69:317-322, February, 1966.

"Pathogenesis of pupillary disorders in various forms of syphilis of the nervous system," by V. D. Kochetkov, et al. VESTN DERM VENER. 44:53-58, March, 1970.

"Penicillin treatment in neurosyphilis," by W. Schubert. MED KLIN. 63:806-810, May 17, 1968.

"Prickle-cell carcinoma of the supra-and infra-clavicular fossa resembling the pancoast-tobias syndrome in a patient with syphilis of the nervous system," by S. Zelazny, et al. PRZEGLAD LEK. 22:514-516, 1966.

"Rapidly progressive cases of neurosyphilitic psychosis," by K. Dewhurst. PSYCHIAT CLIN. 1:320-326, 1968.

"Rapidly progressive deafness caused by syphilitic neuro-labyrinthitis," by G. Pellegrini, et al. REV OTONEUROOPHTAL. 41:203-211, May-June, 1969.

"Recent observations on the treatment of late ocular syphilis and neurosyphilis," by J. L. Smith. TRANS AMER ACAD OPHTHAL OTOLARYNG. 73:1113-1132, November-December, 1969.

"The results of catamnestic examination of 138 patients with neurosyphilis," by M.P. Frishman, et al. VESTN DERM VENER. 40:57-61, February, 1966.

Senile hypophyseal syndromes," by E. Herman. J NEUROL SCI. 4:101-110, January-February, 1966.

Some data on change in the electric activity of the brain in neurosyphilis," by L. A. Brozgol'd. VESTN

SYPHILIS: NEUROSYPHILIS

DERM VENER. 43:58-70, April, 1969.

"Studies on non-inflammatory lesions in neurosyphilis. I. An autopsy case of tabes dorsalis combined with status dysraphicus and Alzheimer's fibrillary changes in the horn of Ammon," by T. Matsuoka, et al. BRAIN NERVE. 20:27-32, January, 1968.

--III. Case of progressive paralysis association with Huntington's chorea." BRAIN NERVE. 20:925-930, 1968.

"Syphilis in current neurology. 1," by G. Moya, et al. ARCH NEUROBIOL. 30:138-166, April-June, 1967+.

"Syphilis of the brain based on data from a psychiatric hospital," by A. P. Tikhonova, et al. VESTN DERM VENER. 40:31-35, December, 1966.

"Syphilis of the nervous system. (The problem as it stands today.)," by M. V. Milich. SOVET MED. 31: 94-99, January, 1968.

"Syphilis of the parents as a cause of several neuropsychic disorders," by L. V. Sazonova, et al. VESTN DERM VENER. 43:57-59, September, 1969.

"Tabetic arthropathy and secondary neurological manifestations," by M. Cardas, et al. NEUROLOGIA. 12: 341-353, July-August, 1967.

"Therapy of neurosyphilis." REV CLIN ESP. 104:425-426, March 15, 1967.

"Therapy of neurosyphilis," by H. Bammer. DEUTSCH MED WSCHR. 92:1280-1283, 1967.

"Treatment of the neurosyphilitic psychoses," by K. Dewhurst. ACTA PSYCHIAT SCAND. 45:62-74, 1969.

"Treponema immobilization and immunofluorescence tests in the cerebrospinal fluid," by L. A. D'iachenko. VESTN DERM VENER. 43:48-53, July, 1969.

"Vascular manifestations in some forms of neurosyphilis," by V. F. Aliferova. VRACH DELO. 6:131-132, June, 1966.

SYPHILIS: OCCURRENCE
"Absence of syphilis in the population of Chipaya

SYPHILIS: OCCURRENCE

(Bolivia)," by P. Cirera, et al. BULL SOC PATH EXOT. 61:849-852, November-December, 1968.

"Analysis of morbidity to venereal diseases in Poland in 1966," by J. Bachurzewski. PRZEGL DERM. 54:641-650, November-December, 1967.

"Aspects of endemic syphilis among the Tuaregs or Niger," by A. Basset, et al. BULL SOC PATH EXOT. 62:80-92, January-February, 1969.

"Congenital syphilis in the Istituto Provinciale Assistenza all' Infanzia of Rome. (Comparison between the decade 1943-1952 and that of 1957-1966). Statistical, clinical, therapeutic and prophylactic considerations," by V. Menichella, et al. MINERVA NIPIOL. 19:35-39, January-February, 1969.

"Current aspect of syphilis in Belem o Pará," by D. Silva, et al. AN BRASIL DERM. 41:213-218, October-December, 1966.

"Current clinical aspects and statistics of early and late syphilis in Poland," by J. Towpik. POL TYG LEK. 22:1477-1480, September 25, 1967.

"Current problems of syphilis," by I. Károlyi. ORV HETIL. 110:225-236, February 2, 1969.

"Data on the incidence of syphilis among the population of Prikarpathia," by P. V. Parashchak. VESTN DERM VENER. 40:68-70, January, 1966.

"Dermatologic diseases observed at an assembly of nomads on the occasion of the salt cure of In Gall (Nigeria)," by A. Basset, et al. BULL SOC FRANC DERM SYPH. 75:820-822, 1968.

"Endemic syphilis in the Karoo," by J. A. Du Toit. S AFR MED J. 43:355-358, March 29, 1969.

"Epidemic in rural Mississippi." SCI N. 94:362, October 12, 1968.

"Epidemiologic aspect of syphilis. City of Santa Maria Rio Grande do Sul (Brazil)," by J. Fogliatto, et al. HOSPITAL. 76:739-746, August, 1969.

"Epidemiologic survey on Chagas' disease and syphilis

SYPHILIS: OCCURRENCE

in Ribeirao Préto," by N. Haddad. REV INST MED TROP S PAULO. 9:333-342, September-October, 1967.

"The epidemiology of infectious syphilis," by C. Lindman. J MAINE MED ASS. 60:237 passim, October, 1969.

"Epidemiology of lues and gonorrhea in Northrhine Westphalia from 1948 to 1968," by K. Gedicke. OEFF GESUNDHEITSWESEN. 32:218-226, May, 1970.

"The epidemiology of syphilis," by C. M. Barnes. J KANSAS MED SOC. 70:59-66, February, 1969.

"Epidemiology of syphilis," by E. Calas, et al. PROPHYL SANIT MORALE. 38:12-21, January, 1966.

"Epidemiology of syphilis," by N. J. Fiumara. MASSACHUSETTS GEN PRACT NEWS. 4 p.p., January-February, 1966.

"Epidemiology of syphilis in Brisbane, 1968-1969," by B. A. Smithurst. MED J AUST. 2:1143-1146, December 6, 1969.

"Epidemiology of syphilitic infection during the past 8 years (1958-1965) according to our clinical material," by R. Ruben, et al. GOD ZBORN MED FAK SKOPJE. 13:185-193, 1966.

"Evolution of syphilis in the region of Suceava in the years 1952 to 1966," by T. Costic. REV MEDICOCHIR IASI. 72:59-62, January-March, 1968.

"Extent and development of late syphilis according to autopsy statistics (1945-1965)," by G. Fromm, et al. DEUTSCH MED WSCHR. 92:1181-1185, June 30, 1967.

"The incidence of lues," by C. H. Beek. NEDERL T GENEESK. 112:614-616, March 30, 1968.

"Incidence of neurosyphilis and its clinical forms in Sao Paulo," by E. Zukerman, et al. REV PAUL MED. 70:270-274, June, 1967.

"Infectious syphilis in South Carolina." J S CAROLINA MED ASS. 62:339, August, 1966.

"Infectious syphilis outbreak in Kentucky," by R. E. Teague. J KENTUCKY MED ASS. 67:22-23, January, 1969.

SYPHILIS: OCCURRENCE

"Juvenile GPI: A case study," by G. C. Kanjilal. NURS TIMES. 65:1066-1067, August 21, 1969.

"The lues curve in Switzerland since World War I," by W. Burckhardt, et al. DERMATOLOGICA. 135:341-344, 1967.

"Neurosyphilis in Uganda: A comparison of two five-year periods," by W. R. Billington. E AFR MED J. 43:469-473, November, 1966.

"1968 survey of treponematosis in the eastern highlands of New Guinea," by M. F. Garner, et al. BRIT J VENER DIS. 46:13-17, February, 1970.

"Nosological and nosographical aspects of syphilis in the province of Cuneo during a 5-year period. Statistical note," by F. Peirone. MINERVA MED. 57:2777-2780, August 25, 1966.

"On the frequency of syphilis in various populations in the Caribbean area," by P. Cirera, et al. BULL SOC PATH EXOT. 61:169-176, 1968.

"Outbreak of syphilis," by J. C. Hedden, et al. J S CAROLINA MED ASS. 62:471-473, December, 1966.

"Primary and secondary syphilis. Country of origin study, 1965," by British Cooperative Clinical Group. BRIT J VENER DIS. 43:89-95, June, 1967.

--1966." BRIT J VENER DIS. 42:167-173, June, 1968.

--1967." BRIT J VENER DIS. 44:307-314, December, 1968.

--1968." BRIT J VENER DIS. 46:69-75, February, 1970.

"Recent trends of syphilis incidence in Korea," by J. Lew, et al. YONSEI MED J. 9:74-80, 1968.

"The rise and fall of the treponematoses. I. Ecological aspects and international trends in venereal syphilis," by O. Idsoe, et al. BRIT J VENER DIS. 43:227-243, December, 1967.

--II. Endemic treponematoses of childhood," by T. Guthe, et al. BRIT J VENER DIS. 44:35-48, March, 1968.

"Studies in syphilis epidemiology," by W. J. Brown.

SYPHILIS: OCCURRENCE

BRIT J VENER DIS. 42:110-115, June, 1966.

"Study of 1,929 cases of primo-secondary syphilis observed in the Clinique des Maladies Cutanées et Syphilitiques of the Faculté de Médecine de Paris," by R. Degos, et al. BULL INST NAT SANTE. 23:549-585, May-June, 1968.

"Survey of serologic evidence for syphilis among the Masai of Tanzania," by G. V. Mann, et al. PUBLIC HEALTH REP. 81:513-518, June, 1966.

"Syphilis epidemic in South Greenland 1965," by G. A. Olsen. UGESKR LAEG. 128:1071-1076, September 15, 1966.

"Treponematosis in the eastern highlands of New Guinea," by M. F. Garner, et al. BULL WHO. 38:189-195, 1968.

"Treponematoses in Ethiopia," by K. F. Schaller. Z HAUT GESCHLECHTSKR. 43:17-28, January 1, 1968.

"Visceral syphilis based on the data of the Moscow District Scientific-Research Institute," by A. R. Zlatkina. VESTN DERM VENER. 40:27-31, December, 1966.

SYPHILIS: OPHTHALMOLOGY

"Argyll Robertson pupil," by D. Leak. NM. 123:ivt, February 17, 1967.

"The Argyll Robertson pupil, 1869-1969, A critical survey of the literature," by I. E. Loewenfeld. SURVEY OPHTHAL. 14:199-200, November, 1969.

"A case of acquired syphilis revealed by unilateral keratitis," by P. Desbordes, et al. MED TROP. 28:230-232, March-April, 1968.

"A case of syphilitic anterior uveitis with posterior chamber hemorrhage," by C. S. Kalidason. J ALL INDIA OPHTHAL SOC. 17:123-124, June, 1969.

"Cerebrospinal fluid findings in ophthalmology. In eye diseases," by S. Shimizu. ACTA SOC OPHTHAL JAP. 71:1825-1845, October, 1967.

"Clinical experience with ampicillin and probenecid in the management of treponeme-associated uveitis," by

SYPHILIS: OPHTHALMOLOGY

by J. N. Goldman. TRANS AMER ACAD OPHTHAL OTOLARYNG. 74:509-514, May-June, 1970.

"Congenital ocular syphilis," by W. G. Nicol, et al. AMER J OPHTHAL. 68:467-471, September, 1969.

"Congenital parenchymal dystrophy of the cornea. (On 2 personal cases)," by A. Scialfa. ANN OTTAL. 92: 383-393, June, 1966.

"Contribution to the problem of ocular syphilis," by S. Merin, et al. CENT AFR J MED. 13:249-251, November, 1967.

"Control of ophthalmia neonatorum. A position statement by the NSPB Committee on Ophthalmia Neonatorum." SIGHTSAV REV. 39:203-204, Winter, 1969.

"The current status of ocular syphilis," by J. L. Smith. SURVEY OPHTHAL. 14:176-178, November, 1969.

"Experimental ocular and neurosyphilis in the primate," by J. A. Wells, et al. BRIT J VENER DIS. 43:10-17, March, 1967.

"Fluorescent antibody staining of treponemes in uveitis," by J. N. Goldman, et al. ARCH OPHTHAL. 79:716-722, June, 1968.

"The fluorescent antibody tissue stain in experimental ocular syphilis," by J. A. Wells, et al. ARCH OPHTHAL. 77:530-555, April, 1967.

"Fluorescent examinations of pupils and pupillary reactions in the early stages of syphilis," by A. V. Braitsev, et al. VESTN DERM VENER. 42:47-51, June, 1968.

"Gumma of the choroid," by F. Soukup. CESK OFTAL. 24: 438-441, November, 1968.

"Histopathologic demonstration of spirochetes in the human eye," by E. N. Montenegro, et al. AMER J OPHTHAL. 67:335-346, March, 1969.

"The importance of the TPI in ophthalmology," by Z. Kumstat, et al. CESK OFTAL. 22:183-186, May, 1966.

"Interstitial keratitis and glaucoma," by P. R. Lichter,

SYPHILIS: OPHTHALMOLOGY

et al. AMER J OPHTHAL. 68:241-248, August, 1969.

"Interstitial keratitis associated with hidradenitis suppurativa," by J. R. Bergeron, et al. ARCH DERM. 95:473-475, May, 1967.

"Intraocular treponemes," by E. H. Christman, et al. ARCH OPHTHAL. 80:303-307, September, 1968.

"Intraocular treponemes in treated congenital syphilis," by J. N. Goldman, et al. ARCH OPHTHAL. 78:47-50, July, 1967.

"Investigation of neonatal conjunctivitis in the Gambia," by S. Sowa, et al. LANCET. 2:243-247, August 3, 1968.

"Late ocular syphilis: transfer of infection from man to experimental animals," by J. L. Smith. TRANS AMER OPHTHAL SOC. 67:658-697, 1969.

"Latent syphilis and cataract," by J. Sédan. BULL SOC OPHTAL FRANC. 67:874-877, October, 1967.

"A luminescent study of pupils and pupillary reactions in the early stages of syphilis," by A. V. Braitsev, et al. VESTN DERM VENER. 42:47-51, June, 1968.

"Nasopharyngeal syphilis with blindness," by W. E. Gager, et al. ARCH OTOLARYNG. 90:641-646, November, 1969.

"Non-tumor causes of the Foster Kennedy syndrome," by N. J. Schatz, et al. J NEUROSURG. 27:37-44, July, 1967.

"Observations on a case of Lilliputian hallucinations in the course of a delirious episode in a patient with an ocular disease," by L. Tremelloni. G PSICHIAT NEUROPAT. 94:625-636, 1966.

"On the recurrence of interstitial keratitis," by J. Sedan. BULL SOC OPHTAL FRANC. 66:432-435, April, 1966.

"Oral disorders associated with ocular disease. II. Disorders affecting dentition," by B. Harcourt. BRIT J OPHTHAL. 51:284-285, April, 1967.

SYPHILIS: OPHTHALMOLOGY

"Pathogenesis of pupillary disorders in various forms of syphilis of the nervous system," by V. D. Kochetkov, et al. VESTN DERM VENER. 44:53-58, March, 1970.

"Pathologic-anatomical ocular findings in fetal lues," by H. J. Thiel, et al. KLIN MBL AUGENHEILK. 154: 712-716, May, 1969.

"Penetrating keratoplasty in interstitial keratitis," by M. F. Rabb, et al. AMER J OPHTHAL. 67:907-917, June, 1969.

"Penicillins and aqueous humor," by E. E. Goldman, et al. AMER J OPHTHAL. 65:717-721, May, 1968.

"Pseudo-retinopathy pigmentosa caused by acquired syphilis," by U. Volpi. ANN OTTAL. 92:408-414, June, 1966.

"Pseudo-retinopathy pigmentosa in congenital syphilis. Description of a case," by M. Santori. MINERVA OFTAL. 8:89-92, May-June, 1966.

"Recent observations on the treatment of late ocular syphilis and neurosyphilis," by J. L. Smith. TRANS AMER ACAD OPHTHAL OTOLARYNG. 73:1113-1132, November-December, 1969.

"Recovery of treponema pallidum from aqueous humor removed at cataract surgery in man by passive transfer to rabbit testis," by J. L. Smith, et al. AMER J OPHTHAL. 65:242-247, February, 1968.

"Recurrent parenchymatous keratitis in 2d generation congenital syphilis," by A. Ullmo. BULL SOC FRANC DERM SYPH. 75:654-656, 1968.

"Relapse of interstitial keratitis," by J. Sedan. BULL SOC OPHTAL FRANC. 66:435-435, April, 1966.

"Results of serologic studies in endogenous ocular inflammations," by W. Paul, et al. KLIN MBL AUGENHEILK. 151:332-344, 1967.

"Spirochetes in the aqueous humor in seronegative ocular syphilis. Persistence after penicillin therapy," by J. L. Smith, et al. ARCH OPHTHAL. 77:474-477, April, 1967.

SYPHILIS: OPHTHALMOLOGY

"Study of late ocular syphilis. Demonstration of treponemes in aqueous humour and cerebrospinal fluid. I. Methods of demonstration of treponemes," by A. E. Wilkinson. TRANS OPHTHAL SOC UK. 88:251-256, 1969.

--II. Ocular findings," by N. S. Rice, et al. TRANS OPHTHAL SOC UK. 88:257-273, 1969.

--III. General and serological findings," by E. M. Dunlop, et al. TRANS OPHTHAL SOC UK. 88:275-294, 1969.

"Symposium on certain forms of infective kerato-uveitis or uveitis: I. An approach to the problem, and the technique of anterior chamber tap," by B. R. Jones, et al. TRANS OPHTHAL SOC UK. 88:235-242, 1969.

"Syphilis and the eye," by W. E. Gager. WISCONSIN MED J. 68:38, May, 1969; also in SIGHT SAVINGR. 39:137-143, Fall, 1969.

"Syphilis and iridocyclitis," by Z. Kumstát, et al. CESK OFTAL. 23:103-108, March, 1967.

"Syphilitic chorioretinitis. A histologic study," by F. C. Blodi, et al. ARCH OPHTHAL. 79:294-296, March, 1968.

"Syphilitic keratitis," by G. M. de Weisenberg, et al. REV FAC CLENC MED CORDOBA. 27:27-35, January-March, 1969.

"Syphilitic ocular manifestations in our clinical experience," by Z. Pavisić, et al. RAD MED FAK ZAGREB. 14:241-252, 1966.

"Syphilitic optic neuritis. A case report," by S. E. Lorentzen. ACTA OPHTHAL, 45:769-792, 1967.

"Traumatic ectopia lentis. Some relationships to syphilis and glaucoma," by L. J. Rosenbaum, et al. AMER J OPHTHAL. 64:1095-1098, December, 1967.

"Treatment of ophthalmic syphilis, with special reference to cephaloridine therapy," by M. Mikuni, et al. OPHTHALMOLOGY. 12:724-731, September, 1970.

"Treponemes in aqueous humor in late seronegative syphilis," by J. L. Smith, et al. TRANS AMER ACAD OPH-

SYPHILIS: OPHTHALMOLOGY

THAL OTOLARYNG. 72:63-75, January-February, 1968.

"Tric agent as a cause of neonatal eye sepsis," by P. G. Watson, et al. BRIT MED J. 3:527-528, August 31, 1968.

"Unusual case of morbid association of parenchymatous keratitis, diffuse choroiditis and Jensen's chorioretinitis in a patient with syphilis," by E. Preste. ANN OTTAL. 92:539-547, July, 1966.

"Uveitis and intraocular treponemes," by R. Whitfield, et al. ARCH OPHTHAL. 84:12-15, July, 1970.

"Uveitis as a presenting sign of acquired syphilis. Report of three cases," by D. H. Pendergrast. J NAT MED ASS. 59:41-42, January, 1967.

SYPHILIS: ORAL

"Atrophic luetic glossitis. Report of a case," by A. M. Captline, et al. ORAL SURG. 30:192-195, August, 1970.

"Diagnosis and differential diagnosis of syphilitic diseases of the mouth mucosa," by K. W. Mach. OEST Z STOMAT. 65:350-357, September, 1968.

"Glossitis interstitialis luetica in the course of late congenital syphilis," by D. Niedzwiecka. PRZEGL DERM. 53:211-212, March-April, 1966.

"Jackson's syndrome (hemiplegia infima alternans) of a luetic basis," by E. Lange, et al. PSYCHIAT NEUROL MED PSYCHOL. 19:32-34, January, 1967.

"Mouth mucosa findings in lues," by H. M. Hofmeier. HNO. 16:73-78, March, 1968.

"On the etiologic relationship between leukoplakia, syphilis and cancer of the oral cavity," by K. Anastassov, et al. REV FRANC ODONTOSTOMAT. 14:1530-1536, November, 1967.

"Oral disorders associated with ocular disease. II. Disorders affecting dentition," by B. Harcourt. BRIT J OPHTHAL. 51:284-285, April, 1967.

"The oral manifestations of acquired syphilis. A study of eighty-one cases," by I. Meyer, et al. ORAL SURG.

SYPHILIS: ORAL

23:45-57, January, 1967.

"Primary syphilis of the gingiva. Report of two cases," by M. Steiner, et al. ORAL SURG. 21:530-535, April, 1966.

"Rare complication after plastic operation in the oral cavity vestibule," by W. Rytlowa, et al. CZAS STOMAT. 19:525-528, May, 1966.

"Secondary oral and laryngeal syphilis," by R. W. Dodd. VIRGINIA MED MONTHLY. 94:229-231, April, 1967.

"The serological diagnosis of syphilis in dental patients," by M. Harris. BRIT J ORAL SURG. 4:235-239, March, 1967

"Syphilitic gumma of the tongue," by F. G. Marill, et al. BULL SOC FRANC DERM SYPH. 74:216-217, 1967.

"2 cases of tertiary syphilis diagnosed in dental field practice," by J. Bukový. CESK STOMAT. 68:297-301, July, 1968.

SYPHILIS: OSSEOUS

"Apropos of a case of osseous syphilis," by M. Ruelle. J BELG RHUM MED PHYS. 21:11-14, January-February, 1966.

"Bone lesions observed in serological treponematosis. Study of 267 patients," by R. P. Delahaye, et al. SEM HOP PARIS. 46:189-194, January 14, 1970.

"Bone marrow inhibition in latent syphilis," by J. Jedličková, et al. VNITRNI LEK. 16:798-801, August, 1970.

"A case of diffuse syphilitic osteoperiostitis," by R. Quilichini, et al. MARSEILLE MED. 107:499-503, June, 1970.

"Circumscribed non-gummous mandibular osteitis as primary organic manifestation of tertiary syphilis," by M. Strassburg. DEUTSCH ZAHNAERZTL Z. 22:1052-1056, August, 1967.

"Multiple osteochondritis due to prenatal syphilis," by J. Mercadal-Peyri, et al. ACTAS DERMOSIF. 58:101-104, March-April, 1967.

SYPHILIS: OSSEOUS

"Secondary syphilis with osteolysis of skull bones," by P. Franceschini, et al. BULL SOC FRANC DERM SYPH. 76:763-764, 1969.

"Syphilitic osteochondritis in congenital late syphilis," by H. Wendler. ARCH KINDERHEILIK. 176:184-190, 1967.

"Syphilitic osteomyelitis of the mandible," by I. H. Heslop. BRIT J ORAL SURG. 6:59-63, July, 1968.

"Syphilitic osteoperiostitis of the orbital apex," by P. Cernea, et al. ANN OCULIST. 201:436-442, April, 1968.

"2 cases of cerebral gummata," by A. Kunicki, et al. MEUROL MEUROCHIR POL. 4:251-254, March-April, 1970.

SYPHILIS: PATHOLOGY

"Cancriform pyoderma," by L. V. Vallejo, et al. PRENSA MED ARGENT. 55:624-627, May 31, 1968.

"Clinicopathologic conference," by E. H. Eigenbrodt, et al. TEXAS MED. 65:84-90, July, 1969.

"Clinicopathologic conference. Case presentation," by V. A. McKusick, et al. BULL HOPKINS HOSP. 119:150-160, August, 1966.

"Electron microscopic observation of syphilid. I. The ultrastructure of treponema pallidum (Nicols strain)," by S. Abe. BULL PHARM RES INST. 60:1-6, January, 1966.

"Histologic structure of the lymph node of recent syphilis," by A. Bazex, et al. BULL SOC FRANC DERM SYPH. 75:140-143, 1968.

"Histopathology of serpiginous skin lesions in late syphilis (lues tubero-ulcero-serpiginosa)," by K. Lejman, et al. PRZEGL DERM. 53:419-423, July-August, 1966.

"Late syphilis in the primate," by F. J. Elsas, et al. BRIT J VENER DIS. 44:267-273, December, 1968.

"Light microscopic observations on the pathology of endolymph," by H. F. Schuknecht, et al. J LARYNG. 80:1-10, January, 1966.

SYPHILIS: PATHOLOGY

"Primary chancre of cervix uteri," by V. Tchertkoff, et al. NEW YORK J MED. 66:1921-1924, July 15, 1966.

"The status of cold reception of the skin (cold spots) in patients with syphilis," by A. A. Shtein. VESTN DERM VENER. 40:44-47, December, 1966.

"Studies on the bone marrow and lymph nodes in primary syphilis," by W. Rasiewicz, et al. Z HAUT GESCHLECHTSKR. 43:351-358, May 1, 1968.

SYPHILIS: PENILE

"Gummous syphilis of the penis refractory to penicillin and bismuth preparations," by A. I. Levykin. VESTN DERM VENER. 43:82-86, January, 1969.

SYPHILIS: PREGNANCY
SEE ALSO: CONGENITAL
SYPHILIS: INFANTS

"Case-finding through ante-natal serological tests for syphilis," by J. A. Burgess. BRIT J VENER DIS. 42:116-118, June, 1966.

"Considerations on a case of primary syphiloma of the cervix uteri in pregnancy, with special reference to the differential diagnosis from cervical carcinoma," by E. Rocco. MINERVA GINEC. 19:30-34, January 15, 1967.

"Current trends in medical care of the pregnant woman," by D. Farina. POLICINICO. 75:1579-1587, November 25, 1968.

"Diagnosis and treatment of syphilis in pregnancy," by M. Kusumoto, et al. SANFUJIN JISSAI. 17:1082-1091, December, 1968.

"Does lues have a role in the intrauterine death today?," by I. Deml. ZBL GYNAEK. 90:240-242, February 17, 1968.

"FTA-ABS test in pregnancy. A probable false-positive reaction," by C. S. Buchanan, et al. ARCH DERM. 102:322-325, September, 1970.

"False-positive serological test for syphilis in pregnancy," by O. P. Salo, et al. ACTA DERMATOVENER. 49:332-335, 1969.

SYPHILIS: PREGNANCY

"Fetal production of immunoglobulins in the course of congenital infections," by G. B. Serra, et al. MINERVA PEDIAT. 19:591-592, March 31, 1967.

"Herxheimer's reaction in maternal milk in early congenital syphilis," by R. Rollier, et al. BULL SOC FRANC DERM SYPH. 74:178-180, 1967.

"Immunologic response of the fetus in congenital syphilis," by B. J. Fogel, et al. J FLORIDA MED ASS. 59:777-779, October, 1969.

"The importance of the fluorescent antibody technic (FAT) as a control of questionable Wassermann reactions in pregnancy," by I. Piacentini. FRACASTORO. 59:615-618, September-October, 1966.

"Incidence of biologic false positive syphilis reactions among pregnant women," by K. Loe. T NORSK LAEGEFOREN. 86:1728-1731, December 15, 1966.

"Interpretation of positive serological tests for syphilis in pregnancy," by A. Adeoba. BRIT J VENER DIS. 43:249-258, December, 1967.

"Microscopic studies on the placenta of a macerated fetus with important clinical implications," by J. C. Stut. NEDERL T VERLOSK. 66:56-64, February, 1966.

"On the routine serology for detection of syphilis in pregnant women treated by the ONMI from 1956-1967," by A. G. Marcozzi. ITAL DERM. 45:185-186, March, 1970.

"On the timing of penicillin treatment of syphilis during pregnancy," by H. Walther. ARCH KLIN EXP DERM. 227:307-308, 1966.

"Pathologic-anatomical ocular findings in fetal lues," by H. J. Thiel, et al. KLIN MBL AUGENHEILK. 154:712-716, May, 1969.

"Recent syphilis in pregnancy and early congenital syphilis in the province of Milan. Statistico-epidemiological findings for 1967 and 1968 (through November, 1968). Considerations and proposals," by C. Ducrey. G ITAL DERM. 45:156-163, March, 1970.

"Serology in gyneco-obstetrics," by Y. Fukuoka. REV

SYPHILIS: PREGNANCY

CHILE PEDIAT. 37:633-648, July, 1966.

"Sero-negative maternal syphilis. Report of a case," by A. E. Tinkler. BRIT J VENER DIS. 42:136-139, June, 1968.

"Some observations on syphilis and pregnancy," by P. C. Brochery, et al. BULL FED GYNEC OBSTET FRANC. 20:45-49, January-March, 1968.

"Syphilis and guidance of expectant mothers," by M. Sumudi. JAP J NURS ART. 8:77-80, August, 1969.

"Syphilis in pregnancy. Diagnosis through VDRL and FTA-200 tests," by C. Krahe, et al. HOSPITAL. 74:975-978, September, 1968+.

"Treatment of pregnant syphilitic as full protection against congenital syphilis," by T. Iwanowska, et al. PRZEGL DERM. 56:753-756, 1969.

SYPHILIS: PREVENTION & CONTROL

"Anti-vaccination and syphilis," by D. Green. MED J AUST. 1:500-501, March 7, 1970.

"Blitz on syphilis in Alabama," by W. H. Smith. J MED ASS ALABAMA. 36:505 passim, November, 1966; also in PUBLIC HEALTH REP. 81:835-841, September, 1966.

"Can syphilis be controlled through treatment and epidemiology," by J. F. Donohue. REV AGRUP ODONT ARGENT. 20:1201-1203, 1968; also in SALUD PUBLICA MEX. 10:607-610, September-October, 1968.

"Certain problems of preventive therapy of syphilis," by L. A. Shteiniukht, et al. VESTN DERM VENER. 41:62-65, September, 1967.

"A combined epidemic of scabies and syphilis. What therapeutic course to follow?," by R. Rollier. LYON MED. 222:953-954, November 23, 1969.

"Contribution to the prophylactic antibiotic treatment of syphilis with special consideration of questionable occupational infections," by K. Wulf. ARCH KLIN EXP DERM. 227:301-307, 1966.

"The control of endemic syphilis of childhood," by T. Guthe, et al. DERM INT. 5:179-199, October-December, 1966.

SYPHILIS: PREVENTION & CONTROL

"Control of infectious syphilis in Detroit," by B. Schwimmer. MICH MED. 65:837-838, October, 1966.

"Critical evaluation of the current system of syphilis control in Poland," by T. Z. Capiński. FOLIA MED CRACOV. 9:521-581, 1967.

"Did you protect the spread?," by E. C. Prather. J FLORIDA MED ASS. 54:1038-1039, November, 1967.

"Domestic eradication of syphilis in Alabama," by W. H. Smith, et al. J MED ASS ALABAMA. 37:1364-1369, June, 1968.

"Environmental indicators and implications for control of infectious syphilis," by W. B. Neser. MISSOURI MED. 64:822-825, October, 1967.

"Eradication of syphilis: the missing element," by W. J. Brown. ANN INTERN MED. 72:278-280, February, 1970.

"For Syphilis Prevention Week," by T. Kawamura. J JAP MED ASS. 56:567-571, September 15, 1966.

"How much does an inadequate syphilis control program cost a country?," by A. E. Callin. SALUD PUBLICA MEX. 10:611-614, September-October, 1968.

"Immunization in the control of syphilis." BRIT MED J. 4:597, December 7, 1968.

"Improved methods of contact tracing," by B. Muspratt, et al. BRIT J VENER DIS. 43:204-208, September, 1967; also in CESK DERM. 45:184-186, August, 1970.

"Is it possible to control syphilis through treatment and epidemiologic measures?," by J. F. Donohue. SALUD PUBLICA MEX. 10:607-610, September-October, 1968.

"Management of chronic diseases and clinical judgment of cure--syphilis," by S. Okamoto. JAP J CLIN MED. 24:2304-2308, December, 1966.

"On the problem of reinfection in early syphilis," by J. Bowszyc. PRZEGL DERM. 54:659-664, November-December, 1967.

SYPHILIS: PREVENTION & CONTROL

"On the problem of re-infection in syphilis," by P. Fritsch, et al. DERM WSCHR. 154:387-393, April 27, 1968.

"On the removal from the register of patients with sero-resistant syphilis," by E. K. Reznikov. SOVET MED. 31:117-120, January, 1968.

"Ounce of prevention; new interest in syphilis research." NEWSWEEK. 70:54, August 28, 1967.

"Physician breaks chain of infectious syphilis." N CAROLINA MED J. 28:107, March, 1967.

"Physician's responsibility in venereal disease control," by C. W. Freeman. MED ANN DC. 35:382, July, 1966.

"Present panorama of syphilis. Basic measurements to control it," by C. Bopp. AN BRASIL DERM. 41:157-164, July-September, 1966.

"Prevention and disinfection of syphilis," by Y. Shimizu. JAP J NURS ART. 8:81-86, August, 1969.

"The prevention of syphilis," by C. W. Freeman. J NAT MED ASS. 59:189-192, May, 1967.

"Results of the control of contagious forms of syphilis in the Chelyabinsk region," by MIa. Trofimova. VESTN DERM VENER. 40:76-78, October, 1966.

"The results of control of venereal and communicable skin diseases in the USSR," by N. M. Turanov, et al. VESTN DERM VENER. 41:21-27, October, 1967.

"The rise in venereal disease: epidemiology and prevention," by R. H. Kampmeier. MED CLIN N AMER. 51:735-751, May, 1967.

"Syphilis control in a southern state," by R. W. Ball. MED TIMES. 94:520-530, May, 1966.

"Syphilis control: joint responsibility of private medicine and public health," by T. J. Friddell, et al. J TENN MED ASS. 59:141-143, February, 1966.

"The syphilis control program in North Carolina." N CAROLINA MED J. 28:32-33, January, 1967.

SYPHILIS: PSEUDO-SYPHILIS

SYPHILIS: PSEUDO-SYPHILIS
"Pseudo-syphilis papulosa naevoides. (Differential diagnostic problems with nevi resembling condylomata lata in the genital region)," by L. Szego, et al. DERM MSCHR. 155:580-585, 1969.

"Pseudosyphilitic pneumonia," by V. I. Pokrovskii, et al. KLIN MED. 47:119-121, June, 1969.

SYPHILIS: PULMONARY
"An additional case of pulmonary syphilis," by J. Horak. VNITRNI LEK. 13:848-852, September, 1967.

"Diagnostic and therapeutic difficulties in late pulmonary syphilis in adults," by W. Kiesz, et al. WIAD LEK. 20:1181-1184, June 15, 1967.

"On the acquired lung syphilis," by H. Stanulla. ZBL CHIR. 93:1503-1504, October 26, 1968.

"On the diagnosis of pulmonary syphilis," by F. Mersch. THORAXCHIRURGIE. 15:456-460, August, 1967.

"Pseudosyphilitic pneumonia," by V. I. Pokrovskii, et al. KLIN MED. 47:119-121, June, 1969.

"Syphilis of the lung. A case report and discussion of its clinical diagnosis," by S. Haim, et al. ACTA DERMATOVENER. 49:97-102, 1969.

"Syphilis of the lungs," by I. I. Pototskii. VRACH DELO. 8:81-84, August, 1967.

"Tuberculosis-syphilis correlations. (Clinical and experimental study)," by P. Cornea, et al. MED INTERN. 20:1387-1398, November, 1968.

SYPHILIS: RENAL
SEE: SYPHILIS: KIDNEY

SYPHILIS: SEROLOGY AND SERODIAGNOSIS
SEE ALSO: DIAGNOSIS
         IMMUNITY

"ABO blood groups and acute biologic false positive serological tests for syphilis," by A. I. Morrison. BRIT J VENER DIS. 42:37-39, March, 1966.

"Absorbed fluorescent treponemal antibody (FTA-ABS) test.

SYPHILIS: SEROLOGY AND SERODIAGNOSIS

Comparison with the FTA-200 and TPI tests on 1,056 problem sera," by N. A. Johnston, et al. BRIT J VENER DIS. 44:287-290, December, 1968.

"Additional information on the TPIT in congenital syphilis," by L. Pospisil, et al. CESK DERM. 41:97-101, April, 1966.

"Advantage of a routine Reiter protein complement-fixation test in the serodiagnosis of syphilis in pregnancy," by C. A. Morris. J CLIN PATH. 21:731-734, November, 1968.

"Ageing and false positive reactions for syphilis," by D. L. Tuffanelli. BRIT J VENER DIS. 42:40-41, March, 1966.

"Agglutination of particulate antigens in agar gel," by F. Milgrom, et al. J IMMUN. 98:102-109, January, 1967.

"Agglutination of Reiter's spirochete in serodiagnosis of syphilis," by G. Mariani. MINERVA MED. 58:3583-3585, October 20, 1967.

"Agglutination of spirochetes in the blood with the Roemer and Schlipkoeter method. Contribution to the serodiagnosis of syphilis," by G. Bratina. MINERVA MED. 58:3245-3247, September 22, 1967.

"An alarming problem in syphilography: the irreductible serologic reactions," by P. Rimbaud. PRESSE MED. 76:2471-2472, December 28, 1968.

"Alfred Klopstock," by W. Pagel. INT ARCH ALLERG. 35:308, 1969.

"Analysis of the antigenic structure of the Reiter strain of treponema pallidum and significance of the strain in the syphilis serologic reaction," by Y. Saijo. JAP J BACT. 22:510-518, September, 1967.

"The antibody pattern in representative groups of Ethiopian village children," by T. Mellbin, et al. ACTA PAEDIAT SCAND. 57:385-394, September, 1968.

"Anticomplement fluorescent antibody technic in experimental studies and serodiagnosis of syphilis," by N. M. Ovchinnikov, et al. VESTN DERM VENER. 42:33-38,

SYPHILIS: SEROLOGY AND SERODIAGNOSIS

December, 1968.

"Anticomplementary activity in serological tests for syphilis as a clue to connective tissue diseases of an auto-immune nature," by A. Lassus, et al. ANN CLIN RES. 1:74-76, May, 1969.

"Anticomplementary reactions and their relation to some auto-immune phenomena in syphilitic infection," by A. Lassus, et al. ACTA DERMATOVENER. 49:519-523, 1969.

"Antigenic characteristics of nucleic acids of cultivable treponemes," by K. Király, et al. Z IMMUNITAETSFORSCH. 131:434-443, December, 1966.

"Antigenic community between the galactodiglyceride of treponema Reiteri and cerebrosides," by P. Dupouey, et al. C R ACAD SCI. 270:1541-1544, March 16, 1970.

"Antigenic relationships of 14 treponemes demonstrated by immunofluorescence," by P. E. Meyer, et al. J BACT. 93:784-789, March, 1967.

"Antigenic structure of treponema pallidum, Nichols strain. II. Extraction of a polysaccharide antigen with 'strain-specific' serological activity," by J. N. Miller, et al. J BACT. 99:132-135, July, 1969.

"Anti-nuclear factors in sera from chronic false positive seroreactors for syphilis," by K. K. Mustakallio, et al. ACTA PATH MICROBIOL SCAND. 69:614-615, 1967.

"Antinuclear factors, rheumatoid factors and Bordet-Wassermann reaction in chronic and systemic lupus erythematosus," by J. Strejcek, et al. ACTA DERMATOVENER. 48:198-202, 1968.

"Antitreponemic immunoglobulins and immunoantibodies. Chromatographic and immunoelectrophoretic preliminary research," by A. Buzzoni. G ITAL DERM. 108:401-410, September-October, 1967.

"Applied immunofluorescence in dermato-venereology," by J. Thivolet, et al. G MAL INFETT. 20:109-118, January, 1968.

"Apropos of false specific serology in a woman presenting habitual abortions," by G. Zographos, et al. BULL FED GYNEC OBSTET FRANC. 18:299-301, June-August, 1966.

SYPHILIS: SEROLOGY AND SERODIAGNOSIS

"Apropos of serological reactivations caused by injection of 'luetin'. Further series of cases," by G. Tramier, et al. BULL SOC FRANC DERM SYPH. 74:596-598, 1967.

"Assessment of the 'luotest' in late syphilis," by S. M. Laird, et al. BRIT J VENER DIS. 42:119-121, June, 1966.

"An assessment of the Reiter Protein Complement Fixation (RPCF) test," by E. Fowler, et al. CANAD J PUBLIC HEALTH. 59:6-9, January, 1968.

"Assessment of various technics of the immunofluorescence test in the serological diagnosis of syphilis," by N. M. Ovchinnikov, et al. VESTN DERM VENER. 42:40-45, February, 1968.

"Attempt at simplification of the TPI test," by S. Stoyanoff, et al. MAROC MED. 45:216-220, March, 1966.

"An attempt to revise the opinion on the sensitivity of Nelson's test and the possibility of its spontaneous rejection," by J. Lesinski. CESK DERM. 41:289-295, October, 1966.

"Attempted simplification of Nelson's test," by S. Stoyanoff, et al. MAROC MED. 45:216-220, March, 1966.

"Attempts at the increase of sensitivity of the treponema pallidum immobilization test," by K. Kiraly. DERM WSCHR. 151:2035-2041, September 25, 1965.

"Atypical serology in neurosyphilis," by K. Dewhurst. J NEUROL NEUROSURG PSYCHIAT. 31:496-500, October, 1968.

"Autoimmune phenomena in patients with old treated syphilis nonreactive to the treponema pallidum immobilization test," by A. Lassus, et al. ACTA PATH MICROBIOL SCAND. 69:613-614, 1967.

"Autoimmune serologic reactions with lipin antigen," by R. L. Kahn. AMER J MED TECHN. 32:57-68, January-February, 1966.

"Automated fluorescent treponemal antibody test: instrument and evaluation," by J. S. Lewis, et al. APPL MICROBIOL. 19:898-901, June, 1970.

SYPHILIS: SEROLOGY AND SERODIAGNOSIS

"Automated instrument for the fluorescent treponemal antibody-absorption test and other immunofluorescence tests," by G. F. Binnings, et al. APPL MICROBIOL. 18:861-868, November, 1969.

"Automated quantitative microhemagglutination assay for treponema pallidum antibodies," by P. M. Cox, et al. APPL MICROBIOL. 18:485-489, September, 1970.

"The automated reagin test: results compared with VDRL and FTA-ABS tests," by R. W. Stevens, et al. AMER J CLIN PATH. 53:32-34, January, 1970.

"Automatic apparatus for Wassermann and Reiter complement-fixation tests utilizing the 'discrete-analysis' principle," by R. E. Trotman. J CLIN PATH. 22:501-503, July, 1969.

"Automation of a flocculation test for syphilis," by B. E. McGrew, et al. AMER J CLIN PATH. 50:52-59, July, 1968.

"Behavior of cardiolipin and protidic antigens toward carate serums," by J. Breuillaud, et al. BULL SOC PATH EXOT. 61:190-194, 1968.

"Behavior of serum mucoproteins in the course of some skin diseases and in early syphilis," by Z. Cygan, et al. PRZEGL DERM. 56:1-5, January-February, 1969.

"Behavior of the VDS test and intradermoreaction with old tuberculin in subjects affected by non-tuberculous pulmonary diseases," by Z. Garnuszewski, et al. CLIN PEDIAT. 48:55-58, February, 1966.

"The biological false positive reaction to serological tests for syphilis," by M. F. Garner. J CLIN PATH. 23:31-34, February, 1970.

"Biologic false-positive reactions and infectious mononucleosis," by H. A. Cabrera, et al. TECHN BULL REGIST MED TECHN. 38:261-263, October, 1968.

"Biologic false-positive reaction for syphilis," by W. L. Palmer. JAMA. 204:833, May 27, 1968.

"The biological false positive reaction to serological tests for syphilis," by M. F. Garner. J CLIN PATH. 23:31-34, February, 1970.

SYPHILIS: SEROLOGY AND SERODIAGNOSIS

"Biological false positive Wassermann reactions in Uganda," by W. D. Foster, et al. BRIT J VENER DIS. 42: 272-275, December, 1966.

"Biologically false-positive serologic tests for syphilis due to smallpox vaccination," by L. J. Grossman, et al. AMER J CLIN PATH. 51:375-378, March, 1969.

"Biologic false-positive yphilis reactions," by L. Kornstad. T NORSK LAEGEFOREN. 86:1724-1828, December 15, 1966.

"A blood bank microscope," by T. E. Allen. AMER J MED TECHN. 32:421, November-December, 1966.

"Blood properidin in recent syphilis," by D. Bubola, et al. G ITAL DERM. 107:223-230, May-June, 1966.

"A brief review of syphilis serology," by W. J. Brown, et al. J AMER OSTEOPATH ASS. 66:1112-1118, June, 1967.

"Cardiolipin antigen in syphilis serodiagnosis according to data of the central dermatologic-venereological institute (1954-1955)," by L. S. Reznikova, et al. VESTN DERM VENER. 41:62-66, November, 1967.

"Case finding through ante-natal serological tests for syphilis," by J. A. Burgess. BRIT J VENER DIS. 42: 116-118, June, 1966.

"A case of (and for) syphilis maligna and negative serology," by D. J. Cripps, et al. ARCH DERM. 100:122-124, July, 1969.

"A case of malignant syphilis," by A. Zanca, et al. MINERVA DERM. 42:462-467, September, 1967.

"Chronic biologic false positive seroreactions for syphilis as a harbinger of systemic lupus erythematosus," by T. Putkonen, et al. ACTA DERMATOVENER. 47:83-88, 1967.

"Clinical significance of chronic biologic false positive Wassermann reaction and 'antinuclear factors'," by S. Berglund, et al. ACTA MED SCAND. 180:407-412, October, 1966.

"Clinical significance of nonspecific syphilis serological reaction," by K. Király, et al. ORV HETIL. 107:1441-1448, July 31, 1966.

"The colored treponemal intradermal test seen from the present immunologic standpoint," by G. Cocuzza, et al. DERM WSCHR. 152:699-702, July 2, 1966.

"Comparative evaluation of serological reactions in syphilis," by F. Osada, et al. JAP J CLIN PATH. 15: 435-438, June, 1967.

"Comparative experiments on syphilis serodiagnosis--results of the 1st and 2nd national quality control of syphilis serodiagnosis at the National University Laboratories," by Y. Fukuoka, et al. JAP J CLIN PATH. 16:365-372, April, 1968.

"Comparative serological diagnosis by classical and specific methods," by G. Elste, et al. DERM MSCHR. 155: 535-544, 1969.

"Comparative studies in syphilis among the RPR (rapid plasma reagin) card test, classical serology, the FTA test and the TPI test," by A. G. Bellone, et al. G ITAL DERM. 107:99-104, March-April, 1966.

"Comparative studies of cardiolipin and lipoid antigens in the diagnosis of syphilis," by D. Naumova. NAUCH TR VISSH MED INST SOFILA. 48:55-62, 1969.

"Comparative studies on the haemolytic and treponema pallidum immobilizing complement activity in the serum of different species," by F. Muller, et al. IMMUNOLOGY. 18:13-18, January, 1970.

"A comparative study of unheated serum reagin (USR) VDRL and CF tests for syphilis," by R. S. Saxena, et al. INDIAN J MED RES. 57:2203-2204, December, 1969.

"Comparison between the results of the Brewer rapid plasma reagin card test and other tests for syphilis," by B. S. Tio. BRIT J VENER DIS. 46:287-289, August, 1970.

"Comparison of fluorescent and conventional darkfield methods for the detection of treponema pallidum in syphilitic lesions," by R. Jue, et al. TECHN BULL REGIST MED TECHN. 37:123-125, May, 1967.

SYPHILIS: SEROLOGY AND SERODIAGNOSIS

"Comparison of the fluorescent treponemal antibody absorption and treponema pallidum immobilization tests on serums from 1182 diagnostic problem cases," by R. M. Wood, et al. TECHN BULL REGIST MED TECHN. 37: 55-58, March, 1967.

"A comparison of results of RPCF and TPHA with those of STS," by H. Usui, et al. BULL PHARM RES INST. 77:9-10, November, 1968.

"Comparison of the TPHA reaction with various syphilis serodiagnostic tests and its clinical significance," by A. Ozawa, et al. JAP J CLIN PATH. 16:911-916, December, 1968.

"Comparison of VDRL, RPCF, and FTA-ABS tests for syphilis," by R. H. Tanimoto, et al. HAWAII MED J. 28: 33-36, September-October, 1968.

"Comparison of the VDRL slide, TPI, and FTA-ABS tests in experimental syphilis in rabbits," by S. M. Mothershed, et al. BRIT J VENER DIS. 43:267-271, December, 1967.

"Comparison of various immunofluorescent procedures in the serological diagnosis of syphilis," by K. Király, et al. DERMATOLOGICA. 135:443-450, 1967.

"Complement and lysozyme requirements for spirochetolysis in guinea pig serum," by T. A. Nevin, et al. J BACT. 1388-1393, November, 1967.

"Complement fixation reaction with antigens prepared from T. pallidum," by K. Király. HAUTARZT. 19:36-42, January, 1968.

"Complement fixation test at cold temperature in the diagnosis of syphilis," by MIa. Gol'dberg. VESTN DERM VENER. 42:41-46, January, 1968.

"Complement-fixing and hemagglutinating antibodies to treponema microdentium," by C. R. Ghosh, et al. PROC SOC EXP BIOL MED. 124:559-562, February, 1967.

"Connective tissue disease and the chronic biologic false-positive test for syphilis (BFP reaction)," by A. M. Harvey, et al. MED CLIN N AMER. 50:1271-1279, September, 1966.

SYPHILIS: SEROLOGY AND SERODIAGNOSIS

"Contribution to the evaluation of immobilisin titre in the serologic diagnosis of syphilis," by I. Orhel. PRZEGL DERM. 53:705-714, November-December, 1966.

"A contribution to staining of treponema pallidum in tissue. IV. Staining of treponema pallidum in tissue of syphilid in test-rabbit and man," by M. Otani. BULL PHARM RES INST. 82:1-10, September, 1969.

"Cooperative studies on the serological tests for syphilis, especially the RPCF," by J. Tanaka. IRYO. 22:86-95, February, 1968.

"Correlation between fluorescent treponemal antibody absorption (FTA-ABS) results and the physicians' diagnoses," by S. S. Lindell, et al. J IOWA MED SOC. 58:1234-1239, December, 1968.

"Correlation between the quantitative F.T.A. test on serum and the qualitative F.T.A. test on dried blood. Preliminary note," by S. Sartoris, et al. MINERVA DERM. 42:14-15, January, 1967.

"A correlative immunologic, microbiologic and clinical approach to the diagnosis of acute and chronic infections in newborn infants," by C. A. Alford, et al. NEW ENG J MED. 277:437-449, August 31, 1967.

"Correspondence. Technique for iridocyclectomy," by M. Frenkel. AMER J OPHTHAL. 66:972-973, November, 1968.

"Critical review of the Chediak test," by G. Moch, et al. DEUTSCH GESUNDH. 21:1719-1722, September 8, 1966.

"Cryoglobulinemia presenting as 'factitial ulceration'," by R. D. Baughman, et al. ARCH DERM. 94:725-731, December, 1966.

"Cryoglobulins and rheumatoid factor in sera from chronic false positive seroreactors for syphilis," by K. K. Mustakalljo, et al. ACTA DERMATOVENER. 47:249-254, 1967.

"Culture and survival of treponema pallidum." WHO CHRON. 21:92-94, March, 1967.

SYPHILIS: SEROLOGY AND SERODIAGNOSIS

"Current concepts in the serological diagnosis of syphilis," by M. J. Allison, et al. VIRGINIA MED MONTHLY. 94:186-187, March, 1967.

"Current methods in the serological diagnosis of syphilis," by J. Delacrétaz. THER UMSCH. 26:67-70, February, 1969.

"Current serodiagnosis and treatment of syphilis," by S. Olansky, et al. JAMA. 198:165-168, October 10, 1966.

"Current serology of syphilis," by K. Király. ORV HETIL. 108:840-841, April 30, 1967.

"Current state of specific syphilis serology and its future perspectives," by L. Pospisil. CESK DERM. 44:102-107, May, 1969.

"Current trends in the clinical diagnosis and therapy of syphilis," by K. Kubec, et al. CESK DERM. 42:306-317, October, 1967.

"Current trends in the Reiter protein complement fixation test," by K. Nonaka, et al. NIPPON IKA DAIG Z. 34:374-375, 1967.

"Justification of serological examinations of lues during systematic examination," by R. Krunic, et al. VOJNOSANIT PREGL. 26:505-506, October, 1969.

"Definitive syphilis serology." S DAKOTA J MED. 20:31, February, 1967.

"Degranulation test of polynuclear basophils in rabbits: Shelley test. Clinical and experimental data," by J. Viallier, et al. ACTA ALLERG. 21:9-16, 1966.

"Demonstration of antibodies by fluorescence in syphilis," by K. D. Gregorczyk. DERMATOLOGICA. 133:327-330, 1966.

"Dermatological don'ts," by K. Riley. J S CAROLINA MED. ASS. 64:239, June, 1968.

"Detection of antitreponemal agglutins in the routine serological tests for syphilis," by G. Lomuto. G ITAL DERM. 109:117-126, March-April, 1968.

SYPHILIS: SEROLOGY AND SERODIAGNOSIS

"The detection of treponema pallidum by a rapid, direct fluorescent antibody darkfield (DFATP) procedure," by D. S. Kellogg, Jr. HEALTH LAB SCI. 7:34-41, January, 1970.

"Determination of hyaluronidase in cultured pale treponema," by N. F. Kalashchnikova. LAB DELO. 2:94, 1969.

"Development of immune haemolytic anaemia and thrombocytopenia in a chronic biologic false-positive reactor for syphilis," by K. Sievers, et al. SCAND J HAEMAT. 5:264-270, 1968.

"Diagnosis of early syphilis," by H. H. Volan. NEW YORK J MED. 66:2908-2912, November 15, 1966.

"Diagnosis of syphilis," by A. Perdrup. NORD MED. 75:483, April 28, 1966.

"The diagnosis of syphilis," by A. H. Wheeler. UNIV MICH MED CENT J. 32:67-76, March-April, 1966.

"Diagnostic significance of the fluorescent treponema antibody test (FTA)," by W. Manikowska-Lesinska. CESK DERM. 41:296-303, October, 1966.

"Dynamic changes in serum transaminases in patients with syphilis," by G. Spirov, et al. BRIT J VENER DIS. 42:129-131, June, 1966.

"Early syphilis: immunoglobulins reactive in immunofluorescence and other serologic tests," by A. J. Julian, et al. J IMMUN. 102:1250-1259, May, 1969.

"The effect of environmental temperature on the reactivity of the VDRL slide test," by J. F. D'Costa, et al. BULL WHO. 39:943-946, 1968.

"The effect of lysozyme and temperature on acceleration of the treponema pallidum immobilization test," by N. M. Ovchinnikov, et al. VESTN DERM VENER. 42:67-69, November, 1968.

"Evaluation of an automated fluorescent treponemal antibody test for syphilis," by E. M. Coffey, et al. BRIT J VENER DIS. 46:271-277, August, 1970.

"Evaluation of an automated serologic test for syphilis,"

by R. C. Bartlett, et al. AMER J CLIN PATH. 53: 494-497, April, 1970.

"An evaluation of the FTA-ABS test for syphilis," by W. E. Beam, Jr., et al. AMER J CLIN PATH. 47:404-407, March, 1967.

"Evaluation of a modified FTA-ABS test, multispot FTA-ABS," by P. O'Neill, et al. BRIT J VENER DIS. 46: 278-283, August, 1970.

"Evaluation of the plasmacrit test for use as a screen test for syphilis in the military," by C. E. Bushbee. MILIT MED. 132:262-264, April, 1967.

"Evaluation of quantitative reaction of immobilization of treponema pallidum by Nelson and Mayer (ITP) in the diagnosis of syphilis," by I. Orhel. MED GLAS. 22:157-160, May, 1968.

"Evaluation of RPCF and FTA in serological reactions of syphilis," by H. Ota, et al. J JAP ASS INFECT DIS. 42:131-135, August, 1968.

"Evaluation of the rapid plasma reagin card test (RPRCT) for serodiagnosis of syphilis," by G. P. Roxas, et al. MISSOURI MED. 66:37 passim, January, 1969.

"Evaluation of some new serological tests for diagnosis of syphilis," by L. D. Butovetskii. VESTN DERM VENER. 40:68-75, September, 1966.

"Evaluation of the sorbents used in the FTA-ABS test," by T. Rathlev. BRIT J VENER DIS. 44:295-298, December, 1968.

"An evaluation of the Technicon Autoanalyzer for automating complement-fixation tests," by C. E. Taylor, et al. J CLIN PATH. 21:521-526, July, 1968.

"An evaluation of the VDRL and FTA-ABS in a general hospital laboratory," by M. J. Allison, et al. TECHN BULL REGIST MED TECHN. 39:42-46, February, 1969.

"Evidence for the presence of circulating antibodies to an oral spirochete in the sera of clinic patients," by A. I. Steinberg. J PERIODONT. 41:213-214, April, 1970.

SYPHILIS: SEROLOGY AND SERODIAGNOSIS

"Experience with the treponema immunofluorescent absorption tests (FTA-ABS test)," by G. Palm. MED MSCHR. 24:58-60, February, 1970.

"Experiences with the fluorescent treponema antibody absorption technic (FTA-ABS) as compared to other serological diagnostic methods for syphilis," by L. Krell, et al. DERM MSCHR. 155:545-553, 1969.

"Experiment of study of immunofluorescent method in serodiagnosis of syphilis," by G. A. Zmechorovskaia, et al. LAB DELO. 1:22-25, 1968.

"Experimental studies on the kinetics of the TPI-test. I. Effect of rabbit homologous antibodies on test-treponema in vivo," by F. Muller, et al. Z IMMUNITAETSFORSCH. 134:54-68, November, 1967.

--II. Effect of rabbit-antibodies bound to the treponema in vivo on the result of the TPI-test and its reproducibility," by M. Pop-Aceva, et al. Z IMMUNITAETSFORSCH. 136:208-217, August-September, 1968.

-III. On the importance of the immobilizing complement activity for the TPI-test and attempts at their standardization," by F. Muller, et al. Z IMMUNITAETSFORSCH. 136:218-229, August-September, 1968.

--IV. On a titrimetic procedure for the exact determination of the endpoint in the immobilization of problem serums," by F. Muller. Z IMMUNITAETSFORSCH. 136:340-346, November, 1968.

--V. Differentiation between in vivo and in vitro presensitization by immobilizing antibodies from infected rabbits," by F. Muller, et al. Z IMMUNITAETSFORSCH. 138:264-272, July, 1969.

"Exploration of some cases of old syphilis by the study of treponema in the CSF, the response of the luo-test and the anamnestic serological reaction," by G. Tramier. BULL SOC FRANC DERM SYPH. 73:392-394, July-August, 1966.

"The FTA-ABS test," by C. H. Okey. J MAINE MED ASS. 57:145-146, July, 1966.

"The FTA-ABS test for syphilis. Performance in 1,033 patients," by J. M. Knox, et al. BRIT J VENER DIS.

42:16-20, March, 1966.

"The F.T.A.-ABS test in the diagnosis of neurogenic bladder," by J. M. Harper, et al. J UROL. 97:862-863, May, 1967.

"The FTA-ABS test in late syphilis. A serological study in 1,985 cases," by R. E. Harner, et al. JAMA. 203: 545-548, February 19, 1968.

"FTA-ABS test in pregnancy. A probably false-positive reaction," by C. S. Buchanan, et al. ARCH DERM. 102: 322-325, September, 1970.

"FTA and lysozyme," by A. Ribuffo, et al. MINERVA DERM. 42:433-434, August, 1967.

"F.T.A. in various stages of syphilis with the use of conjugated antigamma-globulin fractions," by P. Pagnes, et al. MINERVA DERM. 42:431-432, August, 1967.

"FTA test on dried blood. Quantitative evaluation," by S. Sartoris, et al. MINERVA DERM. 42:158-161, May, 1967.

"The FTA test on saliva," by S. Sartoris, et al. MINERVA DERM. 43:409-410, August, 1968.

"F.T.A. test with saliva in primo-secondary syphilis," by S. Sartoris, et al. MINERVA DERM. 43:23-26, January, 1968.

"The false-negative treponema pallidum immobilization test in syphilis. Pseudobiologic false-positive syndrome," by J. L. Smith. JAMA. 199:128-129, January 9, 1967.

"False-positive reaction to VDRL test with prozone phenomena. Association with lymphosarcoma," by K. D. Wuepper, et al. JAMA. 195:868-869, March 7, 1966.

"False-positive reactions for syphilis. Serological abnormalities in relatives of chronic reactors," by D. L. Tuffanelli. ARCH DERM. 98:606-611, December 11, 1968.

"False-positive reactions to the Reiter protein complement fixation (RPCF) test," by L. Forstrom, et al. BRIT J VENER DIS. 45:126-128, June, 1969.

SYPHILIS: SEROLOGY AND SERODIAGNOSIS

"False-positive serologic reactions induced by disinfectant," by R. W. Stevens, et al. AMER J CLIN PATH. 53:110, January, 1970.

"False-positive serological test for syphilis in pregnancy," by O. P. Salo, et al. ACTA DERMATOVENER. 49:332-335, 1969.

"False-positive serology," by W. C. Peterson, Jr. MINN MED. 52:1935-1936, December, 1969.

"False-positive tests for syphilis." BRIT MED J. 2: 394, May 13, 1967.

"Findings and considerations on the behavior of C reactive protein in various stages of syphilitic infection," by M. De Luca, et al. G ITAL DERM. 109:109-116, March-April, 1968.

"5 years of mass serological examinations for syphilis in the province of Arezzo," by E. Ninu, et al. ANN SANIT PUBBLICA. 27:1071-1082, September-October, 1966.

"A fluorescence microscopic study of adsorption onto treponema pallidum of a heat-labile serum factor," by M. Metzger, et al. ARCH IMMUN THER EXP. 15:819-828, 1967.

"Fluorescent antibody test for neonatal congenital syphilis: a progress report," by A. Scotti, et al. J PEDIAT. 75:1129-1134, December, 1969.

"The fluorescent antibody tissue stain in experimental ocular syphilis," by J. A. Wells, et al. ARCH OPHTHAL. 77:530-535, April, 1967.

"Fluorescence serological studies on the morphology of Reiter strain treponemas. I. Demonstration of a heat unstable antigen in the terminal filaments," by W. Bredt. Z MED MIKROBIOL IMMUN. 153:116-121, 1967.

--II. Demonstration of the cell membrane and localisation of group antigens." Z MED MIKROBIOL IMMUN. 153:122-128, 1967.

"Fluorescent-antibody techniques in the diagnosis of syphilis." LANCET. 2:327-328, August 6, 1966.

SYPHILIS: SEROLOGY AND SERODIAGNOSIS

"Fluorescent treponemal absorption and treponema pallidum immobilization tests in syphilitic patients and biologic false-positive reactors," by L. L. Bradford, et al. TECHN BULL REGIST MED TECHN. 37:59-66, March, 1967.

"Fluorescent treponemal antibodies in fractionated syphilitic sera. The immunoglobulin class," by W. G. Atwood, et al. ARCH DERM. 100:763-769, December, 1969.

"The fluorescent treponemal antibody-absorption (FTA-ABS) test. Development, use and present status," by E. F. Hunter, et al. BULL WHO. 39:873-881, 1968.

"Fluorescent treponemal antibody-absorption (FTA-ABS) test for syphilis," by W. E. Deacon, et al. JAMA. 198:624-628, November 7, 1966.

"The fluorescent treponemal antibody-absorption test (FTA-ABS) in treated latent and late syphilis," by L. Forstrom, et al. ACTA DERMATOVENER. 49:326-331, 1969.

"The fluorescent treponemal antibody absorption test for syphilis: a comparison with the treponema pallidum immobilization test and the fluorescent treponemal antibody test," by M. F. Garner, et al. MED J AUST. 1:404-406, March 9, 1968.

"Fluorescent treponemal antibody-absorption test reactions in lupus erythematosus," by S. J. Kraus, et al. NEW ENG J MED. 282:1287-1290, June 4, 1970.

"Fluorescent treponemal-antibody absorption tests. Studies of false-positive reactions to tests for syphilis," by D. L. Tuffanelli, et al. NEW ENG J MED. 276:258-262, February 2, 1967.

"Fluorescent treponemal antibody (FTA) reaction in sera with antinuclear factors," by E. J. Jokinen, et al. ANN CLIN RES. 1:77-80, May, 1969.

"The fluorescent treponemal antibody (FTA-200) test in the serodiagnosis of syphilis," by M. F. Garner, et al. MED J AUST. 1:548-550, March 18, 1967.

"Fluorescent treponemal antibody inhibition test," by A. E. Wilkinson. BRIT J VENER DIS. 43:186-190, September, 1967.

"Fluorescent treponemal antibody test with antihuman immune sera of different specificity," by K. Király, et al. ACTA DERMATOVENER. 48:362-369, 1968.

"Fluorescent treponemal antibody tests. A summary and comparison," by J. Puffer, et al. CALIF MED. 104: 166-167, March, 1966.

"Further studies of an automated flocculation test for syphilis," by B. E. McGrew, et al. AMER J MED TECHN. 34:634-643, November, 1968.

"Gamma-M-fluorescent treponemal antibody in the diagnosis of congenital syphilis," by C. A. Alford, Jr., et al. NEW ENG J MED. 280:1086-1091, May 15, 1969.

"Group antibodies in fluorescent treponemal antibody (FTA) test," by K. Király, et al. J INVEST DERM. 48:98-100, January, 1967.

"Haemagglutination test utilizing pathogenic treponema pallidum for the sero-diagnosis of syphilis," by T. Rathlev. BRIT J VENER DIS. 43:181-185, September, 1967.

"Hemagglutination tests for diagnosis of syphilis. A preliminary report," by T. Tomizawa. JAP J MED SCI BIOL. 19:305-308, December, 1966.

"How to interpret the serologic reactions to lipid antigens in syphilis and outside of it," by J. Delacrétaz. PRAXIS. 55:1497-1498, December 22, 1966.

"Immunoelectrophoretic study of biological false positive serum reactions for syphilis," by K. Király, et al. ACTA DERMATOVENER. 46:506-510, 1966.

"Immunofluorescence anticomplement: Analysis of the antibodies reacting with treponema pallidum," by J. Pillot, et al. C R ACAD SCI. 265:1769-1772, November 27, 1967.

"Immunofluorescence in tubes. Application to serologic study of syphilis," by P. Rimbaud, et al. BULL SOC FRANC DERM SYPH. 76:38-40, 1969.

"An immunofluorescence method for the diagnosis of primary syphilis using an absorption technique," by M. F. Garner, et al. J CLIN PATH. 21:576-577, September, 1968.

"The immunofluorescence reaction in syphilis," by N. M. Ovchinnikov, et al. VESTN DERM VENER. 40:59-63, July, 1966.

"The immunofluorescence reaction of the blood serum of syphilitic patients following therapy with various durable penicillin preparations," by T. V. Vasil'ev, et al. VESTN DERM VENER. 40:40-45, August, 1966.

"Immuno-fluorescence technic for treponema after adsorption of non-specific antibodies with Reiter's ultrasonicate in the diagnosis of syphilis. Apropos of 40000 sera," by A. Fribourg-Blanc, et al. BULL SOC FRANC DERM SYPH. 74:328-339, 1967.

"The immunofluorescence test (FTA-200) in the diagnosis of syphilis. Preliminary note," by A. Rocha, et al. HOSPITAL. 70:617-624, September, 1966.

"The immunofluorescence test for diagnosis of syphilis (FTA-200) performed with sera from lepromatous patients," by R. D. Azulay, et al. HOSPITAL. 71:79-85, January, 1967.

"The immunofluorescence test used in diagnosis of syphilis," by P. Latourelle, et al. MARSEILLE MED. 103:531-535, 1966.

"Immunofluorescent detection of treponema pallidum: a review," by D. S. Kellogg, Jr., et al. JAMA. 207:938-941, February 3, 1969.

"Immunfluorescent reaction in the diagnosis of syphilis," by L. A. D'iachenko. VESTN DERM VENER. 42:38-42, 1968.

"Immunological study on cardiolipin from Escherichia coli," by Y. Kanemasa. ACTA MED OKAYAMA. 22:241-249, October, 1968.

"Importance of the anti-complement immunofluorescence technic in serodiagnosis of experimental treponematoses in various animal species," by A. Vaisman, et al. BULL SOC FRANC DERM SYPH. 74:803-806, 1967.

SYPHILIS: SEROLOGY AND SERODIAGNOSIS

"Importance of serologically positive syphilis in Madagascar," by L. Mathurin, et al. MED TROP. 27:618-628, November-December, 1967.

"Importance of serology for the clinician," by J. Orfila. MAROC MED. 45:204-210, March, 1966.

"The importance of the treponema pallidum immobilization test in ophthalmology," by Z. Kumstat, et al. CESK OFTAL. 22:182-186, May, 1966.

"Incidence of biologic false positive syphilis reactions among pregnant women," by K. Loe. T NORSK LAEGEFOREN. 86:1728-1731, December 15, 1966.

"Incidence of biological false-positive reactions in serological tests for syphilis in 6737 patients with various dermatoses," by E. A. Johansson, et al. ANN CLIN RES. 2:32-41, March, 1970.

"Incidence of reactive VDRL tests in the normal rabbit," by J. S. Pannu, et al. BRIT J VENER DIS. 43:114-116, June, 1967.

"Indirect immunofluorescent test for the diagnosis of syphilis in cerebrospinal fluid," by M. E. Camargo, et al. REV PAUL MED. 69:15-24, July, 1966.

"Influence of treatment of biologic false positive syphilis tests in leprosy," by H. G. Ruge. INT J LEPROSY. 36:328-332, July-September, 1968.

"Initial serological reactions in infectious syphilis," by S. Dandoy. BRIT J VENER DIS. 43:105-110, June, 1967.

"Instant syphilis screening; evaluation of the rapid plasma reagin teardrop card test," by J. Glicksman, et al. TEXAS MED. 63:46-48, January, 1967.

"Interpretation of positive serological tests for syphilis in pregnancy," by A. Adeoba. BRIT J VENER DIS. 43:249-258, December, 1967.

"Interpretation of serologic reactions for syphilis," by J. E. Keilly. NEBRASKA MED J. 52:534-535, December, 1967.

"Intradermal treponemic color reaction (ITC) seen from

the present immunologic standpoint," by G. Cocuzza, et al. DERM WSCHR. 152:699-702, July 2, 1966.

"The intradermal treponemal color reaction in neurosyphilis," by C. Lazzaro, et al. ACTA NEUROL. 21: 287-292, May-June, 1966.

"An investigation of sorbing substances in the FTA-ABS test for syphilis," by G. R. Cannefax, et al. PUBLIC HEALTH REP. 83:411-416, May, 1968.

"Isolation of strains of treponema from endemic syphilis during a survey made in Senegal," by J. Malgras, et al. BULL SOC FRANC DERM SYPH. 76:515-516, 1969.

"It is time to clarify the results of serological reactions in syphilis," by A. I. Kartamyshev. LAB DELO. 2:82-83, 1969.

"Laboratory experience in RPCF, latex, RA, ASO and latex TA tests," by H. H. Chen. J FORMOSAN MED ASS. 67:134-141, April 28, 1968.

"Large-scale screening by the automated Wassermann reaction," by W. Wagstaff, et al. J CLIN PATH. 22: 236-239, March, 1969.

"Latex microreaction in syphilis, the Bordet-Wassermann cardiolipin test and Sachs-Witebski citochol test," by S. Kośmiderski, et al. POL TYG LEK. 24:721-722, May 12, 1969.

"Lipid composition of treponemal strains," by L. Vaczi, et al. ACT MICROBIOL ACAD SCI HUNG. 13:79-84, 1966.

"A logical notation of the degree of positivity of syphilitic sera by measuring the constant of the speed of complement fixation," by R. Vargues, et al. ANN BIOL CLIN. 26:621-631, May-June, 1968.

"Low frequency of chronic biological false positive reactors to serological tests for syphilis in rheumatoid arthritis and ankylosing spondylitis," by O. P. Salo, et al. ANN RHEUM DIS. 27:261-263, May, 1968.

"Management of patients with a positive serologic screening test for syphilis," by M. E. Seay. J FLORIDA MED ASS. 54:457-459, May, 1967.

SYPHILIS: SEROLOGY AND SERODIAGNOSIS

"Medical grand rounds from the University of Alabama Medical Center." SOUTHERN MED J. 61:719-727, July, 1968.

"Methodic and immunologic aspects of current syphilis serodiagnosis," by F. Muller. MUNCHEN MED WSCHR. 109:1591-1595, July 28, 1967.

"Modern methods of serological diagnosis of visceral syphilis," by L. D. Butovetskii. SOVET MED. 30:62-64, September, 1967.

"Modern serology of syphilis," by I. Orhel. RAD MED FAK ZAGREB. 17:103-110, 1969.

"Modifications to the automated Wassermann reaction," by V. W. Pugh, et al. J MED LAB TECHN. 23:126-128, April, 1966.

"Modified preparation of VDRL antigen suspensions," by L. R. Gorczyca. THE FILTER. 38:7-8, March, 1966.

"A modified technic for the complement deviation test in lues," by R. Bruno, et al. MINERVA DERM. 42:637-638, December, 1967.

"Multiple antigenic stimulation in vitro of lymphocytes of syphilis patients in various stages of the disease," by G. C. Chieregato, et al. MINERVA DERM. 43:264-269, June, 1968.

"Mutilative syphilis of the prepuce with positive serologic reaction at an abnormally weak level," by M. Renoux, et al. BULL SOC FRANC DERM SYPH. 75:749-750, 1968.

"Narcotic addiction with false-positive reaction for syphilis. Immunologic studies," by D. L. Tuffanelli. ACTA DERMATOVENER. 48:542-546, 1968.

"The necessity for heating sera for the VDRL slide test," by M. A. Lantz, et al. AMER J MED TECHN. 34:551-556, October, 1968.

"A new method of syphilis serodiagnosis by means of an 'in vivo' test," by P. Pophristov, et al. MAROC MED. 45:211-216, March, 1966.

"A new rapid serologic screening test for syphilis,"

SYPHILIS: SEROLOGY AND SERODIAGNOSIS

by J. E. Stauch, et al. MARYLAND MED J. 15:33-34 passim, June, 1966.

"A new serum reaction test of syphilis," by T. Iizuka. KANGO. 18:203, March, 1966.

"A new simple screening test for syphilis: the Portnoy reaction," by L. Surján, et al. ORV HETIL. 110: 762-764, April 6, 1969.

"New statistical contribution on the relationships between the Nelson-Mayer test and classical serological reactions (13,000) cases," by V. Resta, et al. MINERVA MED. 59:222-228, January 20, 1968.

"Nonspecific positive results of serodiagnostic reactions for syphilis and the possibility of their recognition," by G. Ehrmann. WIEN KLIN WSCHR. 81:213-217, March 21, 1969.

"Non-specific reactions to the quantitative fluorescent antibody test (FTA) in the elderly," by E. I. Grin, et al. BRIT J VENER DIS. 44:216-217, September, 1968.

"A note on the fluorescent treponemal antibody-absorption (FTA-ABS) test," by R. W. Stevens, et al. AMER J CLIN PATH. 47:408-409, March, 1967.

"Occurrence on biologic false-positive reactions with RPR (circle) card test on leprosy patients," by A. Achimastos, et al. PUBLIC HEALTH REP. 85:66-68, January, 1970.

"On an 'in vitro' stimulation of lymphocytes by treponema pallidum. Fluorescence-serological detection of gamma globulins," by H. J. Heitmann. HAUTARZT. 19:556-558, December, 1968.

"On certain properties and behavior of so-called luetic reagins: the problem of biologically false reactions," by M. Miklaszewska, et al. POL TYG LEK. 23:104-106, January 15, 1968.

"On the determination of treponeme immobilizing potency of weakly reactive sera and its suggested interpretation." BULL WHO. 33:705-720, November 5, 1966.

"On the FTA test," by K. Mizuoka, et al. JAP J CLIN

SYPHILIS: SEROLOGY AND SERODIAGNOSIS

PATH. 16:354-359, April, 1968.

"On the frequency of positive unspecific syphilis reactions in mononucleosis infectiosa," by G. Tauchnitz, et al. Z GES INN MED. 23:404-406, July 1, 1968.

"On the hemagglutination reaction using treponema pallidum as an antigen (TPHA)," by T. Tomizawa. JAP J CLIN PATH. 16:360-364, April, 1968.

"On the level of immobilisin in the blood of patients treated for syphilis," by I. Orhel. RAD MED FAK ZAGREB. 14:193-209, 1966.

"On the method of arrangement of the reaction of immobilization of weak treponema," by M. I. A. Goldberg. LAB DELO. 12:735-736, 1967.

"On the practical value of Nelson's test," by U. Boncinelli. MINERVA DERM. 42:618-620, December, 1967.

"On the problems of evaluation of 2 reactive tests in otherwise non-reactive spectrum in routine serology of syphilis," by A. Kern. HAUTARZT. 19:520-555, November, 1968.

"On the provocative effect of the T.P.I. Test Nelson-Mayer and a possibility of the therapeutic modification of the so-called seroresistant lues," by G. Ehrmann. ARCH KLIN EXP DERM. 227:993-1004, 1966.

"On the routine serology for detection of syphilis in pregnant women treated by the ONMI from 1956-1967," by A. Marcozzi. G ITAL DERM. 45:185-186, March, 1970.

"On sensitivity of the treponema pallidum immobilization test in late forms of syphilis," by M. V. Milich. VESTN DERM VENER. 42:62-65, July, 1968.

"On the serologic diagnosis of syphilis," by H. Bornemann. LEBENSVERSICHERUNGSMEDIZIN. 19:16-20, January, 1967.

"On syphilis serodiagnosis using treponema pallidum," by T. Tomizawa, et al. JAP J CLIN MED. 26:1003-1007, April, 1968.

"On the use of protein-polysaccharide complex of cultures of treponema pallidum as an antigen in the complement fixation test," by S. A. Ugrimov. LAB DELO. 10:618-620, 1968.

"The order of appearance of reactivity to treponemal and lipoidal tests in early syphilis," by A. Lassus, et al. ACTA PATH MICROBIOL SCAND. 69:612-613, 1967.

"Our experiences with the use of indirect fluorescence test in the serodiagnosis of syphilis," by P. Schneiderka, et al. CESK EPIDEM. 16:193-198, July, 1967.

"Past and future of the evaluation of syphilis serodiagnosis," by T. Ogata. JAP J CLIN PATH. 16:336-337, April, 1968.

"Pedagogical false-positive test for syphilis?," by A. L. Metzger. ANN INTERN MED. 69:1075-1076, November, 1968.

"Pediatric use of the rapid plasma reagin (circle) card test," by J. C. Herweg, et al. PEDIATRICS. 40:440-443, September, 1967.

"Performance and use of the Reiter protein complement-fixation (RPCF) test," by J. H. Bekker, et al. BRIT J VENER DIS. 42:42-43, March, 1966.

"Persistence of syphilis antibodies in the immunofluorescence reaction of treponema," by M. Hanczakowska, et al. PRZEGL DERM. 56:301-304, May-June, 1969.

"Pitfalls of the treponema pallidum immobilization test," by L. Pospisil, et al. CESK DERM. 45:187-191, August, 1970.

"A polyvalent latex slide test for rapid screening of syphilis in blood donors," by K. Lou, et al. BIBL HAEMAT. 29:1029-1032, 1968.

"The post-treatment disappearance of reactivity to treponemal and lipoidal tests in early syphilis," by A. Lassus, et al. ACTA DERMATOVENER. 50:148-150, 1970.

"Practical use of the auto-analyzer for the serodiagnosis of syphilis (study of 1,009 sera) using a cardiolipid antigen," by R. Gaillon, et al. PATH BIOL. 14:952-954, October, 1966.

SYPHILIS: SEROLOGY AND SERODIAGNOSIS

"The practical value of the immunofluorescence (FTA) test in the diagnosis and prognosis of syphilis," by A. Midana. MINERVA MED. 57:4438-4440, December 22, 1966; also in PANMINERVA MED. 9:181-183, May, 1967.

"The practical value of the Melangeur method of the treponema immobilization test," by S.G. Alieva, et al. VESTN DERM VENER. 42:46-50, January, 1968.

"Preliminary research on the classes of immunoglobulins which are responsible for syphilitic positive serologic reactions," by F. P. Merklen, et al. BULL SOC FRAN DERM SYPH. 75:57-61, 1968.

"Preparation and standardization of the sorbent used in the fluorescent treponemal antibody-absorption (FTA-ABS) test," by G. W. Stout, et al. HEALTH LAB SCI. 4:5-8, January, 1967.

"Preparation of fluorescein-labelled immune glubulin for the identification of treponema pallidum," by S. M. Mothershed, et al. BRIT J VENER DIS. 44:201-207, September, 1968.

"Present status of serological examinations of syphilis," by K. Mizuoka. NAIKA. 24:13-18, July, 1969.

"Preservation of serum antibodies in syphilis," by A. Vaisman, et al. BULL WHO. 34:461-466, 1966.

"The preservation of syphilis serum antibodies subjected to different temperatures," by A. Vaisman, et al. BULL WHO. 40:153-157, 1969.

"Principles and technique of a simple method to automate the complement fixation reactions," by R. Vargues. BIBL HAEMAT. 29:958-967, 1968.

"Problems in the evaluation of syphilis serodiagnosis," by K. Jo. JAP J CLIN PATH. 16:373, April, 1968.

"Proper interpretation of serologic tests for syphilis in the aged," by L. Nicholas. J AMER GERIAT SOC. 15:224-229, March, 1967.

"Properties of fragments of human Wassermann antibodies," by K. Amiraian, et al. IMMUNOLOGY. 10:349-353, April, 1966.

"Protein fractions of blood serum in patients with syphilis during Ecmonovocillin therapy," by T. A. Malygina, et al. VRACH DELO. 11:132-133, November, 1968.

"Provocation of the Nelson-Mayer TPI test and a possibility of therapeutic effect on the so-called seroresistant syphilis. II. Theoretical bases, further results of investigation and treatment," by G. Ehrmann. ARCH KLIN EXP DERM. 230:13-33, 1967.

"Quantitative F.T.A. test made with fluorescent fractionated anti-gamma globulin. I. Primary and secondary syphilis," by S. Sartoris, et al. MINERVA DERM. 43:219-223, May, 1968.

"Quantitative fluorescent treponemal antibody (FTA) studies with balanitis and 'problem' sera," by K. Király. PATH MICROBIOL. 29:75-83, 1966.

"Quantitative fluorescent treponemal antibody test using fluorescent fractionated antigammaglobulins," by S. Sartoris, et al. G ITAL DERM. 110:18-22, January, 1969.

"A quantitative method for the treponema pallidum immobilization test," by L.V. Sazonova, et al. VESTN DERM VENER. 44:63-66, January, 1970.

"Quantitative Reiter protein complement-fixation test," by O. P. Salo, et al. BRIT J VENER DIS. 43:264-266, December, 1967.

"A quick reagin reaction and the TPIT," by L. Pospisil. CESK DERM. 41:102, April, 1966.

"RPC of the month from the AFIP," by R. F. Kilcoyne, et al. RADIOLOGY. 94:687-690, March, 1970.

"RPCF test," by F. Osada. JAP J CLIN PATH. 16:348-353, April, 1968.

"Rapid card test for syphilis diagnosis," by P. Muller. SCHWEIZ MED WSCHR. 97:1196, September 9, 1967.

"A rapid macroscopic screening test for syphilis. II. Further evaluation," by F. M. Lucatorto, et al. J AMER DENT ASS. 73:100-101, July, 1966.

"The rapid plasma reagin card test for the diagnosis

of syphilis," by S. Nolting, et al. MUNCHEN MED WSCHR. 108:845-847, April 15, 1966.

"Rapid staining of treponema pallidum in tissue," by K. Ito, et al. BULL PHARM RES INST. 72:1-6, January, 1968.

"A rapid syphilis test (RPRC-test)," by P. Muller. DERMATOLOGICA. 135:238-242, 1967.

"Rapid technic for the Bordet-Wasserman sero-reaction with hemolytic complex," by P. Cirera. ANN BIOL CLIN 24:709-714, May-June, 1966.

"Rapid test for the diagnosis of syphilis with a treponema antigen," by E. Engelbrecht. PATH MICROBIOL. 29:553-557, 1966.

"Rapid test for syphilis in medical practice," by K. H. Simon. MED MSCHR. 23:466-468, October, 1969.

"Reaction of cardiolipin antigen," by T. Suzuta. JAP J CLIN PATH. 16:341-347, April, 1968.

"Reactions of treponema pallidum, especially to TPI, FTA, TPHA," by T. Tomisawa. JAP J CLIN MED. 26:304-309, February, 1968.

"Reactivations of immunofluorescence in certain cases of old syphilis," by G. Tramier, et al. BULL SOC FRANC DERM SYPH. 73:522-523, September-November, 1966.

"Reactivity in the FTA-ABS test of rabbits hyperimmunized with nonpathogenic treponemes," by G. R. Tringali, et al. BRIT J VENER DIS. 46:313-317, August, 1970.

"Recent progress in the serology of syphilis. Lues: selective rapid tests," by R. Martins, et al. REV BRASIL MED. 23:354-357, May, 1966.

"Recent progress in syphilis serodiagnosis--the complement fixation system (including cardiolipin reaction and RPCF," by F. Osada. JAP J CLIN MED. 26:293-298, February, 1968.

"Recent progress in syphilis serodiagnosis--precipitation and agglutination tests," by K. Mizuoka. JAP

SYPHILIS: SEROLOGY AND SERODIAGNOSIS

J CLIN MED. 26:299-303, February, 1968.

"Recent trends in syphilis," by K. Minami. JAP J CLIN PATH. 16:338-340, April, 1968.

"Reduction of nonspecific background staining in the fluorescent treponemal antibody-absorption test," by M. E. Roberts, et al. J BACT. 96:1500-1506, November, 1968.

"A reevaluation of the chronic biological false positive-phenomenon with the fluorescent treponemal antibody absorption test," by A. Lassus, et al. ACTA PATH MICROBIOL SCAND. 69:159-160, 1967.

"Reiter Protein Complement-Fixation (RPCF) test as a serological test for syphilis. A clinical study," by L. Forstrom. ACTA DERMATOVENER. 47:Suppl:59:1-65, 1967.

"The Reiter protein complement-fixation test using the auto-analyzer," by V. W. Pugh, et al. J CLIN PATH. 19:595-599, November, 1966.

"Reiter's spirochete agglutination reaction (Roemer's test). Correlation with the FTA test and with the classic serologic tests in different stages of lues," by G. F. Strani, et al. MINERVA DERM. 43:329-333, July, 1968.

"Reiter's spirochete agglutination test, Romer and Schilpkoter modification, in syphilis serodiagnosis (clinico-serological contribution)," by T. Cainelli. G ITAL DERM. 108:317-324, July-August, 1967.

"Remarks on lues serology of today. Si duo faciunt idem, non est idem," by H. Ruge. MED WELT. 19:1132-1135, May 10, 1969.

"Repositivation of Nelson's test in a syphilitic, induced by a nonspecific antigenic influence," by A. Bazex, et al. BULL SOC FRANC DERM SYPH. 73:113-116, January-February, 1966.

"Research on treponema in lymph glands of treated serum- and Nelson-negative syphilitics," by U. Boncinelli, et al. MINERVA DERM. 42:259-160, July, 1967.

"Results of the use of the treponema pallidum immobilization test and standard serological tests in syphilis," by G. A. Zmechorovskaia, et al. VESTN DERM VENER. 40:23-27, December, 1966.

"Reversed passive hemagglutination for serodiagnosis of syphilis," by J. M. Biasco-Zuasti, et al. J LAB CLIN MED. 72:670-673, October, 1968.

"The role of serum protein fractions on serologic tests in syphilis," by L. D. Butovetskii. VESTN DERM VENER. 41:67-70, July, 1967.

"Room temperature storage of treponema pallidum on microscope slides for use in the FTA-ABS test," by R. M. Wood, et al. APPL MICROBIOL. 17:335-336, February, 1969.

"Rubber latex in the slide microserological test of syphilis," by S. Kośmiderski. POL TYG LEK. 23:1639-1641, October 21, 1968.

"Search for treponemes in lymph nodes of treated serum- and TPI-negative syphilitics," by U. Boncinelli, et al. MINERVA DERM. 42:259-260, July, 1967.

"Secondary syphilis with negative serology," by F. Blez, et al. LYON MED. 223:860-861, April 19, 1970; also in BULL SOC FRANC DERM SYPH. 77:261-262, 1970.

"Sensitivity to 2-mercaptoethanol of reagins in human syphilis, in B.F.P. reactors and in 'normal rabbits. The macroglobulin nature of B.F.P. reagins," by G. Tringali, et al. RIV IST SIEROTER ITAL. 41:291-298, September-October, 1966.

"Serodiagnosis of syphilis," by W. J. Brown. JAMA. 205:800, September 9, 1968.

"The serodiagnosis of syphilis," by M. F. Garner. MED J AUST. 2:328-331, August 13, 1966.

"Serodiagnosis of syphilis," by L. Nicholas. ARCH DERM. 96:324-328, September, 1967.

"The serodiagnosis of syphilis and automation," by L. C. Norins. SALUD PUBLICA MEX. 10:601-606, September-October, 1968.

"Serodiagnosis of syphilis by fluorescent treponemal

antibody-absorption tests (FTA-ABS)," by K. Oikawa, et al. JAP J CLIN PATH. 17:538-544, July, 1969.

"Serologic control of Hungarian-made VDRL antigens," by L. Surján, et al. ORV HETIL. 109:1755-1757, August 11, 1968.

"Serologic reactivity in consecutive patients admitted to a general hospital. A comparison of the FTA-ABS, VDRL, and automated reagin tests," by P. Cohen, et al. ARCH INTERN MED. 124:364-367, September, 1969.

"Serologic study after inoculation of treponema pallidum in normal mice and mice thymectomized at birth," by J. Thivolet, et al. EXPERIENTIA. 25:304-305, March 15, 1969.

"The serologic syphilis test required for marriage in other states," by R. L. Cavenaugh. MARYLAND MED J. 18:33, May, 1969.

"Serologic testing for syphilis. Report from the Subcommittee on Serology of the Standards Committee of the College of American Pathologists," by M. F. Beeler, et al. AMER J CLIN PATH. 52:300-302, September, 1969.

"Serologic tests for syphilis among narcotic addicts," by W. D. Harris, et al. NEW YORK J MED. 67:2967-2974, November 15, 1967.

"Serologic tests for syphilis and the false-positive reactor," by K. D. Wuepper, et al. ARCH DERM. 94:152-155, August, 1966.

Serologic tests with sera from patients with lepromatous leprosy during the periods of exacerbation," by G. V. Mertslin, et al. VESTN DERM VENER. 40:41-43, October, 1966.

"Serological and epidemiological evaluation of the present methods of examination of blood donors," by S. Jasser, et al. POL TYG LEK. 22:1237-1239, August 14, 1967.

"Serological diagnosis of syphilis," by B. Hederstedt. NORD MED. 77:217-218, February 16, 1967.

"Serological diagnosis of syphilis," by F. Knierim, et

SYPHILIS: SEROLOGY AND SERODIAGNOSIS

al. BOL CHILE PARASIT. 22:21-26, January-March, 1967.

"The serological diagnosis of syphilis in dental patients," by M. Harris. BRIT J ORAL SURG. 4:235-239, March, 1967.

"Serological fluorescence studies on syphilitic veinous changes in animals," by H. J. Heitmann. DERMATOLGICA. 137:129-132, 1968.

"Serological resistance in syphilis and its causes," by M. N. Bucharowicz. PRZEGL DERMATOL. 57:621-630, September-October, 1970.

"A serological review of 156 patients presenting with primary chancres," by M. F. Garner. MED J AUST. 1:672-673, April 20, 1968.

"Serological tests for syphilis." LANCET. 1:1187-1188, June 1, 1968.

"Serological tests for syphilis," by H.R. Cayton. BRISTOL MEDICOCHIR J. 81:32-34, April, 1966.

"Serological tests for syphilis in diseases of the thyroid," by F. S. Ashkar, et al. JAMA. 213:872, August 3, 1970.

"Serological tests for syphilis in the elderly," by E. A. Johansson, et al. ANN CLIN RES. 2:47-50, March, 1970.

"Serological tests for treponemal disease in adults in two Jamaican communities," by M. T. Ashcroft, et al. BRIT J VENER DIS. 43:96-104, June, 1967.

"Serological tests for treponemal infection in leprosy patients. An evaluation of the fluorescent treponemal antibody absorption (FTA-ABS) test," by M. F. Garner, et al. BRIT J VENER DIS. 45:19-22, March, 1969.

"Serology in gyneco-obstetrics," by Y. Fukuoka. REV CHILE PEDIAT. 37:633-648, July, 1966.

"Serology of syphilis," by L. Rouquès. PRESSE MED. 74:1263-1264, May 14, 1966.

"Serology of syphilis and related aspects," by N. Ulker.

SYPHILIS: SEROLOGY AND SERODIAGNOSIS

TURK TIP CEM MEC. 34:277-284, 1968.

"Serology of syphilis in blood transfusion service," by F. Kail. BIBL HAEMAT. 32:247-249, 1969.

"Serology of syphilis in Tassili n'Ajjer (Central Sahara)," by P. Cirera, et al. BULL SOC PATH EXOT. 60:33-43, January-February, 1967.

"Sero-negative maternal syphilis. Report of a case," by A. E. Tinkler. BRIT J VENER DIS. 42:136-139, June, 1968.

"Serum mucoproteins in the course of certain skin disseases and in early syphilis," by Z. Cygan, et al. POL MED J. 8:682-686, 1969.

"The serum reaction to choroid melanin. Henry's reaction. Trensz's technique. 3. Physiopathological significance and practical value," by F. Trensz, et al. ANN BIOL CLIN. 24:1081-1096, October-December, 1966.

"Shelf life of fluorescent treponemal antibody-absorption test reagents," by M. E. Roberts, et al. J BACT. 96:1507-1511, November, 1968.

"The significance of the complement fixation test with protein fraction of treponema pallidum (TPCF) for serodiagnosis of syphilis," by L.D. Butovetskii, et al. VESTN DERM VENER. 40:52-57, November, 1966.

"Significance of the FTA-ABS test in diagnosis of lues. Comparison with the classical TPI test," by P. Schneiderka, et al. CESK EPIDEMIOL MIKROBIOL IMUNOL. 19:225-229, September, 1970.

"Significance of the FTA-test for primary syphilis," by J. Meyer-Rohn. Z HAUT GESCHLECHTSKR. 42:309-312, May 1, 1967.

"Significance of a low-titre V.D.R.L.," by D. G. McLone. J MED ASS GEORGIA. 56:60, February, 1967.

"Significance of a positive serological reaction in a subject originating from a tropical region," by P. Limbos. ACTA ORTHOP BELG. 32:755-764, September-October, 1966.

SYPHILIS: SEROLOGY AND SERODIAGNOSIS

"Significance of S. T. S. in skin diseases and syphilis," by N. C. Bhattacharya. INDIAN J DERM. 14:12-18, October, 1968.

"Simple anaerobic technique for the treponema pallidum immobilization test," by V. Bokkenheuser, et al. HEALTH LAB SCI. 6:162-163, July, 1969.

"A simple procedure for the preparation of diagnostic antigens from culture treponemes," by K. Kiraly, et al. Z IMMUNITAETSFORSCH. 134:32-44, November, 1967.

"Simplified complex of serological syphilis reactions in mass donor examination," by A. M. Chistiakov. LAB DELO. 2:83-86, 1969.

"A simplified method of performing the treponema pallidum immobilization test," by S. Stoianov, et al. VESTN DERM VENER. 41:11-14, April, 1967.

"Simplified method of serum dilutions for performance of the quantitative VDRL test useful for mass examinations," by A. Garlacz. PRZEGL DERM. 56:589-591, September-October, 1969.

"Simplified TPI test. Preliminary report," by T. Ikeda, et al. ACTA DERM. 63:323-327, November, 1968.

"The sixtieth year of the Wassermann Reaction," by T. A. Demchenko. LAB DELO. 1:3-7, 1966.

"Some data on evaluation of treponema pallidum immobilization test in syphilis (TIR)," by Kh N. Khidyrov. VESTN DERM VENER. 42:66-68, July, 1968.

"Some data on the serodiagnosis of syphilis in Surinam. II," by P. Kooy, et al. BULL SOC PATH EXOT. 59:65-70, January-February, 1966.

"Some observations on the sorbing agent used in the absorbed fluorescent treponemal antibody (FTA-ABS) test," by A. E. Wilkinson, et al. BRIT J VENER DIS. 44:291-298, December, 1968.

"Specificity of FTA-ABS and TPHA," by Y. Sasagawa, et al. JAP J CLIN PATH. 16:907-910, December, 1968.

"Specificity of the FTA-ABS test for syphilis," by D. M. Mackey, et al. JAMA. 207:1683-1685, March 3, 1969.

SYPHILIS: SEROLOGY AND SERODIAGNOSIS

"The specificity of various serological tests for syphilis. Further observations on the reactivity of leprosy sera," by H. G. Ruge. GERMAN MED MONTHLY. 12:337-338, July, 1967.

"Spirochaeta antigens," by G. Siefert. ERGEBN MIKROBIOL IMMUNITAETSFORSCH. 39:14-42, 1966.

"Spirochetes in late seronegative syphilis despite penicillin therapy," by J. L. Smith. MED TIMES. 96:611-623, June, 1968.

"Spontaneous deaths among rabbits inoculated with treponema pallidum less than 2 weeks before. Abnormal susceptibility in apparently normal laboratory rabbits indicated by serological tests for human syphilis," by B. B. Jorgensen. Z VERSUCHSTIERK. 10:46-54, 1968.

"Statistical evaluation of syphilis serodiagnosis," by S. Yamamoto, et al. JAP J CLIN PATH. 16:374, April, 1968.

"Status of serological testing for congenital syphilis," by F. D. Hoffmann, et al. J PEDIAT. 71:686-690, November, 1967.

"Studies of false positive serological tests for syphilis following smallpox vaccination," by O. P. Salo, et al. ANN MED EXP FENN. 44:304-306, 1966.

"Studies on the diagnosis of syphilis using the fluorescent antibody technic (absorption method)-FTA-ABS," by M. Murata, et al. JAP J CLIN MED. 26:466-474, February, 1968.

"Studies on durable long term preservation of stained preparations of treponema pallidum. Experiment I. Detection of treponema pallidum in testes of syphilitic rabbits by fluorescent antibody reaction," by H. Furukawa. BULL PHARM RES INST. 61:1-12, March, 1966.

"Studies on fluorescence-microscopy differentiation of antibodies in syphilis," by F. Muller, et al. ARCH HYG BAKT. 152:76-78, January, 1968.

"Studies on the fluorescent treponemal antibody (FTA) test," by A. E. Wilkinson, et al. BRIT J VENER DIS.

42:8-15, March, 1966.

"Studies on the fluorescent treponemal antibody test using fluorescent anti-gamma, anti-alpha, anti-mu, anti-lambda, anti-kappa chains and beta-1CA, E globulin reagents," by T. Matuhasi, et al. BULL WHO. 34: 466-472, 1966.

"Studies on immunofluorescence test for syphilis," by V. K. Gokhale, et al. J POSTGRAD MED. 12:13-25, January, 1966.

"Study of the antigenic relationships between treponema pallidum and borrelia hispancia," by J. Ranque, et al. MED TROP. 27:519-524, September-October, 1967.

"Study of a glycolipidic antigen of treponema reiteri and of the corresponding antibody contained in a human serum," by P. Dupouey, et al. ANN INST PASTEUR. 117:395-407, September, 1969.

"A study of the heat-labile antigen of treponema pallidum," by M. Metzger, et al. ARCH IMMUN THER EXP. 16:888-894, 1968.

"Study of the identification of Neisseria gonorrhoeae by fluorescent antibody technic," by N. Bansho. J JAP OBSTET GYNEC SOC. 20:1437-1445, November, 1968.

"Study on the serological diagnosis of syphilis using the TPHA-test," by T. Kawai, et al. SAISHIN IGAKU. 23:1929-1932, September 10, 1968.

"A study on the serological diagnosis techniques for syphilis," by B. Cacciapuoti, et al. ANN SCLAVO. 8:97-119, February 1, 1966.

"A study on the Wassermann and TPI antibodies in relation to histopathological findings in T. pallidum infected animals and man," by T. Fredriksson, et al. ACTA PATH MICROBIOL SCAND. 72:125-138, 1968.

"Substrates usable for absorption in the reaction of FTA-ABS," by M. Sepetjian, et al. PATH BIOL. 18:393-397, April, 1970.

"Supplementary findings on methods for the serodiagnosis of syphilis. I. Serological specificity of the antigen of treponema pallidum Reiter strain," by T.

SYPHILIS: SEROLOGY AND SERODIAGNOSIS

Tomizawa, et al. JAP J BACT. 21:251-255, May, 1966.

--II. On the specificity of the hemagglutination test and fluorescent antibody technic." JAP J BACT. 22: 607-611, December, 1967.

"Syphilis and serology," by E. E. Vella. MILIT MED. 132:243-251, April, 1967.

"Syphilis: evaluation of blood tests," by V. M. Torres Rodriguez. BOL ASOC MED P RICO. 60:414-421, September, 1968.

"Syphilis latex microreaction, the Bourdet-Wassermann cardiolipin test and the Sachs-Witebsky test," by S. Košmiderski, et al. PRZEGL DERM. Suppl:107-10, 1969.

"Syphilis reactions in leprosy sera. Mass screening tests," by H. Ruge. MED WELT. 48:2620-2627, November 26, 1966.

"Syphilis serodiagnosis: introduction," by N. Matsuhashi, et al. JAP J CLIN PATH. 16:335, April, 1968.

"Syphilis serodiagnostic findings during the course of disease," by J. Meyer-Rohn. DEUTSCH MED WSCHR. 94: 1037, May 9, 1969.

"Syphilis serology today," by A. F. Disalvo. J S CAROLINA MED ASS. 64:503-505, December, 1968.

"Systemic lupus erythematosus with oscillating syphilitic serology," by C. Grupper, et al. BULL SOC FRANC DERM SYPH. 76:497-502, 1969.

"The TPI and FTA-ABS tests in treated late syphilis," by W. G. Atwood, et al. JAMA. 203:549-551, February 19 1968.

"T.P.I. test and blastic transformation of lymphocytes in vitro," by A. Sapuppo, et al. MINERVA DERM. 42: 12-13, January, 1967.

"A technique for detecting treponema pallidum through the use of membrane filters and immunofluorescence staining," by F. W. Chandler, Jr. BRIT J VENER DIS. 45:305-307, December, 1969.

"Technic for the fluorescent treponemal antibody-absorption (FTA-ABS) test." HEALTH LAB SCI. 5:23-30, January, 1968.

"Tests for syphilis in young males. An analysis of a seven-year series from a Central Military Hospital," by O. P. Salo, et al. MILIT MED. 132:258-261, April, 1967.

"Three lipoidal tests in screening for syphilis and biological false-positive reactions in a dermatological series," by E. A. Johansson, et al. ANN CLIN RES. 2:42-46, March, 1970.

"Time saving method for staining treponema pallidum in tissue," by K. Ito, et al. HAUTARZT. 20:85-88, February, 1969.

"Timely serodiagnosis of lues and its evaluation with special reference to quantitative methods," by H. Roser. DEUTSCH MED WSCHR. 93:2017-2019, October 18, 1968.

"Treated late syphilis: immunoglobulin class of antibodies reactive with treponema pallidum," by L. C. Logan, et al. J INVEST DERM. 53:300-301, October, 1969.

"The treponema immunofluorescence absorption test (FTA-ABS). Studies on the technic of quantitative absorption and its significance for the specificity," by G. Schierz, et al. Z HAUT GESCHLECHTSKR. 43:9-16, January 1, 1968.

"Treponema pallidum immobilization reaction with fresh blood," by T. I. Milonova. VESTN DERM VENER. 44:56-58, April, 1970.

"The treponema pallidum immobilization test in oncological diseases," by S. G. Alieva, et al. LAB DELO. 8:484-487, 1966.

"Treponema reactions of syphilis," by K. Aho, et al. DUODECIM. 83:57-59, 1967.

"Treponemal and lipoidal tests in old treated syphilis. A clinical evaluation of 367 cases with special reference to the fluorescent treponemal antibody-absorption (FTA-ABS) test," by A. Lassus. ACTA DERMATOVENER. 48:Suppl:60:1-43, 1968.

SYPHILIS: SEROLOGY AND SERODIAGNOSIS

"Treponemal antibodies in non-syphilitic, positive anti-nuclear factor sera," by T. R. Neblett, et al. J INVEST DERM. 46:84-90, January, 1966.

"Treponemal immobilization tests in leprosy," by H. G. Ruge. BRIT J VENER DIS. 43:191-196, September, 1967.

"2 cases of nonspecific serologic reactions with high titers in patients with toxicodermia," by S. N. Dmitriev. VESTN DERM VENER. 43:85-86, September, 1969.

"2 cases of seronegativity in secondary syphilis," by M. F. Roitburd. VESTN DERM VENER. 42:82-83, August, 1968.

"Use of the auto-analyzer to perform serological tests for syphilis. Study of 1,009 sera using a complement fixation test with the cardiolipidic antigen," by R. Gaillon, et al. INT ARCH ALLERG. 32:278-281, 1967.

"Use of the automatic kinetic technic of complement fixation in the problems of syphilis serology," by R. Vargues, et al. ANN DERM SYPH. 94:265-272, 1967.

"Use of the F.T.A. test as a method of mass screening," by S. Sartoris, et al. MINERVA DERM. 43:18-22, January, 1968.

"Use of the plate micromethod for performance of the Bordet-Wassermann test with blood serum obtained from the finger-tip," by A. Garlacz. PRZEGL DERM. 56:773-777, 1969.

"Use of plate micromethod for studies in Bordet-Wassermann test," by A. Garlacz. PRZEGL DERM. 56:51-55, January-February, 1969.

"Use of slide technics in the mass screening for Bordet-Wassermann test," by A. Garlacz. PRZEGL DERM. 54:483-487, July-August, 1967.

"Usefulness of the hemagglutination test using treponema pallidum antigen (TPHA) for the serodiagnosis of syphilis," by T. Tomizawa, et al. JAP J MED SCI BIOL. 22:341-350, December, 1969.

"The usefulness of a modification of the fluorescent complement fixation test in syphilis diagnosis," by

SYPHILIS: SEROLOGY AND SERODIAGNOSIS

W. Zajac, et al. DERM MSCHR. 155:531-534, 1969.

"The utility of Reiter's complement fixation test in the prognosis of treated syphilis," by J. Lochmannová, et al. DERMATOLOGICA. 139:115-122, 1969.

"Reaction after vaccination against smallpox," by S. Smalik, et al. VNITRNI LEK. 12:152-155, February, 1966.

"The V.D.R.L. test. Significance of 'rough' results," by M. F. Garner, et al. BRIT J VENER DIS. 42:131-133, June, 1968.

"VDRL tests in representative communities of Guyanese adults," by M. T. Ashcroft, et al. BRIT J VENER DIS. 45:140-143, June, 1969.

"Value of the cardiolipin antigen prepared by the Institute 'Dr. I. Cantacuzino' for the flocculation microreaction of VDRL type," by M. Soresco, et al. ARCH ROUM PATH EXP MICROBIOL. 26:573-578, September, 1967.

"The value of the fluorescent treponemal antibody inhibition test for the diagnosis of syphilis," by J. Ruczkowska, et al. POL MED J. 8:497-508, 1969.

"Value of the fluorescent treponemal antibody inhibition test for the diagnosis of syphilitic infection," by J. Ruczkowska, et al. PRZEGL DERM. 55:287-298, May-June, 1968.

"The value of the immunofluorescence reaction in the control of syphilis cures. Reproducibility of the FTA test in dubious cases," by G. Leigheb, et al. MINERVA DERM. 42:261-263, July, 1967.

"Value of the immunofluorescent reaction after absorption of sera by Reiter's treponeme for serodiagnosis of syphilis," by A. Betz. BULL WHO. 34:154-160, 1966.

"The value of routine serological testing for syphilis in a mental hospital," by G. D. Banks. BRIT J PSYCHIAT. 114:113-114, January, 1968.

"Value of serology for the clinician," by J. Orfila. MAROC MED. 45:204-210, March, 1966.

SYPHILIS: SEROLOGY AND SERODIAGNOSIS

"The value of the treponema pallidum immobilization test (T.P.I.) in anomalous syphilis serology," by M. F. Garner. MED J AUST. 2:1101-1103, December 3, 1966.

"The value of treponemic agglutination test," by A. Galliera. FRIULI MED. 23:1-91, January-February, 1968.

"Wassermann." BRIT MED J. 5485:436-437, February 19, 1966.

"What does the Nelson test tell us," by G. Ehrmann. WEIN KLIN WSCHR. 78:6-10, January 7, 1966.

"What information may and may not be provided by the Nelson test?," by J. Langer, et al. CESK DERM. 41:31-32, February, 1966.

"What is the significance of a positive Wassermann or VDRL?," by D. G. Walker. J ORAL SURG. 27:748, September, 1969.

SYPHILIS: SERVICEMEN

"The current clinical aspect of recent syphilis in the navy. (3rd maritime region)," by J. Duluc, et al. REV CORPS SANTE ARMEES. 5:57-67, February, 1964.

SYPHILIS: TREATMENT

"Achievements in Soviet syphilidology," by M. A. Rozentul et al. VESTN DERM VENER. 41:12-20, October, 1967.

"Acute embolic-toxic induced incident in treatment of stomach syphilis with penicillin," by W. Lindheimer. THER GEGENW. 106:755-759, June, 1967.

"Agranulocytosis with monohistiocytosis associated with ampicillin therapy," by M. Graf, et al. ANN INTERN MED. 69:91-95, July, 1968.

"Antibiotics other than penicillin in the treatment of syphilis," by F. P. Merklen, et al. SEM THER. 42:93-95, February, 1966.

"Apropos of an unusual case of penicillin allergy," by M. Zivkovic. SRPSKI ARH CELOK LEK. 95:297-300, May, 1967.

"Behavior of treponema pallidum under the effect of

various antibiotics in the secretion from lesions in early syphilis in man," by K. Lejman, et al. PRZEGL DERM. Suppl:13-27, 1969.

"Bicillin-6 therapy in combination with pyrogenale and prodigiosane of patients with contagious forms of syphilis," by O. K. Loseva, et al. VESTN DERM VENER. 42:71-75, 1968.

"Can syphilis be controlled through treatment and epidemiology," by J. F. Donohue. REV AGRUP ODONT ARGENT. 20:1201-1203, 1968; also in SALUD PUBLICA MEX. 10: 607-610, September-October, 1968.

"Catamnestic studies of syphilis patients treated with arsenobenzene-penicillin-bismuth," by J. Rossberg. DERM WSCHR. 153:161-164, February 18, 1967.

"Cephaloridine in early syphilis," by L. Z. Oller. POSTGRAD MED J. 43:Suppl:43:128-129, August, 1967.

"Cerebrospinal fluid findings after treatment of early syphilis with penicillin. A further series of 80 cases," by W. L. Fernando. BRIT J VENER DIS. 42: 134-135, June, 1968.

"Changes in vaginal microbial flora during treatment with progestational hormones," by B. Ferrari, et al. QUAD CLIN OSTET GINEC. 21:1001-1008, December, 1966.

"Chinaroot in the 'Epistola de radicis Chinae usu' of Andreas Vesalius (1546)," by R. Schmitz, et al. SUDHOFF ARCH. 51:217-228, September, 1967.

"Cholesterol embolism in the course of antiluetic therapy," by P. H. Berghuis, et al. NEDERL T GENEESK. 113:2046-2049, November 15, 1969.

"Chlosterol embolism in the course of antiluetic therapy," by D. J. Vermeer. NEDERL T GENEESK. 114:172, January 24, 1970.

"Clinical criterion of cure in syphilis. Statistical method," by C. Rabito. MINERVA DERM. 42:238-243, July, 1967.

"Clinical picture of syphilitic lesions in 22 men infected by the same female partner," by M. Borkowski. PRZEGL DERM. Suppl:111-114, 1969.

SYPHILIS: TREATMENT

"Clinical relapse in early syphilis: unusual skin lesion following inadequate treatment," by R. H. Kampmeier, et al. J TENN MED ASS. 59:146-150, February, 1966.

"Clinical studies on chewable triacetyloleandomycin," by O. Kitamoto, et al. J ANTIBIOT. 20:410-414, December, 1967.

"Clinical treatment of patients with post-penicillin reactions after early syphilis therapy," by J. Bowszyc. PRZEGL DERM. 54:585-589, September-October, 1967.

"Clinico-laboratory studies of syphilis patients treated with bicillin-6," by A. A. Akovbian, et al. VESTN DERM VENER. 41:63-67, July, 1967.

"Comparative assessment of the treatment of syphilis patients with bacillin-3, -4 and -6," by A. A. Akovbian, et al. VESTN DERM VENER. 43:44-48, November, 1969.

"Congenital luetic hearing impairment. Treatment with prednisone," by M. E. Patterson. ARCH OTOLARYNG. 87:378-382, April, 1968.

"Congenital syphilitic labyrinthitis," by A. G. Kerr et al. ARCH OTOLARYNG. 91:474-478, May, 1970.

"Considerations on cutaneous reactivity in syphilis and its importance in the diagnosis of recovery," by A. Sapuppo. MINERVA DERM. 42:243-247, July, 1967.

"Co-operative evaluation of treatment for early syphilis. Preliminary report with special reference to spectinomycin sulphate (actinospectacin)," by J. B. Lucas, et al. BRIT J VENER DIS. 43:244-248, December, 1967.

"Cure of syphilis," by U. Boncinelli, et al. MINERVA DERM. 42:247-258, July, 11967.

"Current approaches to the problem of 'prophylactic' therapy of syphilis," by F. Ormea. MINERVA MED. 58:1201-1205, April 7, 1967.

"Current status of syphilis therapy," by A. Luger, et al. Z HAUT GESCHLECHTSKR. 43:875-886, November 1, 196

SYPHILIS: TREATMENT

"Current treatment of syphilis, particularly of early syphilis," by S. J. Ramos. REV BRASIL MED. 25:603-604, September, 1968.

"Diagnosis, control of course, and therapy of syphilis," by R. Schroter. THER UMSCH. 26:70-75, February, 1969.

"Diagnostic and therapeutic difficulties in late pulmonary syphilis in adults," by W. Kiesz, et al. WIAD LEK. 20:1181-1184, June 15, 1967.

"Drug treatment of syphilis," by K. Wereide. T NORSK LAEGEFOREN. 86:865-866, June 1, 1966.

"Early diagnosis and treatment of syphilis," by K. Higuchi. NAIKA. 23:1277-1284, June, 1969.

"Effect of debecycline on treponema pallidum," by J. Suchanek, et al. POL TYG LEK. 22:14-16, January 2, 1967.

"Effect of the fluorescein to protein ratio on antitreponema pallidum conjugates," by S. M. Mothershed. APPL MICROBIOL. 18:806-809, November, 1969.

"Effect of gentamicin on the motility of treponema pallidum," by H. Holzmann, et al. HAUTARZT. 20:404-407, September, 1969.

"The effect of specific treatment on the adrenal cortex function in patients with syphilis," by A. A. Shtein, et al. VESTN DERM VENER. 42:58-61, August, 1968.

"Effect of streptomycin on treponema pallidum," by J. Suchanek, et al. POL TYG LEK. 22:89-91, January 16, 1967.

"Effect of 2-mercaptoethanol treatment on anticardiolipin reactivity in sera from syphilitics and false positive reactors," by G. R. Tringali, et al. BRIT J VENER DIS. 45:202-204, September, 1969.

"Effect of V-cillin on treponema pallidum," by J. Suchanek, et al. POL TYG LEK. 22:46-48, January 9, 1967.

"Effects of 2-mercaptoethanol on treponemal antibodies in syphilis," by E. Csermely, et al. MINERVA DERM.

SYPHILIS: TREATMENT

42:418-419, August, 1967.

"Erythromycin in early syphilis," by W. L. Fernando. BRIT J VENER DIS. 45:200-201, September, 1969.

"Evaluation of therapy for early syphilis," by J. Kvicera. CESK DERM. 45:218-221, September, 1970.

"Experience in a shortened period of treatment of contagious forms of syphilis," by I. I. Pototskii, et al. VRACH DELO. 2:85-90, February, 1968.

"Experience of continuous treatment of early forms of syphilis with penicillin and bicillin," by L. A. Rozina. VESTN DERM VENER. 42:62-65, 1968.

"Experience with the treatment of early forms of syphilis in the region of Eastern Slovakia in 1966," by E. Malý, et al. CESK DERM. 44:188-194, October, 1969.

"Experimental studies in vivo on the effect upon treponema pallidum of some antibiotics other than penicillin," by A. Jakubowski, et al. PRZEGL DERM. 55:1-6, January-February, 1968.

"Experimental studies on the masking effect of antibiotics on the course of treponemal infections," by R. Mielech, et al. PRZEGL DERM. Suppl:63-67, 1969.

"Experimental studies on the treatment of syphilis with various antibiotics," by A. Jakubowski, et al. PRZEGL DERM. Suppl:57-61, 1969.

"Experimental under-treatment of early syphilis with probenecid and penicillin in anti-gonorrhoea dosages. A study to assess the best follow-up examination time for syphilis after gonorrhoea treatment in Greenland," by L. Hallinger. ACTA DERMATOVENER. 48:260-267, 1968.

"Fever therapy technique in syphilis and gonococcic infections," by H. W. Kendell, et al. ARCH PHYS MED. 50:503-508, October, 1969.

"Findings on the management of syphilis in military personnel," by A. F. Giordano. REV SANID MILIT ARGENT. 67:38-44, January-June, 1968.

SYPHILIS: TREATMENT

"First observations on the therapy of secondary syphilis with cephaloridine," by F. Flarer, et al. DIS NERV SYST. 27:271-277, September, 1966.

"Follow-up of reverin-treated patients in manifest, primary, secondary, tertiary and latent seropositive lues. IV," by V. Matanič. HAUTARZT. 17:121-123, March, 1966.

"Further findings on the anti-treponemic action in vitro of cephalosporins," by F. Galla, et al. ANTIBIOTICA. 4:309-313, December, 1966.

"Further observations on the persistence of treponema pallidum after treatment in rabbits and humans," by A. R. Yobs, et al. BRIT J VENER DIS. 42:116-130, June, 1968.

"Glitisol in syphilis," by M. Spiezia. ANN MED NAV. 71:247-252, March-April, 1966.

"A graphic guide for clinical management of latent syphilis," by A. J. Pereyra, et al. ARIZONA MED. 27:13-18, May, 1970; also in NORTHWEST MED. 69:Suppl: 13-18, May, 1970.

"Guiding principles for the treatment of early syphilis," by K. Mach. WIEN KLIN WSCHR. 79:97-99, February 10, 1967.

"Histochemical studies of syphilids during treatment with bicillin-4 and bicillin-6," by A. A. Akovbian, et al. VESTN DERM VENER. 42:38-41, December, 1968.

"How is initial syphilis mistreated?," by G. Solente. PRESSE MED. 75:1656, July 1, 1967.

"Immediate and remote results of the treatment of syphilis with antibiotics alone and in combination with bismuth," by G. B. Nesterenko, et al. VESTN DERM VENER. 43:37-40, May, 1969.

"Immediate results of treating patients with contagious forms of syphilis using simultaneously penicillin and bismuth preparations," by T. V. Vasil'ev, et al. VESTN DERM VENER. 44:50-55, April, 1970.

"The immunofluorescence reaction of the blood serum of syphilitic patients following therapy with various durable penicillin preparations," by T. V. Vasil'ev, et al. VESTN DERM VENER. 40:40-45, August, 1966.

"Immunohemolytic anemia following penicillin," by W. Straub. SCHWEIZ MED WSCHR. 97:1294, September 30, 1967.

"In relation to the article by V. N. Ivanov: 'Remote results of preventive treatment of children born of mothers suffering from or having sustained syphilis.' (Vestn Derm Vener No. 1, 1969)," by I. G. Bal'barer. VESTN DERM VENER. 43:63-64, November, 1969.

"Intermediate report of the experiences of the collaborative study group 'Therapy of Syphilis'," by K. Grabner. Z HAUT GESCHLECHTSKR. 44:849-856, September 15, 1969.

"Intravenous injection of reverin in syphilis," by Z. Matanič. MED GLAS. 20:193-198, May-June, 1966.

"The isolation and identification of the urinary oxidative metabolites of metronidazole in man," by J. E. Stambaugh, et al. J PHARMACOL EXP THER. 161:373-381, June, 1968.

"Loco-regional complication after benzathine penicillin," by G. Vasiliu, et al. PEDIATRIA. 17:75-78, January-February, 1968.

"Long-term results in the use of modern therapeutic methods in recent syphilis," by C. L. Meneghini, et al. G ITAL DERM. 108:391-400, September-October, 1967.

"Lupoid hepatitis following administration of penicillin. Case report and immunological studies," by J. P. Girrard, et al. HELV MED ACT. 34:23-35, December, 1967.

"Lytic effect of trypsin, lysozyme, and complement on treponema pallidum," by R. H. Jones, et al. BRIT J VENER DIS. 44:193-200, September, 1968.

"Management of syphilitic patients allergic to penicillin," by J. Lebioda, et al. PRZEGL DERM. 55:311-316, May-June, 1968.

"Meatoplasty," by J. P. Blandy, et al. BRIT J UROL.

SYPHILIS: TREATMENT

39:633, October, 1967.

"Metronidazole and syphilis." BRIT MED J. 4:4-5, October 7, 1967.

"Metronidazole and treponema pallidum." BRIT J VENER DIS. 43:149, September, 1967.

"Metronidazole in human infections with syphilis," by A. H. Davies. BRIT J VENER DIS. 43:197-200, September, 1967.

"Nature and extent of penicillin side effects with special reference to 151 fatal cases after anaphylactic shock," by O. Idsoe, et al. SCHWEIZ MED WSCHR. 99:1190-1197, August 16, 1969; also in BULL WHO. 38:159-188, 1968.

"A note on the effect of metronidazole on the Nichols strain of treponema pallidum in vitro and in vivo," by A. E. Wilkinson, et al. BRIT J VENER DIS. 43:201-203, September, 1967.

"On the antitreponemic action of cephaloridine," by F. Flarer. POSTGRAD MED J. 43:Suppl:43:133-134, August, 1967.

"On the clinical aspects and treatment of syphilis," by M. M. Zheltakov, et al. SOVET MED. 31:65-68, August, 1968.

"On the foundling of the syphilis therapy work team," by H. Weitgasser. Z HAUT GESCHLECHTSKR. 43:887-888, November 1, 1968.

"On the use of benzathine penicillin 'penduran' for the long term therapy of syphilis," by A. Kern. DEUTSCH GESUNDH. 21:1739-1750, September 15, 1966.

"Oral administration of new drugs in the treatment of recent syphilis," by G. Argenziano, et al. MINERVA DERM. 42:396-399, August, 1967.

"Overtreatment in cases with positive serological syphilis reactions," by C. Gjessing, et al. T NORSK LAEGEFOREN. 87:1981-1982, December 1, 1967.

"Parenteral cephaloridine treatment of patients with early syphilis," by J. M. Glicksman, et al. ARCH

SYPHILIS: TREATMENT

INTERN MED. 121:342-344, April, 1968.

"Passive cutaneous anaphylaxis with guinea-pig and rabbit antibodies to penicillin derivatives," by A. E. Cronin. AUST J DERM. 9:65-69, June, 1967.

"Pavilion 8. Dr. Carlos Seminario syphilis and skin services," by O. Dodero. PRENSA MED ARGENT. 55:1980-1983, December 6-13, 1968

"The penetration of bicillin-6 into the cerebrospinal fluid," by O. K. Loseva. VESTN DERM VENER. 41:47-51, August, 1967.

"Penicillin-bicillin treatment of patients with infectious forms of syphilis," by G. I. Egorov. VESTN DERM VENER. 41:42-46, February, 1967.

"Penicillin resistant syphilis," by M. A. Rozentul, et al. VESTN DERM VENER. 40:55-58, April, 1966.

"Persistence of treponemes after treatment of syphilis." LANCET. 2:718-719, September 28, 1968.

"Pimaricin," by J. Bret. SEM THER. 41:427-428, October, 1965.

"Pimaricin, an antibiotic towards fungi and trichomonads," by W. Raab. ARZNEIMITTELFORSCHUNG. 17:538-543, May, 1967.

"Planning and construction of dermato-venereological dispensaries," by N. M. Turanov, et al. VESTN DERM VENER. 43:56-59, February, 1969.

"Preliminary results of penicillin treatment in symptomatic early syphilis in 1959-1963," by J. Towpik. PRZEGL DERM. 53:29-32, January-February, 1966.

"Present state of experimental studies on the effect of antibiotics other than penicillin on treponema pallidum in vitro," by A. Jakubowski. PRZEGL DERM. Suppl:7-12, 1969.

"The problem of cure in syphilis," by F. Flarer. MINERVA DERM. 42:235-236, July, 1967.

"Prognosis in syphilis," by F. E. Rabello. AN BRASIL DERM. 43:243-260, December, 1968.

SYPHILIS: TREATMENT

"The prognosis of syphilitic infection. (Clinical, serological and statistical data)," by U. Boncinelli, et al. G ITAL DERM. 107:463-512, September-December, 1966.

"Prophylactic treatment of syphilis in human carriers of a recent blenorrhagic urethritis," by C. Grupper. SEM THER. 42:239-241, April, 1966.

"Remarks apropos of 5 cases of syphilis of the testis," by F. G. Marill, et al. BULL SOC FRANC DERM SYPH. 77:241-245, 1970.

"Remission possibilities in early seropositive syphilis using high doses of penicillin," by E. Maly, et al. CESK DERM. 45:63-69, April, 1970.

"Remote results of bicillin-3 therapy of patients with active forms of syphilis," by V. A. Rakhmanov, et al. VESTN DERM VENER. 40:43-45, October, 1966.

"Remote results of the continuous treatment of fresh forms of syphilis with penicillin and bicillin," by S. T. Pavlov, et al. VESTN DERM VENER. 41:8-11, April, 1967.

"Remote results of metallo-chemotherapy treatment of recent syphilis," by M. Lancellotti. MINERVA DERM. 42:260-261, July, 1967.

"Remote results of pyro-penicillin therapy of syphilis," by I. I. Pototskii. VESTN DERM VENER. 42:60-62, April, 1968.

"Remote results of the treatment of gonorrhea in girls with sulfanilamide preparations and antibiotics," by V. N. Matveev, et al. VESTN DERM VENER. 41:81-83, April, 1967.

"Remote results of treatment of syphilis patients with bicillin-1 and bicillin-3," by E. P. Nikol'skaia, et al. VESTN DERM VENER. 41:46-48, February, 1967.

"Remote results of the treatment of syphilitic patients with ecmonovocillin and heavy metal salts," by T. V. Vasil'ev. VESTN DERM VENER. 40:52-57, March, 1966.

"Remote results of treatment with metal-chemotherapy in recent syphilis," by M. Lancellotti. MINERVA DERM.

SYPHILIS: TREATMENT

42:28-34, January, 1967.

"Resistance of the manifestations of syphilis to the action of penicillin," by M. N. Bukharovich. SOVET MED. 31:137-138, March, 1968.

"Results of discussions on the treatment of syphilis," by A. A. Studnitsin, et al. VESTN DERM VENER. 42: 48-51, 1968.

"Results of syphilis therapy at the dermatologic clinic in Erfurt," by F. Schiller, et al. Z HAUT GESCHLECHTSKR. 43:691-696, September 1, 1968.

"Results of the treatment of recent syphilids with bismuth alone," by G. Falchi. G ITAL DERM. 107:683-689, September-December, 1966.

"Secondary syphilis after 1 injection of 2,400,000 units of penicillin for primary preserologic syphilis," by R. Degos, et al. BULL SOC FRANC DERM SYPH. 75:289-290, 1968.

"The significance of serum penicillin levels in syphilis therapy," by K. Mach, et al. Z HAUT GESCHLECHTSKR. 44:81-86, February 1, 1969.

"Some current problems of the treatment of syphilis based on data of the inquiry session of the Donets District Scientific Society Dermatovenerologists," by N. A. Torsuev, et al. VESTN DERM VENER. 41:65-69, August, 1967

"Some problems of the treatment of syphilis," by S. S. Gorbulev. VESTN DERM VENER. 40:75-77, September, 1966.

"Some remote results of the treatment of syphilis with bicillin-1, bicillin-3 and bicillin-4," by Kh N. Khidyrov, et al. VESTN DERM VENER. 41:47-50, June, 1967.

"Spinal fluid findings five years or more after infection in patients with early symptomatic syphilis treated with neo-arsphenamine bismuth," by F. M. Haagsma, et al. DERMATOLOGICA. 135:115-120, 1967.

"Statistical findings on the curability of syphilis," by G. Argenziano, et al. MINERVA DERM. 42:630-632,

SYPHILIS: TREATMENT

December, 1967.

"Studies of the value of erythromycin and oxytetracycline in treatment of early syphilis," by J. Bowszyc, et al. POL TYG LEK. 25:1394-1396, September, 1970.

"Studies on the disappearance of treponema pallidum from the eruption of early syphilis under the effect of various antibiotics. Effect of oxyterracine on treponema pallidum," by J. Suchanek, et al. POL TYG LEK. 22:1103-1106, July 17, 1967.

"Studies on the effect of most frequently used antibiotics on the course of syphilitic infection," by R. Mielech, et al. PRZEGL DERM. 55:143-149, March-April, 1968.

"Study of the therapeutic effectiveness of bicillin-6 in patients with communicable forms of syphilis," by O. K. Loseva. VESTN DERM VENER. 41:59-62, May, 1967.

"Study on the persistance of treponema pallidum in the lymph nodes of treated luetics," by U. Boncinelli, et al. G ITAL DERM. 107:1-14, January-February, 1966.

"Susceptibility of common pathogenic bacteria to seven tetracycline antibiotics in vitro," by N. H. Steigbigel, et al. AMER J MED SCI. 255:179-195, March, 1968.

"Symptoms 20 years after treatment of secondary syphilis," by S. Olansky. JAMA. 207:961, February 3, 1969.

"Syphilis therapy 1967," by W. T. Linton. APPL THER. 9:529, June, 1967.

"TPI and FTA tests in the evaluation of effectiveness of the oral treatment of early symptomatic syphilis with detreomycin, erythromycin and oxytetracycline with considerations of the clinical picture," by J. Lebioda, et al. PRZEGL DERM. Suppl:39-51, 1969.

"Therapy of early syphilis," by O. Braun-Falco. DEUTSCH MED WSCHR. 95:1611-1613, July 31, 1970.

"Therapy of early syphilis during the last 21 years at

the dermatologic clinic of Wiesbaden," by F. Nemec. Z HAUT GESCHLECHTSKR. 45:561-575, August 1, 1970.

"Therapy of early syphilis--review of the literature," by M. Pacenovska, et al. CESK DERM. 45:171-180, August, 1970.

"Therapy of early syphilis with cephaloridine," by O. A. González, et al. REV INVEST SALUD PUBLICA. 27: 201-214, July-September, 1967.

"Therapy of syphilis," by J. Obrtel. CESK DERM. 45: 154-159, August, 1970.

"Therapy of syphilis with penicillin with special consideration of the time factor," by A. Kern, et al. Z AERZTI FORTBILD. 60:1201-1206, November 15, 1966.

"Treatment of early and latent syphilis," by A. Steppert. THER GEGENW. 105:314-322, March, 1966.

"The treatment of early lues with oxtetracycline," by K. Bosse. HAUTARZT. 17:306-309, July 16, 1966.

"Treatment of early symptomatic syphilis with tetraverin 'Polfa'," by D. Janicka. PRZEGL DERM. Suppl:53-55, 1969.

"The treatment of early syphilis with cephaloridine," by O. A. González, et al. POSTGRAD MED J. 43:Suppl: 43-134-135, August, 1967.

"The treatment of early syphilis with vibramycin. Preliminary communication," by P. Wodniansky, et al. Z HAUT GESCHLECHTSKR. 44:571-574, September 1, 1969.

"Treatment of latent syphilis with jasomycin," by R. Osako, et al. J JAP ASS INFECT DIS. 43:44-48, May, 1969.

"Treatment of recent syphilis in the adult," by W. M. Stewart. SEM THER. 41:156-158, March, 1965.

"Treatment of syphilis," by G. Garnier. MAROC MED. 45:199-203, March, 1966.

"The treatment of syphilis," by D. H. Rasmussen. SURVEY OPHTHAL. 14:184-197, November, 1969.

SYPHILIS: TREATMENT

"Treatment of syphilis," by E. Skog. NORD MED. 76: 814-815, July 14, 1966.

"Treatment of syphilis," by T. H. Sternberg. WESTERN MED. Suppl:1:32-33, February, 1967.

"Treatment of syphilis," by V. A. Tomari. REV CORPS SANTE ARMEES. 7:533-553, August, 1966.

"Treatment of syphilis in 1967," by G. Leclere. UN MED CANADA. 96:833-836, July, 1967.

"Treatment of syphilis with antibiotics other than penicillin," by J. Towpik. POL TYG LEK. 25:1033-1036, July 13, 1970.

"Treatment of syphilis with demethyltetracycline (ledermycin)," by S. Nolting. MED KLIN. 61:2043-2044, December 23, 1966.

"Treatment of syphilitic patients with a single course of penicillin," by G. I. Egorov. VESTN DERM VENER. 40:68-71, May, 1966.

"Trial treatment of primo-secondary syphilis with intravenous perfusion of penicillin. Long persistence of seropositivity in favor of actual clinical penicillin resistance of treponema," by M. Bolgert, et al. BULL SOC FRANC DERM SYPH. 74:325-328, 1967.

"Use of doxycycline in the treatment of syphilis," by L. H. Paschoal, et al. HOSPITAL. 75:1965-1967, June, 1969.

"The use of pyrogenal in the treatment of late forms of syphilis," by A. K. Shcherbakova. VESTN DERM VENER. 41:43-47, June, 1967.

"Value and possibility of long-lasting penicillin therapy in early syphilis," by A. Kern. PRZEGL DERM. 54: 95-101, January-February, 1967.

"Value and security of a weekly injection interval in dispensing doses of 1.8 mega units of benzathine penicillin (penduran-AWD) during long-term therapy of early syphilis," by A. Kern. DERM WSCHR. 154: 608-616, June 29, 1968.

"Various experimental studies on the behavior of 3

SYPHILIS: TREATMENT

strains of treponema pallidum (Nichols strain, cortisone treated Nichols strain and Gand strain)," by P. Collart, et al. ANN DERM SYPH. 95:59-68, 1968.

"Venereal diseases. Introduction," by S. Hellerstrom. NORD MED. 76:797-799, July 14, 1966.

"Violent Herxheimer-Lukasiewicz reaction in the course of congenital syphilis," by A. Garlicka, et al. WIAD LEK. 21:1261-1264, July 15, 1968.

SYPHILIS: VOCAL CHORDS

"Gumma of the vocal cord. (Clinical record)," by H. K. Ismail. J LARYNG. 80:638-639, June, 1966.

TABES

SEE ALSO: SYPHILIS: ARTHRITIC
SYPHILIS: ARTHROPATHY

"An anatomo-clinical case of tabes and syphilitic aneurysm of the aorta. Its course under treatment," by M. Giroud, et al. LYON MED. 215:1603-1609, June 5, 1966.

"Carbamazepine for tabetic pain," by D. Alarcon-Segovia, et al. JAMA. 203:57, January 1, 1968.

"A case of tabetic mandibular fracture," by J. F. Laroche, et al. REV STOMAT. 71:74-76, January-February, 1970.

"Current status of tabes in Algeria," by F. G. Marill, et al. BULL SOC FRANC DERM SYPH. 77:245-248, 1970.

"Diagnostic difficulties in a case of tabes dorsalis as a cause of several operative procedures," by M. Kozik. POL PRZEGL CHIR. 38:801-803, August, 1966.

"Has the clinical picture of tabes dorsalis changed due to therapy," by H. Ley, et al. MUNCHEN MED WSCHR. 110:1924-1930, August 30, 1968.

"On a case of parafemoral ossification in a patient with tabes dorsalis," by G. Rava. ARCH SCI MED. 121:228-234, April, 1966.

"Segmental exzema reaction in a tabetic patient in the area of lancinating back pains," by G. W. Korting, et al. MED WELT. 45:2440, November 5, 1966.

TABES

"Studies on non-inflammatory lesions in neurosyphilis. 1. An autopsy case of tabes dorsalis combined with status dysraphicus and Alzheimer's fibrillary changes in the horn of Ammon," by T. Matsuoka, et al. BRAIN NERVE. 20:27-32, January, 1968.

"Surgical problems associated with tabes dorsalis," by M. T. Hoerner. INDUSTR MED SURG. 35:483-488, June, 1966.

"Tabes dorsalis," by C. L. Gerard. PROC MINE MED OFFICERS ASS. 46:23-26, May-July, 1966.

"Tabes dorsalis of sudden onset associated with possible transverse myelitis," by A. S. Wigfield. BRIT J VENER DIS. 46:262-263, June, 1970.

"The tabetic spine," by A. Passerini, et al. RADIOL. MED. 52:23-29, January, 1966.

"Tegretol, a new therapy of tabetic lightning pains. Preliminary report," by K. Ekbom. ACTA MED SCAND. 179:251-252, February 2, 1966.

"2 cases of spinal disease due to tabes dorsalis," by K. Fuse, et al. ORTHOP SURG. 19:518-523, June, 1968.

TEGRETOL

"Tegretol, a new therapy of tabetic lightning pains. Preliminary report," by K. Ekbom. ACTA MED SCAND. 179:251-252, February 2, 1966.

TERRAMYCIN

"Acute vaginitis and its treatment by a gynecologic terramycin foam. Clinical study and therapeutic results," by P. Magnier. GYNEC PRAT. 17:315-334, 1966.

"Individual prophylaxis in venereal diseases. Trial of a prophylactic silicon-terramycin ointment," by J. Duluc, et al. REV CORPS SANTE ARMEES. 8:91-98, February, 1967.

"Trial of a terramycin foam for local usage in treatment of vaginitis of bacterial and parasitic (trichomonas) origin," by M. Levrier, et al. GYNEC PRAT. 18:381-389, 1967.

TETRACYCLINE

TETRACYCLINE
SEE ALSO: DOXYCYCLINE
OXYTETRACYCLINE

"Gonococcal urethritis in males in Vietnam: three penicillin regimens and one tetracycline regimen," by L. H. Maurer, et al. JAMA. 207:946-948, February 3, 1969.

"Gonorrhoea in females treated with one oral dose of tetracycline," by D. G. McLone, et al. BRIT J VENER DIS. 44:218-219, September, 1968.

"Non-specific urethritis treated with pyrrolidinomethyl tetracycline nitrate," by C. B. Schofield, et al. BRIT J VENER DIS. 45:47-49, March, 1969.

"On the immunological reactivity of penicillin, cephalosporin and tetracycline antibiotics," by J. Lochmannova, et al. J HYG EPIDEM. 14:201-210, 1970.

"Oral tetracycline phosphate complex (tetrex) in the treatment of non-specific urethritis," by E. B. Wijetunga, et al. BRIT J VENER DIS. 45:50-51, March, 1969

"Possible mycoplasma hominis urethritis revealed by differing responses of 'abacterial urethritis' to treatment with tetracycline and erythromycin," by A. S. Grimble. BRIT J VENER DIS. 44:230-231, September, 1968.

"Relationships between the sensitivities in vitro of Neisseria gonorrhoeae to spiramycin, penicillin, streptomycin, tetracycline and erythromycin," by A. Reyn, et al. BRIT J VENER DIS. 45:223-227, September, 1969.

"Rolitetracycline by injection and tetracycline phosphate complex by mouth given in a single session in the treatment of gonorrhoea in males," by R. R. Wilcox. ACTA DERMATOVENER. 50:154-158, 1970.

"Six-city study of treatment of gonorrhoea in men using single oral doses of 1.5 or 3 G tetracycline hydrochloride," by C. E. Cornelius, 3rd. BRIT J VENER DIS. 46:303-333, August, 1970.

"Studies of venereal disease. I. Probenecid-procaine

TETRACYCLINE

"penicillin G combination and tetracycline hydrochloride in the treatment of penicillin-resistant gonorrhea in men," by K. K. Holmes, et al. JAMA. 202: 461-473, November 6, 1967.

"Susceptibility of common pathogenic bacteria to seven tetracycline antibiotics in vitro," by N. H. Steigbigel, et al. AMER J MED SCI. 255:179-195, March, 1968.

"Susceptibility of Neisseria gonorrhoeae to penicillin and tetracycline," by A. R. Ronald, et al. ANTIMICROB AGENTS CHEMOTHER. 8:431-434, 1968.

"Treatment of chancroid. A comparison of tetracycline and sulfisoxazole," by R. E. Kerber, et al. ARCH DERM. 100:604-607, November, 1969.

"Treatment of gonorrhoea with double doses of demethylchlortetracycline," by R. R. Willcox. ACTA DERMATOVENER. 49:103-105, 1969.

"Treatment of 'penicillin-resistant' gonorrhea in military personnel in SE Asia: a cooperative evaluation of tetracycline and of penicillin plus probenecid in 1263 men," by K. K. Holmes, et al. MILIT MED. 133: 642-646, August, 1968.

TETRAVERIN

"Results of treatment of gonorrhoea with tetraverin," by E. Chodyń, et al. PRZEGL DERM. Suppl:69-73, 1969.

"Treatment of early symptomatic syphilis with tetraverin 'Polfa'," by D. Janicka. PRZEGL DERM. Suppl: 53-55, 1969.

TETROID LACTIC

"Treatment of gonococcia with tetroid lactic," by H. Thiers, et al. LYON MED. 222:1172-1173, December 14, 1969.

THIAMPHENICOL

"Clinical experimentation with a new urinary antibiotic: thiamphenicol," by L. Timmermans, et al. ACTA UROL BELG. 34:349-353, July, 1966.

"On the effectiveness of low doses of thiamphenicol in the treatment of urethritis," by A. Riboldi. MINERVA DERM. 41:35-37, January, 1966.

THIOPHENICOL

THIOPHENICOL
"Notes on the treatment of gonorrhea with injectable thiophenicol," by H. Thiers, et al. LYON MED. 217: 589-591, February, 1967

THRUSH COLPITIS
SEE: MINOR VENEREAL DISEASES & INFECTION

THYADIONE
"Treatment of trichomonas colpitis with thyadione," by E. Vartiainen, et al. DUODECIM. 82:755-757, 1966.

THYROID
"Serological tests for syphilis in diseases of the thyroid," by F. S. Ashkar, et al. JAMA. 213:872, August 3, 1970.

TINIDAZOLE
"Tinidazole and metronidazole pharmacokinetics in man and mouse," by J. A. Taylor, et al. ANTIMICROB AGENTS CHEMOTHER. 9:267-270, 1969.

"Tinidazole, a new antiprotozoal agent: Effect on trichomonas and other protozoa," by H. L. Howes, Jr., et al. ANTIMICROB AGENTS CHEMOTHER. 9:261-266, 1969.

TREATMENT
"Advances in the treatment of venereal diseases," by C. B. Schofield. PRACTITIONER. 119:506-512, October, 1967.

"Clinical experience with sigmamycin in skin- and venereal diseases," by E. Heinke. MED WELT. 5:265-269, February 4, 1967.

"Clinical experimentation with rifomycin in dermatologic and venereal diseases," by L. Rasponi. G CLIN MED. 50:896-903, October, 1969.

"Consent for care," by D. A. Dukelow. J SCH HEALTH. 40:223, May, 1970.

"Current therapy of gonorrhea and syphilis," by A. C. Kind. WISCONSIN MED J. 69:218-219, September, 1970.

"Dermatologic-venereologic service in the BSSR," by O. P. Komov. VESTN DERM VENER. 43:79-81, June, 1969.

"Dermato-venerological service in Tadzhikistan," by

TREATMENT:

B. R. Rakhmatov, et al. VESTN DERM VENER. 42:63-66, April, 1968.

"How can venereal disease care be improved?," by V. Starck. LAKARTIDNINGEN. 65:2356-2359, June 5, 1968.

"National survey of venereal disease treated by physicians in 1968," by W. L. Fleming, et al. JAMA. 211:1827-1830, March 16, 1970.

"New viewpoints in the management of vaginal discharge," by H. Spitzbart. Z AERZTL FORTBILD. 61:117-119, February 1, 1967.

"On the therapy of skin and venereal diseases. Review of the literature 1965-1966," by H. Walther. DEUTSCH MED J. 19:171-176, March 5, 1968+.

"On the therapy of venereal diseases according to the current status," by W. Undeutsch. HIPPOKRATES. 39:89-97, February 15, 1968.

"On the treatment of bacterial skin infections and venereal diseases," by A. Steppert. WIEN MED WSCHR. 118:599-602, June 22, 1968.

"Prodigiozane in the therapy of skin and venereal diseases," by M. A. Rozentul, et al. VESTN DERM VENER. 40:46-47, October, 1966.

"Rifampicin in dermatology. Clinical trial," by E. Cappelli. ARCH MARAGLIANO PAT CLIN. 25:397-401, September-October, 1969.

"Rifampicin in dermatology and venereology," by L. Ayala. G ITAL DERM. 44:665-672, December, 1969.

"Syphilis and gonorrhea in general practice," by R. Schmitz. MED WELT. 11:434-437, March 14, 1970.

"Therapy of skin and venereal diseases. Review of the literature of 1967-1968," by H. Walther. DEUTSCH MED J. 20:480-485, August, 1969.

"Treatment of dermato-venereal diseases with chlorocide injections," by G. Maramarosi. THER HUNG. 14:11-15, 1966.

"The treatment of syphilis and gonorrhea," by E. J.

TREATMENT:

Gillespie. MED ANN DC. 35:372-374, July, 1966.

"Treatment of venereal diseases in The Royal Navy," by F. E. Willmott. J ROY NAV MED SERV. 54:254-257, Winter, 1968.

"Use of hetacillin in urogenital infections," by L. H. Rodriguez-Diaz. REV VENEZ UROL. 19:163-180, January-June, 1967.

"Viewpoints on the clinical aspects and therapy of venereal diseases," by J. Soltz-Szots. WIEN KLIN WSCHR. 77:1001-1003, December 24, 1965.

TRIACETYLOLEANDOMYCIN
"Clinical studies on chewable triacetyloleandomycin," by O. Kitamoto, et al. J ANTIBIOT. 20:410-414, December, 1967.

TRICHO-KOLPICORTIN
"Results of studies of a new local antitrichomonal agent 'tricho-kolpicortin'," by L. Kiss. PRAXIS. 58:58-59 January 14, 1969.

TRICHOMONIASIS
SEE ALSO: BEDSONIAE
MINOR VENEREAL INFECTIONS & DISEASES

"Apropos of the pathogenesis of trichomonas vaginitis," by D. Cazzola, et al. ANN OSTET GINEC. 88:683-691, September, 1966.

"Association of carcinoma of the uterine cervix and trichomonas vaginalis infestations. Frequency of trichomonas vaginalis in preinvasive and invasive cervical carcinoma," by O. Berggren. AMER J OBSTET GYNEC. 105:166-168, September, 1969.

"A clinical and laboratory study of trichomoniasis of the female genital tract," by H. E. Hughes, et al. J OBSTET GYNAEC BRIT COMM. 73:821-827, October, 1966.

"Clinical course of gonorrhea combined with trichomoniasis in males," by Ia I. Khasin, et al. VESTN DERM VENER. 41:69-70, December, 1967.

"Clinical studies of alimentary system disorders in trichomonas infections in women," by C. Todea. PRZEGL LEK. 23:565-568, July, 1967.

TRICHOMONIASIS

"Clinical studies on trichomonas vaginalis," by A. Motobayashi. J JAP OBSTET GYNEC SOC. 20:199-203, March, 1968.

"Clinical studies on trichomonas vaginitis," by S. Nohara. J ANTIBIOT. 19:253-268, August, 1966.

"Comparative cyto-histological studies on the precancerous and early stages of cervix carcinoma with simultaneous trichomonas vaginitis," by E. Boquoi. Z GEBURTSH GYNAEK. 169:59-74, 1968.

"Current aspects of vaginal trichomoniasis and candidiasis," by R. Bourg. BRUXELLES MED. 47:443-452, April 23, 1967.

"Current problems of urogenital trichomoniasis in males," by S. Scultety, et al. Z UROL. 60:311-316, May, 1967.

"Current views on vaginal trichomoniasis," by G. Leone. MINERVA MED. 61:913-918, March 7, 1970.

"Cystoscopic changes and trichomoniasis," by B. Zivkovic, et al. LIJECNVJESN. 91:1175-1178, 1970.

"Cytological and histochemical study of the epithelium in trichomonas colpitis," by E. I. A. Brezhneva. AKUSH GINEK. 45:13-16, August, 1969.

"Cytological, colposcopic and histological changes of the uterine cervix associated with vaginal trichomoniasis," by B. Azocar. REV OBSTET GINEC VENEZ. 26:129-140, 1966.

"Data on the clinical pathomorphological characteristics of post-trichomonas urethritis," by N. S. Liakhovitskii. UROL NEFROL. 32:40-43, January-February, 1967.

"Evolution of the 'problem' of trichomoniasis in the past 5 years," by G. Chappaz, et al. GYNAECOLOGIA. 161:36-48, 1966.

"Evolution of vaginal trichomoniasis from 1957 to 1964. Statistical discussion," by M. Gaudefroy, et al. J SCI MED LILLE. 84:409-422, September-October, 1966.

"Findings on trichomonas vaginitis--from the view of uterine cancer examination," by Y. Yokoyama, et al. SAISHIN IGAKI. 21:1585-1591, July, 1966.

TRICHOMONIASIS

"Fine structure of chromatic granules in trichomonas vaginalis Donne," by F. Filadoro. EXPERIENTIA. 26: 213-214, 1970.

"Genitourinary trichomoniasis," by F. Lillo. REV CHILE OBSTET GINEC. 33:367-374, 1968.

"Grave form of trichomoniasis and lambliasis," by N. Mosora, et al. MED INTERN. 18:857-864, July, 1966.

"Histopathologic studies of the vaginal mucosa in chronic trichomoniasis," by J. Plonski, et al. GINEK POL. 38:887-892, August, 1967.

"Hormonal function of the ovary in genitourinary trichomoniasis according to the urocytogram," by V. I. Kleban. PEDIAT AKUSH GINEK. 5:49-51, September-October, 1966.

"The incidence of trichomonas vaginalis in cases of pre-invasive and invasive cervical cancer. Relationship between cervical cancer and trichomonas vaginalis," by O. Berggren. LAKARTIDNINGEN. 64:3335-3340, August 31, 1967.

"Influence of trichomonas vaginalis on preinvasive non-radical treatment of carcinoma of the cervix uteri," by M. Wawrzkiewicz, et al. WIAD PARAZYT. 16:195-197, 1970.

"Latent trichomoniasis in men with gonorrhea," by M. A. Zelikman. VESTN DERM VENER. 40:55-58, January, 1966.

"Location of trichomonas vaginalis in the female genital tract," by E. Grys. POZNAN TWO PRZYJAC NAUK WYDZ LEK. 36:5-23, 1967.

"Male urethritis caused by trichomonas," by R. Fioccardi. MINERVA MED. 57:3189-3191, October 3, 1966.

"Male urogenital trichomoniasis," by M. De Luca, et al. MINERVA DERM. 41:315-340, September, 1966.

"Occurrence of trichomonas in the male urethra," by M. L. Antunes. REV ASS MED BRASIL. 11:213-214, May, 1965.

"Occurrence of vaginal trichomoniasis and mycosis in our material," by M. Valent, et al. BRATISL LEK LISTY.

53:573-577, May, 1970.

"On the transmission of trichomoniasis by thermal water," by G. Catar, et al. BRATISL LEK LISTY. 47: 196-204, February 28, 1967.

"Phagocytic capability of the vaginal trichomonas and its role in female infertility," by A. P. Kolesov. UKRANIAN PEDIAT AKUSH GINEK. 2:63, March-April, 1966.

"Pleuro-pulmonary localization of trichomonas," by L. Abed, et al. BULL SOC PATH EXOT. 59:962-964, November-December, 1966.

"Present aspects of urogenital trichomoniasis," by L. Scarpellini, et al. MINERVA GINEC. 19:668-681, July 15, 1967.

"Present status of female trichomoniasis in Okinawa," by T. Okawa, et al. SANFUJIN JISSAI. 19:201-203, February, 1970.

"The present status of urogenital trichomoniasis. A general review of the literature," by Z. Gallai, et al. APPL THER. 8:773-778, September, 1966.

"Psychosomatic aspects of female genital trichomoniasis," by G. Pinoli, et al. MINERVA GINEC. 21:508-511, April 30, 1969.

"Relation of TRIC agent to 'non-specific genital infection'," by E. M. Dunlop, et al. BRIT J VENER DIS. 42:77-87, June, 1966.

"Relations between trichomoniasis and male infertility. Preliminary note," by G. Argenziano, et al. MINERVA DERM. 42:388-391, August, 1967.

"Relative incidence of corynebacterium vaginale (haemophilus vaginalis), Neisseria gonorrhoeae, and trichomonas spp. among women attending a venereal disease clinic," by W. E. Dunkelberg, Jr., et al. BRIT J VENER DIS. 46:187-190, June, 1970.

"Role of the male in reinfestation of the female with trichomonas vaginalis," by L. Dao. GYNEC PRAT. 15: 25-28, 1964.

"Studies on immunity and allergy in ectopic infections

TRICHOMONIASIS

with trichomonas vaginalis," by A. Westphal, et al. Z TROPENMED PARASIT. 19:60-73, March, 1968.

"Studies on the occurrence and the frequency of various microorganisms (anaerobic bacteria, trichomonads, mycoplasms and yeasts) in the human vagina in vaginitis," by W. A. Muller, et al. ARCH HYG BAKT. 151:609-621, November, 1967.

"Studies on the risk of trichomonas infection in swimming pools," by J. Sarosiek. WIAD PARAZYT. 13:37-39, 1967.

"Studies on trichomonas vaginalis," by M. S. Grewal. INDIAN PRACT. 19:403-410, June, 1966.

"Studies on trichomonas vaginalis donne. IV. Size of the population of trichomonads in the vaginal secretions of women," by A. Kurnatowska. ACTA MED POL. 9:175-182, 1968.

"Studies on trichomonas vaginalis in the urological field. 1," by N. Kawamura. JAP J UROL. 60:15-24, January, 1969.

--2." JAP J UROL. 60:25-28, January, 1969.

"A study of 183 cases of leucorrhea: incidence of trichomonas vaginalis, candida spp., and hemophilus vaginalis," by Z. D. Desai, et al. J POSTGRAD MED. 12:91-98, April, 1966.

"The terrain favorable for trichomoniasis," by G. Chappaz. GYNEC PRAT. 17:391-396, 1966.

"Transmission of trichomonas," by R. D. Catterall, et al. BRIT MED J. 1:765, June 21, 1969.

"Trichomonas invasion and intraepithelial cancer of the cervix uteri," by R. M. Sokolovskii, et al. VOP ONKOL. 12:37-43, 1966.

"Trichomonas vaginalis and trichomoniasis," by O. Jirovec, et al. ADVANCES PARASIT. 6:117-188, 1968.

"Trichomonas vaginalis in general practice," by F. Bruhn-Petersen. UGESKR LAEG. 130:648-650, April 11, 1968.

TRICHOMONIASIS

"Trichomonas vaginalis, a review," by J. F. O'Sullivan. IRISH J MED SCI. 6:207-212, May, 1967.

"Trichomonas vaginitis and accompanying microflora," by H. Walecki, et al. WIAD PARAZYT. 15:307-308, 1969.

"Trichomonas vaginitis and sex circles," by T. Morita, et al. J JAP OBSTET GYNEC SOC. 21:1417-1423, December, 1969.

"Trichomoniasis and gonorrhea," by D. F. Hawkins. BRIT MED J. 2:116, April 12, 1969.

"Trichomoniasis and gonorrhoea," by W. Tsao. BRIT MED J. 1:642-643, March 8, 1969.

"Trichomoniasis-genitourinary disease and urological problem," by A. Drazancic. LIJECN VJESN. 91:1203-1207, 1970.

"Trichomoniasis, sterility and abortion," by G. Carvalho, et al. VIRGINIA MED MONTHLY. 96:444-448, August, 1969.

"Urogenital trichomoniasis in the daily consultation of the dermato-venereologist," by A. Kraus. DERM WSCHR. 152:97-103, June 29, 1966.

"Urogenital trichomoniasis in dermatologic practice," by H. Walther. DERM MSCHR. 155:988-989, 1969.

"Vaginal implantation of flagellates of trichomonas strains from the intestine and the effects on these flagellates to adapt," by P. Georges, et al. ANN PARASIT HUM COMP. 43:121-130, March-April, 1968.

TRICHOMONIASIS: CHILDREN & INFANTS

"A case of trichomonas vulvovaginitis in the newborn," by B. I. Bondarenko. PEDIAT AKUSH GINEK. 5:62-63, September-October, 1966.

"Clinical studies on trichomonas infections in girls," by I. Sipowicz, et al. WIAD PARAZYT. 15:337-339, 1969.

"Genital trichomoniasis in girls," by V. I. Rubnikov. VOP OKHR MATERIN DETS. 13:43-46, March, 1968.

TRICHOMONIASIS: CHILDREN & INFANTS

"The problems of urogenital trichomoniasis in prepubertal girls," by B. Beric, et al. GYNEC PRAT. 21:217-222, 1970.

"Trichomonas infection in an infant," by E. Grys, et al. PEDIAT POL. 41:969-971, August, 1966.

"Trichomonas infections in children," by A. Stolyhwo-Suchanek, et al. PEDIAT POL. 45:319-322, March, 1970.

"Trichomonas vaginalis infection in a newborn infant," by R. J. Blattner. J PEDIAT. 71:608-610, October, 1967.

"Trichomonas vaginalis: Urinary infection in a boy," by J. R. Harper. PROC ROY SOC MED. 60:897, September, 1967.

"Trichomonas vaginitis in young girls," by O. Jirovec, et al. GYNEC PRAT. 18:351-353, 1967.

"Urinary tract infection by trichomonas vaginalis in a newborn baby," by J. M. Littlewood, et al. ARCH DIS CHILD. 41:693-695, December, 1966.

TRICHOMONIASIS: COMPLICATIONS

"Abnormal bleeding in women with trichomonas vaginalis infection," by G. Terzano, et al. WIAD PARAZYT. 15:331-332, 1969.

"Dysplasias caused by trichomonas infections and dyskaryoses," by P. D'Alessandro, et al. QUAD CLIN OSTET GINEC. 21:1318-1328, December, 1966.

"Epididymitis due to trichomonas vaginalis," by I. Fisher, et al. BRIT J VENER DIS. 45:252-253, September, 1969.

"Genital and extragenital complications of trichomoniasis in men," by I. I. Iljin. DERM WSCHR. 154:294-300, March 30, 1968.

"Genital trichomoniasis and conjugal sterility," by G. Nicora, et al. GYNEC PRAT. 19:309-327, 1968.

"On the role of trichomonas infection of the sperm in sterility," by E. B. Bank. ZBL GYNAEK. 88:566-569, April 30, 1966.

TRICHOMONIASIS: CHILDREN & INFANTS

"The role of trichomonas urogenitalis in the development of adnexitis and its treatment," by B. Pejtsik, et al. Z GEBURTSH GYNAEK. 170:68-72, 1969.

"Role of trichomonas vaginalis in sterility," by P. Kostie. GYNEC PRAT. 15:467-469, 1964.

"The role of trichomoniasis in the development of portio uteri preblastomoses," by I. Szell, et al. ZBL GYNAEK. 89:312-323, March 4, 1967.

"The role of trichomoniasis in the development of precancerous state of the uterine cervix," by I. Szell, et al. ORV HETIL. 108:150-156, January 22, 1967.

"The role of urogenital trichomonas in the genesis of changes in the portio epithelium," by B. Toth, et al. ZBL GYNAEK. 91:547-551, April 26, 1969.

"The role of urogenital trichomonas infections in the incidence of changes in the cervix epithelium," by B. Toth, et al. ORV HETIL. 108:924-926, May 14, 1967.

"Studies on the pathogenic significance of female urogenital trichomoniasis with special reference to its effects of fertility," by D. Hofmann, et al. ARCH GYNAEK. 203:1-19, 1966.

"Trichomonal erosive-ulcerative balanoposthitis," by A. A. Avanesov. VESTN DERM VENER. 42:84-85, June, 1968.

TRICHOMONIASIS: DIAGNOSIS

"Active detection of patients with trichomoniasis," by L. M. Korik, et al. VESTN DERM VENER. 42:90-92, January, 1968.

"Attempts to standardize the trichomonas laboratory diagnosis," by W. A. Muller. DEUTSCH GESUNDH. 23:2041-2043, October 24, 1968.

"A biomathematical model for prevalence of trichomonas vaginalis," by J. Ipsen, et al. AMER J EPIDEM. 91:175-184, February, 1970.

"The changes in the pH levels of the vagina in infections with trichomonas vaginalis and candida," by H. Spitzbart. ZBL GYNAEK. 88:1680-1683, December 3, 1966.

TRICHOMONIASIS: DIAGNOSIS

"Characteristics of the colpo-cytological changes in women infested with trichomonas vaginalis Donne," by J. Teras, et al. WIAD PARAZYT. 15:327-329, 1969.

"Clinical and laboratory studies on vaginal trichomoniasis," by C. N. Nagesha, et al. AMER J OBSTET GYNEC. 106:933-935, March 15, 1970.

"Clinical picture of trichomonas hominis colitis and its differential diagnosis," by L. Cziraki, et al. ORV HETIL. 108:1850-1852, September 24, 1967.

"Colposcopic examination of patients with and after infection with trichomonas vaginalis," by K. J. Verschoof. NEDERL T VERLOSK. 68:269-272, August, 1968.

"Colposcopy and photo-colposcopy in the diagnosis of trichomonal colpitis," by F. A. Syrovatko, et al. AKUSH GINEK. 9:27-35, 1970.

"Colposcopy in the diagnosis of trichomonas vaginitis," by P. G. Kalov. AKUSH GINEK. 45:17-21, August, 1969.

"Comparative assessment of various methods of laboratory diagnosis of trichomonas infections," by G. A. Voskresenskaia. VESTN DERM VENER. 40:48-53, December, 1966.

"Comparative studies on the value of culture media Roiron, diamond and CPLM modified by Stepkowski in laboratory diagnosis of trichomoniasis," by B. Hoffmann, et al. WIAD PARAZYT. 15:271-274, 1969.

"Comparison of culture media for the growth of trichomonas vaginalis," by C. F. Rayner. BRIT J VENER DIS. 44:63-66, March, 1968.

"Detection of T. vaginalis in women. Comparison of 'wet smear' results with those of two cervical cytological methods," by R. N. Thin, et al. BRIT J VENER DIS. 45:332-333, December, 1969.

"Detection of trichomonas vaginalis in chronic urethritis in men," by J. Darewicz, et al. WIAD PARAZYT. 15:357-358, 1969.

"Determining trichomonas antigen for diagnosing trichomonas infection of the accessory sexual organs," by L. M. Korik. VESTN DERM VENER. 43:48-50, May, 1969.

TRICHOMONIASIS: DIAGNOSIS

"Diagnostic methods in human trichomoniasis," by I. V. Boldescu. REV MEDICOCHIR IASI. 71:397-402, April-June, 1967.

"Diagnostic methods for trichomonas vaginitis. (Microscopic examination before and after staining, culture examination, examination by fluorescence microscopy)," by G. Ortolani, et al. NUOVI ANN IG MICROBIOL. 17: 539-549, November-December, 1966.

"Diagnostic staining of dry smears for trichomonas," by R. G. Capet, et al. OBSTET GYNEC. 33:564-573, April, 1969.

"Direct microscopical examination of tube cultures for the detection of trichomonads," by G. I. Barrow, et al. J CLIN PATH. 23:91, February, 1970.

"The efficiency of microscopic, culture and serological diagnostic methods in the different clinical forms of genito-urinary trichomonadosis," by J. Teras, et al. WIAD PARAZYT. 15:359-361, 1969.

"Efficiency of microscopic examination of fresh smears and cultures in diagnosis of trichomonas vaginalis," by I. De Carneri, et al. AMER J OBSTET GYNEC. 100: 299-301, January 15, 1968.

"Evaluation of laboratory methods for detecting acute TRIC agent infection," by J. Schachter, et al. AMER J OPHTHAL. 70:375-380, September, 1970.

"Experience with the diagnosis of trichomonas vaginitis," by L. Grunner, et al. BRATISL LEK LISTY. 53:578-580, May, 1970.

"Immunofluorescence demonstration of antibodies in urogenital trichomoniasis. A preliminary report," by J. Kramar, et al. J HYG EPIDEM. 10:85-88, November 1, 1966.

"Importance of mass colpocytological examination in the diagnosis of uterine tumors in preclinical phases, of vaginal trichomoniasis and of prolonged pregnancy," by S. DeLeo, et al. MINERVA MED. 58:2821-2822, August 11, 1967.

"Improvement of culture media of trichomonas for rapid diagnosis," by R. G. Capet. CANAD J PUBLIC HEALTH.

TRICHOMONIASIS: DIAGNOSIS

   59:201-203, May, 1968.

"Inhibitory and toxic effect of various antibiotics on trichomonas and their practical use in the laboratory diagnosis of trichomoniasis," by B. Hoffmann, et al. WIAD PARAZYT. 15:425-428, 1969.

"Intradermal allergic reaction for the recognition of trichomoniasis," by L. M. Korik. UROL NEFROL. 31: 43-45, September-October, 1966.

"Intradermal allergic reaction in trichomonas infections in males," by K. Liubimova, et al. VESTN DERM VENER. 41:56-58, August, 1967.

"Isolation, cultivation, low temperature preservation, and infectivity titration of trichomonas vaginalis," by W. H. Lunsden, et al. BRIT J VENER DIS. 42:145-154, September, 1966.

"The laboratory diagnosis of vaginal infections caused by trichomonas and candida (monilia) species," by D. A. Eddie. J MED MICROBIOL. 1:153-159, August, 1968.

"Morphological study of vaginal trichomonas in cultures," by A. Noda. J JAP OBSTET GYNEC SOC. 20:1589-1598, December, 1968.

"New methods of diagnosis and treatment of vaginal trichomoniasis," by K. L. Keburlia, et al. VESTN DERM VENER. 43:55-57, January, 1969.

"New possibilities for the cultivation of trichomonas," by M. Valent, et al. CESK GYNEK. 32:414-416, August, 1967.

"Observations on the versatile symptomatology of trichomonas infections in women in gynecological practice," by H. Deis. MED WELT. 39:2095-2099, September 28, 1968.

"On the diagnosis of trichomonas infection," by V. Grunberger. WIEN KLIN WSCHR. 79:551-553, June 30, 1967.

"On the diagnosis of trichomonas invasion on dry smears by the method of luminescent microscopy," by I. A. Fridman, et al. LAB DELO. 1:14-16, 1968.

TRICHOMONIASIS: DIAGNOSIS

"On the distribution, incidence and laboratory diagnosis of trichomoniasis in Bulgaria," by N. Iankov, et al. AKUSH GINEK. 5:188-191, 1966.

"On the immunological diagnosis of trichomoniasis," by L. M. Korik. LAB DELO. 4:230-233, 1967.

"On the protective effect of blood sera of persons infested with trichomonas vaginalis Donne," by J. Teras, et al. WIAD PARAZYT. 15:481-483, 1969.

"On the value of the complement fixation test in the laboratory diagnosis of trichomoniasis," by N. Iankov, et al. AKUSH GINEK. 7:187-189, 1968.

"Pathogenicity of fresh isolates of trichomonas vaginalis; 'the mouse assay' versus clinical and pathologic findings," by B. M. Honigberg, et al. ACTA CYTOL. 10:353-361, September-October, 1966.

"Pitfalls in the diagnosis of trichomonas vaginalis by the Papanicolaou smear," by G. Perl. MT SINAI J MED. 37:632-634, September-October, 1970.

"Practical value of cytological and cytochemical diagnosis in trichomoniasis," by A. Marconato, et al. MINERVA GINEC. 18:954-955, September 15, 1966.

"Probable trichomonas vaginalis epididymitis," by A. D. Amar. JAMA. 200:417-418, May 1, 1967.

"The relationship of propagation of trichomonas vaginalis to the amount of inoculating material," by E. Grys. WIAD PARAZYT. 15:275-276, 1969.

"Review of current methods for the detection of trichomonas in clinical material," by J. Hess. J CLIN PATH. 22:269-272, May, 1969.

"Rosette-like variety of trichomonadosis granulocytica," by M. Z. Kwoczynski, et al. POL TYG LEK. 21:744-745, May 16, 1966.

"Serological studies on trichomonads," by E. Mannweiler, et al. Z TROPENMED PARASIT. 19:308-316, September, 1968.

"A simple diagnostic method in uro-genital trichomoniasis," by A. Pandele, et al. RUM MED REV. 12:70-73,

TRICHOMONIASIS: DIAGNOSIS

April-June, 1968.

"Simultaneous isolation of trichomonas vaginalis and collection of vaginal exudate," by D. H. Robertson, et al. BRIT J VENER DIS. 45:42-43, March, 1969.

"Some methods of serological proof of trichomonas infections in women," by J. Krupova. CESK EPIDEM. 17:162-168, May, 1968.

"Trichomonads and other flagellates from the vaginal secretion," by E. Dyner. WIAD PARAZYT. 15:309, 1969.

"Trichomonas and candida albicans as a cause of conjugal sterility. Proposal of a new fundic test," by S. Gaffuri, et al. MINERVA GINEC. 20:1260-1268, July 31, 1968.

"Trichomonas and haematospermia," by H. C. Walton. BRIT MED J. 1:514, May 24, 1969.

"Trichomonas infection and its importance to the cytological smear diagnosis," by J. A. Ruiz-Moreno, et al. GEBURTSH FRAUENHEILK. 26:231-243, February, 1966.

"Trichomonas vaginalis and accompanying microflora," by C. Zwierz. WIAD PARAZYT. 15:305-306, 1969.

"Trichomonas vaginalis in gram-stained smears," by G. E. Cree. BRIT J VENER DIS. 44:226-227, September, 1968.

"Usefulness of the addition of an antimycotic agent in the culture medium for trichomonas vaginalis," by D. Patrono, et al. NUOVI ANN IG MICROBIOL. 19:361-363, September-October, 1968.

"Vaginal trichomonas infections and sensitization of small laboratory animals," by A. Westphal, et al. Z TROPENMED PARASIT. 20:60-66, March, 1969.

"Vaginal trichomoniasis and cervix uteri changes," by A. Drazancic, et al. GEBURTSH FRAUENHEILK. 29:914-919, October, 1969.

"Vaginal trichomoniasis and lesions of cervical epithelium," by E. Guerresi. RIV ITAL GINEC. 52:819-

TRICHOMONIASIS: DIAGNOSIS

837, December, 1968.

"Vaginal trichomoniasis as a cause of false cytologic positivity," by G. C. Tosolini, et al. FRIULI MED. 23:807-817, November-December, 1968.

"The vitamin C concentration in the cervical mucus in women with and without trichomonas vaginitis," by B. Hoffman, et al. GINEK POL. 40:773-778, July, 1969.

TRICHOMONIASIS: EXPERIMENTAL

"Experimental studies on trichomonas vaginalis and trichomonacidal agents," by M. Nakae. NIPPON IKA DAIG Z. 34:269-284, 1967.

TRICHOMONIASIS: OCCURRENCE

"Epidemiologic study of trichomoniasis in normal women," by S. M. Naguib, et al. OBSTET GYNEC. 27: 607-616, May, 1966.

"Epidemiological study of vaginal trichomoniasis in the province of Udine," by G. C. Tosolini, et al. FRIULI MED. 23:723-744, September-October, 1968.

"Epidemiology of trichomoniasis in girls," by E. Gorzedowska. WIAD PARAZYT. 15:353-354, 1969.

"Frequence of treponematosis in various populations in Bolivia," by P. Cirera, et al. BULL SOC PATH EXOT. 61:184-190, 1968.

"Frequency of human trichomoniasis in relation to the seasons," by G. M. Jerzy. GYNEC PRAT. 15:227-238, 1964.

"On the distribution, incidence and laboratory diagnosis of trichomoniasis in Bulgaria," by N. Iankov, et al. AKUSH GINEK. 5:188-191, 1966.

"Present status of trichomoniasis in women in Fukushima prefecture," by T. Okawa, et al. J JAP OBSTET GYNEC SOC. 21:1360-1353, November, 1969.

"Results of a study on the occurrence of trichomoniasis in the Ostrava region," by J. Asmera, et al. CESK EPIDEM. 19:199-205, July, 1970.

"Status of trichomonas vaginitis among 15,000 women in Fukushima prefecture," by T. Okawa, et al. OBSTET

TRICHOMONIASIS: OCCURRENCE

GYNEC SOC. 19:93-96, January, 1967.

"Study of seasonal variations and general development of trichomonas vaginitis from 1957 to 1966," by M. Gaudefroy, et al. GYNEC PRAT. 18:355-379, 1967.

"A survey of trichomonal and Neisserian infection in antenatal patients," by R. Gaal, et al. MED J AUST. 1:634-635, April 13, 1968.

"A survey of trichomonal and Neisserian infection in antenatal patients," by R. A. Osborn, et al. MED J AUST. 2:92, July 13, 1968.

"Trichomonas infections in the province of Verona, social implications of their diffusion," by L. Caldera, et al. FRACASTORO. 61:289-292, May-June, 1968.

TRICHOMONIASIS: PREGNANCY
"Gonorrhoea, trichomoniasis and yeast infection in late pregnancy in an unselected series of gravidae," by E. Purola, et al. ANN CHIR GYNAEC FENN. 56:95-98, 1967.

"Importance of mass colpocytological examination in the diagnosis of uterine tumors in preclinical phases, of vaginal trichomoniasis and of prolonged pregnancy," by S. Deleo, et al. MINERVA MED. 58:2821-2822, August 11, 1967.

"The role of trichomonas and candida albicans as the principal cause of rupture of some perineorrhaphies after delivery," by D. Maroudi, et al. GYNEC OBSTET. 65:651-654, November-December, 1966.

"Treatment of trichomoniasis during puerperium," by R. Wawryk, et al. WIAD PARAZYT. 15:467-468, 1969.

"Trichomoniasis in pregnant women and its treatment with RP 8823," by M. Glowinski, et al. GYNEC PRAT. 15:239-246, 1964.

TRICHOMONIASIS: TREATMENT
"Action and secondary action of metronidazol in the therapy of trichomoniasis," by K. Wiesner, et al. FORTSCHR ARZNEIMITTELFORSCH. 9:361-391, 1966.

"Alpha-chloromethyl-2-methyl-5-nitro-1-imidazole ethanol (RO 7-0207), a substance exhibiting antiparasitic activity against amoebae, trichomonads, and pinworms," by E. Grunberg, et al. PROC SOC EXP BIOL MED. 133: 490-492, February, 1970.

"Ambulatory treatment of trichomonas infections in industrial and rural population," by T. Lopatecki. WIAD LEK. 22:11-13, January 1, 1969.

"The amoebicidal, trichomonicidal, and antibacterial effects of niridazole in laboratory animals," by F. Kradolfer, et al. ANN NY ACAD SCI. 160:740-748, October 6, 1969.

"Balneotherapy in trichomonas vaginitis," by R. Dionigi. QUAD CLIN OSTET GINEC. 21:1258-1268, December, 1966.

"Behavior of trichomonas vaginalis in women treated with radiation energy and cytostatic drugs," by J. Zawadzki, et al. WIAD PARAZYT. 13:729-732, 1967.

"Certain problems of dispensarization and treatment of trichomoniasis in males," by M. G. Manikhas, et al. VESTN DERM VENER. 43:60-62, November, 1969.

"Changes in the nuclear ultrastructure observed in trichomonas vaginalis after treatment with metronidazole," by D. Panaitescu, et al. MICROBIOLOGIA. 15: 43-48, January-February, 1970.

"Changes occurring in the composition of the vaginal bacterial flora accompanying trichomonas vaginalis in women treated with gamma- and x-rays," by E. Slowakiewicz, et al. WIAD PARAZYT. 15:449-451, 1969.

"Chemotherapy of trichomoniasis," by R. M. Michaels. ADVANCES CHEMOTHER. 3:39-108, 1968.

"Clinical evaluation of metronidazole 'Polfa' in the treatment of trichomoniasis in women," by C. Zwierz, et al. WIAD PARAZYT. 15:387-388, 1969.

"Clinical investigations on a new treatment of vaginal trichomoniasis," by F. Destro, et al. HOSPITAL. 75:1065-1072, March, 1969.

"A clinical study of the efficacy of levorin in urogenital trichomoniasis," by I. I. Il'in. VESTN DERM VENER. 41:87-88, September, 1967.

TRICHOMONIASIS: TREATMENT

"Clinical test of a drug: nitroimidazine (1-N-Beta-ethylmorpholin-5-nitroimidazole) in genital trichomoniasis," by J. E. Zuniga, et al. REV COLUMBIA OBSTET GINEC. 21:193-196, March-April, 1970.

"Clinical tests using iodopovidone in patients with vaginal trichomoniasis," by A. A. Rustrian, et al. GINEC OBSTET MEX. 27:467-470, April, 1970.

"Comparative assessment of the treatment of trichomonad-urethritis in males with iodinol and ACD preparations," by L. M. Korik, et al. VESTN DERM VENER. 40:62-65, March, 1966.

"Comparative efficacy of the use of metronidazole of diverse manufacture in the treatment of patients with trichomoniasis," by M. M. Dadashzade. UROL NEFROL. 32:39-41, July-August, 1967.

"Contribution to the resistance of trichomonas vaginalis to metronidazole," by M. Valent, et al. BRATISL LEK LISTY. 52:58-61, July, 1969.

"Determination of therapeutic effects and therapeutic standards of anti-trichomonal agents," by S. Mizuno, et al. J JAP OBSTET GYNEC SOC. 21:198-203, February, 1969.

"Determination of trichomonas antigen in trichomoniasis," by L. M. Korik. VESTN DERM VENER. 40:50-55, January, 1966.

"Drug resistance of trichomonas vaginalis," by L. Slucki. WIAD LEK. 21:541-544, April 1, 1968; also in WIAD PARAZYT. 15:477-478, 1969.

"Effect of albothyl in trichomonas vaginalis infection on the changes in vaginal environment," by J. Fidler, et al. WIAD PARAZYT. 15:453-454, 1969.

"Effect of an anti-fungal agent, pimaricin, on trichomonas vaginalis in vitro," by K. Asami, et al. J ANTIBIOT. 20:344-346, October, 1967.

"Effect of desiccation of the vaginal contents on the vitality of trichomonas vaginalis," by E. Grys. WIAD PARAZYT. 15:285-286, 1969.

"Effect of high doses of antibiotics on the course of

trichomoniasis in women," by W. Jacyk, et al. WIAD PARAZYT. 15:423-424, 1969.

"The effect of metronidazole on the inflammatory changes in trichomonas vaginitis," by J. Mleziva, et al. ZBL GYNAEK. 90:425-431, March 23, 1968.

"The effect of metronidazole therapy on cervical histology in trichomoniasis," by B. Gray, et al. J OBSTET GYNAEC BRIT COMM. 74:98-103, February, 1967.

"Effect of new chlorosulfonamides on the female vagina. Considering trichomoniasis complicated by mycosis. Experimental part," by A. Kurnatowska. WIAD PARAZYT. 15:19-33, 1969.

"Effect of pimaricin on vaginal trichomoniasis," by H. Wada, et al. J ANTIBIOT. 20:281-284, August, 1967.

"Effect of temperature and environment on the vitality of the trichomonas vaginalis," by E. Grys. WIAD PARAZYT. 15:281-283, 1969.

"Evaluation of the nitrimidazine activity in giardiasis and genital trichomoniasis," by J. M. Salles, et al. HOSPITAL. 1689-1697, May, 1970.

"Experience in the dispensarization and treatment of trichomoniasis with flagyl," by I. I. Shkliar. VESTN DERM VENER. 41:67-70, May, 1967.

"Experience in the treatment of trichomonas urogenital infection in males with flagyl," by M. M. Dadash-Zade. VESTN DERM VENER. 41:87-89, August, 1967.

"Experience in the treatment of trichomoniasis in women with flagyl," by A. M. Mezhebovskii, et al. AKUSH GINEK. 42:45-46, February, 1966.

"Experience with therapy of urogenital trichomoniasis in males with a new indigenous preparation, chlomizole," by F. B. Potapnev. VESTN DERM VENER. 42:41-46, December, 1968.

"Experience with the use of furadonin in trichomoniasis," by B. I. Il'In. UROL NEFROL. 32:40-43, March-April, 1967.

"Experiences with atricana in the treatment of trichomoniasis," by J. C. Aure, et al. T NORSK LAEGEFOREN. 89:1792-1794 passim, December 1, 1969.

"Experiences with pimafucin in candida and trichomonas vaginitis," by T. Ozbay, et al. MED WELT. 50:2741-2743, December 13, 1969.

"Flagyl in the therapy of trichomoniasis. (Results of a complex work)." VESTN DERM VENER. 40:88-92, November, 1966.

"Furazolidone in the therapy of trichomonas urethritis in men," by A. I. Poliakov, et al. VESTN DERM VENER. 40:70, July, 1966.

"Furazolidone in the therapy of trichomoniasis in men," by S. A. Artem'ev, et al. SOVIET MED. 29:128-130, October, 1966.

"Further observations on strain sensitivity of trichomonas vaginalis to metronidazole," by J. A. McFadzean, et al. BRIT J VENER DIS. 45:161-162, June, 1969.

"Further studies on the occurrence and treatment of trichomoniasis in connection with the problem of erosion of the cervix uteri," by J. Zawadzki. PRZEGL LEK. 22:689-694, 1966.

"Immediate and remote results of the treatment of male trichomonas infections with trichomonas vaccine," by L. M. Korik, et al. VESTN DERM VENER. 42:80-84, March, 1968.

"The importance of organized prophylaxis in the control of trichomoniasis," by J. Kiss. ORV HETIL. 107:2229-2231, November 20, 1966.

"Is paromomycin appropriate for the treatment of trichomona infection in women. II. Clinical experiences," by H. Spitzbart, et al. ZBL GYNAEK. 88:563-566, April 30, 1966.

"Leucorrhoea due to trichomonas vaginalis--clinical trial with hamycin," by D. Ganju, et al. HINDUSTAN ANTIBIOT BULL. 9:69-75, November, 1966.

"Levorin in the therapy of trichomoniasis in men, and in post-trichomonas secondary infections," by L. M. Korik, et al. UROL NEFROL. 34:48-49, July-August, 1969.

TRICHOMONIASIS: TREATMENT

"Levorin in the treatment of women with trichomoniasis and candidiasis of the sexual organs," by V. A. Lenartovich, et al. VESTN DERM VENER. 43:39-43, February, 1969.

"Long-term treatment of trichomonas infections with a diiodine derivative of oxyguinoline," by M. Arnold. PRAXIS. 57:1663-1666, November 26, 1968.

"Macmiror in the therapy of vaginal trichomoniasis," by A. Baron. MINERVA GINEC. 22:269-271, February 28, 1970.

"Management of trichomonas vaginitis with pimaricin," by A. Papaloukas, et al. Z HAUT GESCHLECHTSKR. 43:343-348, April 15, 1968.

"Metronidazole in the treatment of trichomoniasis in men," by A. I. Poliakov, et al. VESTN DERM VENER. 42:86-87, November, 1968.

"Metronidazole treatment of trichomonal vaginitis. A comparison of cure rates in 1961 and 1967," by J. C. Aure, et al. ACTA OBSTET GYNEC SCAND. 48:440-445, 1969.

"Metronidazole treatment of vaginal trichomoniasis. II. Oral vs. vaginal therapy," by S. Porapakkham. OBSTET GYNEC. 29:213-216, February, 1967.

"A new anti-trichomonal agent: negative clinical results," by U. Larsson-Cohn, et al. LAKARTIDNINGEN. 67:914-915, February 25, 1970.

"A new trichomonicide. Experimental work done under Prof. Rosaldo Cavalcanti, gynecology clinic of F.M. U.F.P.," by N. P. De Almeida, et al. HOSPITAL. 77:1581-1585, May, 1970.

"Nifuratel compared with metronidazole in the treatment of trichomonal vaginitis," by B. A. Evans, et al. BRIT MED J. 1:335-336, May 9, 1970.

"Nifuratel for trichomonal vaginitis," by M. Arnold. BRIT MED J. 2:792, June 27, 1970.

"Nifuratel for trichomonal vaginitis," by A. Grimble, et al. BRIT MED J. 2:542, May 30, 1970.

TRICHOMONIASIS: TREATMENT

"Nifuratel for trichomonal vaginitis," by S. M. Laird. BRIT MED J. 2:731, June 20, 1970.

"Nifuratel for trichomonal vaginitis," by I. Sagone. BRIT MED J. 2:792, June 27, 1970.

"Nifuratel (magmilor) in trichomonal vaginitis," by W. Fowler, et al. BRIT J VENER DIS. 44:331-333, December, 1968.

"Nitrimidazone, a new systemic trichomonacide," by A. Cantone, et al. G MAL INFETT PARASSIT. 21:954-958, December, 1969.

"Observations and problems in the treatment of trichomonas vaginitis," by M. Arnold. THER UMSCH. 23:356-359, September, 1966.

"Observations on the problem of trichomoniasis and its systemic treatment with nitrimidazine," by I. Signorelli, et al. MINERVA GINEC. 21:1649-1654, December 15, 1969.

"On the clinical use of a new antibiotic, pimaricin, in the therapy of vaginitis caused by candida albicans and by trichomonas," by B. Ferrari, et al. QUAD CLIN OSTET GINEC. 21:929-945, November, 1966.

"On evaluation of systemic trichomonacide activity," by R. Giannone. MINERVA GINEC. 18:900-906, August 31, 1966.

"On the sensitivity of trichomonas vaginalis strains to metronidazole," by E. Kovacs, et al. ORV HETIL. 110:66-68, January 12, 1969.

"On the therapeutic value of flagyl in trichomoniasis in the male," by L. M. Rozhinskii. VESTN DERM VENER. 40:59-60, April, 1966.

"On the use of a new drug in the treatment of vaginal trichomona infections," by A. Segre. HOSPITAL. 75:1483-1492, April, 1969.

"Pimaricin in the treatment of trichomoniasis and vaginal moniliasis," by H. Zorn. Z ALLGEMEINMED. 45:1640-1643, December 10, 1969.

"The pitfalls of trichomonas," by A. Lieveaux. REV

TRICHOMONIASIS: TREATMENT

FRANC GYNEC OBSTET. 65:433-436, July-August, 1970.

"Pregnancy, trichomoniasis, and metronidazole. A novel dose schedule," by R. X. Sands. AMER J OBSTET GYNEC. 94:350-353, February 1, 1966.

"Preliminary clinical findings using nifuratel in vaginal trichomoniasis," by C. G. de Netto, et al. REV BRASIL MED. 26:190-192, March, 1969.

"Preliminary observations on the use of pimaricin in vaginitis due to candida albicans, trichomonas vaginalis and in aspecific vaginitis," by B. I. De Luca. MINERVA GINEC. 18:840-846, August 15, 1967.

"Prevention of complications after gynecological operations in cases with trichomonas vaginalis," by J. Starzyk, et al. PRZEGL LEK. 23:446-448, 1967.

"Purulent vulvovaginitis in a newborn girl as a rare form of a trichomonas vaginalis infection and its treatment," by C. Sander. Z KINDERHEILK. 98:364-369, 1967.

"Results of complex treatment and clinical-laboratory examinations of men with trichomoniasis," by E. R. Gordon. VESTN DERM VENER. 42:46-49, December, 1968.

"Results of studies of a new local antitrichomonal agent 'tricho-kilpicortin'," by L. Kiss. PRAXIS. 58:58-59, January 14, 1969.

"A semester experience at the Bari University obstetric and gynecologic clinic on the incidence and therapy of trichomonas vaginalis (in 3313 patients examined)," by G. Giocoli, et al. MINERVA GINEC. 19:740-745, July 31, 1967.

"Sequential therapy and trichomoniasis," by A. Calugi, et al. QUAD CLIN OSTET GINEC. 22:551-556, August, 1967.

"Significance of the treatment of trichomoniasis in gynecology and obstetrics," by J. Zawadzki, et al. WIAD PARAZYT. 15:473-475, 1969.

"625 cases of trichomoniasis treated with metronidazole (statistical discussion)," by M. Gaudefroy, et al. GYNEC PRAT. 19:339-362, 1968.

TRICHOMONIASIS: TREATMENT

"Studies on the trichomonacidal effects of various nitrofuran preparations," by H. Birnbaum. ZBL GYNAEK. 89:1303-1313, September 9, 1967.

"Studies on the value of atrican (TC 109) in the treatment of trichomonal and monilial infections," by W. Kilczewski, et al. PRZEGL DERM. 55:531-535, July-September, 1968.

"A study of the trichomonicidal activity of the association of chloramphenicol and 1-hydroxyethyl-2methyl-5nitro-imidazole," by F. Filadoro. ANTIBIOTICA. 5: 105-113, June, 1967.

"Symptomatology and therapy of female and male trichomoniasis," by H. Walther. THER GEGENW. 105:886-889, July, 1966.

"Therapeutic and diagnostic problems of vaginal trichomoniasis treated with imidazole (klion)," by B. Toth, et al. ORV HETIL. 108:452-455, March 5, 1967.

"Therapeutic problems of trichomoniasis of the urogenital apparatus in men," by J. Darewicz, et al. POL PRZEGL CHIR. 42:Suppl:6A:969+, 1970.

"Therapy of trichomonas and thrush colpitis using nifuratel," by A. Weidenbach, et al. MUNCHEN MED WSCHR. 110:343-345, February 6, 1968.

"Therapy of trichomoniasis," by R. M. Baker, et al. WISCONSIN MED J. 66:370-371, August, 1967.

"Tinidazole and metronidazole pharmacokinetics in man and mouse," by J. A. Taylor, Jr., et al. ANTIMICROB AGENTS CHEMOTHER. 9:267-270, 1969.

"Tinidazole, a new antiprotozoal agent: Effect on trichomonas and other protozoa," by H. L. Howes, et al. ANTIMICROB AGENTS CHEMOTHER. 9:261-266, 1969.

"Treatment of female and male trichomoniasis with metronidazol," by W. Lapuszek. POL TYG LEK. 24:533-534, April, 1969.

"Treatment of genital trichomonas using a new drug: nitrimidazine," by M. A. Fonngera, et al. REV COLUMBIA OBSTET GINEC. 21:141-146, March-April, 1970.

TRICHOMONIASIS: TREATMENT

"Treatment of trichomonas colpitis," by G. Zwerenz. Z ALLGEMEINMED. 45:1590-1591, November 30, 1969.

"Treatment of trichomonas colpitis with thyadione," by E. Vartiainen, et al. DUODECIM. 82:755-757, 1966.

"Treatment of trichomonas infection," by W. Raab. THER GEGENW. 108:967-974, July, 1969.

"Treatment of trichomonas infection in males with metronidazole," by M. E. Babichenko. VESTN DERM VENER. 41:86, August, 1967.

"The treatment of trichomonas infestations with klion," by P. Salacz, et al. Z AERZTL FORTBILD. 60:805-808, July 1, 1966.

"Treatment of trichomonas vaginitis," by T. Okawa. SANFUJIN JISSAI. 19:623-631, June, 1970.

"Treatment of trichomonas vaginitis in the pregnant woman with metronidazole (8 823 RP0). Absence of teratogenic effects," by P. Magnin, et al. REV FRANC GYNEC OBSTET. 61:861-867, December, 1966.

"Treatment of trichomonas vaginitis with nifuratel," by H. Gjonnaess, et al. ACTA OBSTET GYNEC SCAND. 48:85-94, 1969.

"Treatment of trichomoniasis during puerperium," by R. Wawryk, et al. WIAD PARAZYT. 15:467-468, 1969.

"Treatment of trichomoniasis in men with antibiotics-sodium salt of usnic acid," by I. I. Shkliar. VESTN DERM VENER. 42:89-91, April, 1968.

"Treatment of trichomoniasis in women with flagyl," by J. Zawadzki, et al. PRZEGL LEK. 22:367-369, 1966.

"Treatment of trichomoniasis in women with Macmiror," by A. Baron. WIAD PARAZYT. 15:379-380, 1969.

"Treatment of trichomoniasis of the urogenital organs with the 2nd fraction of ASD preparation," by E.P. Eganov, et al. VESTN DERM VENER. 44:71-73, January, 1970.

"Treatment of trichomoniasis with citral," by V. I. Danilin. SOVET MED. 31:139-140, May, 1968.

TRICHOMONIASIS: TREATMENT

"Treatment of trichomoniasis with complications," by E. Szule. THER HUNG. 14:30-33, 1966.

"Treatment of urogenital trichomoniasis," by V. I. Zhukov. VESTN DERM VENER. 42:51-55, June, 1968.

"Treatment of urogenital trichomoniasis with flagyl," by L. Slucki. WIAD LEK. 19:855-1158, June 1, 1966.

"Treatment of vaginal trichomoniasis using a new drug. Results using naxogin (K-1900)," by F. V. Rodrigues, et al. HOSPITAL. 77:417-424, February, 1970.

"Treatment of vaginal trichomoniasis with metronidazole flagyl in gel form. Preliminary results," by C. G. De Netto, et al. HOSPITAL. 70:447-449, August, 1966.

"Treatment of vaginal trichomonadosis with nifuratel," by H. Schmidt, et al. WIAD PARAZYT. 15:373-376, 1969.

"Treatment of vaginal trichomoniasis with nitrofurazone," by Z. Malachowski, et al. POL TYG LEK. 24: 1823-1824, October 24, 1969.

"Trial of a terramycin foam for local usage in treatment of vaginitis of bacterial and parasitic (trichomonas) origin," by M. Levrier, et al. GYNEC PRAT. 18:381-389, 1967.

"Tric agent. Characteristics and detection by laboratory methods," by I. A. Harper. BRIT J VENER DIS. 42:71-76, June, 1966.

"The trichomonacidal action of flagyl," by G. A. Voskresenskaia. VESTN DERM VENER. 39:54-58, October, 1965.

"Trichomonal vaginitis: Epidemiology and therapy," by W. F. Peterson, et al. AMER J OBSTET GYNEC. 97:472-478, February 15, 1967.

"Trichomonas vaginalis. A pathogen of prostatitis," by P. H. Van Laarhoven. ARCH CHIR NEERL. 19:263-273, 1967.

"Trichomonas vaginitis, its treatment and colposcopic findings before and after treatment," by W. Konopada.

TRICHOMONIASIS: TREATMENT

POL TYG LEK. 22:2020-2021, December 25, 1967.

"Trichomonas vaginalis: resistance to metronidazole," by A. W. Diddle. AMER J OBSTET GYNEC. 98:583-585, June 15, 1967.

"Trichomoniasis in women. A personal method of treatment," by A. Senra. HOSPITAL. 76:245-283, July, 1969.

"Trichomoniasis in women treated at the Ciechocinek Resort," by D. Kozlowska, et al. GINEK POL. 40:407-412, 1969.

"Trichomoniasis urogenitalis and metronidazol therapy in dermato-venerologic practice," by G. Elste. DERM WSCHR. 152:263-266, March 12, 1966.

"Trichopol in the treatment of trichomoniasis in women," by F. V. Potapnev, et al. AKUSH GINEK. 45:66-68, August, 1969.

"Trichopol in trichomoniasis infections," by F. V. Potapnev. VESTN DERM VENER. 42:55-60, June, 1968.

"Use of metronidazole in trichomonas vaginitis," by R. J. Moreno. REV OBSTET GINEC VENEZ. 28:275-290, 1968.

"Use of metronidazole in vaginal trichomoniasis," by R. J. Moreno. REV OBSTET GINEC VENEZ. 29:275-290, 1968.

"The use of a new drug (deflamon) in the treatment of vaginal trichomoniasis," by A. Segre. MINERVA GINEC. 20:52-59, January 15, 1968.

"The use of urotropin for artificial activation of trichomonas infection in men," by V. I. Zhukov. VESTN DERM VENER. 40:45-52, August, 1966.

TRICHOPOL

"Trichopol in the treatment of trichomoniasis in women," by F. V. Potapnev, et al. AKUSH GINEK. 45:66-68, August, 1969.

"Trichopol in trichomoniasis infections," by F. V. Potapnev. VESTN DERM VENER. 42:55-60, June, 1968.

TRIMETHOPRIM-SULPHONAMIDE

TRIMETHOPRIM-SULPHONAMIDE

"The possible scope of trimethoprim-sulphonamide treatment," by L. P. Garrod. POSTGRAD MED J. Suppl:45: 52-55, November, 1969.

"Therapeutic trial of trimethoprim as a potentiator of sulphonamides in gonorrhoea," by G. W. Csonka, et al. BRIT J VENER DIS. 43:161-165, September, 1967.

"Trimethoprim mixture," by D. J. Wright, et al. BRIT MED J. 1:637, March 8, 1969.

"Trimethoprim-sulphamethoxazole in the treatment of non-gonoccal urethritis and gonorrhoea," by B. R. Carroll, et al. BRIT J VENER DIS. 46:31-33, February, 1970.

2-MERCAPTOETHANOL

"Effect of 2-mercaptoethanol treatment on anticardiolipin reactivity in sera from syphilitics and false positive reactors," by G. R. Tringali, et al. BRIT J VENER DIS. 45:202-204, September, 1969.

"Effects of 2-mercaptoethanol on treponemal antibodies in syphilis," by E. Csermely, et al. MINERVA DERM. 42:418-419, August, 1967.

"Sensitivity to 2-mercaptoethanol of reagins in human syphilis in BFP reactors and in 'normal' rabbit. The macroglobulin nature of BFP reagins," by G. Tringali, et al. RIV IST SIEROTER ITAL. 41:291-298, September-October, 1966.

URETHRITIS: NON-GONOCOCCAL AND/OR NON-SPECIFIC
SEE ALSO: MINOR VENEREAL DISEASES & INFECTIONS
MYCOPLASMAS

"Cephaloridine in the treatment of non-gonococcal urethritis," by G. W. Csonka, et al. POSTGRAD MED J. 43:Suppl:43:123-124, August, 1967.

"Clinical application of methyldichlorophenylisoxazolyl penicillin (dicloxacillin, staphcillin A) for urinary tract infections, especially for non-gonorrheal urethritis," by J. Ishigami, et al. J ANTIBIOT. 19:354-357, October, 1966.

"Contribution to the etiology of nonspecific urethritis," by J. Frantoz, et al. LIJECN VJESN. 90:1173-1181, 1968.

URETHRITIS: NON-GONOCOCCAL AND/OR NON-SPECIFIC

"Controlled study of the prevalence of T-strain mycoplasmata in males with non-gonococcal urethritis," by H. R. Ingham, et al. BRIT J VENER DIS. 42:269-271, December, 1966.

"Diagnosis and therapy of nongonorrheal urethritis and prostatitis," by G. Elste. Z AERZTL FORTBILD. 60:619-621, May 15, 1966.

"Erythromycin in the treatment of non-gonococcal urethritis," by R. R. Willcox. BRIT J VENER DIS. 44:157-159, June, 1968.

"The etiology of non-gonococcal urethritis," by G. Furness. S DAKOTA J MED. 20:39-42, December, 1967.

"Evaluation of different therapeutic regimens in the treatment of acute urethritis (707 cases)," by P. L. Stebbins. MILIT MED. 132:535-538, July, 1967.

"Gonorrhea-like urethritis due to mima polymorpha var oxidans. Patient summary and bacteriological study," by W. R. Kozub, et al. ARCH INTERN MED. 122:514-516, December, 1968.

"Gonorrheal and non-gonorrheal urethritis," by J. Bonelli, et al. HOSPITAL. 70:921-935, October, 1966.

"Kanamycin in non-gonococcal urethritis," by G. W. Csonka. POSTGRAD MED J, London. 63:64, May, 1967.

"Lincomycin, non-gonococcal urethritis, and mycoplasmata," by G. W. Csonka, et al. BRIT J VENER DIS. 45:52-54, March, 1969.

"Mycotic diseases of the male genital organs with specific reference to non-gonorrheal or mycotic urethritis," by J. Rossberg. CESK DERM. 43:168-170, June, 1968.

"Non-gonococcal urethritis acquired concomitantly with gonorrhoea in males," by J. D. Mahony. ULSTER MED J. 38:148-149, Summer, 1969.

"Non-gonococcal urethritis and Reiter's syndrome: personal experience with etiological studies during 15 years," by D. K. Ford. CANAD MED ASS J. 99:900-910, November 9, 1968.

"Non-gonococcal urethritis associated with human strains

of 'T' mycoplasmas," by M. C. Shepard. JAMA. 211: 1335-1340, February 23, 1970; also in US NAVAL MED FIELD RES LAD. 18:1-17, September, 1968.

"Non-gonorrheal urethritis," by C. H. Beek. NEDERL T GENEESK. 111:533-554, March 25, 1967.

"Non-gonorrheal urethritis in men," by G. Rajka. LAKARTIDNINGEN. 63:4613-4620, November 30, 1966.

"Nonspecific urethritis in females," by S. Marshall, et al. NORTHWEST MED. 69:9-10, June, 1970.

"Non-specific urethritis treated with purrolidinomethyl tetracycline nitrate," by C. B. Schofield, et al. BRIT J VENER DIS. 45:47-49, March, 1969.

"Occurrence of T-strains and other mycoplasmata in non-gonococcal urethritis," by F. T. Black, et al. BRIT J VENER DIS. 44:324-330, December, 1968.

"Oral tetracycline phosphate complex (tetrex) in the treatment of non-specific urethritis," by E. B. Wijetunga, et al. BRIT J VENER DIS. 45:50-51, March, 1969.

"Outbreak of non-specific urethritis associated with the presence of complement-fixing antibodies to the LB4 strain of TRIC agent," by T. Pasieczny, et al. BRIT J VENER DIS. 42:191-194, September, 1966.

"Penicillin and urethritis," by H. N. De Carvalho. HOSPITAL. 76:763-768, August, 1969.

"Possible mycoplasma hominis urethritis revealed by differing responses of 'abacterial urethritis' to treatment with tetracycline and erythromycin," by A. S. Grimble. BRIT J VENER DIS. 44:230-231, September, 1968.

"Problems of diagnosis and therapy of acute and chronic nonspecific urethritis," by H. D. Jung. ZUROL. 59: 865-871, December, 1966.

"Pyrogenal in the therapy of nongonococcal urethritis and its complications," by A. M. Kukushkin. VESTN DERMATOL VENEROL. 44:80-83, March, 1970.

"Relationships between mycoplasma and the etiology of

URETHRITIS: NON-GONOCOCCAL AND/OR NON-SPECIFIC

nongonococcal urethritis and Reiter's syndrome," by D. K. Ford. ANN NY ACAD SCI. 143:501-504, July 28, 1967.

"Role of mycoplasma in nongonococcal urethritis," by J. Thivolet, et al. PRESSE MED. 76:1755-1776, October 5, 1968.

"Role of mycoplasma in urethritis. I. Mycoplasma hominis type 1," by M. Sepetjian, et al. PATH BIOL. 17:953-959, November, 1969.

"T-strain mycoplasma in nongonococcal urethritis," by G. W. Csonka, et al. ANN NY ACAD SCI. 143:794-798, July 28, 1967.

"T-strain mycoplasma in non-gonococcal urethritis. Pathogen or commensal?," by W. Fowler, et al. BRIT J VENER DIS. 45:287-293, December, 1969.

"T-strain mycoplasmas in non-specific urethritis," by A. Shipley, et al. MED J AUST. 1:794-796, May 11, 1968.

"Trimethoprim-sulphamethoxazole in the treatment of non-gonococcal urethritis and gonorrhea," by B. R. Carroll, et al. BRIT J VENER DIS. 46:31-33, February, 1970.

USNIC ACID
"Treatment of trichomoniasis in men with antibiotics--sodium salt of usnic acid," by I. I. Shkliar. VESTN DERM VENER. 42:89-91, April, 1968.

UVEITIS
SEE: OPHTHALMOLOGY

VACCINATION
"Anti-vaccination and syphilis," by D. Green. MED J AUST. 1:500-501, March 7, 1970.

"Jonathan Hutchinson on vaccination syphilis," by C. T. Nelson. ARCH DERM. 99:529-535, May, 1969.

"The search for a vaccine for syphilis. An epidemiological approach," by R. W. Thatcher. BRIT J VENER DIS. 45:10-12, March, 1969.

"Toward a syphilis vaccine," by F. Marley. SCI N.

VACCINATION

92:356, October 7, 1967.

V-CILLIN
"Effect of V-cillin on treponema pallidum," by J. Suchanek, et al. POL TYG LEK. 22:46-48, January 9, 1967.

VENEREAL DISEASE
"Activities of the Minsk dermatologists," by AIa. Prokopchuk. VESTN DERM VENER. 43:3-6, May, 1969.

"Attempt at classification of skin and venereal diseases," by J. Danda. CESK DERM. 42:167-172, June, 1967.

"The British venereal diseases service, 1916-1966." BRIT J VENER DIS. 42:223-224, December, 1966.

"C-reactive protein in skin and venereal diseases (a review of the literature," by V. N. Mikhailov, et al. VESTN DERM VENER. 40:48-53, October, 1966.

"Cervical cytology of patients attending a venereal disease clinic," by A. J. Lucas, et al. J OBSTET GYNAEC BRIT COMM. 74:104-110, February, 1967.

"Changing pattern of morbidity at Groote Schuur Hospital, 1939-1965," by J. F. Brock. S AFR MED J. 41:739-747, August 12, 1967.

"Considerations on the failure to eradicate gonorrhoea and syphilis," by N. Danbolt. TRIANGLE. 8:2-6, 1967.

"Crisis in venereology," by R. D. Catterall, et al. BRIT MED J. 3:699-701, September 19, 1970.

"Current problems of venereal diseases in females," by A. Wiedmann. MUNCHEN MED WSCHR. 108:1837-1843, September 23, 1966.

"Current problems of venereal diseases in women," by A. Wiedmann. MINERVA MED. 57:3415-3419, October 20, 1966.

"Current problems of venereology," by R. Schuppli. PRAXIS. 57:1368-1372, October 8, 1968.

"Current problems of venereology abroad," by N. M. Turanov, et al. VESTN DERM VENER. 42:59-63, May, 1968.

VENEREAL DISEASE

"Current recrudescence of gonococcia," by A. Siboulet. J UROL NEPHROL. 75:Suppl:12-557+, December, 1969.

"The current status and perspectives of development of Soviet dermatovenereology," by M. M. Zheltakov, et al. SOVET MED. 30:3-12, September, 1967.

"Current status of venereal diseases," by K. Takeuchi, et al. SANFUJIN JISSAI. 17:131-137, February, 1968.

"Current venereal diseases. Transition in the diseases as seen from the microbiological aspect," by Y. Onoda. JAP J NURS ART. 8:87-96, August, 1969.

"Current venereologic problems," by R. Staps. DEUTSCH GESUNDH. 21:503-508, March 17, 1966.

"Dermato-venereological trends," by L. Texier, et al. J MED BORDEAUX. 143:1621-1632, October, 1966.

"Effects on the public health of the incidence of venereal and skin diseases during the last quarter of the century," by C. Huriez. BULL ACAD NAT MED. 153:396-406, 1969.

"Facts about venereal disease." BRIT MED J. 1:67-68, January 11, 1969.

"Five years of research on the treponematoses and venereal diseases." WHO CHRON. 24:53-60, February, 1970.

"5 years of studies on treponematosis and venereal diseases." PRENSA MED ARGENT. 57:585-591, May 22, 1970.

"Form the experience of the work of a dermatovenereologist in Yemen," by M. P. Vil'chinskii. VESTN DERM VENER. 40:82-85, July, 1966.

"Getting involved with V.D.," by J. A. Yacenda. J SCH HEALTH. 40:43-45, January, 1970.

"The growing menace of VD," by J. Block. PARENTS'. 45:86+, November, 1970.

"In a specialist's office," by A. Skriver. T SYGEPI. 67:217-221, May, 1967.

"The intimate evil." WORLD HLTH. 22:38+, July, 1969.

VENEREAL DISEASE

"Main results of fulfilling plans for scientific studies on the problem 'Scientific bases of dermatology and venereology' for 1968," by N. M. Turanov, et al. VESTN DERM VENER. 43:7-12, September, 1969.

"Main results of scientific studies on the problem of 'scientific principles of dermatology and venereology' during 1967," by N. M. Turanov, et al. VESTN DERM VENER. 42:3-9, August, 1968.

"New venereal disease: vibrio fetus infections." TIME. 87:62, February 25, 1966.

"On the participation of Soviet dermato-venereologists in the development of international scientific relations," by N. M. Turanov, et al. VESTN DERM VENER. 41:3-10, June, 1967.

"Perspectives in verereology-1965," by R. R. Willcox. BULL HYG. 41:1033-1056, October, 1966.

--1966." BULL HYG. 42:1169-1200, November, 1967.

"Plan of scientific research during 1968 on the problem: 'scientific foundations of dermatology and venereology'," by N. M. Turanov, et al. VESTN DERM VENER. 42:3-6, March, 1968.

"Present problems of venereal diseases in women," by A. Wiedmann. REV CLIN ESP. 103:429-435, December 31, 1966.

"Present status of venereal disease," by S. Mizuno. J JAP OBSTET GYNEC SOC. 18:871-872, August, 1966.

"Present status of venereal diseases," by Y. Onoda. J JAP MED ASS. 60:1081-1095, December 1, 1968.

"Present tasks and possibilities of the Polish health services in the field of venereal disease control," by T. Z. Capinski. PRZEGL DERM. Suppl:85-91, 1969.

"The prevalence of infectious syphilis in patients with acute gonorrhea," by R. C. Brown. SOUTHERN MED J. 61:98-100, January, 1968.

"Prevention of venereal disease' quackery'?," by G. Lomholt. LAKARTIDNINGEN. 65:2156-2158, May 22, 1968.

VENEREAL DISEASE

"The problem of syphilis and gonorrhea today," by W. L. Fleming. ARCH ENVIRON HEALTH, Chicago. 13:357-366, September, 1966.

"Rapid panorama of the most frequent dermato-venerological diseases. Their importance for the public health," by C. Huriez. BULL SOC FRANC DERM SYPH. 76:803-813, 1969.

"The reported and actual morbidity of syphilis and gonorrhea," by A. C. Curtis. ARCH ENVIRON HEALTH, Chicago. 13:381-384, September, 1966.

"Revision of the concept of venereal vaginal infection," by R. Peter. CESK GYNEK. 31:290-293, May, 1966.

"Selected aspects of syphilis and gonorrhoea. Research in the United States, 1967," by L. C. Norins. BRIT J VENER DIS. 42:103-108, June, 1968.

"Sexually transmitted diseases. Part 1.," by J. Ribeiro, DISTRICT NURS. 12:201+, January, 1970.

--Part 2." DISTRICT NURS. 12:225+, February, 1970.

--Part 4. Minor infections," by J. K. Oates. NURS MIRROR. 128:38-39, February 21, 1969.

"The sexually-transmitted diseases and marriage," by J. R. Seale. BRIT J VENER DIS. 42:31-36, March, 1966.

"Shocking facts about VD," by P. Deutsch, et al. PARENTS MAG. 42:44-45, January, 1967

"A study in New Zealand mortality. 7. Infectious diseases (concluded)," by J. W. Donovan. NEW ZEAL MED J. 71:143-147, March, 1970.

"Time to put an end to venereal disease care," by H. Moller. LAKARTIDNINGEN. 65:987-990, March 6, 1968.

"Upgrading V.D. departments," by A. King. BRIT MED J. 3:46, July 4, 1970.

"'V.D.', as a diagnosis." BRIT MED J. 3:630-631, September 14, 1968.

"V.D. a disease with a sorry stigma," J W AUST NURSES.

VENEREAL DISEASE

35:20+, August, 1969.

"VD is more than a dirty word," by F. Field. FAMILY HLTH. 2:43+, June, 1970.

"VD: a major health problem," by S. D. Furst, Jr. PARENTS MAG. 42:104, November, 1967.

"VD menace alarming," by P. McBroom. SCI N. 90:402, November 12, 1966.

"VD: a national problem that can no longer be ignored," SR. SCHOL. 88:11-14, February 25, 1966.

"VD on the increase: gonorrhea cases climb as promiscuity rises and drugs lose effect," by R. R. Leger. WALL ST J. 171:1+, June 18, 1968.

"V.D., the unconquered menace," by S. Golub. RN. 33:38+, March, 1970.

"Venereal disease." LANCET. 2:250-251, August 1, 1970.

"Venereal disease," by T. H. Bierre. OCCUP HEALTH. 4:3-4, December, 1970.

"Venereal disease," by J. Jefferiss. LANCET. 2:673, September 26, 1970.

"Venereal disease," by Z. Sternadel. PIELEG POLOZ. 9:9-10, September, 1969+.

"Venereal disease," by L. Watt. LANCET. 2:364, August 15, 1970.

"Venereal disease: society's stigma," by M. Kamp. AM COUNTY GOVT. 32:44-45+, May, 1967.

"Venereal disease: this hazard to public health could be eliminated; instead, it grows worse." CONSUMER REPTS. 35:118-123, February, 1970.

"Venereal disease today," by H. Shryock. LIFE AND HLTH. 83:16+, July, 1968.

"Venereal disease today," by J. R. Spencer. LIFE AND HLTH. 85:18+, October, 1970.

"Venereal disease: the unmentionable menace." SR SCHOL.

VENEREAL DISEASE

90:10-11, May 12, 1967.

"Venereal diseases." LYON MED. 223:287-317, February 1, 1970.

"Venereal diseases." MONTHLY BULL MINIST HEALTH. 25:170, August, 1966.

"Venereal diseases." MONTHLY BULL MINIST HEALTH. 26:31, February, 1967.

"Venereal diseases." WORLD HLTH. 22:26, June, 1969.

"The venereal diseases," by J. L. Breen. J AMER COLL HEALTH ASS. 15:Suppl:26-34, May, 1967.

"Venereal diseases," by P. J. De Amorim. HOSPITAL. 70:1739-1745, December, 1966.

"Venereal diseases are reappearing," by C. D. Carrillo; ACTAS DERMOSIF. 59:487-489, July-August, 1968.

"Venereal diseases. Extract from the Annual Report of the Chief Medical Officer of the Department of Health and Social Security for the year 1968." BRIT J VENER DIS. 46:76-83, February, 1970.

"Venereal diseases to date," by E. Mach. DEUTSCH ZBL KRANKENPFI. 12:624-626, November, 1968.

"The venereological scene," by A. S. Grimble. BRIT J CLIN PRACT. 22:243-247, June 6, 1968.

"Venereology ought to be a subspecialty," by M. Skogh. LAKARTIDNINGEN. 65:1296-1297, March 27, 1968.

"Venereology today. Part 1," by W. V. Macfarlane. NM. 124:229+, June 9, 1967.

--Part 2." NM. 124:261+, June 16, 1967.

"What's new in venereal disease?," by V. G. Cave. RHODE ISLAND MED J. 52:519-522, September, 1969.

"You & VD. (Editorial)," by C. B. Kanterman. DENT STUD MAG. 44:379-380, February, 1966.

VENEREOLOGICAL INSTITUTES
SEE: CLINICS

VETERINARY

VETERINARY
"Equine coital exanthema," by K. Petzoldt. BERLIN MUNCHEN TIERAERZTL WSCHR. 83:93-95, March, 1970.

"Transmissible venereal tumour in a boxer bitch," by J. B. Tutt. VET REC. 84:13, January 4, 1969.

"Treatment of venereal sarcoma in a bitch by vulvo-vagino-ovario-hysterectomy with perineal urethrostomy. (A case report)," by P. J. Philip. INDIAN VET J. 45: 874-877, October, 1968.

VIBRAMYCIN
"The treatment of early syphilis with vibramycin. Preliminary communication," by P. Wodniansky, et al. Z HAUT GESCHLECHTSKR. 44:571-574, September 1, 1969.

VIRUSES
"A search for viruses in smegma, premalignant and early malignant cervical tissues. The isolation of herpesviruses with distinct antigenic properties," by W. E. Rawls, et al. AMER J EPIDEM. 87:647-655, May, 1968.

VULCACYCLINE
"Note on the treatment of male gonococcic urethritis with vulcacycline," by F. Labouche, et al. BULL SOC FRANC DERM SYPH. 74:665-667, 1967.

YAWS
"Early yaws," by L. Fry, et al. BRIT J VENER DIS. 42: 28:30, March, 1966.

"Experimental method for the differentiation of several treponemal infections: venereal syphilis, endemic syphilis and yaws," by A. Paris-Hamelin, et al. BULL WHO. 38:808-809, 1968.

"Fluorescent treponemal antibody absorption (FTA-ABS) test in yaws," by M. F. Garner, et al. BRIT J VENER DIS. 46:284-286, August, 1970.

"Late yaws," by J. L. Fluker, et al. BRIT J VENER DIS. 46:264, June, 1970.

"The radiologic aspects of the osseous lesions of yaws," by R. P. Delahaye, et al. J RADIOL ELECTR. 49:41-48, January-February, 1968.

"Tertiary form of frambesia with localization in the

YAWS

spine," by V. Benes. ACTA CHIR ORTHOP TRAUM CECH. 33:440-442, October, 1966.

"The x-ray picture of bone changes in yaws," by K. Chmel. CESK RADIOL. 21:185-192, May, 1967.

"Yaws: Clinical manifestations and criteria for diagnosis. (Based on a study in Dudhi Tehsil of District Mirzapur, U.P., India in 1954-1956)," by B. L. Taneja. INDIAN J MED RES. 56:100-113, January, 1968.

YAWS: OCCURRENCE

"Epidemiological study of yaws," by K. C. Sahu. INDIAN J DERM. 11:119-122, July 4, 1966.

"Frambesia in Indonesia (Clinical manifestations and treatment)," by M. D. Tverskoi. VESTN DERM VENER. 43:59-67, September, 1969.

"Infectious and active yaws in a midland city," by F. M. Lanigan-O'Keeffe, et al. BRIT J DERM. 79:325-330, June, 1967.

"Serologic yaws in Paris," by G. Solente. PRESSE MED. 74:1681-1682, June 25, 1966.

"Yaws--incidence and epidemiology (study in Dudhi Tehsil of district Mirzapur, Uttar Pradesh, India)," by B. L. Taneja. J TROP MED HYG. 70:215-223, September, 1967.

YAWS: PREVENTION & CONTROL

"Campaign for eradication of yaws in Indonesia," by M. D. Tverskoi. MED PARAZIT. 36:103-106, January-February, 1967.

YAWS: TREATMENT

"Clinical manifestations and treatment of frambesie," by S. N. Strakhov. KLIN MED. 44:120-127, November, 1966.

"Clinical, serological and epidemiological features of framboesia tropica (yaws) and its control in rural communities," by T. Guthe. ACTA DERMATOVENER. 49:343-368, 1968.

YOUTH
SEE ALSO: EDUCATION
SOCIOLOGY

YOUTH

"Adolescent coitus and cervical cancer: associations of related events with increased risk," by I. D. Rotkin. CANCER RES. 27:603-617, April, 1967.

"The adolescent's crisis today. Sex and the adolescent," by G. B. Blaine. NEW YORK J MED. 67:1967-1975, July 15, 1967.

"Attitudes of college students in East Africa to sexual activity and venereal disease," by O. P. Arya, et al. BRIT J VENER DIS. 44:160-166, June, 1968.

"Considerations in counselling teen-agers on sexual matters," by H. P. Coppolillo. MED TIMES. 95:580-585, May, 1967.

"Considerations on some helpful measures in the propaganda against venereal diseases. (On experiences in the high schools of the Province of Venezia)," by A. Serena. ARCH ITAL DERM VENER. 34:395-398, 1966.

"A doctor speaks of college students and sex," by W. Dalrymple. J AMER COLL HEALTH ASS. 15:279-286, 1967.

"Evaluation of venereal disease information campaign for adolescents," by D. Rosenblatt, et al. AMER J PUBLIC HEALTH. 56:1104-1115, July, 1966.

"Experiences of a doctor sexologist with youth," by Z. L. Starowicz. WIAD LEK. 23:1359-1362, August 1, 1970.

"Genital infection in young delinquent girls," by E. Gallagher. BRIT J VENER DIS. 46:129-131, April, 1970.

"Health education and spreading of venereal diseases among youth," by L. Dyskin, et al. PRZEGL DERM. 55:273-280, May-June, 1968.

"Health in a rural hippie commune," by D. L. Palmer, et al. JAMA. 213:1307-1310, August 24, 1970.

"Highest venereal disease rates for United States and Georgia in younger age groups." J MED ASS GEORGIA. 56:300-302, July, 1967.

"Information on venereal diseases in Los Angeles' county schools," by W. H. Smartt. BOL OFIC SANIT PANAMER.

66:226-230, March, 1969.

"Juvenile GPI: a case study," by G. C. Kanjilal. NURS TIMES. 65:1066-1067, August 21, 1969.

"Law, medicine and minors. I," by D. H. Russell. NEW ENG J MED. 278:35-36, January 4, 1968.

--II." NEW ENG J MED. 278:265-266, February 1, 1968.

"Medical and legal problems in the treatment of delinquent girls in Scotland. I. Girls in custodial institutions," by D. H. Robertson. BRIT J VENER DIS. 45:129-139, June, 1969.

--II. Sexually transmitted disease in girls in custodial institutions." BRIT J VENER DIS. 46:46-53, February, 1970.

"Prescribing contraception for teenagers--a moral compromise," by R. J. Pion. OBSTET GYNEC. 30:752-755, November, 1967.

"Reported patterns of venereal diseases in adolescents," by H. C. Faigel. CLIN PEDIAT. 8:620, November, 1969.

"Research on lues in children and juveniles," by L. Pospisil. CESK PEDIAT. 25:462-263, September, 1970.

"Sex attitudes of young people: London, England," by M. Holmes, et al. ED RES. 11:38-42, November, 1968.

"Sex behavior of adolescent patients," by U. Sprafke. DERM MSCHR. 155:554-568, 1969.

"The sexual behavior of young people. Practical implications of the C.C.H.E. report," by A. J. Dalzell-Ward. ROY SOC HEALTH J. 86:167-170, May-June, 1966.

"Sexual morality: Campus dilemma," by D. L. Farnsworth. INT PSYCHIAT CLIN. 7:133-151, 1970.

"Social problems of venereal diseases among New York youth," by W. Curth. ARCH KLIN EXP DERM. 227:637-640, 1966.

"Sociomedical study of young gonorrhea patients," by B. H. Hatt. NORD MED. 76:816, July 14, 1966.

YOUTH

"Sociopsychiatric investigation of teenage girls with gonorrhea," by L. Palmgren. ACTA PSYCHIAT SCAND. 42:295-314, 1966.

"Students as special clinic patients," by R. S. Morton. BRIT J VENER DIS. 42:280-282, December, 1966.

"The teenager and VD," AMER J PUBLIC HEALTH. 59:898-899, June, 1969.

"A U.S. youngster is infected with VD every two minutes," by N. Keifetz. N Y TIMES MAG. p85+, March 9, 1969.

"VD and the teenager," by A. Stitt. EMERGENCY MED. 1:60+, October, 1969.

"VD: the greatest threat to teen-age health," by A. Lake. SEVENTEEN. 28:146-147+, May, 1969.

"VD--protect children against venereal disease," by F. H. Richardson. LIFE AND HLTH. 83:18+, August, 1968.

"Vaginal discharge in puberty. A survey of 1000 adolescents," by J. Orley, et al. GYNAECOLOGIA. 168:191-202, 1969.

"Venereal disease and the young woman. Part 1," by J. L. Fluker. NM. 121:633+, March 4, 1966.

--Part 2." NM. 121:663+, March 11, 1966.

"Venereal disease in adolescence," by J. A. Knowles. MED ARTS SCI. 22:45-48, 1968.

"Venereal disease in an elite group (University students) in east Africa," by O. P. Arya, et al. BRIT J VENER DIS. 43:275-279, December, 1967.

"The venereal disease problem in schools, rural areas, and among juveniles," by J. L. Logan. ARCH ENVIRON HEALTH, Chicago. 13:385-387, September, 1966.

"Venereal disease problems and adolescent health," by A. King. CLIN PEDIAT. 5:597-603, October, 1966.

"Venereal disease rates and student attitudes," by I. E. Robinson, et al. J MED ASS GEORGIA. 56:298-299, July, 1967.

YOUTH

"Venereal diseases among adolescents in the agrarian district Neubrandenburg sociological study," by G. G. Bartschies, et al. DEUTSCH GESUNDH. 25:455-460, March 13, 1970.

"Venereal diseases in adolescents," by P. Baribeau. INFIRM CANAD. 11:17-21, July, 1969.

"What our kids don't know about health," by T. Irwin. TODAY'S HLTH. 44:19+, May, 1966.

"Young should know more about V.D.," by M. Binyon. TIMES ED SUP. 2792:1154, November 22, 1968.

AUTHOR INDEX

Abe, S., 67, 438, 477
Abed, L., 156, 545
Abelli, G., 85
Abrams, A.J., 121, 336
Abudsametov, Rkh, 111, 275
Achimastos, A., 138, 334, 504
Achten, M.G., 211
Ackerman, A.B., 18, 97, 286, 287
Ackerman, B.D., 43, 434
Acres, S.B., 130, 156, 305
Adams, A., 240, 361
Adeoba, A., 111, 479, 501
Adinolfi, G., 147, 270
Afanas'ev, B.A., 72, 278, 311
Aho, K., 117, 200, 225, 426, 519
Aiuti, F., 105, 197, 436
Akovbian, A.A., 37, 38, 98, 255, 524, 527
Alarcon-Segovia, D., 24, 261, 536
Alergant, C.D., 60, 273
Alexander, L., 230, 276, 358
Alford, C.A., Jr., 48, 87, 355, 435, 491, 499
Alieva, S.G., 157, 225, 507, 519
Aliferova, V.F., 239
Allen, E.S., 101, 305
Allen, T.E., 23, 488
Allinne, M., 58, 347
Allison, M.J., 50, 74, 492, 494

Almard, G., 137, 426
Altchek, A., 69, 290, 367
Altman, R.D., 169, 284
Altucci, P., 128, 352
Altucci, P.L., 129, 353
Aluigi, A., 197, 349
Amar, A.D., 162, 553
Amies, C.R., 57, 64, 184, 290, 296, 318, 368, 373
Amiraian, K., 164, 507
A'mor, B., 55, 253, 403
Amos, H.E., 153, 399
Anatassov, K., 142, 259, 335, 475
Andelman, S.L., 47, 379
Anderson, K., 183, 318
Anderson, L., 191, 319
Andre, R., 48, 257
Andrew, G.S., 37, 267, 309
Andrews, E.M., 242, 277
Antunes, M.L., 139, 544
Arans, M.I., 123, 266
Ardouin, M., 178, 364
Argenziano, G., 148, 173, 199, 332, 414, 529, 532, 545
Aricò, M., 67, 417
Aristova, V.N., 58, 289
Arnold, M., 120, 134, 137, 355, 365, 561, 562
Aronson, S.M., 34, 268
Artemev, S.A., 86, 279, 560
Arya, O.P., 13, 18, 221, 240, 307, 323, 409, 580, 582
Asami, K., 64, 376, 558
Ascari, W.Q., 97, 369
Ashamalla, G., 170, 317
Ashcroft, M.T., 188, 236, 513, 521
Ashkar, F.S., 187, 513, 540
Asmera, J., 177, 555
Atwood, W.G., 83, 213, 498, 518

Aure, J.C., 76, 252, 343, 560, 561
Avanesov, A.A., 226, 549
Aviosor, M.L., 138, 387, 398
Avksent'Eva, T.A., 25, 377, 393
Ayala, L., 179, 405, 541
Azar, H.A., 68
Azocar, B., 53, 543
Azulay, R.D., 104, 500
Azure, J.C., 125

Babaiants, R.S., 35, 151, 195, 267, 270, 360
Babichenko, M.E., 223, 344, 565
Babudieri, B., 233, 271
Bachwyzewski, J., 10
Baer, R.L., 183, 401
Bafverstedt, B., 42, 346
Bailey, A., 28, 262
Baker, H., 110, 265, 313, 385
Baker, R.M., 217, 564
Bakker, P.M., 197, 231, 437, 438
Bal'barer, I.G., 107, 436, 528
Balcar, Z., 11, 387
Baldwin, D.S., 175, 387, 400
Baledent, M., 61
Ball, R.W., 208, 246, 362, 482
Bammer, H., 216
Banerjee, D., 129, 397
Bank, E.B., 145, 414, 548
Bankl, H., 190, 401
Banks, G.D., 238, 521
Bansho, N., 204, 517
Baptista, O.R., 148, 279, 364
Baribeau, P., 242, 583
Barlow, D.E., 182, 358
Barnes, C.M., 70
Baron, A., 122, 223, 338, 561, 565
Baron, F., 54, 421, 435

Barondess, J.A., 195, 427
Barrow, G.I., 60, 551
Barsam, P.C., 197, 302
Bartholomew, L.E., 246, 354
Bartlett, R.C., 73, 494
Bartschies, G.G., 242, 583
Bartunek, J., 159, 293
Bashforth, D., 235, 267
Bashakova, M.A., 88, 254, 351
Bashforth, D., 383
Bashmakova, M.A., 112, 351, 377
Basset, A., 17, 55
Batchelor, F.R., 195, 401
Batko, B., 26
Bauch, K., 61, 431
Bauer, M.F., 149, 432
Baughman, R.D., 49, 491
Bazex, A., 99, 176, 477, 510
Beam, W.E., Jr., 73, 494
Beardwell, A., 208, 444
Beauchamp, F., 233, 364
Becker, W., 16, 333, 379
Beek, C.H., 40, 108, 135, 298, 306, 570
Beeler, M.F., 186, 512
Beilby, J.O., 98, 286, 326
Bekker, J.H., 153, 506
Belda, W., 134, 315
Bellone, A.G., 39, 489
Benell, F.B., 100, 149, 274, 275
Benes, V., 215, 579
Beniak, M., 150, 295
Beniaková, J., 57, 358
Bénichou, C., 194, 444
Benner, E.J., 175, 388, 389
Berger, J., 34, 309, 334
Berger, U., 8, 176, 282, 287
Bergeron, J.R., 112, 472
Berggren, O., 17, 108, 258, 259, 542, 544
Berghuis, P.H., 31, 424, 523
Berglund, S., 35, 488
Beric, B., 163, 264, 548
Berndt, J., 140
Bernfeld, W.K., 101, 339
Berni, C.M., 141, 406
Berry, E.B., 221, 323

Best, E.J., 23
Bethenod, M., 171, 437
Betz, A., 238, 521
Bhattacharyya, N.C., 188, 191, 382, 407, 515
Bialski, R., 72, 278, 311
Biasco-Zuasti, J.M., 178, 511
Biehler, H., 193, 216, 319, 321, 373, 416
Bien, K., 65, 390
Bierre, T.H., 239, 576
Bijerk, H., 108, 359
Billington, W.R., 132
Binnings, G.F., 19, 487
Binyon, M., 246, 583
Birnbaum, H., 202, 357, 564
Biro, L., 183, 443
Bischoff, A., 198, 445
Bjornberg, A., 21, 22. 285, 287
Black, F.T., 139, 353, 570
Blaine, G.B., 8, 580
Blanco Gutierrez, L.A., 218, 321
Blandy, J.P., 123, 528
Blatner, R.J., 227, 548
Blez, F., 183, 511
Bloch, C., 167
Block, V., 95, 573
Blodi, F.C., 211, 474
Blumberg, N., 153, 316, 371
Bohnstedt, R.M., 85, 254
Bohorquez, A., 123, 442
Bokkenheuser, V., 192, 515
Boldescu, I.V., 60, 551
Bolgert, M., 164, 226, 230, 375, 439, 535
Boncinelli, U., 144, 163, 176, 182, 205, 413, 505, 510, 511, 524, 531, 533
Bondarenko, B.I., 27, 547
Boneff, A., 132
Bonelli, J., 94, 312, 569
Boñu, G., 138, 405
Bopp, C., 159, 482

Boquoi, E., 39, 258, 543
Borchardt, K.A., 192, 264
Borisenko, A.M., 69, 277
Borkowski, M., 35, 523
Borman, J.B., 132, 398
Bornemann, H., 146, 505
Bornemann, K., 7, 391, 402
Bosse, K., 219, 366, 534
Botsov, P., 44, 270
Boulle, S., 26, 416
Bourg, R., 50, 543
Bowszyc, J., 11, 36, 145, 149, 200, 278, 366, 387, 394, 481, 524, 533
Boyle, G.L., 112, 262, 364
Brachwitz, R., 143, 328
Bradenburg, A., 147, 348
Bradford, L.L., 83, 498
Braitsev, A.V., 83, 121, 441, 471, 472
Branger, F., 58, 346
Bratina, G., 8, 484
Brauer, U., 95, 279, 325
Braun, P., 28, 125, 262, 352, 378
Braun-Falco, O., 216, 533
Braunstein, G.D., 131
Braun-Vallon, S., 16, 345
Bravo, O.J., 20, 287
Bredt, W., 82, 497
Breen, J.L., 241, 577
Brehm, G., 59, 394
Breier, M., 116
Breslin, A.B., 20, 295, 393
Breslow, L., 166, 382
Bret, J., 155, 376, 530
Breuillaud, J., 21, 487
Breyer, U., 29, 429
Brezhneva, E.I.A., 53, 543
British Cooperative Clinical Group, 93, 160
Brochery, P.C., 196, 480
Brock, J.F., 30, 572
Brooks, J.C., Jr., 42, 252, 288, 403
Brown, R.C., 160, 574
Brown, W.J., 23, 71, 77, 91, 93, 106, 166, 176, 185, 196, 200, 232, 236, 240, 242, 299, 304, 359, 381, 382, 383, 384, 409, 411, 481, 488, 511

Brown, W.M., Jr., 90, 297, 302
Browne, G., 119
Browne, S.G., 45, 346
Brozgol'd, L.A., 195
Bruhn-Petersen, F., 227, 546
Brundin, G., 46, 304
Brunner, F.P., 100, 396
Bruno, R., 126, 503
Brzin, B., 236, 350
Bubola, D., 23, 488
Buchanan, C.S., 79, 478, 496
Bucharowicz, M.N., 187, 513
Bukharovich, M.N., 176, 372, 532
Bukový, J., 230, 476
Bunn, P.A., 14, 251, 392
Burckhardt, W., 120
Burgess, J.A., 25, 478, 488
Burgess, S.C., 32, 345
Burmeister, R.E., 237, 350
Bushbee, C.E., 73, 494
Butovetskii, L.D., 66, 74, 126, 180, 191, 274, 494, 503, 511, 514
Buzzoni, A., 15, 485

Cabrera, H.A., 22, 350, 487
Cacciapuoti, B., 205, 517
Cagianut, B., 68, 395
Cainelli, T., 172, 510
Calabro, J.J., 89, 283, 324
Calas, E., 70
Caldera, L., 147, 227, 442, 556
Califano, A., 216, 321, 405
Callin, A.E., 100, 245, 384, 481
Calugi, A., 184, 563
Camargo, M.E., 109, 501

Campos, S.A., 158, 159, 360, 381
Canby, J.P., 164, 302
Candela, G., 239, 350
Canet, L., 26, 420
Cannefax, G.R., 105, 113, 502
Cantone, A., 135, 356, 562
Capet, R.G., 60, 107, 551
Capiński, K., 193, 329
Capiński, T.Z., 48, 151, 160, 238, 275, 383, 481
Cappelli, E., 179, 405, 541
Caprilli, F., 176, 361
Captine, A.M., 18, 475
Cardas, M., 214, 421
Caron, J., 244, 429
Carrillo, C.D., 242, 577
Carrion, A.L., 155, 349
Carroll, B.R., 228, 323, 568, 571
Carruthers, M.M., 25, 366
Carton, F.X., 162, 400
Carvalho, G., 228, 379, 414, 547
Castaigne, P., 34, 376
Catalano, G., 114, 351
Catalano, P.M., 72
Catar, G., 147, 545
Catterall, R.D., 21, 24, 48, 59, 218, 260, 268, 289, 410, 546, 572
Caubet, P., 15, 416
Cave, V.G., 92, 134, 164, 184, 245, 299, 302, 303, 318, 373, 418, 577
Cavenaugh, R.L., 186, 333, 512
Cayton, H.R., 187, 513
Cazzola, D., 16, 542
Cazzola, R., 121
Cernea, P., 212, 477
Chacko, C.W., 6, 29, 185, 206, 287, 294, 320, 374, 446
Chaika, N.A., 71, 441
Chambers, R.W., 218, 258
Chandler, F.W., Jr., 214, 518
Chappaz, G., 74, 215, 543, 546

Charles, J., 9, 392
Charpin, J., 152, 398
Chassagne, P., 169, 360, 413
Chastikova, A.V., 32, 153, 280, 316, 371
Chaudhury, D.S., 27, 334, 345
Chen, H.H., 117, 502
Cherubin, C.E., 185, 272, 326, 337, 386, 418
Chichinadze, Z.S., 26, 423
Chieregato, G.C., 121, 127, 503
Chistiakov, A.M., 192, 257, 515
Chmel, K., 246, 579
Chmielecki, A., 164, 437
Chodyn, E., 178, 318, 539
Christensen, A.W., 5, 416
Christensen, E.F., 68, 347
Christman, E.H., 112, 472
Christmas, B.W., 155, 339
Churcher, G.M., 111, 313, 355
Cicera, P., 5, 85, 142, 168, 188, 509, 514, 555
Ciecierski, L., 97, 392, 395
Clark, J.F., 46, 342, 346
Clark, J.W., Jr., 137, 187, 418
Clark, L., 118, 281
Clauberg, G., 178, 400
Cleere, R.L., 155, 339, 381
Clutton, H.H., 207
Cobbold, R.J., 127, 148, 221, 316, 323, 348, 371, 384, 405
Coblentz, D.R., 179
Cocuzza, G., 37, 112, 489, 502
Coffey, E.M., 72, 493
Cohen, I.R., 13, 130, 189, 295, 296, 297, 331
Cohen, J.A., 119, 426
Cohen, L., 110, 155, 287

Cohen, P., 185, 512
Cohill, D.F., 28, 393
Colavita, D., 37, 346, 376
Collart, P., 117, 150, 170, 177, 239, 404, 536
Collomb, H., 87, 366, 430, 431
Collum, E.W., 182, 275, 358
Combe, P., 174, 437
Comstock, G.W., 69
Conant, M.A., 183, 443
Conraths, H.J., 27, 305
Consbruch, U., 45, 429
Contreras, D.F., 99, 330
Cook, I., 114, 337
Coombs, L.C., 158, 378, 410
Cooper, C.E., 215, 249, 430
Cooperman, R.S., 235, 409
Coppolillo, H.P., 44, 580
Cornea, P., 229, 483
Cornelius, C.E., 3d, 193, 198, 319, 411, 538
Costic, T., 74
Cottini, G.B., 158, 443
Cowan, J.A., 199, 340, 383
Cowan, L., 90, 307
Cox, P.M., 20, 487
Cozza, G., 81
Craig, M.W., 44, 346
Cree, G.E., 227, 554
Cremin, B.J., 118, 436
Cripps, D.J., 25, 209, 488
Cristiana, R., 183, 433
Cronin, A.E., 150, 398, 530
Crosby, A.W., Jr., 63
Csermely, E., 67, 525, 568
Csonka, G.W., 28, 116, 119, 183, 213, 216, 262, 321, 335, 336, 352, 354, 415, 568, 569, 571
Curth, W., 194, 411, 581
Curtis, A.C., 175, 245, 341, 575
Cvejić, S., 243, 362
Cygan, Z., 21, 189, 487, 514
Cziraki, L., 35, 550

Dadashzade, M.M., 39, 75, 341, 342, 558, 559

D'Agostino, S., 203, 205, 338
D'Alessandro, P., 63, 548
Dairymple, W., 61, 580
Dalzell-Ward, A.J., 85, 189, 274, 581
Danbolt, N., 44, 572
Danda, J., 18, 133, 151, 275, 314, 572
Dandoy, S., 111, 501
Dang, R.W., 90, 306
Danielsson, D., 59, 289, 290
Danielsson, D.G., 14, 306
Danielsson, D.L., 89
Danilin, V.I., 223, 265, 565
Dantsig, I.I., 144, 398, 403
Dao, L., 180, 545
Darewicz, J., 56, 216, 550, 564
Das, P.C., 131, 420
Datey, K.K., 114, 426
Datta, A., 211, 433
David, L., 100, 417
David-Chausse, J., 114, 420
Davidoff, P., 97, 432
Davies, A.H., 125, 342, 529
Davis, C.M., 95, 324
Davis, L., 93, 139, 312
Davis, R.B., 115, 390
Davis, W.M., 95
Dawkins, R.S., 199, 422, 437
Dawson-Butterworth, K., 192, 444
D'Costa, J.F., 65, 493
Deacon, W.E., 83, 498
De Almeida, N.P., 134, 561
De Amorim, P.J., 241, 577
de Andrade, D.F., 131
de Barros, J.M., 148, 250, 316
De Camillus, L., 63, 435
De Carneri, I., 15, 67, 357, 551

De Carvalho, H.N., 152, 371, 570
De Girolami, E., 154
Degos, R., 63, 182, 188, 204, 372, 417, 427, 470, 532
de Huerta, N.H., 61, 269
Deis, H., 138, 552
Delacrètaz, J., 50, 60, 100, 431, 492, 499
Delahaye, R.P., 23, 167, 476, 578
Del Bianco, C., 129, 353
Delektorskii, V.V., 68
DeLeo, S., 106, 377, 551, 556
Delhanty, J.J., 104
Deliagina, E.M., 26, 388
DeLuca, B.I., 157, 261, 376, 563
De Luca, M., 81, 123, 172, 404, 497, 544
Delvecchio, E., 213, 421
Delzant, O., 10, 12, 419
Dembicki, E.L., 165, 272, 281
Demchenko, T.A., 193, 515
Deml, I., 61, 478
de Murillo, G.G., 209
De Netto, C.G., 157, 224, 344, 356, 563, 566
Dennerstein, G.J., 59, 290
Dennis, R.H., 246, 365
Dennison, W.L., 82, 395
de Oliveira, P.P., 78, 264
Desai, S.C., 229, 329
Desai, Z.D., 204, 261, 349, 546
Desbordes, P., 25, 431, 470
Despierres, G., 238, 388
Destro, F., 34, 557
Deutsch, P., 191, 229, 383, 575
DeWald, W., 85, 327
De Weck, A.I., 180, 401
De Weck, A.L., 9, 84, 369, 392
de Weisenberg, G.M., 212, 474
Dewhurst, K., 19, 37, 42, 132, 168, 221, 445, 486
Diabalovà, H., 93, 302

D'iachenko, L.A., 104, 224, 500
Diddle, A.W., 227, 344, 567
Dietz, O., 50
Dillon, M.L., 12, 422
DiMatteo, J., 97, 425
Dionigi, R., 20, 557
Disalvo, A.F., 210, 518
Di Virgilio, G., 138
Divis, J., 35, 285
Djankov, I., 102
Dmitriev, S.N., 230, 520
Dobrovol'skii, IuN, 143, 305
Dodd, R.W., 182, 476
Dodero, O., 151, 530
Dogliotti, M., 111, 396
Domescik, G., 233, 272, 323
Donatelli, R., 154, 427
Donohue, J.F., 24, 113, 480, 481, 523
Donovan, J.W., 203, 575
Dougherty, R.L., 224, 349
Dowzenko, A., 132, 173
Drazancic, A., 228, 237, 547, 554
Dressler, W., 42, 424
Dreyfus, B., 62, 431
Driscoll, A.M., 190, 349
Driscoll, S.G., 110, 351
Druian, KhL, 85, 435
Drusin, L.M., 68
Drutz, D.J., 152, 398
Ducrey, C., 170, 413, 479
Dudley, S., 160, 408
DuFlorey, C.V., 175, 407
Duhamel, J., 134, 337
Dukelow, D.A., 44, 235, 383, 540
Duluc, J., 50, 109, 522, 537
Dumont, M., 223
Dunkelberg, W.E., Jr., 124, 174, 203, 301, 348, 349, 545
Dunlop, E.M., 56, 109, 129, 173, 188, 204, 252, 253, 349, 352, 364, 403, 404, 430, 445, 474, 545

Dunn, J.H., 149, 398
Duperrat, B., 117, 127, 417, 432
Dupouey, P., 14, 203, 485, 517
Durel, P., 57, 168, 296, 343
DuToit, J., 68
Duverne, J., 231, 433
Dvorak, V., 144, 355
Dyer, N.H., 93, 312
Dyner, E., 226, 554
Dyskin, L., 96, 274, 580
Dzioba, A., 66
Dzioba, H., 61, 425

Eaglestein, W.H., 53, 438
Eddie, D.A., 117, 552
Edmundson, W.F., 37, 346
Edwards, C.C., 5, 416
Eganov, E.P., 223, 565
Egorov, G.I., 152, 222, 256, 371, 375, 530, 535
Ehrlich, P., 67, 85, 327
Ehrmann, G., 135, 143, 145, 164, 245, 504, 505, 508, 522
Eigenbrodt, E.H., 37, 268, 424, 477
Ekbom, K., 215, 537
Ekstrom, K., 148, 151, 301, 306, 410
Elebute, E.A., 156, 286
Elliott, H., 235, 267, 383
Ellner, P.D., 139, 291
Elsas, F.J., 118, 477
Elste, G., 39, 57, 63, 111, 172, 228, 344, 380, 489, 567, 569
Enfors, W., 54, 310, 334, 368
Engelbrecht, E., 168, 509
Engleman, E.P., 172, 404
Erber, B., 158, 360
Ermol'eva, Z.V., 139, 203, 315, 320, 362, 363
Ernst, G., 135, 398
Etcheverry, J.A., 118, 417
Evans, A.J., 172, 318, 372, 415

Evans, A.S., 130, 408
Evans, B.A., 134, 343, 355, 561

Faigel, H.C., 176, 581
Faigel, H., 218, 264
Falchi, G., 178, 257, 532
Falk, V., 61, 290
Farber, E.R., 69, 347
Farber, I., 128, 352
Farina, D., 52, 478
Farnsworth, D.L., 190, 581
Farrell, L., 116
Fazio, M., 33, 308
Fegeler, F., 130, 292
Feinberg, J.G., 9, 390, 392
Feizi, T., 109, 396
Fellner, M.J., 9, 54, 62, 101, 105, 123, 331, 387, 391, 395, 396, 397
Fenner, O., 171, 378
Ferinden, W.E., Jr., 240, 277
Fernando, W.L., 29, 71, 278, 368, 429, 526
Ferrari, B., 30, 141, 261, 376, 523, 562
Ferrea, E., 233, 323, 341
Festenstein, H., 181
Fidler, J., 64, 249, 558
Field, F., 235, 576
Fikuoka, Y., 39
Filadoro, F., 81, 205, 265, 544, 564
Filatov, G.I., 246, 362
Filho, N.S., 150
Filina, E.I.A., 108, 359
Filipp, G., 105, 331, 396
Finger, A., 10, 250, 307
Fioccardi, R., 123, 544
Fioresi, B., 22, 430
Fischnaller, J.E., 116
Fisher, D.A., 120, 254, 439
Fisher, I., 71, 548
Fiumara, N.J., 70, 94, 190, 239, 285, 303, 383

Flarer, F., 81, 140, 162, 262, 263, 527, 529, 530
Fleming, W.L., 129, 162, 541, 575
Fluker, J.L., 98, 118, 170, 240, 250, 313, 330, 369, 578, 582
Fogel, B.J., 105, 479
Fogliatto, J., 69
Fonngera, M.A., 219, 356, 564
Ford, D.K., 115, 135, 173, 347, 353, 404, 569, 571
Ford, J.B., 225
Forkman, A., 110, 249, 313
Forshaw, J., 152, 399
Forssell, J., 178, 318
Forstrom, L., 80, 83, 172, 496, 498, 510
Foster, W.D., 22, 488
Foulkes, J.F., 197, 266
Fowinkle, E., 234, 323
Fowler, E., 17, 486
Fowler, W., 135, 213, 354, 356, 562, 571
Franceschini, P., 183, 229, 433, 477
Francini, A., 105, 396
Francois, R., 211, 437
Frank, H.D., 87
Frantoz, J., 45, 568
Frater, R.W., 212, 428
Fredriksson, T., 205, 517
Freedman, A., 109, 253, 364, 403
Freeman, C.W., 25, 29, 155, 160, 379, 482
Freiman, I., 217, 438
Frenkel, M., 48, 491
Fribourg-Blanc, A., 103, 500
Frichot, B.C., 3rd, 91, 284, 285
Friddell, T.J., 208, 482
Fridman, I.A., 141, 552
Friedebold, G., 17, 420
Friedman, B., 211, 428
Friedrich, E., 25, 54, 308, 310, 367, 368
Friendly, D.S., 89, 92, 291, 297, 301, 303
Frishman, M.P., 45, 175, 176, 424, 427

Fritsch, P., 145, 482
Fromm, G., 78, 413
Fry, L., 64, 578
Fuga, G.C., 167, 293
Fujita, K., 231
Fukuoka, Y., 188, 479, 489, 513
Fuld, G.L., 90, 284, 302
Furness, G., 72, 569
Furst, S.D., Jr., 235, 576
Furukawa, H., 201, 516
Fuse, K., 230

Gaal, R., 206, 264, 301, 556
Gaffuri, S., 226, 261, 414, 554
Gager, W.E., 129, 158, 208, 366, 372, 472
Gaillon, R., 157, 232, 506, 520
Galegov, G.A., 232, 338
Galla, F., 86, 263, 527
Gallai, Z., 159, 254, 545
Gallagher, E., 87, 580
Gallanis, T.C., 116, 284, 291
Galliera, A., 239, 522
Gallwey, J.M., 104, 291
Ganju, D., 118, 325, 560
Garagnani, A., 173, 432
Garcia, J.A., 133
Garlacz, A., 192, 233, 515, 520
Garlicka, A., 244, 536
Garner, L.M., 64, 273
Garner, M.F., 22, 63, 83, 84, 103, 135, 185, 187, 188, 225, 236, 238, 334, 441, 442, 470, 487, 498, 500, 511, 513, 521, 522, 578
Garnier, G., 222, 534
Garnuszewski, Z., 21, 487
Garrachon, J., 131
Garrod, L.P., 156, 316, 568
Gastrin, B., 106, 291
Gate-Lyon, J., 137, 328

Gatti, A., 12, 422
Gaudefroy, M., 74, 193, 204, 343, 413, 543, 556, 563
Gavrilescu, M., 120, 292
Gedicke, K., 70, 142, 298, 360
Geelhoed, G.W., 28, 262
Geizer, E., 45, 139, 288, 291
Gelfand, M., 60, 425
Geller, L.I., 189, 401
Georges, P., 237, 547
Gerard, C.L., 213, 537
Ghosh, C.R., 41, 490
Giannone, R., 142, 569
Gianotti, F., 231
Gilbert, D.N., 244, 409
Gilchrist, R.K., 5, 336
Gillespie, E.J., 222, 542
Gilpin, C.A., 176, 349
Giocoli, G., 184, 563
Giordano, A.F., 81, 408, 526
Gip, L., 74, 92, 299, 311
Giroud, M., 11, 422, 536
Girrard, J.P., 121, 397, 528
Gjessing, C., 150, 529
Gjessing, H.C., 112, 148, 265, 314, 316, 370, 371
Gjonnaess, H., 223, 356, 565
Glaser, S., 89, 254, 283, 297
Glass, L.H., 10, 306
Glewski, M.J., 85, 555
Glicksman, J., 111, 501
Glicksman, J.M., 90, 150, 263, 285, 529
Glowinski, M., 228, 378, 556
Goffinet, D.R., 183, 443
Gokhale, V.K., 202, 517
Goldberg, J., 201, 260, 325
Gol'dberg, MIa, 41, 143, 490, 505
Golden, B., 105, 225, 363
Goldman, E.E., 153, 400, 472
Goldman, J.N., 33, 83, 112, 250, 384, 436, 471, 472
Golebiowska-Podgorczyk, 196, 333, 383
Golovinskii, M.P., 11, 392
Golub, S., 236, 576
Goncalves, A.P., 105, 347

Gonzalez, C.L., 195, 382
Gonzales, O.A., 216, 219, 263, 534
Goodwill, C.J., 225, 419
Gorbovitskii, S.E., 182, 194, 329, 411
Gorbulev, S.S., 196, 532
Gorbunova, M.I., 32, 424
Gorczyca, L.R., 126, 503
Gordon, E.R., 176, 563
Gorlick, H.S., 24
Gorzedowska, E., 70, 555
Gosset, O.G., 57, 68, 346, 347
Gostin, L., 210
Gould, W.M., 95, 324
Gourlay, E., 343, 379
Govers, J., 34, 271
Grabner, K., 111, 242, 379, 528
Grady, S.A., 41, 287
Graf, M., 8, 250, 522
Grandbois, J., 209
Grant, M., 235, 383
Granz, W., 232, 270
Grauer, I., 44, 424
Gravatt, A.E., 31, 273
Gray, B., 65, 342, 559
Gray, O.P., 215, 249, 430
Greaves, A.B., 57, 289, 310
Green, D., 15, 480, 571
Greenberg, J.H., 166, 382, 408
Gregorczyk, K.D., 55, 492
Gregory, J.E., 128, 352
Grewal, M.S., 202, 546
Grewel, F., 165, 360
Griffith, R.S., 71, 277
Grigor'ev, V.E.196,319,350
Grigoriou, D., 24, 261
Grimble, A., 134, 355, 561
Grimble,A.S., 156, 243, 278, 353, 538, 570, 577
Grimmer, H., 24, 244, 261, 326
Grin, E.I., 136, 280, 504
Groshev, V.N., 11, 392
Grossman, J., 94, 284

Grossman, L.J., 22, 488
Groth, O., 148, 251, 316
Grunberg, E., 10, 249, 557
Grunberger, V., 141, 552
Grunner, L., 75, 551
Grupper, C., 154, 164, 213, 303, 518, 531
Grys, E., 65, 66, 120, 173, 227, 544, 548, 553, 558, 559
Gudjònsson, H., 65, 377, 390
Guerresi, E., 237, 554
Guest, W.J., 102
Guillen, T.J., 199, 388, 401
Guilmet, D., 27, 424
Gundersen, T., 220, 250, 322, 385
Gunn, A.D.G., 193, 282
Guthe, T., 35, 47, 69, 242, 361, 430, 480, 579
Gwinn, J.L., 167, 432

Haagsma, F.M., 198, 257, 430, 532
Haavelsrud, O.I., 58, 95, 289, 325
Haddad, N., 70, 264
Haddad, N.A., 21, 252, 355
Hadden, S.B., 221, 330
Hadida, E., 96, 442
Haim, S., 90, 209, 302, 483
Hall, G.E., 118, 333
Hallinger, L., 78, 311, 368, 384, 526
Hallis, N.O.J., 343, 362
Hallock, J., 43, 434
Halverson, C.W., 107, 313
Hanczakowska, M., 154, 506
Hansen, T., 94, 302
Hantschke, D., 13, 307
Harcourt, B., 148, 437, 472, 475
Hardy, J.B., 79, 369
Hardy, P.H., 137
Hare, M.J., 129, 353
Harner, R.E., 78, 496
Harper, I.A., 109, 226, 253, 364, 403, 566
Harper, J.M., 78, 496

Harper, J.R., 227, 548
Harris, M., 187, 476, 513
Harris, W.D., 186, 272, 512
Hart, M., 43, 434, 439
Hartgill, J.C., 58, 347
Hartmen, A.A., 190, 411
Hartsock, R.J., 118, 120
Harvey, A.M., 44, 490
Harwick, H.J., 128, 352, 378
Hasegawa, T., 66, 68, 446
Hatos, G., 220, 322, 385
Hatt, B.H., 194, 301, 307, 581
Hausnerova, S., 184, 319
Hawkins, D.F., 228, 282, 547
Haye, R., 117
Hayes, G.S., 214, 240, 361, 383
Hayman, C.R., 189, 411
Heathfield, K.W., 131
Heberer, G., 15, 57, 423, 425
Hedden, J.C., 149
Hederstedt, B., 186, 512
Hegyi, E., 10, 78, 141, 298, 300, 388
Heimans, A.L., 49, 282, 288
Heine, H., 85
Heinke, E., 33, 198, 309, 320, 409, 412, 540
Heitmann, H.J., 55, 112, 143, 187, 387, 397, 406, 440, 504, 513
Hejzlar, M., 130, 215, 314, 321
Heller, R.H., 245, 264, 350
Hellerstrom, S., 241, 536
Henderson, R.A., 75, 290
Herman, E., 184
Hertoft, P., 113, 410
Herweg, J.C., 151, 430, 506
Herzberg, J.J., 122, 337
Heslop, I.H., 212, 477
Hess, E.V., 185, 294

Hess, J., 178, 553
Heuillet, G., 15
Hewitt, A.B., 148, 191, 211, 268, 293, 319, 433
Heyl, U., 232, 294
Higoumenakis, K.G., 98, 435, 441
Higuchi, K., 63, 441, 525
Hill, B.H., 91, 285
Hill, D., 69, 281
Hiltenbrand, C., 25, 423
Hirai, H., 110, 347
Hirsch, H.A., 49, 174, 288, 293
Hirth, R.S., 88, 351
Hobs, A.R., 86
Hoerner, M.T., 206, 537
Hoffmann, B., 39, 111, 244, 552, 555
Hoffmann, F.D., 199, 437, 516
Hofmann, D., 202, 332, 549
Hofmeier, H.M., 127, 442, 475
Hogarth, W.P., 94, 324
Holder, A.R., 119, 333, 397
Holmes, K.K., 72, 200, 222, 286, 298, 320, 323, 373, 375, 384, 385, 408, 539
Holmes, M., 189, 411
Holt, S., 115, 352
Holzegel, B., 146, 301
Holzegel, K., 59, 290, 310
Holzmann, H., 65, 525
Honigsberg, B.M., 151, 553
Hooton, W.F., 116
Horácek, J., 163, 360
Horak, J., 7, 483
Hori, M., 169
Howes, H.L., Jr., 218, 540, 564
Hrncir, Z., 35, 179
Huber, A., 163, 378
Hudson, E.H., 31, 225
Huffman, G., 131
Hughes, G.R., 115, 390, 425
Hughes, H.E., 32, 542
Hughes, M.K., 156, 270, 407
Hunder, G.G., 156
Hunter, E.F., 83, 498
Huriet, C., 62
Huriez, C., 67, 168, 573, 575

Hutchinson, R.I., 230, 294
Hutfield, D.C., 98, 99, 286, 326

Iankov, N., 141, 147, 553, 555
Ianushkevich, N.I., 129, 426
Idsoe, O., 130, 179, 398, 529
Ieri, A., 56
Ignat'ev, M.V., 11, 389
Iizuka, T., 133, 504
Ikeda, T., 64, 173, 192, 262, 264, 446, 515
Il'In, B.I., 76, 279, 559
Il'in, I.I., 36, 71, 234, 244, 276, 278, 335, 337, 340, 350, 557
Iljin, I.I., 87, 548
Imazu, K., 97, 274, 357
Ingham, H.R., 47, 569
Ionescu, E., 239, 445
Ipsen, J., 22, 549
Irwin, T., 245, 583
Ishigami, J., 32, 368, 568
Ishiwata, Y., 20, 434
Ismail, H.K., 95, 536
Ito, I., 15, 423, 509
Ito, K., 168, 217, 519
Iudin, I.A.L., 194, 266
Ivanov, V.N., 174, 430
Iversen, S., 216, 349
Iwanowska, T., 222, 480

Jacobs, P.H., 126, 348
Jacobson, L., 137, 348
Jacobson, S., 165, 400
Jacyk, W., 65, 559
Jakubowski, A., 76, 77, 122, 159, 526
Janicka, D., 219, 534, 539
Jarrett, W.H., II, 61, 363
Jarvis, J.F., 19, 421

Jasser, S., 186, 257, 512
Jawetz, E., 31, 345
Jeansson, S., 87, 326
Jedlicková, J., 23, 476
Jefferis, F.J., 99, 330
Jefferiss, J., 239, 576
Jekel, J.F., 179
Jin, M., 207, 260
Jina, Z., 150, 366, 427
Jirovec, O., 227, 546, 548
Jo, K., 162, 507
Johansson, E.A., 108, 187, 217, 280, 501, 513, 519
Johnson, A.H., 88, 283
Johnson, A.N., 240, 340
Johnson, D.W., 73, 193, 290, 319
Johnston, N.A., 5, 484
Jokinen, E.J., 84, 498
Jones, B.R., 109, 207, 253, 364, 403, 416, 474
Jones, D., 37, 268
Jones, D.M., 128, 352, 378
Jones, R.H., 122, 277, 528
Jorgensen, B.B., 198, 516
Josey, W.E., 244, 350
Jouglard, J., 152, 399
Jouhar, A., 28, 262, 308
Jozsa, L., 29, 424
Jubelin, J., 78, 395
Jue, R., 40, 489
Juhlin, I., 152, 161, 316, 317, 371
Juhlin, L., 63, 79, 110, 274, 287, 295, 298, 299, 300, 306, 410, 435
Julian, A.J., 63, 493
Jung, E.G., 126, 314, 370
Jung, H., 210
Jung, H.D., 141, 162, 381, 570

Kabatova, A., 38, 287
Kagwa-Nyanzi, J.A., 107, 364
Kahn, G., 184, 294
Kahn, M.F., 205, 433
Kahn, R.L., 19, 486
Kail, F., 188, 257, 514
Kaiser, W., 21, 55, 273, 327

Kakusu1, K., 102
Kalashchnikova, N.F., 56, 493
Kalbarczyk, K., 69, 298
Kalidasan, C.S., 26, 470
Kaliner, B.S., 150, 316, 367
Kallings, L.O., 60, 290
Kalov, P.G., 38, 550
Kamel, S., 7, 363
Kamp, M., 241, 576
Kampmeier, R.H., 35, 179, 482, 524
Kanemasa, Y., 105, 500
Kanjilal, G.C., 27, 115, 581
Kanterman, C.V., 246, 577
Kaouzny, J., 26, 363
Karik, L.M., 6
Karmi, G., 17, 254, 265
Karmody, C.S., 54, 421, 435
Károlyi, I., 51
Kartamyshev, A.I., 115, 149, 275, 339, 502
Kasik, J.E., 9, 388
Katsilabors, L., 221, 331, 374, 402
Kaufer, R., 68, 395
Kaufman, W.H., 208, 418
Kaupas, V., 220, 321
Kawai, T., 205, 517
Kawamura, N., 202, 546
Kawamura, T., 84, 481
Keburlia, K.L., 116, 133, 291, 552
Keifetz, N., 230, 582
Keilly, J.E., 111, 501
Keiser, H., 34, 283
Kelley, J.H., 237, 350
Kellock, I.A., 208
Kellogg, D.S., Jr., 56, 104, 130, 244, 282, 292, 493, 500
Kendell, H.W., 80, 311, 526
Kenéz, J., 245, 330
Kennedy, H.K., 47, 379
Kerber, R.E., 219, 264, 415, 539
Kercull, R.G., 76, 250, 311, 407

Kerk, L., 121, 337
Kern, A., 145, 147, 217, 237, 370, 375, 505, 529, 534, 535
Kerr, A.G., 44, 435, 524
Keys, T.F., 193, 319
Khasin, IaI, 33, 281, 542
Kheifets, S.N., 199, 357
Khidyrov, KhN, 195, 196, 256, 515, 532
Khozeniuk, D.I., 9, 392
Kierland, R.R., 12
Kiesewalter, D., 27, 308
Kiesewetter, R., 218, 402
Kiesz, W., 59, 440, 483, 525
Kilcoyne, R.F., 167, 508
Kilczewski, W., 203, 252, 564
Kimata, S., 239, 429
Kimball, M.W., 90, 295, 312
Kind, A.C., 52, 540
Kinda, K., 137, 315
King, A., 79, 231, 241, 380, 575, 582
Kingsley, H.J., 151, 325
Kinsella, F.J., 97, 359
Kinsella, T.D., 42, 253, 403, 412
Kirai, K., 178, 254
Kiraly, K., 14, 18, 35, 41, 51, 84, 95, 103, 166, 192, 485, 486, 489, 490, 492, 499, 508, 515
Kirch, A., 45
Kirchheim, D., 151, 277
Kirjakov, I., 208
Kirkpatrick, D.J., 62, 324
Kirsner, A.B., 88, 283
Kislova, T.A., 139, 315, 362
Kiss, J., 106, 560
Kiss, L., 177, 542, 563
Kitamoto, O., 36, 524, 542
Kleban, V.I., 99, 544
Klein, J.O., 37, 351
Klein, P., 143, 328
Klimenko, A.V., 145, 286
Knapikowa, D., 67, 425
Knierim, F., 187, 512
Knowles, J.A., 240, 582
Knox, J.M., 78, 495

Kober, P., 88, 297
Kochetkov, V.D., 150, 212, 340, 473
Kochura, O.D., 215, 267
Kodandapani, C., 247, 439
Kodlová, E., 231, 428
Kody, P., 23
Kolankowski, J., 218, 301
Kolesov, A.P., 154, 332, 545
Komorowski, J., 199, 427
Komov, O.P., 55, 540
Konopada, W., 228, 566
Konopik, J., 162, 360
Konopka, Z., 27, 423
Kooy, P., 195, 358, 406, 515
Kop, P., 34, 439
Kopczynski, S., 112, 425
Kopéc, W., 128
Kopecký, K., 92, 299
Korepanov, A.M., 30, 393
Korik, L.M., 38, 57, 101, 112, 119, 143, 249, 332, 335, 549, 550, 552, 553, 558, 560
Kornstad, L., 23, 488
Korte, C., 113, 432
Korting, G.W., 183, 536
Kösmiderski, S., 118, 181, 209, 502, 511, 518
Kostanecki, W., 96
Kostie, P., 180, 414, 549
Kovacs, E., 146, 343, 562
Kozakiewicz, J., 162, 257
Kozerski, J., 221, 322, 374
Kozhevnikov, P.V., 197, 267
Kozik, M., 59, 536
Kozin, S.L., 133, 215, 256, 321, 380
Kozina, W., 59, 420
Kozlowska, D., 228, 567
Kozub, W.R., 92, 569
Kradolfer, F., 10, 356, 557
Krahe, C., 209, 480
Kramar, J., 103, 551
Kraubig, H., 80, 377

Kraus, A., 232, 547
Kraus, G.W., 91, 303
Kraus, N., 45, 424
Kraus, S.J., 19, 84, 345, 498
Kraus, Z., 109, 300
Kravchuk, P.A., 117, 397
Krell, L., 76, 495
Kresbach, H., 141, 220, 322, 442
Krezel, T., 149, 421
Krich, A., 409
Krishna, K.S., 243, 362
Krishnan, M.U.
Krook, G., 156, 317
Kropfl, A., 181, 427
Krunic, R., 115, 492
Krupova, J., 196, 554
Kubec, K., 52, 492
Kuhn, U.S., 347
Kukushkin, A.M., 166, 570
Kumstát, Z., 106, 208, 471, 474, 501
Kundsin, R.B., 128, 332, 352
Kunicki, A., 229, 477
Kuntsevich, L.D., 71, 184, 277, 311, 318, 362, 373
Kuptsov, V.V., 11, 388
Kurnatowska, A., 66, 202, 265, 347, 546, 559
Kuroda, K., 36, 412
Kushner, I., 88, 283
Kusumoto, M., 58, 478
Kutscher, E., 35, 309
Kuvaldina, O.A., 30, 389
Kuwuhara, S., 28, 262, 446
Kuznetsova, M.K., 126, 292
Kvicera, J., 57, 74, 144, 289, 310, 381, 526
Kwalick, D.S., 182, 294
Kwoczynski, M.Z., 181, 553

Labouche, F., 136, 161, 315, 439, 578
Lagerholm, B., 53, 153, 288, 316, 400
Lahiri, K.D., 230, 286
Laird, S.M., 17, 135, 355, 486, 562

Lake, A., 235, 582
Lamar, C.G., 8, 304
Lamb, A.M., 133, 380
Lancellotti, M., 174, 175, 531
Lancucki, J., 18, 358, 407
Landes, E., 245, 350
Lang, W.R., 236, 350
Lange, E., 115, 475
Lange, P.K., 89, 290
Langer, J., 245, 522
Laugier, P., 26, 416
Lanigan-O'Keeffe, F.M., 110, 579
Lantis, L.R., 182, 260, 433
Lantz, M.A., 130, 503
Lapuszek, W., 219, 343, 564
Laroche, J.F., 27, 536
Larsson-Cohn, U., 132, 561
Lassus, A., 10, 13, 19, 57, 62, 149, 156, 171, 221, 225, 243, 271, 272, 311, 322, 336, 361, 386, 440, 485, 486, 506, 510, 519
Latourelle, P., 104, 500
Laurell, A.B., 98, 189, 258
Lawson, B.J., 100
Lazar, M., 132, 292
Lazzaro, C., 112, 502
Leak, D., 16, 363, 470
Lebioda, J., 123, 213, 269, 279, 366, 397, 528, 533
Leclerc, G., 222, 535
Le Coulant, P., 11, 134, 337, 438
Ledvina, M., 102, 396
Lee, H.Y., 210
Leger, R.R., 236, 576
Leigh, D.A., 184, 319, 373
Leigheb, G., 238, 521
Lejman, K., 6, 21, 99, 149, 162, 211, 327, 391, 433, 438, 477, 523

Lemercier, G., 31
Lenartovich, V.A., 119, 335, 561
Le Noc, P., 159, 317
Lentini, J., 12, 251
Lenz, P.E., 47, 273
Leone, G., 53, 543
Lesinski, J., 18, 486
Levene, G.M., 171
Levine, B., 102, 396
Levine, B.B., 157, 400
Levine, B.M., 188, 236, 407
Levrier, M., 226, 537, 566
Levy, B., 30
Levykin, A.I., 96, 256, 369, 478
Lew, J., 170
Lewis, J.S., 19, 486
Ley, H., 96, 536
Liakhovitskii, N.S., 54, 543
Liashuk, P.M., 11, 392
Lichter, P.R., 111, 471
Liden, S., 94, 300
Lieveaux, A., 155, 562
Lillo, F., 88, 544
Limbos, P., 191, 514
Lind, I., 38, 101, 287, 291
Lindell, S.S., 48, 491
Lindheimer, W., 7, 212, 391, 522
Lindman, C., 70, 92, 281
Linguiti, L., 20, 345
Linken, A., 164, 203, 268, 272
Linton, W.T., 210, 533
Lip, J., 29, 345
Lipskii, I.A., 84, 327
Litchfield, J.T., Jr., 62, 355, 377
Littlewood, J.M., 232, 548
Litinova, N.N., 75
Liubimova, L.K., 112, 552
Livshits, M.L., 213, 421
Lochmannova, J., 143, 234, 263, 331, 521, 538
Lockyer, J.W., 210, 444
Lodin, A., 92, 299
Loe, K., 108, 479, 501
Loesch, D., 34
Loewenfeld, I.E., 16, 253, 363, 470

Logan, J.L., 240, 582
Logan, L.C., 73, 218, 441, 519
Lohr, E., 12, 422
Lomholt, G., 93, 160, 299, 574
Lomuto, G., 56, 492
Lopatecki, T., 10, 557
Lopatin, A.I., 144, 286
Lorentzen, S.E., 212, 474
Loseva, O.K., 22, 152, 205, 255, 256, 385, 386, 523, 530, 533
Lospalluti, M., 104
Lou, K., 156, 506
Loughlin, M.J., 92, 299
Lourie, R.S., 124
Lozada, E., 198, 338
Lucas, J.B., 47, 220
Lucas, A.J., 29, 572
Lucas, J.B., 58, 132, 263, 289, 305, 310, 322, 411, 524
Lucatorto, F.M., 168, 508
Luckerath, I., 217, 402
Ludwig, G., 146, 315, 370
Luger, A., 52, 126, 380, 524
Luise, A., 15, 423
Lunsden, W.H., 114, 552
Lupovitch, A., 120, 397
Lur'e, S.S., 40, 309
Lynch, P.J., 127, 348
Lyon, L.J., 47, 395, 431

McBroom, P., 235, 576
McCall, C.E., 119, 335
McCracken, J.D., 131
McDonald, R., 43, 434
McFadzean, J.A., 86, 342, 560
Macfarlane, W.V., 243, 577
McGill, M.I., 116
McGrew, B.E., 20, 86, 166, 443, 487, 499
Mach, E., 243
Mach, K.W., 57, 95, 191, 373, 440, 475, 527, 532, 577

Maciejowska, E., 39, 125, 134, 180, 394, 397, 398, 400, 401
Mack, L.W., Jr., 215
McKenzie-Pollock, J.S., 155 339, 381
Mackey, D.M., 197, 515
McKusick, V.A., 37, 268, 424, 477
Macleod, C.A., 12, 422
McLone, D.G., 28, 92, 94, 191, 250, 262, 308, 312, 313, 365, 514, 538
McNeel, D.P., 30, 420
Maeland, J.A., 13, 14, 102, 186, 187, 294, 296, 305
Magnier, P., 7, 345, 537
Magnin, P., 223, 344, 378, 565
Mahapatra, S.B., 87, 366
Maheras, M.G., 152, 399
Mahoney, J.D., 135, 286, 569
Majima, E., 217
Maksimov, V.F., 22, 308
Makuch, M., 211, 421
Malachowski, Z., 224, 357, 566
Maleville, 49, 417
Malgras, J., 115, 502
Malý, E., 75, 138, 163, 174, 360, 372, 436, 526, 531
Malygina, T.A., 164, 272, 508
Mamunes, P., 63, 441
Mandal, S.B., 108, 438, 442
Manikhas, M.G., 29, 557
Manikowska-Lesinska, W., 60, 493
Mann, G.V., 206, 470
Mannweiler, E., 187, 553
Manser, H., 113, 275
Many, P., 200, 276
Maramarosi, G., 219, 265, 541
Marchi, A.G., 43, 231, 254, 434, 438
Marconato, A., 157, 553
Marcondes, R.S., 97, 385, 408
Marcozzi, A., 146, 479, 505
Marcus, D.F., 88, 283

Mardh, P.A., 229, 354
Mariani, G., 8, 484
Marill, F.G., 52, 61, 174, 176, 212, 264, 433, 476, 531, 536
Marks, M.I., 132, 398
Marley, F., 218, 571
Maroudi, D., 180, 261, 378, 556
Marquez-Monter, H., 24, 258, 336
Marquis, Y., 61, 425
Marshall, M.J., 193, 264, 319
Marshall, S., 136, 570
Martin, J.E., Jr., 107, 161, 293, 313
Martin-Bouyer, G., 53, 358
Martini, G.A., 198
Martini, J., 218, 279, 321
Martins, R., 170, 509
Maslenikov, V., 127, 426
Matanič, V., 84, 404, 527
Matanič, Z., 84, 113, 528, 84
Mathesius, V.J., 96, 269, 297
Mathurin, L., 106, 501
Matner, T., 194, 401
Matsuda, T., 124, 385
Matsuhashi, N., 210, 518
Matsuoka, T., 202, 204, 367, 537
Matthews, L.J., 32, 334
Matuhasi, T., 104, 201, 517
Matveev, V.N., 175, 415, 531
Maurer, H.J., 16, 420
Maurer, L.H., 90, 306, 312, 369, 538
Mausner, J.S., 175, 301
Mavrov, I.I., 75, 311, 362
Mayer, R.F., 137
Mayer, H.G., 219, 284
Mazzacuva, D., 107
Mbanefo, S.E., 68, 306

Meade, R.H., 92, 312
Mechie, A.M., 243, 280
Medebach, H., 144, 292
Melanowski, W.H., 7, 363
Mellbin, T., 13, 484
Meloni, C., 178, 329
Mendel, L., 115
Meneghini, C.L., 72, 120, 261, 528
Menichella, V., 43, 413, 434
Mercadal-Peyri, J., 127, 436, 476
Merin, S., 45, 471
Merklen, F.P., 13, 157, 507, 522
Mersch, F., 141, 442, 483
Mertslin, G.V., 186, 334, 512
Meshaka, J.M., 19, 416
Metzger, A.L., 89, 151, 283, 303, 506
Metzger, M., 17, 82, 104, 203, 417, 446, 497, 517
Meyer, A., 16, 50, 423
Meyer, I., 149, 475
Meyer, P.E., 14, 485
Meyer-Rohn, J., 27, 159, 191, 210, 317, 372, 514, 518
Mezhebovskii, A.M., 75, 342, 559
Michaels, R.M., 31, 557
Michalowski, B., 156, 328
Michaud, P., 212, 428
Michelazzi, L., 109
Midana, A., 157, 507
Miedziński, F., 162, 317
Mielech, R., 77, 201, 526, 533
Mierzejewski, W., 69, 261
Migliano, L., 123, 314
Mikhail, G.R., 84
Mikhailov, V.N., 24, 572
Miklaszewska, M., 140, 504
Mikuni, M., 221, 263, 474
Mildner, T., 158, 328
Milgrom, F., 8, 484
Milich, M.V., 146, 209, 505
Miljkovic, M., 45, 288
Miller, J.N., 14, 102, 485
Milonova, T.I., 225, 519
Milor, J.H., 64, 274

Minami, K., 170, 510
Minkin, W., 98, 108, 220, 231, 321, 322, 326, 374, 396, 438
Mirsagatov, M.U., 22, 255, 308
Misgeld, V., 60, 270, 385, 406, 440
Mizuno, S., 56, 159, 558, 574
Mizuoka, K., 142, 159, 170, 504, 507, 509.
Mleziva, J., 65, 342, 559
Moch, G., 48, 491
Modde, H., 89, 281
Mofty, A.M., 193, 325
Moghissi, K.S., 70, 258
Moiseev, S.G., 229, 428
Moisseev, S.G., 61, 425
Molin, L., 92, 161, 299, 317
Molina Leguizamon, E.B., 123, 419
Moller, H., 217, 246, 575
Montenegro, E.N., 99, 471
Montes, J., 67, 277
Moore, M.B., Jr., 32, 270
Mora, Z.P., 82, 254, 380
Morel, P., 53, 440
Moreno, R.J., 233, 344, 567
Morenz, J., 142, 406
Morita, T., 227, 547
Morris, C.A., 8, 377, 484
Morrison, A.I., 5, 483
Morrison, G.D., 219, 321, 374
Mortada, A., 7, 363
Morton, R.S., 12, 64, 91, 96, 122, 124, 200, 274, 281, 314, 341, 349, 582
Mosora, N., 95, 544
Mothershed, S.M., 41, 65, 158, 490, 507, 525
Motobayashi, A., 36, 543
Motomiya, M., 31
Mouton, R.P., 58, 289
Mowat, A.G., 172, 404
Moya, G., 209

Muller, F., 39, 77, 82, 102, 125, 141, 201, 429, 445, 489, 495, 503, 516
Muller, P., 168, 220, 321, 508, 509
Muller, W.A., 18, 202, 546, 549
Murata, M., 201, 516
Murphy, J.E., 6, 345, 355
Muspratt, B., 107, 481
Mustakallio, K.K., 14, 19, 49, 485, 491
Mustala, O., 191, 388
Muth, H., 145, 332

Naess, K., 37, 394
Nagay, B., 32, 368
Nagele, E., 194, 444
Nagesha, C.N., 32, 550
Naguib, S.N., 173, 259, 555
Nahmias, A.J., 87, 134, 326
Najafi, H., 15, 423
Nakae, M., 77, 555
Nanjiani, M.R., 139, 427, 442
Nathan, D.L., 165, 381, 408
Naumann, G., 110
Naumova, D., 18, 39, 78, 446, 489
Nazarian, L.F., 50, 284
Neblett, T.R., 225, 520
Negreiros, E.B., 9, 392
Negulici-Baliff, E., 71, 277
Nelson, C.Y., 115, 330, 571
Nelson, M., 40, 309
Nemec, F., 216, 221, 323, 374, 534
Neser, W.B., 18, 69, 106, 273, 409, 481
Nesmith, L.W., 97, 395
Nesterenko, G.B., 101, 256, 527
Neves, J., 205, 272, 338
Nevin, T.A., 41, 490
New York City Board of Education, 176
Nexmand, P.H., 182

Nicholas, L., 59, 117, 118, 164, 185, 280, 422, 440, 442, 507, 511
Nicol, C.S., 162, 317
Nicol, W.G., 43, 471
Nicolau, S.G., 154
Nicora, G., 88, 414, 548
Niedner, A., 134, 387
Niedzwiecka, D., 88, 435, 475
Nielsen, A., 17, 94, 252, 282, 284, 291, 303, 305
Nielsen, R., 184
Nikitina, N.V., 122, 380
Nikol'skaia, E.P., 175, 256, 531
Niles, J.H., 89, 283, 303
Nilsson, L., 96, 313
Ninu, E., 81, 497
Nishida, M., 28, 251, 262
Nishida, S., 68
Noda, A., 127, 552
Nohara, S., 36, 543
Nolting, S., 168, 222, 334, 509, 535
Nonaka, K., 52, 492
Nordin, K., 80, 395, 441
Norins, L.C., 183, 185, 511, 575
Norn, M.S., 69, 363
Novotný, F., 69, 72, 81, 246, 251, 358, 380

Oates, J.K., 190, 329, 349, 575
Ober, W.B., 23, 280, 296
Oberhauser, E., 40, 429
O'Brien, J.T., 116, 291
Obrtel, J., 33, 42, 47, 138, 139, 174, 199, 214, 216, 268, 276, 296, 301, 308, 340, 359, 413, 534
Oda, T., 169
Odegaard, K., 49, 113, 288, 296, 310
Oganesian, E.N., 117, 436

Ogata, M., 218
Ogata, T., 150, 506
Oikawa, K., 185, 512
Okamoto, S., 123, 481
Okawa, T., 159, 199, 223, 545, 555, 565
Okey, C.H., 78, 495
Okuma, H., 92, 299
Olansky, S., 51, 58, 194, 207, 210, 382, 418, 440, 492, 533
Oliver, M., 31, 424
Oller, L.Z., 28, 79, 86, 160, 171, 250, 262, 263, 298, 312, 337, 343, 523
Olsen, G.A., 93, 209, 312, 369, 384, 470
Olszewska, Z., 113
Ondrejicka, M., 99, 395
O'Neill, P., 73, 494
Oner, A., 113
Onisk, Z.
Onoda, Y., 52, 160, 573, 574
Orfila, J., 106, 238, 106, 501, 521
Orhel, I., 10, 45, 73, 126, 143, 446, 491, 494, 503, 505
Orley, J., 236, 582
Ormea, 49, 524
Oros, M., 179, 437
Ortolani, G., 60, 551
Osada, F., 39, 167, 170, 489, 508
Osako, R., 221, 332, 534
Osborn, R.A., 206, 264, 301, 556
Osoba, A.O., 98, 326
Osofsky, H.J., 189
Ostendorf, P., 124, 426
Osterlund, K., 139, 298, 302
Osti, A., 231, 421
Ostrovskii, A.G., 25, 391, 393
O'Sullivan, J.F., 227, 547
Ota, H., 73, 494
Otani, M., 46, 491
Ovchinnikov, N.M., 13, 17, 65, 68, 86, 87, 103, 186, 230, 312, 329, 369, 484, 486, 493, 500

Oxelius, V.A., 104, 430
Ozawa, A., 41, 490
Ozbay, T., 76, 261, 375, 560

Pacenovská, M., 215, 255, 534
Pagel, W., 9, 484
Pagnes, P., 79, 496
Pait, C.F., 171, 293
Pallidum, T., 41
Palm, G., 76, 495
Palmer, D.L., 97, 580
Palmer, W.L., 22, 487
Palmgren, L., 194, 307, 582
Panaitescu, D., 30, 341, 557
Pandele, A., 192, 553
Pankov, B.S., 29, 100, 432, 438
Pannu, J.S., 108, 501
Papaloukas, A., 123, 376, 561
Parashchak, P.V., 54
Pariser, D.M., 161, 293
Pariser, H., 58, 991, 220, 263, 289, 299, 322
Parish, L.C., 150, 349
Paris-Hamelin, A., 76, 441, 578
Parker, E.W., 89, 303
Parker, R.T., 10, 365
Partain, J.O., 16, 251, 282
Paschoal, L.H., 55, 232, 271, 272, 324, 535
Pashkov, B.M., 6, 214, 255, 266
Pasieczny, T., 149, 570
Passerini, A., 214, 537
Passoni, M., 140, 436
Patrono, D., 234, 554
Patterson, M.E., 43, 377, 421, 524
Paul, W., 177, 443, 473
Pautrat, J., 58, 425
Pavisic, Z., 212, 474
Pavlov, S.T., 174, 256, 531

Peacock, W.L., Jr., 125, 292
Peck, S., 94, 324
Pedder, J.R., 165, 206, 386
Pedersen, A.H., 167, 293
Pedersen-Bjergaard, J., 33, 156, 194, 197, 393, 400, 401, 407
Peirone, E., 136
Peisert, E., 98, 269, 390
Pejtsik, B., 180, 549
Pekowski, M., 131, 314, 414
Pellegrini, G., 168, 421
Pendergrast, D.H., 235, 475
Perdrup, A., 59, 65, 298, 493
Pereyra, A.J., 95, 527
Perl, G., 155, 553
Perti, E., 180, 339, 382
Pesina, Z.A., 13, 307
Peter, R., 92, 178, 284, 575
Petersen, K.F., 206, 407
Peterson, W.C., Jr., 80, 497
Peterson, W.F., 125, 226, 342, 378, 566
Petzoldt, K., 71, 578
Phelps, L.N., 114
Philip, P.J., 224, 260, 578
Philip, R.N., 185, 337
Philipp, E., 99, 330
Phillips, I., 13, 107, 307, 313
Philips, L., 107, 265, 278, 335
Piacentini, I., 106, 479
Pickett, G., 208, 444
Pillot, J., 103, 499
Pinoli, G., 165, 386, 545
Pinter, M., 20, 345
Pion, R.J., 158, 268, 581
Pippione, M., 102, 189
Platts, W.M., 240, 361
Plauchu, G., 230, 429
Plintovic, V., 138, 296
Plonski, J., 99, 407, 544
Płoński, K., 47, 380
Podair, S., 190, 276
Podesta, H.A., 98, 390
Pokrovskii, V.I., 165, 483
Poliakov, A.I., 86, 125, 139, 279, 315, 343, 362, 560, 561

Poliakova, Z.P., 146, 305
Pollingher, 46, 417
Pollner, P., 131, 436
Ponting, L.I., 62, 272
Pop-Aceva, M., 77, 495
Pophristov, P., 133, 503
Porapakkham, S., 126, 343, 561
Porter, W.L., 19, 64, 100, 162, 274, 317, 339, 409
Porudominskii, I.M., 6, 16, 51, 288, 304, 308, 310
Poske, R.M., 88, 283
Pospisil, L., 7, 51, 155, 167, 176, 195, 484, 492, 506, 508, 581
Potapnev, F.B., 75, 559
Potapnev, F.V., 22, 228, 255, 308, 567
Pototskii, I.I., 75, 174, 182, 209, 329, 372, 483, 526, 531
Potuznik, V., 55, 58, 164, 183, 192, 195, 289, 293, 294, 340, 382
Powrozny, W., 189, 391
Prakken, J.R., 212, 419
Prandini, N.M., 33, 309
Prather, E.C., 60, 481
Preste, E., 231, 475
Prevosti, L., 72, 425
Prewitt, T.A., 211, 280, 428
Privat, Y., 244, 386, 402
Prochacki, H., 238, 402
Prokopchuk, AIa., 6, 572
Prorok, I., 94, 300
Puccinelli, V., 53, 438
Puffer, J., 84, 499
Pugh, V.W., 126, 172, 503, 510
Purola, E., 93, 303, 556
Putkonen, T., 31, 80, 152, 316, 371, 390, 488
Pytel-Dabrowska, T., 26, 393

Quilichini, R., 26, 476

Raab, W., 155, 223, 565
Rabb, M.F., 151, 473
Rabello, F.E., 163, 530
Rabito, C., 33, 523
Racz, I., 99, 330
Raj, B., 204, 388
Rajka, G., 135, 220, 322, 570
Rakhmanov, V.A., 6, 29, 81, 139, 145, 163, 174, 177, 195, 256, 266, 275, 328, 339, 381, 418, 439, 531
Rakhmatov, B.R., 55, 541
Ramos, S.J., 52, 525
Rampini, E., 161, 204, 414
Rangiah, P.N., 27, 324
Ranque, J., 03, 517
Rasiewicz, W., 201, 478
Rasmussen, D.H., 222, 534
Rasponi, L., 34, 405, 540
Raszeja-Kotelba, B., 181, 318, 405
Rathlev, T., 74, 96, 494, 499
Rava, G., 140, 146, 432, 536
Ravenholt, O., 240, 384
Rawlins, D.C., 62, 272
Rawls, N.B., 119, 281
Rawls, W.E., 17, 182, 260, 325, 578
Rayner, C.F., 40, 550
Reddy, D.B., 211, 428
Reddy, K.S., 212
Redmond, A.P., 54, 394
Rees, E., 89, 90, 91, 284, 290
Reichenberger, M., 215, 402
Reifferscheid, M., 179, 259, 349
Reinig, E., 23, 273
Reising, G., 169, 317, 387
Renkonen, O.V., 52, 310, 368
Renoux, M., 128, 503

Resl, V., 15, 35, 297 301, 379
Resta, V., 86, 133, 413, 504
Restivo, Manfridi, M.L., 163, 364
Restrepo, C., 136, 426
Retel-Laurentin, A., 28, 358
Reyn, A., 12, 170, 173, 204, 278, 279, 293, 307, 318, 320, 372, 373, 412, 415, 538
Reynaud, G., 140, 436
Reznikov, E.K., 125, 145, 275, 582
Reznikova, L.S., 24, 177, 218, 488
Ribeiro, J., 190, 575
Riboldi, A., 141, 315, 539
Ribuffo, A., 79, 496
Rice, N.S., 55, 204, 430, 440, 474
Richardson, D.R., 210, 418
Richardson, F.H., 236, 582
Riley, K., 55, 492
Rimbaud, P., 8, 103, 484, 499
Ritter, G., 119
Roberts, M.E., 171, 190, 510, 514
Roberts, R.S., 81, 327
Robertson, D.H., 124, 192, 215, 333, 431, 554, 581
Robinson, I.E., 241, 582
Robinson, M.H., 234, 295
Robinson, O.P., 39, 394
Robinson, R.C., 43, 434
Rocco, E., 44, 258, 440, 478
Rocco, P.U., 50, 385
Rocha, A., 103, 500
Rochet, M.E., 6, 331, 344, 376
Rockl, H., 101, 339
Roder, H., 141, 242, 337, 361

Rodovský, J., 177, 318, 372
Rodrigues, F.V., 224, 354, 566
Rodriguez, D.C., 38, 40, 250, 309, 326, 327, 333
Rodriguez Diaz, L.H., 233, 327, 542
Rodriquez-Arias, B., 132
Roepstorff, S.O., 75, 282, 290
Roeth, C.L., 90, 285
Roitburd, M.F., 230, 520
Roland, J., 6
Rollier, R., 38, 98, 390, 405, 435, 479, 480
Ronald, A., 13, 307, 374
Ronald, A.R., 207, 320, 539
Roper, P., 67, 330
Rosenbaum, L.J., 218, 474
Rosenblatt, D., 64, 74, 273, 580
Rosenblum, A.H., 152, 399
Roser, H., 217, 519
Rossberg, J., 27, 129, 348, 367, 523, 569
Rossi, D., 165, 443
Rossiter, M.A., 153, 399
Roth, W.G., 229, 386, 444
Rotkin, I.D., 7, 258, 580
Rotta, C., 50, 385
Rouquès, L., 188, 513
Roussel, A., 163, 360
Rovinescu, I.A., 118, 432
Rowntree, F.S., 165, 275
Roxas, G.P., 73, 494
Royston, I., 17, 258, 325
Rozentul, M.A., 6, 51, 153, 163, 371, 385, 438, 522, 530, 541
Rozhinskii, L.M., 146, 343, 562
Rozina, L.A., 75, 255, 368, 526
Ruben, R., 70
Rubnikov, V.I., 88, 547
Ruczkowska, J., 237, 238, 521
Ruelle, M., 15, 476
Ruge, H., 174, 210, 335, 510, 518

Ruge, H.G., 110, 197, 225, 334, 335, 501, 516, 520
Ruiz-Moreno, J.A., 226, 554
Rumbolt, Z., 20, 393
Russell, D.H., 118, 333, 581
Russo, E., 169, 293
Russo, V., 42, 346
Rustrian, A.A., 36, 332, 558
Ruys, A.C., 114, 351
Rykowski, H., 121, 426
Rytlowa, W., 169, 476

Saadi, J.F., 12, 422
Sabes, W.R., 238, 365
Sagone, I., 135, 356, 562
Sahu, K.C., 70, 579
Saijo, Y., 10, 484
Saito, I., 56, 289
Salacz, P., 223, 331, 565
Salazar, E., 154
Salem, M.R., 54
Salembier, Y., 26
Salim, A.R., 114, 336
Salles, J.M., 73, 280, 356, 559
Salo, O.P., 59, 80, 120, 167, 200, 215, 326, 408, 409, 419, 478, 497, 502, 508, 516, 519
Samenius, B., 12, 161, 419
Samsonov, V.A., 53, 431
Sander, C., 166, 563
Sands, R.X., 157, 343, 378, 563
Sanford, D., 244, 267
Santini, R., 133, 315
Santori, M., 165, 473
Santos, J.M., 124, 325, 341
Sapuppo, A., 44, 213, 518, 524
Sarosiek, J., 202, 546
Sarrel, P.M., 207, 304

Sartoris, S., 48, 79, 166, 167, 233, 491, 496, 508, 520
Sasagawa, Y., 197, 515
Sasaki, M., 186, 349, 407
Savin, J.A., 109, 194, 411, 432
Saxena, R.S., 40, 489
Saxoni, F., 43, 434
Sazonova, L.V., 167, 210, 508
Scandellari, C., 217, 428
Scarpellini, L., 158, 545
Schabinski, G., 191, 354
Schachter, J., 21, 41, 73, 121, 243, 252, 336, 337, 363, 365, 551
Schaller, K.F., 225, 229, 350, 470
Schatz, N.J., 136, 472
Schellen, A.M., 60, 377
Schepers, G.W., 117, 270
Scherbakova, A.K., 87
Schierz, G., 224, 519
Schiller, F., 99, 177, 330, 532
Schilliro, R., 125, 341
Schirren, C.G., 51
Schmale, J.D., 114, 137, 185, 292, 294, 296
Schmid, A.H., 207, 419, 444
Schmid, P., 193, 319, 405
Schmidt, H., 105, 188, 224, 331, 334, 356, 366, 407, 566
Schmidt, W., 144, 337
Schmitz, R., 31, 208, 523
Schneiderka, P., 149, 191, 506, 514
Schofield, C.B., 5, 8, 124, 136, 220, 298, 322, 406, 410, 415, 538, 540, 570
Schoning, W.F., 121, 336
Schopf, E., 121, 387
Schrive, V., 211, 428
Schroeter, A.L., 91, 281
Schroter, R., 58, 440, 525
Schubert, W., 153, 371
Schuknecht, H.F., 119, 477
Schuppli, R., 51, 572
Schwartz, W.F., 236, 276

Schwimmer, B., 47, 230, 438, 481
Sciafani, G., 140
Scialfa, A., 43, 471
Scott, J., 196, 282
Scotti, A., 83, 335, 497
Scotti, A.T., 197, 208, 444
Scultety, S., 51, 543
Seale, J.R., 190, 575
Seamans, K.B., 153, 399
Seay, M.E., 123, 502
Sebek, V., 92, 281
Sedan, J., 118, 145, 172, 437, 472, 473
Sedlacek, V., 30, 50, 281, 306
Segre, A., 147, 233, 269, 562, 567
Seidler, E., 136, 357
Semmola, L., 45, 331
Semràdovà, V., 163, 285
Senra, A., 228, 567
Sepetjian, M., 113, 180, 205, 354, 517, 571
Serafino, X., 232
Serdiuk, M.P., 230
Serena, A., 45, 242, 273, 330, 580
Seropian, E., 37, 394
Serra, G.B., 80, 479
Serre, H., 131, 167, 420, 421
Seycek, V., 162, 381
Seze, S.D.E., 16, 420
Sgarbi, G., 169, 421
Shanholtz, M.I., 236, 383
Shapiro, L.H., 33, 81, 116, 117, 308, 312, 314, 365, 370
Shaposhnikov, O.K., 148, 328
Sharp, J.T., 36, 128, 252, 283, 352, 403
Shaw, D.J., 193, 388
Shchepin, A.P., 240, 361
Shcherbakova, A.K., 233, 386, 535
Sheeley, W.F., 189, 340
Shepard, M.C., 135, 213, 279, 353, 354, 570

Sheppe, W.M., Jr., 189, 340
Shestakov, S.V., 140, 427
Shifrin, L.A., 27
Shiman, G.V., 7, 266
Shimizu, S., 29, 429, 470
Shimizu, Y., 160, 482
Shipley, A., 213, 354, 571
Shipton, E.A., 59, 347
Shkliar, I.I., 74, 220, 223, 256, 322, 559, 565, 571
Shnaider, E.B., 26, 423
Shorr, N., 71, 277
Short, D.H., 105
Short, G.D., 132, 370
Shripkin, IuK, 196, 267
Shryock, H., 241, 576
Shtein, A.A., 66, 132, 199, 305, 478, 525
Shteinlukht, L.A., 29, 480
Siboulet, A., 15, 50, 51, 124, 126, 300, 314, 345, 346, 573
Sidaravichius, BIu., 54, 387
Siefert, G., 198, 516
Sievers, K., 57, 493
Signorelli, I., 138, 356, 562
Sikes, O.J., 3rd, 171, 382
Sil. L., 122
Silva, D., 49
Silverio, J., 8, 391
Simao, C., 63, 434
Simberkoff, M.S., 107, 370
Simon, C., 103, 144, 291, 436
Simon, K.H., 168, 509
Simon, N., 234, 445
Singh, J., 95, 420
Singh, K., 165, 408, 410
Sipowicz, I., 36, 547
Skencic, M., 25, 46, 94, 285, 302, 309
Skog, E., 46, 65, 140, 222, 257, 271, 391, 535
Skogh, M., 243, 577
Skokh, B.P., 146, 389
Skriver, A., 107, 573
Skrocka, M.B., 41, 406
Slowakiewicz, E., 30, 557
Slucki, L., 62, 224, 344, 558, 566

Sluis, I., 61, 324
Smálik, S., 82, 236, 441, 521
Smartt, W.H., 110, 580
Smirnov, B.V., 11, 392, 402
Smith, D., 137, 359
Smith, D.O., Jr., 71, 278, 311
Smith, E.B., 10, 28, 250, 263, 307, 308
Smith, J.A., 148, 364
Smith, J.L., 52, 79, 117, 158, 170, 171, 198, 212, 225, 373, 428, 437, 471, 472, 473, 474, 496, 516
Smith, W.H., 23, 61, 480, 481
Smithurst, B.A., 70, 163, 381
Smoler, J., 209, 444
Soares, J.P., 42
Sobbe, A., 212, 419
Socransky, S.S., 127, 175
Sohn, D., 120, 426
Sokolovskii, R.M., 227, 260, 546
Solente, G., 100, 186, 579
Soltz-Szots, J., 42, 144, 244, 286, 309, 542
Somkuti, G.A., 14, 251
Somogyi, Z., 101, 339
Sonnichsen, N., 34, 142, 393, 442
Soresco, M., 237, 521
Soukup, F., 95, 471
Soullard, J., 12, 282
Soumrov, I., 179
Southern, P.M., Jr., 7, 307, 375
Sowa, S., 113, 472
Spaeth, G.L., 221, 302, 374
Sparling, P.F., 37, 297
Spellberg, M.A., 221
Spencer, J.R., 241, 576
Spiezia, M., 88, 280, 527
Spirov, G., 62, 492

Spitzbart, H., 30, 113, 134, 367, 541, 549, 560
Spitzer, R.J., 199, 320, 415
Sprafke, U., 189, 581
Stach, J., 246, 362
Stambaugh, J.E., 114, 342, 528
Stammová, E., 138, 436
Stangalini, A., 107, 351
Stanulla, H., 139, 483
Staps, R., 53, 573
Starck, V., 42, 100, 232, 285, 295, 541
Starowicz, Z.L., 76, 580
Starzyk, J., 160, 563
Starzycki, Z., 152, 333, 387, 391, 399
Statham, R., 91, 286
Stauch, J.E., 133
Stebbins, P.L., 73, 569
Steigbigel, N. ., 207, 533, 539
Steinberg, A.I., 74, 494
Steiner, M., 161, 476
Steppert, A., 147, 219, 534, 541
Sternadel, Z., 239, 576
Sternberg, T.H., 222, 535
Sternberger, L.A., 231, 444
Sterner, J.H., 5, 416
Stevens, R.W., 20, 80, 136, 487, 497, 504
Stewart, D.B., 229, 325
Stewart, G.T., 9, 32, 100, 152, 166, 251, 368, 389, 391, 399
Stewart, R.H., 49, 388, 394
Stewart, W.M., 222, 534
Stien, R., 131, 420
Stitt, A., 235, 582
Stocki, E., 8, 296, 355
Stockli, A., 134, 348
Stoianov, S., 192, 515
Stoinova, O.A., 116
Stojiljkovic, S., 163, 328, 367
Stoller, A., 87, 366
Stolyhwo-Suchanek, A., 227, 548
Stone, O.J., 172, 404

Storck, H., 51, 90, 126, 297, 310, 312, 369
Storer, J., 123, 426
Storey, G.O., 31, 420
Stout, G.W., 158, 507
Stoyanoff, S., 18, 486
Straczkowski, W., 26, 431
Strakhov, S.N., 34, 579
Strani, G.F., 172, 510
Strassburg, M., 31, 476
Strassmann, H., 200, 255, 401
Straub, W., 105, 396, 528
Strauss, A.J., Jr., 43, 434
Strejcek, J., 14, 485
Studnitsin, A.A., 6, 29, 86, 122, 143, 177, 266, 328, 379, 532
Sturde, H.C., 70, 358
Sturzbecher, M., 138, 359
Stut, J.C., 126, 479
Suchanek, J., 65, 66, 201, 269, 365, 414, 525, 533, 572
Suchenwirth, R., 23, 423
Sulutiu, E., 106, 194, 274, 382
Sul'zhenko, A.I., 182, 339
Sumudi, M., 208, 480
Sunder-Plassmann, P., 34, 394
Surján, L., 133, 185, 504, 512
Sutherland, J.M., 11, 439
Suvorova, K.N., 126, 417
Suzuta, T., 169, 509
Svanbom, M., 90, 285
Svindland, H.B., 93, 296
Swierczewski, J.A., 85, 285
Sylvester, E., 5, 249, 390
Sylvestre, L., 111, 148, 271, 314, 315, 366, 412
Syrovatko, F.A., 38, 550
Szabó, J., 97, 431, 435
Szarmach, H., 52, 310
Szego, L., 165, 483
Szell, I., 181, 259, 549
Szodoray, L., 101
Szule, E., 224, 566

Takase, S., 166, 445
Takasugi, K., 127
Takeuchi, K., 52, 573
Tala, P., 12, 422
Tanaka, J., 48, 491
Taneja, B.L., 34, 246, 579
Tanimoto, R.H., 41, 490
Tanzer, A., 131
Tarel, A., 229, 433
Tatochenko, V.K., 108, 359
Tauchnitz, G., 142, 505
Tawes, R.L., Jr., 95, 286, 313
Taylor, C.E., 74, 187, 407, 494
Taylor, G.J., 194, 437
Taylor, H.A., 89, 283, 303
Taylor, J.A., Jr., 217, 540, 564
Taylor-Robinson, D., 128, 129, 352, 353
Tchertkoff, V., 161, 478
Teague, R.E., 110
Telfer, J.G., 129, 416
Teokharov, B.A., 42, 101, 135, 342, 346, 348
Teras, J., 30, 67, 145, 550, 551, 553
Tereschenko, I.U.A., 11, 388
Terminello, V., 198, 320, 412
Terzano, G., 5, 548
Terzi, I., 20, 273, 409
Texier, L., 55, 573
Thatcher, R.W., 17, 94, 182, 287, 313, 344, 571
Thayer, J.D., 106, 291
Thew, M.A., 10, 250, 324
Thiebaut, F., 124
Thiel, H.J., 151, 473, 479
Thiers, H., 136, 219, 315, 321, 539, 540
Thin, R.N., 56, 104, 190, 270, 291, 550

Thivolet, J., 15, 180, 196, 353, 485, 512, 571
Thomas, B.A., 12, 336
Thomas, M.E., 128, 352
Thompson, A.F., 44
Thomsen, K., 133, 275, 339
Thomson, K.D., 181, 361
Thurel, R., 167, 421
Tikhonova, A.P., 209
Timakov, V.D., 144, 353
Timmermans, L., 33, 539
Tinkler, A.E., 188, 480, 514
Tio, B.S., 40, 489
Tobia, L., 199, 413
Todea, C., 36, 542
Tolchin, S., 64, 274
Tomari, V.A., 222, 535
Tomaszunas, S., 239, 361
Tomizawa, T., 97, 142, 146, 169, 202, 206, 234, 239, 499, 505, 509, 518, 520
Tompsett, R., 164, 400
Toporovskii, L.M., 60, 71, 440, 441
Torre, J.M., 129, 426
Torres Rodriguez, V.M., 209, 518
Torsuev, N.A., 195, 196, 267, 276, 340, 532
Tosolini, G.C., 70, 237, 555
Toth, B., 181, 215, 259, 260, 330, 549, 564
Tottie, M., 242, 411
Towpik, J., 30, 50, 51, 136, 157, 180, 222, 358, 371, 380, 381, 382, 413, 416, 530, 535
Tramièr, G., 16, 44, 78, 169, 417, 486, 495, 509
Tremelloni, L., 137, 472
Trensz, F., 189, 514
Triapichnikov, P.F., 25, 420
Tringali, G., 119, 184, 202, 511

Tringali, G.R., 66, 169, 509, 525, 568
Trinka, C., 128, 352
Trofimova, MIa., 176, 482
Trotman, R.E., 20, 487
Truksa, Z., 46, 288
Trussell, R.R., 229, 350
Tsao, W., 228, 282, 547
Tselischeva, A.D., 160, 259, 317
Tsiura, I.G., 75, 338
Tsuchiya, K., 69, 277
Tsugami, H., 159, 418
Tuffanelli, D.L., 8, 80, 84, 129, 272, 484, 496, 498, 503
Tullett, G.L., 206, 402
Tumasheva, N.I., 64, 173, 269, 297, 429, 443
Tuna, I., 116
Turanov, N.M., 51, 122, 144, 155, 177, 482, 530, 572, 574
Turanova, E.N., 71, 203, 278, 294, 311
Turbessi, G., 231
Turk, J.L., 62, 395
Turner, T.B., 110, 442
Turro, O.R., 63, 435
Tursunov, N.T., 177, 328
Tuszkiewicz, A.R., 238, 402
Tutt, J.B., 218, 578
Tverskoi, M.D., 24, 85, 579
Tyrrell, D.A., 36, 351

Ueda, H., 15, 423
Ugrimov, S.A., 140, 147, 506
Ulker, N., 188, 513
Ullal, S.R., 152, 399
Ullmo, A., 171, 473
Undeutsch, W., 147, 541
Usmanov, T.U., 143
Usui, H., 41, 490
Utley, P.M., 7, 391
Utrilla, A., 203, 257, 418

Vachtenheim, J., 217
Vaczi, L., 119, 502
Vaisman, A., 106, 160, 500, 507
Valent, M., 46, 133, 139, 341, 348, 544, 552, 558
Vallejo, L.V., 24, 477
Van Arsdel, P.P., Jr., 179, 400
Van Dellen, R.G., 153, 399
van Doesschate, J., 48, 297
Van Laarhoven, P.H., 227, 566
Van Wymeersch, H., 238, 271
Varela, G., 76, 347
Vargues, R., 120, 161, 232, 502, 507, 520
Vartiainen, E., 223, 540, 565
Vasil'ev, T.V., 101, 103, 104, 175, 225, 257, 273, 369, 370, 375, 445, 500, 527, 528, 531
Vasiliu, G., 120, 397, 528
Vella, E.E., 208, 518
Venkoba, R.A., 175, 367
Verbov, J., 21, 131, 280
Vergara, L., 114, 347
Verjat, R., 207, 433
Vermeer, D.J., 31, 424, 523
Verschoof, K.J., 38, 550
Vessal, K., 122, 337
Viallier, J., 54, 492
Victoria, R.V., 114, 291
Vietzke, W.M., 89, 284
Vilches, A.M., 180, 270
Vil'chinskii, M.P., 85, 573
Vilenskii, M.M., 144, 300
Vilotte, J., 70, 251
Vivas, S.E., 211, 374, 428
Vogt, H., 49, 310, 389, 394

Voight, G.C., 89, 284
Volan, H.H., 58, 493
Volosceanu, D.I., 46, 446
Volpi, U., 165, 473
Von Fischer, F., 215
Von Wasserman, A., 19
Vora, M.P., 80, 338
Voskresenskaia, G.A., 38, 226, 344, 550, 566
Vosmik, F., 53, 440
Vukotich, D., 25, 423
Vuori, E.E., 142, 300, 408
Vymola, F., 18, 308, 367

Wada, H., 66, 376, 559
Wade, M.E., 32, 345
Wagner, G., 224, 411
Wagstaff, W., 117, 502
Wainstock, J., 33, 346, 355
Walecki, H., 227, 547
Walker, D.G., 245, 522
Wallace, A.L., 171, 254, 404
Wallace, D.R., 21, 365
Wallmann, K., 25, 420
Walsh, F.A., 136, 357, 381
Walther, H., 146, 147, 207, 216, 232, 254, 255, 370, 479, 541, 547, 564
Walton, H.C., 226, 554
Ward, M.E., 91, 297
Warner, J.H., 89, 283
Warot, P., 96
Warren, R.M., 108, 300
Watanabe, T., 211, 428
Waters, J.R., 90, 303
Watson, P.G., 226, 475
Watt, L., 239, 576
Watt, P.J., 80, 281
Wawryk, R., 42, 223, 346, 378, 556, 565
Wawrzkiewicz, M., 110, 259, 544
Weberschinke, J., 191, 443
Webster, B., 214, 245, 276, 277, 340
Wechselberg, K., 127
Wehling, H., 60, 207, 425, 427

Weidenbach, A., 217, 356, 564
Weinstein, E.G., 121, 336
Weise, H.J., 62, 324
Weisman, A.I., 211
Weitgasser, H., 142, 529
Welborn, J.F., 87, 431
Wells, B.P., 214, 276
Wells, B.W., 154, 410
Wells, J.A., 76, 83, 471, 497
Wendland, K.L., 234, 295
Wendler, H., 212, 477
Wereide, K., 62, 525
Werner, H.P., 125, 397
Wertlake, P.T., 184
Westenfielder, G.O., 119, 397
Westphal, A., 202, 237, 546, 554
Whalen, J.P. 68, 347
Wheeler, A.H., 59, 493
White, D.L., 234, 267
White, J.M., 153, 399
White, P.C., Jr., 240, 409
Whitfield, R., 234, 475
Wiedmann, A., 51, 159, 572, 574
Wiek, H.H., 146
Wierer, A., 49, 288
Wiesner, K., 6, 341, 556
Wigfield, A.S., 213, 537
Wijetunga, E.B., 149, 538, 570
Wik, R., 56, 351
Wilkinson, A.E., 84, 116, 136, 196, 201, 204, 343, 430, 445, 474, 498, 515, 516, 529
Willcox, R.R., 45, 54, 72, 102, 130, 154, 161, 170, 179, 181, 206, 220, 229, 278, 304, 310, 317, 318, 320, 322, 334, 339, 348, 359, 375, 405, 538, 539, 569, 574
Williams, W.J., 101
Willmott, F.E., 224, 408, 542
Winslow, D.J., 121

Wiskemann, A., 96, 268
Witzleb, W., 56, 351
Wodniansky, P., 113, 145, 219, 314, 315, 370, 534, 578
Wojas, K., 162, 360
Wolff, C.B., 94, 285
Wood, J.K., 150, 432
Wood, R.M., 40, 181, 490, 511
Wray, P.M., 21, 345
Wren, B.G., 91, 305
Wright, D.J., 9, 132, 206, 228, 246, 320, 323, 415, 418, 431, 568
Wuepper, K.D., 80, 171, 186, 258, 443, 496, 512
Wulf, K., 46, 480
Wysham, D.N., 19, 423

Yacenda, J.A., 88, 573
Yamamoto, S., 199, 414, 516
Yano, T., 127
Yarington, C.T., Jr., 208, 444
Yobs, A.R., 66, 357, 446, 527
Yokoyama, Y., 81, 258, 543
Yoshida, O., 201, 260, 414
Yu, F.C., 34, 434

Zaborowski, Z., 168, 427
Zackler, J., 157, 293
Zadjelovic, J., 38, 439
Zajac, W., 234, 521
Zanca, A., 26, 488
Zawadzki, J., 21, 86, 192, 223, 344, 378, 557, 560, 563, 565
Zelazny, S., 160, 259
Zelenkova, L., 56, 289
Zelger, J., 128, 387, 397
Zelikman, M.A., 118, 544
Zellmann, H.E., 63
Zenin, A.S., 178, 329
Zheltakov, M.M., 52, 140, 529, 573

Zhodzishskii, I.A., 142, 348
Zhukov, V.I., 146, 224, 234, 315, 566, 567
Zivkovic, B., 53, 543
Zivkovic, M., 16, 393, 522
Zlatkina, A.R., 244, 470
Zmechorovskaia, G.A., 76, 178, 495, 511
Znamenucek, K., 48, 269
Zographos, G., 16, 377, 485
Zorn, H., 155, 376, 562
Zuber, E., 109, 327
Zuch, A., 214, 428
Zukerman, E., 108
Zuniga, J.E., 36, 357, 558
Zwahr, C., 147, 292
Zwerenz, G., 222, 565
Zwierz, C., 33, 227, 341, 554, 557